Fungal Pathogenicity
and the
Plant's Response

Third Long Ashton Symposium 1971

Fungal Pathogenicity and the Plant's Response

Proceedings of a Symposium held at
Long Ashton Research Station
University of Bristol
22-24 September 1971

Edited by R. J. W. BYRDE *and* C. V. CUTTING

1973

ACADEMIC PRESS · London · New York

ACADEMIC PRESS INC. (LONDON) LTD.
24/28 Oval Road,
London NW1

United States Edition published by
ACADEMIC PRESS INC.
111 Fifth Avenue
New York, New York 10003

Library of Congress Catalog Card Number: 70-189938
ISBN: 0-12-148850-0

Printed in Great Britain by
The Whitefriars Press Ltd., London and Tonbridge

Participants in the Symposium

ABBOTT, Dr A. J. Long Ashton Research Station, University of Bristol, England.

ALCORN, J. W. S. Department of Botany, West of Scotland Agricultural College, Ayr, Scotland.

ANN, D. Plant Pathology Department, ADAS, West Midland Region, Wolverhampton, England.

ARCHER, S. A. Long Ashton Research Station, University of Bristol, England.

AYRES, P. G. Department of Biological Sciences, University of Lancaster, England.

BAILEY, Dr. J. A. ARC Plant Growth Substance and Systemic Fungicide Unit, Wye College, Kent, England.

BEYERSBERGEN, Dr J. C. M. Laboratorium voor Bloembollenonderzoek Lisse, Netherlands.

BLAKEMAN, Dr J. P. Department of Botany, University of Aberdeen, Scotland.

BRACKER, Dr C. E. Department of Botany and Plant Pathology, Purdue University, Indiana, U.S.A.

BRIAN, Professor P. W. F.R.S. School of Botany, University of Cambridge, England.

BROKENSHIRE, T. Department of Biological Sciences, University of Exeter, England.

BROWN, Dr Averil E. Department of Plant Pathology, Queen's University of Belfast, Northern Ireland.

BURNETT, Professor J. H. Department of Agricultural Science, University of Oxford, England.

BUTCHER, Dr D. N. Unit of Developmental Botany, Cambridge, England.

BUTLER, Professor E. E. Department of Plant Pathology, University of California, Davies, U.S.A.

BYRDE, Dr R. J. W. Long Ashton Research Station, University of Bristol, England.

CALONGE, Dr F. D. Department de Botanica, Universidad de Madrid, Spain.

CASEBY, W. R. Shellstar Ltd., Stonehaven Nurseries, Berrick Salome, Oxford, England.

CHALLICE, J. S. Long Ashton Research Station, University of Bristol, England.

CLIFFORD, Dr B. C. Welsh Plant Breeding Station, Aberystwyth, Wales.

CLIFFORD, D. R. Long Ashton Research Station, University of Bristol, England.

CODNER, R. C. School of Biological Sciences, University of Bath, Somerset, England.

COLE, Dr A. L. J. Department of Botany, University of Hull, Yorkshire, England.

COLEY-SMITH, Dr J. R. Department of Botany, University of Hull, Yorkshire, England.

COPELAND, R. Plant Pathology Field Station, Belfast, Northern Ireland.

CORKE, Dr A. T. K. Long Ashton Research Station, University of Bristol, England.

CRONSHAW, D. K. Department of Biological Sciences, Wye College, University of London, England.

CROWDY, Professor S. H. Department of Botany, University of Southampton, England.

CURTIS, Dr R. F. Chemistry Division, Food Research Institute, Norwich, England.

CUTTING, Dr C. V. Long Ashton Research Station, University of Bristol, England.

DALLAS-NEWTON, J. Department of Microbiology, University College of South Wales and Monmouthshire, Cardiff, Wales.

DAVENPORT, R. R. Long Ashton Research Station, University of Bristol, England.

DAVIES, Dr D. L. G. ADAS, Northern Regional Office, Newcastle-upon-Tyne, England.

DEKHUIJZEN, Dr H. M. Organisch Chemisch Instituut TNO, Wageningen, Netherlands.

DEVERALL, Dr B. J. ARC Plant Growth Substance and Systemic Fungicide Unit, Wye College, University of London, England.

DIJKMAN, A. van Organisch Chemisch Instituut TNO, Wageningen, Netherlands.

DRYSDALE, Dr R. B. Department of Microbiology, University of Birmingham, England.

EVANS, Dr E. J. ADAS, East Midland Regional Office, Shardlow, Derby, England.

EVANS, Dr R. L. Department of Botany, Westfield College, University of London, England.

FARRELL, Dr G. M. I.C.I. Ltd., Jealott's Hill Research Station, Bracknell, Berks., England.

FEAKIN, Mrs Susan D. Centre for Overseas Pest Research, London, England.

FIELDING, A. H. Long Ashton Research Station, University of Bristol, England.

FISHER, Dr D. J. Long Ashton Research Station, University of Bristol, England.

FRIEND, Professor J. Department of Botany, University of Hull, England.
GALPIN, Mrs Mary F. J. Department of Biological Sciences, University of Exeter, England.
GOOD, Dr N. Department of Botany and Plant Pathology, Michigan State University, U.S.A.
HALL, Dr Josephine A. Water Pollution Research Laboratory, Stevenage, Herts., England.
HARROWER, K. M. Department of Biological Sciences, University of Exeter, England.
HAWKER, Professor Lilian E. Department of Botany, University of Bristol, England.
HEWITT, Dr E. J. Long Ashton Research Station, University of Bristol, England.
HIGNETT, Dr R. C. East Malling Research Station, Maidstone, Kent, England.
HILL, S. A. ADAS, South Western Regional Office, Bristol, England.
HILL-COTTINGHAM, Dr D. G. Long Ashton Research Station, University of Bristol, England.
HISLOP, Dr E. C. Long Ashton Research Station, University of Bristol, England.
HOAD, Dr G. V. Long Ashton Research Station, University of Bristol, England.
HOWELL, Mrs Hazel, Long Ashton Research Station, University of Bristol, England.
HOWELL, Dr P. J. Department of Agriculture and Fisheries for Scotland, Edinburgh, Scotland.
HUDSON, Professor J. P. Long Ashton Research Station, University of Bristol, England.
INGRAM, Dr D. S. ARC Unit Of Developmental Botany, University of Cambridge, England.
JACOBS, Dr L. School of Biological Sciences, University of Bath, Somerset, England.
JOHNSON, Dr R. Plant Breeding Institute, Cambridge, England.
JONES, P. Department of Biological Sciences, University of Lancaster, England.
KAMERBECK, Dr G. A. Laboratorium voor Bloembollenonderzoek, Lisse, Netherlands.
KAVANAGH, Professor J. A. University College, Dublin, Ireland.
KEETON, Miss I. P. Long Ashton Research Station, University of Bristol, England.
KELMAN, Professor A. University of Wisconsin, Madison, Wisconsin, U.S.A.
KIRKHAM, Dr D. S. East Malling Research Station, Maidstone, Kent, England.
KLIFFEN, C. Instituut voor Plantenziektenkundig Onderzoek, Wageningen, Netherlands.
LANGCAKE, Dr P. Shell Research Ltd., Woodstock Agricultural Research Centre, Sittingbourne, Kent, England.
LEGGE, S. H. Long Ashton Research Station, University of Bristol, England.

LITTLEFIELD, Dr L. J. Department of Plant Pathology, North Dakota State University, Fargo, North Dakota, U.S.A.

LIYANAGE, A. de S. Department of Hop Research, Wye College, University of London, England.

LONG, Dr P. E. School of Biology, University of Leicester, England.

LUCAS, J. A. Department of Biological Sciences, University of Exeter, England.

LUCKWILL, Dr L. C. Long Ashton Research Station, University of Bristol, England.

LUND, Dr Barbara M. ARC Food Research Institute, Norwich, England.

MARSH, R. W. Long Ashton Research Station, University of Bristol, England.

MARTIN, Dr J. T. Long Ashton Research Station, University of Bristol, England.

MYERS, Dr A. Department of Botany, University of Southampton, England.

O'BRIEN, Miss F. Department of Botany, Imperial College, University of London, England.

OLIVIER, J. M. Station de Pathologie Vegetale, Beaucouze, France.

PITT, Dr D. Department of Biological Sciences, University of Exeter, England.

PRICE, Dr D. Glasshouse Crops Research Institute, Littlehampton, Sussex, England.

PRING, R. J. Long Ashton Research Station, University of Bristol, England.

REYNOLDS, S. B. Department of Botany, University of Hull, England.

RICHMOND, Dr D. V. Long Ashton Research Station, University of Bristol, England.

ROBERTSON, Professor N. F. School of Agriculture, University of Edinburgh, Scotland.

ROBINSON, T. J. Department of Botany, Imperial College, University of London, England.

ROYLE, Dr D. J. Department of Hop Research, Wye College, University of London, England.

RUSSELL, Dr G. E. Plant Breeding Institute, Cambridge, England.

SARGENT, Dr J. A. ARC Unit of Developmental Botany, Cambridge, England.

SIJPESTEIJN, Dr A. Kaars. TNO Biochemical Department, Utrecht, Netherlands.

SMITH, Dr I. M. Department of Botany, Imperial College, University of London, England.

SPENCER, Dr D. M. Glasshouse Crops Research Institute, Littlehampton, Sussex, England.

STAHMANN, Professor M. A. Department of Biochemistry, University of Wisconsin, Madison, Wisconsin, U.S.A.

STEAD, D. E. Imperial College Field Station, Ascot, Berks., England.

STURDY, M. L. Department of Botany, University of Hull, England.

SWINBURNE, Dr T. R. Ministry of Agriculture, Plant Pathology Division, Queen's University of Belfast, Northern Ireland.

TOMMERUP, Dr. Inez C. ARC Unit of Developmental Botany, University of Cambridge, England.

TUCKWELL, Miss S. V. Department of Biological Sciences, University of Exeter, England.

VERHOEFF, Professor K. Phytopathologisch Laboratorium, Baarn, Netherlands.

WICKINS, Miss S. Shell Research Ltd., Woodstock Agricultural Research Station, Sittingbourne, Kent, England.

WAARD, M. A. de Laboratory of Phytopathology, Wageningen, Netherlands.

WILKINS, P. W. Plant Pathology Department, Welsh Plant Breeding Station, Aberystwyth, Wales.

WILLIAMS, Professor P. H. Department of Plant Pathology, University of Wisconsin, Madison, Wisconsin, U.S.A.

WOOD, Professor R. K. S. Department of Botany, Imperial College, University of London, England

WOODCOCK, Dr D. Long Ashton Research Station, University of Bristol, England.

Preface

Topics for the biennial Long Ashton Symposia are decided for their importance to Agriculture and Horticulture, and also for the timeliness of a critical review of current thinking and future developments in the subject selected. Although many plant pathologists are still occupied with diagnosis and eradication of diseases, the diagnostic stage of plant pathology may be considered to be well advanced. We are now in an era of physiological plant pathology, and the theme of this book is therefore ideally appropriate.

We were fortunate in having Professor R. K. S. Wood, President of the International Society for Plant Pathology, to present the inaugural lecture, in which he emphasized the importance and specificity of the hypersensitive response (using the term in its botanical context). Originally applied to the death of cells in an incompatible relation between an obligate pathogen and a resistant host, it is now clear that the general concept may be more widely applicable.

The Symposium benefited from the presence of European participants and also, by timing it to follow the 1st International Mycological Congress, we had additional contributors from America. This has enabled us to present a comprehensive text with a wide coverage of current research.

A valuable feature of this text is the inclusion of the extensive discussion which developed, for which we appreciate the enthusiasm of the participants who had clearly made full use of the pre-circulated papers.

This book should therefore give research workers, teachers and students a comprehensive review with some original data and speculative comment on host-parasite contact. As Professor Brian stated in his perceptive summing-up, we may also 'hope that in the future we can base more logical approaches to control on our growing knowledge of the host–parasite relationship'.

We wish to thank all the contributors who complied so freely with our timetable for preparation of their papers, and also the Chairmen of the respective Sessions. Drs Bracker and Littlefield eventually combined their contributions to produce an extensive survey of host–pathogen interfaces, giving a presentation not available elsewhere. This took longer to produce than was originally planned, and some delay has therefore occurred in the appearance of this volume. The editors trust, however, that the value of the Proceedings will have been enhanced by the inclusion of this material.

Although prepared stencils were submitted by each author, we wish to thank those who assisted in the final preparation of this book, especially Miss C. Hoyle who also transcribed the discussion from the tape recording, and Mr E. G. R. Chenoweth who prepared most of the final diagrams for publication.

Acknowledgement is also made of the permission granted by the Journals concerned for reproduction of diagrams and tables, as indicated in the respective captions.

December 1972

R. J. W. Byrde
C. V. Cutting

Contents

SECTION V

Altered Metabolism

Chairman: Professor P. W. Brian F.R.S.

INAUGURAL LECTURE

Specificity in Plant Diseases

R. K. S. WOOD

Department of Botany and Plant Technology
Imperial College of Science and Technology
London, England

In biology, as I suppose in other sciences, it is usually dangerous and certainly difficult to start a lecture such as this by defining what one is going to talk about. So I shall not attempt to do so with any precision. Instead, I shall assume that you all have a good idea of what is meant by specificity and merely ask you to regard it as that part of plant pathology which seeks to explain why one micro-organism is able to parasitize one plant, or group of plants, but not another. As such, the problem of specificity dominates much of plant pathology because, although plant pathologists are preoccupied with plant diseases, we cannot remind ourselves too often that disease is a relatively rare phenomenon and that particular pathogens are able to parasitize only a very small proportion of the plants available to them. This applies even to pathogens such as *Botrytis cinerea* usually described as unspecialized because, although they do have many more hosts than one such as *Phytophthora infestans,* the number of species parasitized is in fact quite small and even these are susceptible only under somewhat special conditions. This specialization of parasitism is coupled with the fact that in culture plant pathogens grow perfectly well on relatively simple media; even the rust fungi that can be cultured have no very special requirements in this respect. Superficially, therefore, because plants contain all the substances that micro-organisms need for growth, and because dead plants are actively colonized by micro-organisms, we should be surprised that almost all of them cannot grow on living plants, and that it is virulence, the ability to do so, that is so exceptional. It might be as well, therefore, to start from this much rarer phenomenon of virulence and see how far specificity of parasitism can be explained in terms of toxins, produced by a parasite, that damage only those host species colonized by it, on the assumption that virulence can be equated with the capacity to damage and kill the plant. Specificity would be explained as follows. Micro-organism *X* (but not others) produces substance *Y* which damages plant or plant group *A* but not others, and only *A* is parasitized by *X*. The classic example of such a substance *Y*, is, of course, HV-toxin produced by *Helminthosporium victoriae*, the subject of outstanding work by Scheffer, Pringle, Wheeler and their colleagues over many years and now summarized in recent reviews (Scheffer and Samaddar, 1970; Scheffer and Yoder, 1972; Pringle, 1972). HV-toxin is a low molecular weight peptide linked with a base, victoxinine (mol. wt. 264) which is probably a N-containing sesquiterpene. The peptide contains one molecule each of aspartic and glutamic acids, glycine, valine and leucine. There is now much good evidence that implicates HV-toxin in diseases caused by *H. victoriae*. Thus, there is the remarkable agreement between susceptibility of plants to the parasite and to the toxin; between pathogenicity of strains of the parasite and their capacity to produce the toxin; and between the many types of changes in host tissues caused by both toxin and parasite (Scheffer and Pringle, 1961; Scheffer *et al.*, 1964; Luke and Wheeler, 1964; Scheffer and Pringle, 1967; Kuo, 1968). HV-toxin is active at remarkably low concentrations preventing growth of susceptible roots at 0.0002 μg/ml whereas 4×10^5 times this concentration is needed to prevent growth of resistant roots (Kuo, 1968).

Further striking evidence about its specificity comes from crosses between *H. victoriae*—pathogenic to oats—and *H. carbonum*—pathogenic to corn—which also produces a host-specific toxin (HC-toxin) (Pringle and Scheffer, 1967). Progeny of crosses segregate in equal numbers for capacity to produce HV-toxin, HC-toxin, both toxins, or no toxin. Pathogenicity to oats, corn, oats and corn, or to neither, segregates in the same way implying that production of toxin and pathogenicity is controlled by two gene pairs segregating independently (Scheffer *et al.*, 1967).

HV-toxin affects intact cells in many ways. It increases oxygen uptake and permeability to electrolytes, and inhibits a wide range of other cellular activities. But the primary effect seems to be on the integrity and function of the plasma membranes because the toxin is much less active on fractions isolated from cells, e.g. on electron transport and phosphorylation in isolated protoplasts.

It has been suggested that HV-toxin first acts upon some component in susceptible cells to disrupt surface membranes, with many consequential effects that can be regarded as secondary and that cells are resistant when they lack the susceptible component. In this connexion it may be significant that degraded HV-toxin will protect cells from intact toxin, possibly by occupying susceptible sites of action (Scheffer and Pringle, 1964).

Preliminary work suggests that PC-toxin from *Periconia circinata*, pathogenic on grain sorghum, has effects similar to those of HV-toxin, whereas HC-toxin shows points of similarity and difference because it is not toxic to seedlings in a nitrogen atmosphere and because low concentrations stimulate growth.

Alternaria kikuchiana, parasitic on certain cultivars of pears, probably produces a host specific toxin (Hiroe *et al.*, 1958) and recently Steiner and Byther (1971) have reported that *Helminthosporium sacchari* produces a host-specific toxin, helminthosporoside, identified as the simple compound 2-hydroxycyclopropyl-α-D-galactopyranoside (Steiner and Strobel, 1971). This is the first to be characterized completely.

All this, and much other evidence, strongly implicates host-specific toxins as primary determinants of specificity in these five diseases. And the view has been expressed that further work will reveal host-specific toxins in many other diseases though they may act less spectacularly than those already studied and may, therefore, be even more difficult to work with (Scheffer and Samaddar, 1970). There are, however, a number of difficulties still to be resolved before these and similar toxins can be accepted as the sole determinants of specificity. Thus, take the behaviour of *H. victoriae* and *H. carbonum* on resistant and susceptible plants (Jennings and Ullstrup, 1957). It is similar to that of fungal pathogens in many other diseases in which host-specific toxins have not yet been implicated. The fungi infect resistant plants but then grow only to a limited extent, killing a few cells in the process. In susceptible plants, death of cells is delayed though the pathogen does grow through the tissue. Later, many cells are killed and a lesion is produced, presumably because dead cells are a substrate suitable for production of the toxin and because sufficient accumulates to kill them. This can explain continued growth of the parasite through susceptible tissues. But the parasite also kills the first cells of the resistant plant that it encounters though these cells are not affected by the toxin or, rather, are affected only by much higher concentrations. Why then does the pathogen not continue to kill cells because this is what the virulent pathogen does in susceptible plants although, of course, the mechanism of killing may be different. A similar argument would apply to the behaviour of avirulent mutants that have lost the capacity to produce toxin. It seems to me that some explanation other than insensitivity of host cells, or inability to produce toxin must be invoked to explain why the avirulent pathogen does not continue to grow and kill cells in plants that it infects.

An essential feature of specificity based on host-specific toxins is, of course, the sensitivity of susceptible cells. But in other attempts to explain specificity, the sequence of events in susceptible (compatible), and resistant (incompatible) reactions between host and parasite have been interpreted quite differently. We may now revert to the early growth of avirulent and virulent pathogens on and in plants. There is not much difference until the outer wall of surface cells is penetrated and contact is made with the plasmalemma. Then, although there are differences in detail particularly in the speed with which the reactions occur, the sequence is somewhat as follows. Resistant cells react very much more quickly in ways that lead to disorganization and death of the cytoplasm. Susceptible cells also react to the pathogen but they do not die, at least not for a considerable time. There are, however, striking changes in the cells. Thus, a remarkable feature for fungi such as *Colletotrichum lindemuthianum* is that hyphae grow through living, susceptible cells and invaginate the plasmalemma, or by-pass it in other ways, a behaviour more reminiscent of that of obligate parasites (Mercer, 1970; Skipp, 1971). This apparently benign relationship between parasite and host cells does not last long. I shall return later to what happens when it ends. But for the present I want to emphasize that now the sign of susceptibility is the insensitivity of host cells to damage by substances produced by the pathogen in its early growth. In contrast, it is the resistant cell that is excessively sensitive to these products. Note, too, that *H. victoriae* and *H. carbonum* also kill resistant cells more quickly in the earliest stages of infection.

The rapid death of cells in response to infection is usually described as hypersensitivity. It first attracted attention as a typical response of plants resistant to obligate parasites. Here its significance is obvious because such parasites do not grow continuously on dead substrates (*pace* Williams *et al.*, 1966 and subsequently). Only later has the significance of hypersensitivity for facultative parasites become apparent. Even now it is not realized often enough that for these parasites death of cells in response to infection does not itself explain why a parasite does not continue to grow in resistant plants. Death must also be accompanied by changes in dead cells, or in others around them that prevent growth of the parasite.

For some diseases, it is now clear that tissue killed in response to infection does come to contain sufficient of substances toxic to the pathogen to prevent its growth, substances now, of course, called phytoalexins, a number of which have now been characterized chemically (Cruickshank *et al.*, 1971). Thus we have pisatin, 3-hydroxy-7-methoxy-4′, 5′-methylenedioxy-chromanocoumarane, from peas (Perrin and Bottomley, 1962); phaseollin, 6b,12b-dihydro-3,3-dimethyl-3H,7H-furo [3,2-C:5,4-f^1] bis [1] benzopyran-10-ol from French beans (Perrin, 1964), ipomeamarone, 2-methyl-2-(4 methyl-2-oxypentyl)-5-(3 furyl)-tetrahydrofuran, from sweet potato (Akazawa, 1960); orchinol, 9,10-dihydro-2,4-dimethoxy-6-hydroxy-phenanthrene, from tubers of *Orchis militaris* (Böller *et al.*, 1957); an isocoumarin, 3-methyl-6-methoxy-8-hydroxy-3,4-dihydroxy-isocoumarin, from carrots (Condon and Kuć, 1962); medicarpin, (−)-3-hydroxy-9-methoxypterocarpan from alfalfa (Higgins and Millar, 1968; Smith *et al.*, 1971); wyerone acid, an acetylenic furanoid keto ester, from broad bean (Deverall and Vessey, 1969; Letcher *et al.*, 1970); rishitin, a bicyclic sesquiterpene alcohol, from potato tubers and tomato fruit (Tomiyama *et al.*, 1968; Katsui *et al.*, 1968; Sato *et al.*, 1968); rishitinol, another bicyclic sesquiterpene alcohol, from potato (Katsui *et al.*, 1971); hydroxy-phaseollin from soybean (Klarman and Sanford, 1968; Keen, 1971); safynol a polyacetylene diol from safflower (*Carthamus tinctorius*) (Thomas and Allen,

1970); gossypol and related compounds from cotton (Adams *et al.*, 1960; Bell, 1967). One can predict that many other phytoalexins will be isolated and identified as successive diseases are studied from this point of view. But it will be a great pity if this type of work is not followed, at least in some diseases, by studies in depth which seek to establish the precise role of phytoalexins in resistance. There is for example, the difficult but important problem of determining whether phytoalexins are produced and accumulate in the killed cells, in adjacent living cells, or in both. There is certainly good evidence that the adjacent cells are important in the hypersensitive response because it is greatly delayed, or does not occur, unless the infected cell is supported by a group of cells that are not infected (Tomiyama *et al.*, 1958, 1967; Skipp, 1971). In contrast, however, certain phytoalexins are very localized. Thus, rishitin is confined to the outer 1-2 layers of potato slices infected by *P. infestans* (Sato and Tomiyama, 1969).

Not much is known about the relation between death of hypersensitive cells and the accumulation of toxic substances. Clearly, if accumulation always followed death then one should be able to induce resistance by killing a small group of cells and waiting a short time before adding a potential pathogen. This simple sort of experiment does not seem to have been done very often but one suspects that in many diseases it would not lead to resistance. On the contrary, dead cells are a prerequisite for infection by typical wound parasites. Also, there is the fact that only certain types of damage lead to the production of phytoalexins, though one must admit that for peas the range of treatments that results in the formation of pisatin is remarkably wide (Schwochau and Hadwiger, 1968; Bailey, 1969; T. J. Robinson, 1970, personal communication). Are we to assume that cells can be killed in different ways that also cause different changes in adjacent cells, and that a special type of damage and death is necessary before phytoalexins are produced? The hypersensitive response would, of course, be one of these special types. For this and many other reasons the nature of the hypersensitive response is central to hypotheses about specificity, especially any based on phytoalexins, if only because these substances are non-specific in toxicity to different pathogens. Unfortunately, comparatively little is known about the response itself except in terms of somewhat gross biochemical changes and alterations in sub-cellular structure. In spite of excellent work by Tomiyama (1971) on potato and *P. infestans,* and on beans and *C. lindemuthianum* by Mercer (1970) and Skipp (1971), the visual changes, though striking and interesting, are difficult to interpret at the present time. I cannot refer to them in detail but I should like to contrast the immediate response of infected cells and the subsequent effects on adjacent cells; the marked difference between the structureless disorganization of a hypersensitive cell containing a hypha of *C. lindemuthianum,* and the apparently healthy cells around it, though such cells are changed in quite striking ways. Thus in the cell adjacent to the one infected, the layer of cytoplasm is 2-3 times as thick as that in unaffected cells, the endoplasmic reticulum is orientated parallel to the anticlinal wall of the epidermal cell, and the nucleus is larger and lobed (Mercer, 1970). Another striking feature is the way in which the gross changes in the infected cell are confined by the middle lamella separating it from adjacent cells. The significance of these changes is not clear but it would be most interesting to know if they are related to the accumulation of phytoalexins in the zone of tissue that contains the altered cells.

This is a suitable point at which to refer to induction of resistance by the use of avirulent pathogens because it may tell us something about the hypersensitive response. This type of resistance is well known for a number of diseases and has recently been studied in detail for potato and *P. infestans,* and beans and *C. lindemuthianum.* Infection of tissue by an avirulent race leads to hypersensitive responses and also makes the tissues resistant to a race that is virulent on uninfected tissue. The obvious explanation for this resistance is the one upon which the concept of phytoalexins was based, that the hypersensitive response results in the accumulation of phytoalexins to concentrations that prevent growth of the virulent form inoculated later. But it is obvious that if this is the explanation then resistance cannot be confined to cells that have reacted hypersensitively. Adjacent cells must also have changed so that they now also contain phytoalexins. This, however, conflicts with the proposal given earlier that phytoalexins are very localized. An alternative explanation is that the hypersensitive response of an infected cell induces changes in adjacent cells such that they will now react in a hypersensitive manner to a virulent parasite whereas unchanged cells would not have done so (Skipp, 1971; Varns and Kuć, 1971). An interesting point in this connexion is that cells around those that have been killed by an avirulent race also become more sensitive to forms of damage other than those caused by pathogens (Skipp, 1971).

This explanation of induced resistance implies that phytoalexins are, in fact, largely confined to infected cells where their function is, presumably, to prevent growth of the pathogen out of the cells; it also poses the question as to what prevents movement of phytoalexins from infected cells especially when there is evidence that large amounts are produced.

All this and much other work emphasizes the subtlety and flexibility of the response of the host to infection the nature of which is still largely a matter for speculation. One view starts from the fact that in some diseases there is a gene-for-gene relationship between resistance in the host and avirulence in the pathogen, both controlled by dominant genes, frequently allelic in the host but at independent loci in the pathogen. Avirulence depends on production by the pathogen of a factor that induces the hypersensitive response in host cells that contain a system that can react to this factor. I need not proceed to show how such a hypothesis can be extended to explain the additive and effective type of resistance based on genes which acting independently in different hosts contribute little to resistance. For certain diseases there is some evidence for this hypothesis along the following lines. Pathogen *X* induces a hypersensitive response in host *A* but not *B*. Pathogen *Y* does the reverse. Metabolic products from cultures of *X* and *Y* behave in the same way (Raa and Kaars Sijpesteijn, 1968; van Dijkman and Kaars Sijpesteijn, 1971). At a different level, dead cells of *X* and *Y* do likewise, though here the effects can be more subtle because specific induction of the hypersensitive response seems to depend in some undetermined way on how the cells are killed. In other diseases, such as anthracnose of beans and blight of potato, it has not yet been possible to reproduce the specific responses other than by using living cells. For bean, even the liquid in which spores have germinated does not act specifically; contact between hypha and plasmalemma seems essential. Nevertheless, one must assume that sooner or later, with improved techniques, substances will be isolated that reproduce the specific reactions caused by the pathogens.

Another way of looking at this problem has superficial (and I stress this) similarities to the immune and surveillance phenomena in mammals. It predicts that plant cells in some way 'recognize' cytoplasm (or certain of its products) that are 'not-self', and that this recognition is followed by a series of reactions that end in the hypersensitive response. The further implication is that the response is a general one to foreign substances and would, therefore, be invoked by all micro-organisms, except those that are virulent, that can make contact with the plasmalemma.

Now one asks whether all avirulent micro-organisms invoke the response in the same way or whether this can be done in different ways, all with the same end result. What is the connexion between the pattern of highly specific responses controlled by gene-for-gene relations in systems such as the one involving R-genes in potato and *P. infestans*, and the thousands of potentially incompatible reactions of potato with parasites of other species, because presumably these also result in hypersensitive death of cells. This, however, is a presumption because we are in fact remarkably ignorant about how plants react when challenged in this way as they must be continually in the field.

There is, of course, also another range of problems relating to the reaction, or rather, the lack of reaction, to the virulent parasite. Does this depend on failure of the host cell to recognize the pathogen or its products, or does the pathogen prevent or delay the hypersensitive response from developing? Recent work by Tomiyama (1966) is relevant here because he has shown that potato cells infected by a virulent race of *Phytophthora infestans* respond much more slowly than uninfected cells to later infection by an avirulent race.

Another puzzling feature is that although the virulent parasite does grow for some time before it kills cells, the fact that it is virulent means that after this delay it kills very many more cells than does the avirulent parasite. What then is the difference between death of hypersensitive cells which prevents further growth of avirulent pathogens, and the killing of cells by the virulent pathogen which apparently stimulates its growth? Is the difference primarily one of scale, in that the delayed response to the virulent pathogen allows it to develop so that by the time host cells are killed, adjacent cells have no time to contribute towards the production of the toxic substances that characterize the resistant reaction? If this were so, then the hypersensitive response might be nullified by the use of large inocula. This can happen in some diseases.

Another problem, at least in bean anthracnose, relates to the behaviour of enzymes that degrade cell walls. These are very active in lesions in susceptible plants. But there are few signs of their activity during the early growth of virulent pathogens in susceptible tissues. Is synthesis not induced, or is it repressed? Or, if the enzymes are synthesized and secreted, why do they have so little effect? This is especially relevant because apart from effects on cell walls, certain of these enzymes rapidly decrease the permeability of protoplasts and kill them (Mount *et al.,* 1970; Hall and Wood, 1970). The wall-degrading enzymes have usually been regarded as what Scheffer would call secondary determinants of pathogenicity but, recently, Albersheim and his colleagues (1969) have sought to implicate them directly in specificity. Their hypothesis is based on the following:

(i) the cell wall (and for convenience I shall assume that this includes the middle lamella) contains a wide variety of complex polysaccharide polymers the types and composition of which characterize species, plant parts and age of tissues. There is, however, striking similarity in neutral sugar analyses of wall polysaccharides of cultivars of the same species;
(ii) the polysaccharide-degrading enzymes are very highly substrate specific, e.g. β-1,3 glucanases degrade β-1,4-glucans slowly if at all, and β-1,4-glucanases have little effect on β-1,3-glucans;
(iii) some groups of wall-degrading enzymes are complex; in particular the pectic enzymes differ in one or more of the following ways; end or random cleavage of polymers, action on methyl esterified galacturonosyl linkages, or on those with free carboxyl groups, linkages broken by hydrolysases or lyases, very different pH optima, requirement for calcium, isoenzymes;
(iv) it is well established for a range of other systems that sugar and sugar-containing molecules can be very sensitive to specific recognition by protein;
(v) production by pathogens is highly inducible or repressible by polysaccharides or products of their degradation.

Because of the complexity of these enzymes, and because all fungal pathogens are associated with cell walls in all but the earliest stages of infection, it is proposed that the multitude of possible interactions between cell walls of plants and the enzymes that degrade them could decide specific reactions between host and parasite. Key factors would be induction or repression of the various enzymes by cell-wall polysaccharides.

This is an attractive hypothesis but there are a number of difficulties in accepting it as the sole explanation of specificity, especially for anthracnose of beans, the disease upon which it is mainly based. Thus, an earlier paper claimed that α-galactosidase, an enzyme considered important in cell-wall degradation, was produced much more abundantly when *C. lindemuthianum* was grown on cell walls from susceptible plants than when grown on resistant cell walls (English and Albersheim, 1969). But later work has not substantiated this claim (English *et al.*, 1971). There are similar disagreements for other diseases.

There are also difficulties if one compares the behaviour of avirulent and virulent strains on the same host, or the behaviour of one strain in a susceptible and resistant plant. It is then clear that the avirulent fungus does penetrate the wall of the first cell invaded and then its growth is stopped, whereas the virulent form continues to grow and penetrate cell walls though at this stage it does not degrade them extensively. In these critical stages, growth seems to be determined by cytoplasmic reactions and not by the cell wall. Indeed, one wonders whether penetration of the outer cell wall in these early stages is not largely a mechanical process.

It is also important that resistance can be greatly altered by treatments that undoubtedly affect the cytoplasm but are much less likely to affect the cell wall. Also, it is difficult to explain resistance induced by an avirulent strain in terms of cell wall changes. At present, the evidence is against cell walls as primary determinants of specificity along the lines I have mentioned. But it would be rash to assume that cell walls, and the enzymes that degrade them, play no part in resistance in other ways. There is, for example, good evidence that the resistance that develops as tissues get older depends on cell wall changes (Bateman and Lumsden, 1965). Also, there are a number of treatments of plants that affect resistance by altering the composition of cell walls. And, one cannot ignore the fact that products of cell wall breakdown often appear very soon after infection, that there are subtle relationships between such products and the induction and repression of cell wall-degrading enzymes, and that isolated insoluble cell walls are remarkably effective inducers of pectic enzymes (R. Cooper, personal communication), of α-galactosidase and many other enzymes. Also, certain pectic enzymes cause protoplasts to lose solutes and water rapidly and this is soon followed by death. Could this be important in hypersensitivity?

There is, too, the recent work on protein and enzymes of cell walls which may implicate pectic enzymes in various ways. I refer to the studies of Lamport (1965, 1967, 1969) on the structural protein of cell walls and its complex with carbohydrate through O-glycosidic linkages between hydroxyproline and arabinose; the fact that cell walls contain covalently-bound peroxidase and that ethylene increases both the peroxidase activity and hydroxyproline content of cell walls (Ridge and Osborne, 1970, 1971); and the intriguing discovery that infection of tissues by a soft rot bacterium greatly stimulates production of ethylene by the tissues (Lund and Mapson, 1970). Yet another way in which cell walls may be involved in specificity is suggested by the recent work of Albersheim and Anderson (1971) who isolated glycoproteins with properties similar to the phytoagglutinins well known in seeds of higher plants. These proteins are remarkably active inhibitors of the polygalacturonases which have a key role in cell wall breakdown. In contrast, they have little effect on cellulase, xylanase, α-galactosidase or α-arabinofuranosidase. Inhibitors have been obtained from bean hypocotyls, tomato stems and sycamore cells. The preliminary evidence suggests that they have different capacities to inhibit the polygalacturonases of *C. lindemuthianum, Fusarium oxysporum* f. sp. *lycopersici* and *Sclerotium rolfsii,* that different species contain different inhibitors, and that there may be more than one in a single species.

It is premature to make too much of the significance of this recent work for specificity but perhaps I could add that the ethylene so readily produced by damaged cells is now regarded as an important regulator of cell growth and development (Pratt and Goeschl, 1969); that chain-splitting pectic enzymes do kill cells rapidly and must alter the structure of cell walls and, therefore, the availability and activity of cell wall-bound proteins and enzymes; and that pronounced changes in peroxidase enzymes and peroxidase activity are well known as early symptoms in many plant diseases. It would, therefore, be rash to dismiss these and possibly other cell wall-degrading enzymes as unimportant in specificity as some have been inclined to do.

The host-specific toxins and the cell wall-degrading enzymes are the two groups of substances produced by parasites that are known to damage and kill cells and for which there is evidence for a role in specificity. What about the large number of other substances produced by pathogens, such as wildfire toxin of *Pseudomonas tabaci,* which damage plants at low concentrations, but which affect resistant and susceptible plants in much the same way. Such substances have been called 'secondary determinants of pathogenicity' by Scheffer and Pringle (1967) in that they contribute to the virulence of the pathogen but play no part in determining whether it will be able to establish itself in a plant in the first place, i.e. to be pathogenic in the sense that this word is used by these authors. Be that as it may, one would presumably not be very much concerned with *P. tabaci* and many other micro-organisms as pathogens were it not for these 'secondary determinants'. It would be possible to develop arguments for these non-specific toxins along lines similar to those for cell wall-degrading enzymes which are also not specific on substrates derived from different hosts. On this basis, specificity would be determined by factors that affect production of the toxins rather than their activity.

I must now refer to the provocative work on common antigens first reported some years ago by Doubly *et al.* (1960) for *Melampsora lini* and flax, and more recently by DeVay and his colleagues for a number of diseases.

For four races of *M. lini* and four lines of flax differing essentially only in genes which condition reaction to the rust, it was claimed that races shared a common antigen with susceptible but not with resistant lines. This work was reported only in a preliminary way and, so far as I know, no fuller account of it has appeared, but results along similar lines have been described for two races of *Xanthomonas malvacearum* and three cultivars of cotton (DeVay *et al.*, 1967). Surprisingly, serological relationships between *X. malvacearum* and susceptible cotton were closer than those between it and other species of *Xanthomonas.* Also, leaves of resistant cotton gave a hypersensitive reaction with antigen of an avirulent race but not with antigen of a virulent race, that is, lack of a common antigen was associated with a hypersensitive response. There is similar evidence for common antigens for *Ceratocystis fimbriata* and a susceptible but not a resistant cultivar of sweet potato, *Ipomoea batatas.* However, more recently, DeVay has reported that a strain of *Fusarium oxysporum* f. sp. *vasinfectum,* virulent to cotton and two avirulent mutants had common antigens with resistant and susceptible cultivars, and that loss of virulence did not markedly change the serological relationships between host and parasite (DeVay *et al.*, 1971). Similar work with *Verticillium albo-atrum* revealed at least one common antigen which was the same as the one shared by cotton and *F. oxysporum. Ustilago maydis* had a common antigen with corn and an 'unusually strong antigenic relationship' with three-day-old oat seedlings but much less with six-week-old seedlings, and no common antigens with barley. The older oat plants and barley seedlings were not affected by *U. maydis* whereas the young oat seedlings were rapidly killed (Wimalajeewa and DeVay, 1971).

I need hardly stress the interest of this work, puzzling though its significance may be. Thus, there is the lack of clear relationships for certain vascular wilt fungi that are, nevertheless, highly specific in their parasitism, and certain anomalies in the results for *U. maydis* where there are common antigens between it and corn, a compatible relationship, at least for some time, and between it and oat seedlings, a highly incompatible relationship which rapidly kills the host, presumably in the manner of a hypersensitive response. In other words, there are common antigens in what could be regarded as typical susceptible and resistant responses. Another puzzling feature is that usually it is avirulence and hypersensitivity that are controlled by a dominant gene. Does this imply that the gene for avirulence mutates to one that gives a product antigenically similar to one in the host and that this is what delays recognition in the compatible reaction? If so then it would be of great interest to isolate the homologue of the common antigen to see if it can cause the hypersensitive response.

I shall end by returning to an aspect of specificity I have already referred to, namely, the relation between resistance expressed as a hypersensitive response of a cultivar to an avirulent race of a pathogen, and its resistance to pathogens of other host species. For certain bacteria it seems that both types of resistance are expressed as hypersensitive responses (Klement and Goodman, 1967). But in a system such as the *P. infestans*/R-gene cultivars of potato, resistance is under the control of a number of genes that can act independently to produce the same final response. Does this mean that a very much larger number of genes control the response of potato to the multitude of micro-organisms that are pathogenic to other species but not to potato? Also, how does the behaviour of the saprophyte fit into this scheme, because saprophytic bacteria do not invoke the hypersensitive response and multiply little, if at all, when introduced into the plant. What is the nature of the reaction that prevents growth of saprophytes in these conditions because one must, I think, regard it as an active response. In this connexion, too, there is the recent work of Lozano and Sequeira (1970) to consider. Here, infiltration of heat-killed cells of *Pseudomonas solanacearum* into tobacco leaves prevented the hypersensitive response that would be expected when leaves were inoculated later with an avirulent strain. Nevertheless, the numbers of avirulent bacteria decreased after inoculation. This means that growth of the bacterium was prevented by factors not associated with the necrosis that characterizes the hypersensitive response. How valid, therefore, is the distinction between saprophytes and avirulent pathogens? The fact that one can ask such a deceptively simple question and be certain that the question is rhetorical is evidence again, if any more were needed, of how very little we know about specificity of parasitism.

You will notice that no mention has yet been made of field resistance, adult plant resistance, horizontal resistance and minor-gene resistance (or call it what you will), a type of resistance now becoming more popular because of the failure in practice of the specific types of resistance based on major genes.

An excuse for avoiding this topic may be made as it is outside the scope of my lecture because field resistance is supposedly non-specific. But this would not be a very convincing reason because field resistance is in many respects as specific as the types I have been talking about. But you will be spared yet another series of questions from me which would, I fear, do little more than demonstrate certainly my and, I think, our ignorance of the nature of field resistance as, indeed, of any other type of disease resistance.

References

Adams, R., Geissman, T. A. and Edwards, J. D. (1960). Gossypol, a pigment of cotton seed. *Chem. Rev.* **60**, 555-574.

Akazawa, T. (1960). Chromatographic isolation of pure ipomeamarone and reinvestigation of its chemical properties. *Archs Biochem. Biophys.* **90**, 82-89.

Albersheim, P. and Anderson, Anne J. (1971). Host-pathogen interactions. III. Proteins from plant cell walls inhibit polygalacturonases secreted by plant pathogens. *Proc. natn. Acad. Sci. U.S.A.* **68**, 1815-1819.

Albersheim, P., Jones, T. M. and English, Patricia D. (1969). Biochemistry of the cell wall in relation to infective processes. *A. Rev. Phytopathol.* 7, 171-194.

Bailey, J. A. (1969). Effects of antimetabolites on production of the phytoalexin pisatin. *Phytochemistry* 8, 1393-1395.

Bateman, D. F. and Lumsden, R. D. (1965). Relation of calcium content and nature of pectic substances in bean hypocotyls of different ages to susceptibility to an isolate of *Rhizoctonia solani. Phytopathology* **55**, 734-738.

Bell, A. A. (1967). Formation of gossypol in infected or chemically irritated tissues of *Gossypium* species. *Phytopathology* **57**, 759-764.

Böller, A., Corrodi, H., Gäumann, E., Hardegger, E., Kern, H. and Winterhalter-Wild, N. (1957). Über induzierte Abwehrstoffe bei Orchideen. *Helv. chim. Acta.* **40**, 1062-1066.

Condon, P. and Kuć, J. (1962). Confirmation of the identity of a fungitoxic compound produced by carrot root tissue. *Phytopathology* **52**, 182-183.

Cruickshank, I. A. M., Biggs, D. R. and Perrin, Dawn R. (1971). Phytoalexins as determinants of disease reaction in plants. *J. Indian bot. Soc. Golden Jubilee Vol.* **50A**, 1-11.

DeVay, J. E., Schnathorst, W. C. and Foda, M. S. (1967). Common antigens and host-parasite interactions. *In* 'The dynamic role of molecular constituents in plant-parasite interaction' (eds C. J. Mirocha and I. Uritani). Bruce Publishing Co., St. Paul, Minnesota.

DeVay, J. E., Charudattan, R. and Wimalajeewa, D. L. S. (1971). Common antigenic determinants as a possible regulator of host-pathogen compatibility. *Am. Nat.* In press.

Deverall, B. J. and Vessey, J. C. (1969). Role of a phytoalexin in controlling lesion development in leaves of *Vicia faba* after infection by *Botrytis* spp. *Ann. appl. Biol.* **63**, 449-458.

van Dijkman, A. and Kaars Sijpesteijn, A. (1971). A biochemical mechanism for the gene-for-gene resistance of tomato to *Cladosporium fulvum. Neth. J. Pl. Path.* 77, 14-24.

Doubly, J. A., Flor, H. H. and Clagett, C. O. (1960). Relation of antigens of *Melampsora lini* and *Linum usitatissimum* to resistance and susceptibility. *Science, N.Y.* **131**, 229.

English, Patricia D. and Albersheim, P. (1969). Host-pathogen interactions: I. A correlation between α-galactosidase production and virulence. *Pl. Physiol. Lancaster* **44**, 217-224.

English, Patricia D., Jurale, J. B. and Albersheim, P. (1971). Host-pathogen interactions: II. Parameters affecting polysaccharide-degrading enzyme secretion by *Colletotrichum lindemuthianum* grown in culture. *Pl. Physiol. Lancaster* **47**, 1-6.

Hall, Josephine A. and Wood, R. K. S. (1970). Plant cells killed by soft rot parasites. *Nature, Lond.* **227**, 1266-1267.

Higgins, Verna J. and Millar, R. L. (1968). Phytoalexin production by alfalfa in response to infection by *Colletotrichum phomoides, Helminthosporium turcicum, Stemphylium lotii,* and *S. botryosum. Phytopathology* **58**, 1377-1383.

Hiroe, I., Nishimura, S. and Sato, M. (1958). Pathochemical studies on black spot disease of Japanese pear. 1. On leaf necrotic toxins produced by the causal fungus. *Trans. Tottori Soc. agr. Sci.* **11**, 291-299.

Jennings, P. R. and Ullstrup, A. J. (1957). A histological study of three *Helminthosporium* leaf blights of corn. *Phytopathology* **47**, 707-714.

Katsui, N., Murai, A., Takasugi, M., Imaizumi, K., Masamune, T. and Tomiyama, K. (1968). The structure of rishitin, a new antifungal compound from diseased potato tubers. *Chem. Commun.* No. 1, 43-44.

Katsui, N., Matsunaga, A., Imaizumi, K. and Mazazume, T. (1971). The structure and synthesis of rishitinol, a new sesquiterpene alcohol from diseased potato tubers. *Tetrahedron Lett.* **2**, 83-86.

Keen, N. T. (1971). Hydroxyphaseollin production by soybeans resistant and susceptible to *Phytophthora megasperma* var. *sojae*. *Physiol. Pl. Pathol.* **1**, 265-275.

Klarman, W. L. and Sanford, J. B. (1968). Isolation and purification of an antifungal principle from infected soybeans. *Life Sci.* **7**, 1095-1103.

Klement, Z. and Goodman, R. N. (1967). The hypersensitive reaction to infection by bacterial plant pathogens. *A. Rev. Phytopathol.* **5**, 17-44.

Kuo, M. S. (1968). Comparative effects of *Helminthosporium carbonum* and *Helminthosporium victoriae* toxins on susceptible plant tissues. Ph.D. Thesis, Michigan State University, East Lansing.

Lamport, D. T. A. (1965). The protein component of primary cell walls. *Adv. bot. Res.* **2**, 151-218.

Lamport, D. T. A. (1967). Hydroxyproline-O-glycosidic linkage of the plant cell wall protein extensin. *Nature, Lond.* **211**, 1322-1324.

Lamport, D. T. A. (1969). The isolation and partial characterization of hydroxyproline-rich glycopeptides obtained by enzymic degradation of primary cell walls. *Biochemistry* **8**, 1155-1163.

Letcher, R. M., Widdowson, D. A., Deverall, B. J. and Mansfield, J. W. (1970). Identification and activity of wyerone acid as a phytoalexin in broad bean (*Vicia faba*) after infection by Botrytis. *Phytochemistry* **9**, 249-252.

Lozano, J. C. and Sequeira, L. (1970). Prevention of the hypersensitive reaction in tobacco leaves by heat-killed bacterial cells. *Phytopathology* **60**, 875-879.

Luke, H. H. and Wheeler, H. (1964). An intermediate reaction to victorin. *Phytopathology* **54**, 1492-1493.

Lund, Barbara M. and Mapson, L. W. (1970). Stimulation by *Erwinia carotovora* of the synthesis of ethylene in cauliflower tissue. *Biochem. J.* **119**, 251-263.

Mercer, P. C. (1970). Infection of *Phaseolus vulgaris* by *Colletotrichum lindemuthianum* and *Corticium praticola*. Ph.D. Thesis, University of London.

Mount, M. S., Bateman, D. F. and Basham, H. G. (1970). Induction of electrolyte loss, tissue maceration and cellular death of potato tissue by an endopolygalacturonate transeliminase. *Phytopathology* **60**, 921-931.

Perrin, Dawn R. (1964). The structure of phaseolin (phaseollin). *Tetrahedron Lett.* **1**, 28-35.

Perrin, Dawn R. and Bottomley, W. (1962). Studies on phytoalexins. V. The structure of pisatin from *Pisum sativum* L. *J. Am. chem. Soc.* **84**, 1919-1922.

Pratt, H. K. and Goeschl, J. D. (1969). Physiological roles of ethylene in plants. *A. Rev. Pl. Physiol.* **20**, 541-584.

Pringle, R. B. (1972). Chemistry of host-specific phytotoxins. *In* 'Phytotoxins in plant diseases' (eds R. K. S. Wood, A. Ballio, A. Graniti). Academic Press, London and New York.

Pringle, R. B. and Scheffer, R. P. (1967). Isolation of the host-specific toxin and a related substance with non-specific toxicity from *Helminthosporium carbonum. Phytopathology* **57**, 1169-1172.

Raa, J. and Kaars Sijpesteijn, A. (1968). A biochemical mechanism of natural resistance of apple to *Venturia inaequalis. Neth. J. Plant Path.* **74**, 229-231.

Ridge, Irene and Osborne, Daphne J. (1970). Hydroxyproline and peroxidases in cell walls of *Pisum sativum*: regulation by ethylene. *J. exp. Bot.* **21**, 843-856.

Ridge, Irene and Osborne, Daphne J. (1971). Role of peroxidase when hydroxyproline-rich protein in plant cell walls is increased by ethylene. *Nature, Lond.* **229**, 205-208.

Sato, N. and Tomiyama, K. (1969). Localized accumulation of rishitin in the potato-tuber tissue infected by an incompatible race of *Phytophthora infestans. Ann. phytopath. Soc. Japan* **35**, 202-217.

Sato, S., Tomiyama, K., Katsui, N. and Masamune, T. (1968). Isolation of rishitin from tomato plants. *Ann. phytopath. Soc. Japan* **34**, 344-345.

Scheffer, R. P. and Pringle, R. B. (1961). A selective toxin produced by *Periconia circinata. Nature, Lond.* **191**, 912-913.

Scheffer, R. P. and Pringle, R. B. (1964). Uptake of *Helminthosporium victoriae* toxin by oat tissue. *Phytopathology* **54**, 832-835.

Scheffer, R. P. and Pringle, R. B. (1967). Pathogen produced determinants of disease and their effects on host plants. *In* 'The dynamic role of molecular constituents in plant-parasite interaction' (eds C. J. Mirocha and I. Uritani). The Bruce Publishing Co., St. Paul, Minnesota.

Scheffer, R. P. and Samaddar, K. R. (1970). Host-specific toxins as determinants of pathogenicity. *Recent Adv. Phytochem.* **3**, 123-142.

Scheffer, R. P. and Yoder, O. C. (1972). Host-specific toxins and selective toxicity. *In* 'Phytotoxins in Plant Diseases' (eds R. K. S. Wood, A. Ballio and A. Graniti). Academic Press, London and New York.

Scheffer, R. P., Nelson, R. R. and Pringle, R. B. (1964). Toxin production and pathogenicity in *Helminthosporium victoriae. Phytopathology* **54**, 602-603.

Scheffer, R. P., Nelson, R. R. and Ullstrup, A. J. (1967). Inheritance of toxin production and pathogenicity in *Cochliobolus carbonum* and *Cochliobolus victoriae. Phytopathology* **57**, 1288-1291.

Schwochau, M. E. and Hadwiger, L. A. (1968). Stimulation of pisatin production by actinomycin D and other compounds. *Archs Biochem. Biophys.* **126**, 731-733.

Skipp, R. A. (1971). Factors affecting the resistance and susceptibility of *Phaseolus vulgaris* to races of *Colletotrichum lindemuthianum.* Ph.D. Thesis, University of London.

Smith, D. G., McInnes, A. G., Higgins, V. J. and Millar, R. L. (1971). Nature of the phytoalexin produced by alfalfa to fungal infection. *Physiol. Pl. Pathol.* **1**, 41-44.

Steiner, G. W. and Byther, R. S. (1971). Partial characterization and use of a host-specific toxin from *Helminthosporium sacchari* on sugar cane. *Phytopathology* **61**, 691-695.

Steiner, G. W. and Strobel, G. A. (1971). Helminthosporoside, a host-specific toxin from *Helminthosporium sacchari. J. biol. Chem.* **246**, 4350-4357.

Thomas, C. A. and Allen, E. H. (1970). An antifungal polyacetylene compound from *Phytophthora*-infected safflower. *Phytopathology* **60**, 261-263.

Tomiyama, K. (1966). Double infection by an incompatible race of *Phytophthora infestans* of a potato cell which has been previously infected by a compatible race. *Ann. phytopath. Soc. Japan* **32**, 181-185.

Tomiyama, K. (1971). Cytological and biochemical studies of the hypersensitive reaction of potato cells to *Phytophthora infestans. In* 'Morphological and biochemical events in plant-parasite interaction' (eds S. Akai and S. Ouchi). The Phytopathological Society of Japan, Tokyo.

Tomiyama, K., Takakuwa, M. and Takase, N. (1958). The metabolic activity in healthy tissue neighbouring the infected cells in relation to resistance to *Phytophthora infestans* (Mont.) de By in potatoes. *Phytopath. Z.* **31**, 237-250.

Tomiyama, K., Sakai, R., Sakuma, T. and Ishizaka, N. (1967). The role of polyphenols in the defense reaction in plants induced by infection. *In* 'The dynamic role of molecular constituents in plant-parasite interaction' (eds C. J. Mirocha and I. Uritani). Bruce Publishing Co., St. Paul, Minnesota.

Tomiyama, K., Sakuma, T., Ishizaka, N., Sato, N., Katsui, N., Takasugi, M. and Masamune, T. (1968). A new antifungal substance isolated from resistant potato tuber tissue infected by pathogens. *Phytopathology* **58**, 115-116.

Varns, J. L. and Kuć, J. (1971). Suppression of rishitin and phytotuberin accumulation and the hypersensitive response in potato by compatible races of *Phytophthora infestans. Phytopathology* **61**, 178-181.

Williams, P. G., Scott, K. J. and Kuhl, J. L. (1966). Vegetative growth of *Puccinia graminis* f. sp. *tritici in vitro. Phytopathology* **56**, 1418-1419.

Wimalajeewa, D. L. S. and DeVay, J. E. (1971). The occurrence and characterization of a common antigen relationship between *Ustilago maydis* and *Zea mays. Physiol. Pl. Pathol.* **1**, 523-535.

A. FUNGAL PATHOGENICITY

Section I

Direct Involvement of Fungal Proteins

I. 1 The Killing of Plant Cells by Pectolytic Enzymes

JOSEPHINE A. HALL* AND R. K. S. WOOD
Department of Botany and Plant Technology,
Imperial College of Science and Technology, London, England

INTRODUCTION

This study was undertaken to compare the rots in potato tubers caused by the bacterium *Erwinia atroseptica* (*Erwinia carotovora* var. *atroseptica*) or by the fungus *Corticium praticola* to obtain evidence on the mechanisms by which these very different pathogens cause cell separation and cell death, and on the relation between these two effects on tuber tissue. From the information already available it seemed likely that the cell separation caused by the two pathogens would result from the activity of different types of enzymes. It would, therefore, be of interest to see whether cell death was also closely related to the activities of the different enzymes responsible for cell separation. This, if established, would provide strong–if indirect–evidence for the role of cell-separating enzymes in cell death–a long standing problem in plant pathology and one still incompletely resolved (Brown, 1965).

When conditions are right, *E. carotovora* causes a rapidly spreading, cream-coloured, soft rot in potato tubers. Rotted tissue was obtained from whole tubers inoculated with the bacterium and incubated at 25° C for 3 days; it was mixed with an equal volume of 0.85% NaCl solution and homogenized in a Kenwood blender at full speed for 1 min. The mixture was strained through two layers of nylon cloth and made cell-free by centrifuging at 12 000 *g* 4°C before storing at –20° C.

C. praticola causes only a very slowly developing rot when introduced into whole tubers. To obtain large amounts of rot, tuber slices (10 mm thick) were inoculated with single disks (5 mm dia.) taken from cultures of the fungus grown on a nutrient agar. The slices were incubated for three days at 25° C above a film of water in a plastic box. The rotted tissue was then removed and treated in the way described above.

The extracts from the two types of rot were then compared for their effects on pectic substances *in vitro,* for their capacity to cause cell separation and cell death, and for their effects on the permeability of cells to electrolytes.

* Now at the Water Pollution Research Laboratory, Stevenage, Herts.

EFFECT OF ROT EXTRACTS ON PECTIC SUBSTANCES *IN VITRO*

Activity was measured in three ways: (*i*) inverse of the time required to cause a given loss of viscosity of solutions; (*ii*) release of reducing groups following break of α-1,4 glycosiduronic linkages; (*iii*) increase in absorption of reaction mixtures at 230 nm.

Methods *i* and *ii* measure polygalacturonase and transeliminase activity whereas method *iii* measures only the latter. Under appropriate conditions activity measured in each way is linear against enzyme concentration.

Use of the viscosity and reducing-group methods showed that the *C. praticola* extract degraded polypectate only slightly more rapidly than pectin whereas the *E. atroseptica* extract was twice as active on polypectate. The pH optimum for the *C. praticola* extract was *c.* 5.0, and 9.0-10.0 for the *E. atroseptica* extract.

The *E. atroseptica* extract was most active with Ca^{2+} at 0.001 M. At this concentration calcium added with *C. praticola* rot extract to a solution of pectate caused a firm gel which did not disperse after incubation.

Use of the ultraviolet light absorption method showed that the *E. atroseptica* extracts contained a pectate transeliminase with properties similar to those described above. Treatment of reaction mixtures with thiobarbituric acid confirmed pectate lyase activity. No transeliminase was detected in *C. praticola* extracts though this enzyme was found in extracts from cultures. It is very probable, therefore, that the chain-splitting, pectic enzyme in *C. praticola* extracts is a polygalacturonase and that it and the lyase from *E. atroseptica* extracts are endo-type enzymes.

EFFECT OF ROT EXTRACTS ON CELL SEPARATION AND CELL DEATH

Cell separation was assessed by estimating the time at which disks of potato tuber tissue (7 mm dia., 0.5 mm thick) lost coherence. Inverse of this time is linear against log (enzyme concentration). Death of cells was assessed by the neutral red method (Tribe, 1955). Disks were transferred to 2 ml of a solution containing M KNO_3, 0.1% neutral red, 0.1 M phosphate buffer at pH 7.5 (85 : 15 : 5 by vol.). After 20 min the neutral red solution was replaced by a solution containing 0.9 M KNO_3 and 0.1 M phosphate buffer at pH 7.5. Cells considered to be still alive retained the neutral red whereas cells considered dead became colourless.

For both extracts, cell separation and cell death corresponded closely at different pH values. Thus for the *E. atroseptica* extract, cell separation took *c.* 20 min and about half of the cells were dead in 30 min at pH 9, whereas at pH 5 most cells separated within 90 min and about half the cells were dead in 90-120 min. In contrast, for the *C. praticola* extract at pH 9 there was loss of coherence after *c.* 180 min when somewhat over half the cells were dead whereas at pH 5 similar effects occurred after 70 min.

Cell separation and cell death also corresponded at intermediate values. In each of the many tests there was some killing of cells before cell separation. Very few cells died in the water controls during the 180 min of the experiments.

Effects of Rot Extracts on Permeability of Cells

Changes in permeability were assessed by using a conductivity meter to measure increase in conductivity as electrolytes moved out of cells into water. Disks from tubers were exposed to rot extracts under defined conditions, removed, washed rapidly in water, then transferred to water and the increase in conductivity during 15 min was measured. This method was used because of the high background activity of the mixtures containing rot extracts. But it has certain disadvantages because of the loss of electrolytes before the disks are transferred for conductivity measurements. Nevertheless, it was a convenient method to use and gave results that could be interpreted readily. Representative figures are shown in Table I for disks kept for different times in the following mixtures before transfer to water.

E. atroseptica 1.5 ml rot extract, 2 ml 0.1 M tris-HCl buffer pH 9.0, 6.5 ml water; control, water or heat-inactivated extract.
C. praticola 5.0 ml rot extract, 2.0 ml 0.1 M citrate buffer pH 5.0, 3 ml water; control, water or heat-inactivated extract.

TABLE I

Effect of rot extracts on permeability of potato tuber cells

Time (min)	Increase in conductivity (μmhos/15 min) *E. atroseptica*	*C. praticola*
0	1.2	1.2
10	3.6	14.7
20	7.7	26.0
30	11.5	26.3
40	18.6	25.5
50	18.5	24.3[a]
60	17.5[a]	22.5
90	15.5	5.0
120	11.0	3.1
150	11.0	5.8
180	9.1	3.2

[a] Time for loss of coherence.

Heat treated *C. praticola* extracts caused increases of *c.* 4.0 μmhos at each measurement; corresponding value for *E. atroseptica*, *c.* 1.7; and for water 0.7.

These, and many other results, illustrate the striking effects of the rot extracts on the permeability of tuber cells to electrolytes and that only a small part of this effect can be attributed to thermostable substances in the rot extracts though in this respect the *C. praticola* extracts are the more active. Perhaps the most surprising effect is the rapidity of the increase in permeability; marked changes are detectable within 10-20 min for tissues which remain coherent for another 40 min, and loss of electrolytes continues at the same high level until coherence is lost and for some time afterwards in the *E. atroseptica* extracts.

Rot extracts tested over a wide range of pH values had much the same effect on increasing permeability as on cell separation with optima of *c.* 5.0 and 9.0 for *C. praticola* and *E. atroseptica* respectively.

The effect of calcium on the activity of *E. carotovora* rot extracts was established by comparing extracts dialysed against calcium chloride or water and by measuring the effect of calcium added to extracts dialysed against water. In each case, loss of electrolytes was about twice as great in solutions containing the greater concentrations of calcium. Failure to obtain larger differences is probably explained by calcium in the cells and cell walls of the disks used in the permeability tests.

It is known from the work of Tribe (1955) and others, and we have confirmed that plasmolysis of cells greatly delays killing in solutions that cause cell separation. Plasmolysis in glucose solutions also decreases the rate of loss of electrolytes from cells though the effects are much more striking for *C. praticola* extracts at pH 5.0 than for *E. atroseptica* extracts at pH 9.0. This corresponded with the more pronounced effect of plasmolysing solutions in delaying killing of cells by *C. praticola* extracts.

It was suggested by Friedman and Jaffe (1960) that liberation of ions from middle lamella could account for some of the increase in conductivity similar to that described above. This was investigated by killing disks by placing them in 30% ethanol for 10 min and then washing them in water for 3 h at room temperature. They were then immersed in untreated or autoclaved *C. praticola* extracts for 0-120 min before loss of electrolytes was measured. Both extracts had similar effects with no increase in efflux of electrolytes with time of treatment. There was also no increase in conductivity over 30 min when the washed disks were placed in glass-distilled water. This suggests that the large increases in conductivity obtained with fresh disks did not originate in the walls or middle lamella. It was also of interest to find that the treatment of disks with 30% ethanol had much the same effect on conductivity as did the extracts.

All the above evidence and other results not cited here strongly suggest that chain-splitting pectic enzymes, polygalacturonase of *C. praticola* and pectate transeliminase of *E. atroseptica* are primarily responsible for cell separation and cell death and that these enzymes also cause profound changes in the permeability of cells to electrolytes that parallel their other effects on cells. This correspondence between the different effects was now investigated in other ways.

Fractionation of Rot Extracts

AMMONIUM SULPHATE FRACTIONATION

The rot extracts were fractionally precipitated with $(NH_4)_2SO_4$ at 10-90% saturation at room temperature, and the precipitates were collected by centrifuging. *E. atroseptica* precipitates were dissolved in water, and dialysed against 0.002 M $CaCl_2$ at 4° C before use. *C. praticola* precipitates were dissolved in a minimum volume of 0.5 mM phosphate buffer at pH 7.0 and dialysed against water at 4° C before use. Solutions of the precipitates were assayed for: (*i*) protein; (*ii*) chain-splitting pectic enzyme activity by the viscosity method; (*iii*) ability to cause loss of electrolytes from disks of tuber tissue; (*iv*) phosphatidase activity by the lecithin-cup plate assay of Doery *et al.* (1965). *E. atroseptica* preparations were tested in the presence of 0.001 M $CaCl_2$. For the *E. atroseptica* extracts there was very good correspondence between pectic enzyme activity and effects on permeability with most of the activity associated with the 60-80% fraction. But almost all the phosphatidase activity was associated with the fractions precipitated at 10-50% saturation with no activity in the 60-80% fraction. Clearly, therefore, phosphatidases do not account for the permeability changes caused by *E. atroseptica* extracts.

With the *C. praticola* fractions the results were less conclusive. Most of the pectic enzyme activity was in the 60-70% and 70-90% fractions and these fractions were also among the most active in causing loss of electrolytes. They had no phosphatidase activity. But fractions precipitating at 20-60% which had much less effect on pectic substrates did cause loss of electrolytes at rates similar to those obtained with higher fractions and these fractions were also as active in the phosphatidase tests. For *C. praticola* extracts, therefore, these experiments did not exclude a role for phosphatidases in causing electrolyte loss.

GEL FILTRATION

A solution of the fraction precipitated from *E. atroseptica* rot extracts by 60-90% saturation with $(NH_4)_2SO_4$ with no activity on phosphatides was fractionated by passing through a column of Sephadex G75 gel. Fractions were assayed for pectic enzyme activity by the reducing-group method, for ability to cause electrolyte loss, and for ability to kill cells as assessed by the neutral red method. These activities were essentially confined to fractions 12-15 (inclusive) of the 25 fractions collected. The active fractions accounted for *c.* 25% of the total protein. This experiment was repeated with fractions of *C. praticola* rot extract precipitated with $(NH_4)_2SO_4$ at 60-90% saturation and which had no effect on phosphatides, and with the fraction precipitated at 30-60% saturation which did degrade lecithin. For the 60-90% batch there was again a very striking correspondence between hydrolysis of pectate, almost entirely confined to fractions 10-13 (inclusive out of 25), and ability to cause electrolyte loss which was virtually confined to fractions 11, 12 and 13; fractions 10-13 accounted for some 30% of the total protein.

For the 30-60% batch almost all the phosphatidase activity was contained in fractions 9-14 with *c.* 60% in fractions 9 and 10 whereas the ability to cause electrolyte loss was largely confined to fractions 12-14. There was, therefore, a substantial separation between the two activities. Pectic enzyme activity was evenly spread over fractions 9-15 and did not correspond to the sharp peak for electrolyte loss. Some 60% of the protein occurred in fractions 9 and 10.

The results for the fractionation experiments are summarized in Table II.

TABLE II

Fractionation of rot extracts

Activity	% Saturation $(NH_4)_2SO_4$ for bulk of activity: *E. atroseptica*	*C. praticola*
Pectic enzyme[a]	60-80	70-90
Electrolyte loss	60-80	40-90
Phosphatidase	30-50	20-60

Sephadex G75 fractions (1-25) with bulk of activity

Activity	*E. atroseptica*	*C. praticola*	
% Saturation $(NH_4)_2SO_4$	60-90	30-60	60-90
Pectic enzyme[b]	12-15	9-15	10-13
Electrolyte loss	12-15	12-14	11-13
Cell killing	12-15	—	—
Phosphatidase	—	9-14	—

[a] Estimated by viscosity method.
[b] Estimated by reducing-group method.

In summary, therefore, for the enzymes in *E. atroseptica* and *C. praticola* rots precipitating between 60-90% saturation with $(NH_4)_2SO_4$, there is good evidence that it is the pectic enzymes that cause loss of electrolytes and that phosphatidases are unimportant in this respect. But for *C. praticola* extracts and the fraction precipitating at 30-60% saturation with $(NH_4)_2SO_4$ while loss of electrolytes again cannot be attributed to phosphatidase activity neither can it be unequivocally attributed to pectic enzyme activity unless there are more than one of these enzymes with similar effects on pectic substrates but different effects on cell membranes.

Effect of Rot Extracts on Oxygen Uptake

We are indebted to Miss Frances O'Brien for the following data.

Oxygen uptake by disks of potato tubers in *E. atroseptica* rot extract was much higher (x3-4) than was uptake by disks in water or heat inactivated extract. Dialysis decreased oxygen uptake by about 10-15%. But the results obtained with fractions precipitated with $(NH_4)_2SO_4$ were unexpected. The fraction precipitating at 40-50% saturation had most effect and increased uptake 2-3 fold. In contrast the fraction precipitating at 70-90% saturation had little effect on oxygen uptake although it was the fraction with the bulk of the pectic enzyme activity and the one that caused the most rapid loss of electrolytes.

Essentially similar results were obtained with the *C. praticola* extracts.

Triton X100 (0.1 ppm) and nigericin (10^{-6}M) also caused very rapid loss of electrolytes from tuber disks but these agents also increased oxygen uptake particularly during the first 45 min. Thereafter, uptake by nigericin-treated disks continued to increase for another 60 min when it stopped, whereas uptake by Triton-treated disks stopped after 45 min.

These results can be interpreted in a number of ways. Thus for both rot extracts, the factor increasing oxygen uptake may be the one that causes loss of electrolytes but its effect is masked because it rapidly kills an increasing proportion of the cells. But the more likely explanation is that loss of electrolytes and changes in oxygen uptake are caused by different factors.

Discussion

A body of reasonably conclusive evidence is thus available to show that the main enzymes responsible for cell separation in rots of potato tubers caused by *Erwinia atroseptica* is a pectate transeliminase and that the corresponding enzyme in *Corticium praticola* rots is a polygalacturonase; both are endo-type enzymes.

For both rots there is a close relation between the activity of the cell separating enzyme, loss of electrolytes from cells and cell death so far as the latter is reflected by inability of protoplasts to retain neutral red. We know, too, that it is associated with rapid loss of water (Webb, 1970; D. K. Cronshaw, 1971, personal communication).

It has been tentatively suggested elsewhere that phosphatidases may be involved in cell death (Tseng and Bateman, 1968) but our work shows that phosphatidases degrading lecithin play no part in the permeability changes and cell death caused by extracts of *E. atroseptica* rots. Our results do not exclude phosphatidases of *C. praticola* as causes of permeability changes and cell death but their role, if any, is probably a minor one. We shall assume, therefore, that for both rots, phosphatidases are not important and that it is the transeliminase of *E. atroseptica* and the polygalacturonase of *C. praticola* that are primarily responsible for increasing the permeability and the killing of potato tuber cells.

Similar conclusions were reached in related work with *E. carotovora* (Mount *et al.,* 1970), and with *E. chrysanthemi* (Garibaldi and Bateman, 1971).

We shall now speculate on how chain-splitting pectic enzymes cause cell death and we should begin by emphasizing that most of what is known about these enzymes is based on studies with soluble and, therefore, degraded pectic substances extracted by arbitrary methods from plant tissues, whereas cell separation involves degradation of substances in the middle lamella/cell wall that are insoluble. The relation between the two remains to be elucidated and will not be discussed now although we should like to mention in this connexion the recent work by Albersheim and his colleagues (Nevins *et al.,* 1967; Karr and Albersheim, 1970; English *et al.,* 1971). It has already done much to explain the key role of the pectic enzymes in the degradation of cell walls by plant parasites.

In considering how cell-separating enzymes cause cell death the following points may be considered.

(i) The chain-splitting pectic enzymes are highly substrate specific, a property shared with enzymes that degrade other polysaccharide polymers in cell walls and one repeatedly emphasized by many workers, notably Albersheim and his colleagues (Albersheim *et al.,* 1969). In this respect these enzymes differ from those attacking other types of polymers such as proteins.

(ii) The substrates for pectic enzymes are usually regarded as confined largely to middle lamella and matrix of the primary cell wall with much lower concentrations in the matrix of the secondary cell wall which abuts on the plasmalemma (Northcote, 1958; Roelofsen, 1965).

(iii) The plasmalemma plays an important and critical role in the control of the movement of solutes and water in and out of protoplasts and, therefore, in the permeability of the protoplast and its ability to plasmolyse, properties by which the activity of cell-separating enzymes have been assessed in our work and that of others. Although the composition and structure of the plasmalemma is still somewhat conjectural no one so far as we know has proposed that it contains pectic substances though Albersheim and Killias (1963) have reported that cytoplasmic particles in onion cells stain with the ferric iron-hydroxylamine reagent developed by them for the detection of esterified pectic substances.

(iv) Very little is known about the relation between plasmalemma and the inner layers of the cell wall matrix. Again, so far as we are aware, no one has produced evidence for a role for pectic substances in this connexion. There are, however, indications from studies of fine structure that the relation between plasmalemma and matrix is not so simple as is often assumed.

On the basis of the above, the problem would, in the first place, seem to resolve itself as follows. First, do the cell-separating enzymes act by affecting the plasmalemma directly and by causing some change in the hypothetical relationship between this membrane and the matrix of the secondary cell wall? Along these lines, Mount *et al.* have suggested that because plasmolysed cells are less readily killed by pectic enzymes, the limiting cell membrane may contain a substrate for them and that this is less exposed when the membrane is in a contracted condition. They suggest as another possibility that the cytoplasm contains such a substrate and that contraction of the membrane greatly retards penetration by the enzyme so that the substrate is protected. It remains to be seen whether plasmalemma or cytoplasm contains substrates for these enzymes but in emphasizing the effects of plasmolysis it should also be noted that killing of protoplasts is delayed when the plasmolyticum is such that protoplasts are only just plasmolysed so that there would, in effect, be very little contraction of the plasmalemma. There may, of course, be all sorts of subtle effects once plasmalemma and cytoplasm begin to retract from the cell wall but until such effects are demonstrated it may be as well also to consider the possibility that protoplasts die because pectic enzymes affect substrates in the middle lamella and matrix not directly connected either with plasmalemma or ground cytoplasm. To do this we return again to the delay in the killing of cells kept in a plasmolyticum while they are being separated from one another, and afterwards. This is why cell-separating enzymes, followed by cellulases, can be and are used for the isolation of protoplasts that remain alive in a plasmolyticum until they have produced a new cell wall (Takebe *et al.*, 1968; Schenk and Hildebrandt, 1969; Power and Cocking, 1970). The use of this technique suggests that killing of cells by pectic enzymes may be an osmotic effect in which the plasmalemma is ruptured at one or a number of points following degradation of substrates within the middle lamella/cell wall. Thus, it is a matter of observation that pectic enzymes cause cells to separate along the line of the middle lamella the bulk of the cell wall remaining coherent for some time—this is why cellulases are used to obtain isolated protoplasts. It follows that substances within the middle lamella or adjacent matrix become soluble so that a solution replaces the stiff gel that formerly held the cells together. However, so long as they are not separated deliberately, the cells remain in their original position relative to one another if only because the corners between cells where the middle lamella is generally much better developed usually remains long after the very thin layers between cells have been degraded. One now wonders what happens in these circumstances to the many plasmodesmata which connect adjacent parenchyma cells; numbers of the order of 6000 to 24 000/cell are quoted (Strugger, 1957; Krull, 1960). And one thinks of the characteristic 'puffing' or proliferation of membraneous structures that so often appears in good sections of plasmodesmata at the plane of the middle lamella. If this layer is degraded from the ambient solution inwards, and, therefore, from the intercellular spaces into the planes of partitions between cells, presumably the plasmodesmata become successively exposed to the solution that replaces the gel between cells. This means that the plasmalemma which is continuous through the plasmodesmata also becomes exposed to this solution. What happens then is conjectural but if the solution is hypotonic to the cell then the plasmalemma between cell walls could be ruptured by osmotic forces. But what happens even if it does rupture? Does it merely retract and reform within the lumen of the cell and if so, does it remain susceptible to osmotic rupture? And could this happen successively as plasmodesmata become exposed and so explain the rapidity with which pectic enzymes increase permeability to solutes and to water culminating in loss of capacity to plasmolyse?

In this connexion we refer to the neutral red method of Tribe (1955) which is so widely used to assess cell death. This stain is believed to accumulate within vacuoles which are, of course, limited by the tonoplast. Release of neutral red would, therefore, be expected to be associated with rupture of this membrane which is, however, described as having properties quite different from those of the plasmalemma. Thus, the tonoplast remains as a coherent, semipermeable membrane in conditions in which the plasmalemma becomes non-functional (Robards, 1970). The neutral red method probably needs to be re-examined in relation both to the changes in permeability that precede loss of stain from cells and for what it may reveal about the mechanism of killing.

By postulating a role for plasmodesmata in cell death there is the difficulty of explaining what happens when washed disks cut from tubers are placed in water. The surface of these disks are covered by ruptured cells on the inner surfaces of which the plasmodesmata are, presumably, in a condition similar to that described above. Nevertheless, such disks lose solutes only slowly and the undamaged cells immediately below the damaged cells remain alive for long periods. Consider too the cells that remain alive when the epidermis is removed from the scale leaf of an onion bulb. This behaviour is not what one would expect if pectic enzymes kill cells by exposing plasmodesmata which then rupture, unless damaged cells have mechanisms of repair which do not operate when the middle lamella or adjacent matrix is brought into solution. Also, Calonge *et al.* (1969) state that *Sclerotinia fructigena* may kill cells without destroying the physical integrity of the plasmalemma.

There remains another possibility, that pectic enzymes alter the structure of middle lamella and matrix in other ways that allow osmotic effects to rupture the plasmalemma. Here it may be significant that hydroxyproline-rich proteins in cell walls are now believed to be part of a structural complex with carbohydrates through O-glycosidic linkages between hydroxyproline and sugars, mainly arabinose (Lamport, 1965, 1967, 1969). Arabinose and other sugars are integral parts of pectic polymers (Albersheim, 1965; Barrett and Northcote, 1965). Rupture of glycosidic linkages between the uronic acid residues of pectic substances by polygalacturonases and transeliminases may, therefore, affect the integrity of the complex with the protein in ways that could expose the plasmalemma to the ambient solution and lead to rupture and release of cell contents. In this connexion it may be relevant that when intact cells containing neutral red are exposed to cell-separating enzymes, darker-staining, well-defined circular zones appear in the outer layers of the cytoplasm. These expand rapidly and then appear to burst to release the stain contained within them. This happens at a number of points and as a result the cell rapidly loses its stain, the cytoplasm shrinking away from the cell wall like a collapsed balloon (Margaret Dean, 1966, personal communication). This observation would be worth pursuing particularly in view of the fact that stains such as neutral red are supposed to accumulate within vacuoles.

Against the idea that pectolytic enzymes can affect the integrity of cell walls in this way is the fact that Lamport (1969) has shown that of a range of enzymes tested, including a commercial pectinase, only cellulases released significant amounts of hydroxyproline-rich material from cell walls and even for the cellulase there was evidence that this was due to proteolytic enzymes present as contaminants because pronase was also active in this respect.

The results from two other lines of work may also bear on the killing of and post-mortem changes in protoplasts. The first relates to the effect of ethylene in increasing both the hydroxyproline associated with proteins bound covalently to cell walls and the content of wall-bound peroxidase (Ridge and Osborne, 1970, 1971), and the second to the marked increase in synthesis of ethylene when cauliflower is infected by *Erwinia carotovora* (Lund and Mapson, 1970). Also, there is the marked increase in peroxidase activity as one of the earliest effects of infection in many plant diseases. Whether these changes are the consequence of the killing of cells or an integral part of the process remains to be established. But the rather striking confluence of so many factors in ways that were hardly considered a few years ago certainly suggests a number of interesting, if highly speculative, possibilities.

We have not yet mentioned the part that lysosomes (or spherosomes) may play in the killing of cells by pectic enzymes though we could have done so when referring to the observations of Margaret Dean. With a few notable exceptions (e.g. Pitt and Combes, 1968; Wilson *et al.*, 1970) plant pathologists have not concerned themselves greatly with these structures though in the animal field they have long been investigated as agents of cell death. We do not know of any hypothesis that connects the degradation of a pectic substrate with rupture of the membrane of lysosomes to release the hydrolytic enzymes they contain. And there would, of course, be the problem of how the enzyme in the ambient solution gets to the surface of the lysosome although here, perhaps, one should be cautious in view of recent work on the movement of large molecules through membranes (Seear *et al.*, 1968).

In summary, therefore, our view is that until there is some evidence that pectic substances occur in and are critical for the structure of membranes or components within the cytoplasm, it may be more profitable to explore how pectic enzymes can affect protoplasts by acting upon substrates where they are known to occur, within the middle lamella and the matrix of the cell wall.

REFERENCES

Albersheim, P. (1965). Biogenesis of the cell wall. *In* 'Plant Biochemistry' (ed. J. Bonner and J. E. Varner), 298-321. Academic Press, New York and London.

Albersheim, P. and Killias, U. (1963). Histochemical localisation at the electron microscope level. *Am. J. Bot.* **50**, 732-745.

Albersheim, P., Jones, T. M. and English, Patricia D. (1969). Biochemistry of the cell wall in relation to infective processes. *A. Rev. Phytopathol.* 7, 171-194.

Barrett, A. J. and Northcote, D. H. (1965). Apple fruit pectic substances. *Biochem. J.* **94**, 617-627.

Brown, W. (1965). Toxins and cell-wall dissolving enzymes in relation to plant disease. *A. Rev. Phytopathol.* **3**, 1-18.

Calonge, F. D., Fielding, A. H., Byrde, R. J. W. and Akinrefon, O. A. (1969). Changes in ultrastructure following fungal invasion and the possible relevance of extracellular enzymes. *J. exp. Bot.* **20**, 350-357.

Doery, H. M., Magnusson, B. J., Gulasekharam, J. and Pearson, J. E. (1965). The properties of phospholipase enzymes in staphylococcal toxins. *J. gen. Microbiol.* **40**, 283-296.

English, Patricia D., Jurale, J. B. and Albersheim, P. (1971). Host pathogen interactions. II. Parameters affecting polysaccharide-degrading enzyme secretion by *Colletotrichum lindemuthianum* grown in culture. *Plant Physiol., Lancaster* **47**, 1-6.

Friedman, B. A. and Jaffe, M. J. (1960). Effect of soft rot bacteria and pectolytic enzymes on electrical conductance of witloof chicory tissue. *Phytopathology* **50**, 272-274.

Garibaldi, A. and Bateman, D. F. (1971). Pectic enzymes produced by *Erwinia chrysanthemi* and their effects on plant tissue. *Physiol. Pl. Path.* **1**, 25-40.

Karr, A. L. and Albersheim, P. (1970). Polysaccharide degrading enzymes are unable to attack plant cell walls without prior action by a 'wall modifying' enzyme. *Pl. Physiol., Lancaster* **46**, 69-80.

Krull, R. (1960). Untersuchungen über den Bau und die Entwicklung der Plasmodesmen in Rindenparenchyma von *Viscum album. Planta* **55**, 598-629.

Lamport, D. T. A. (1965). The protein component of primary cell walls. *Adv. bot. Res.* 2, 151-218.

Lamport, D. T. A. (1967). Hydroxyproline-O-glycosidic linkage of the plant cell wall glycoprotein extension. *Nature, Lond.* **216**, 1322-1324.

Lamport, D. T. A. (1969). The isolation and partial characterization of hydroxyproline-rich glycopeptides obtained by enzymic degradation of primary cell walls. *Biochemistry* **8**, 1155-1163.

Lund, Barbara M. and Mapson, L. W. (1970). Stimulation by *Erwinia carotovora* of the synthesis of ethylene in cauliflower tissue. *Biochem. J.* **119**, 251-263.

Mount, M. S., Bateman, D. F. and Basham, H. G. (1970). Induction of electrolyte loss, tissue maceration, and cellular death of potato tissue by an endopolygalacturonate transeliminase. *Phytopathology* **60**, 924-931.

Nevins, D. J., English, Patricia D. and Albersheim, P. (1967). The specific nature of plant cell wall polysaccharides. *Pl. Physiol., Lancaster* **42**, 900-906.

Northcote, D. H. (1958). The cell walls of higher plants. *Biol. Rev.* **33**, 53-102.

Pitt, D. and Combes, C. (1968). The disruption of lysosome-like particles of *Solanum tuberosum* during infections by *Phytophthora erythroseptica* Pethybr. *J. gen. Microbiol.* **53**, 197-204.

Power, J. B. and Cocking, E. C. (1970). Isolation of leaf protoplasts: macromolecule uptake and growth substance response. *J. exp. Bot.* **21**, 64-70.

Ridge, Irene and Osborne, Daphne J. (1970). Hydroxyproline and peroxidases in cell walls of *Pisum sativum;* regulation by ethylene. *J. exp. Bot.* **21**, 843-856.

Ridge, Irene and Osborne, Daphne J. (1971). Role of peroxidase when hydroxyproline-rich protein in plant cell walls is increased by ethylene. *Nature, Lond.* **229**, 205-208.

Robards, A. W. (1970). 'Electron microscopy and plant ultrastructure.' McGraw-Hill, London.

Roelofsen, P. A. (1965). Ultrastructure in the wall of growing cells and its relation to the direction of growth. *Adv. bot. Res.* **2**, 67-149.

Schenk, R. U. and Hildebrandt, A. C. (1969). Production of protoplasts from plant cells in liquid culture using purified commercial cellulases. *Crop Sci.* **9**, 629-631.

Seear, Joan, Bradfute, O. E. and McLaren, A. D. (1968). Uptake of proteins by plant roots. *Physiologia Pl.* **21**, 979-989.

Strugger, S. (1957). Der elektron mikroscopische Nachweis von Plasmodesmen mit Hilfe der Uranylimprägnierung an Wurzel-meristem. *Protoplasma* **48**, 231-236.

Takebe, I., Otsuki, Y. and Aoki, S. (1968). Isolation of tobacco mesophyll cells in intact and active state. *Pl. Cell Physiol.* **9**, 115-124.

Tribe, H. T. (1955). Studies in the physiology of parasitism. XIX. On the killing of plant cells by enzymes from *Botrytis cinerea* and *Bacterium aroideae. Ann. Bot.* **19**, 351-371.

Tseng, T. C. and Bateman, D. F. (1968). Production of phosphatidases by phytopathogens. *Phytopathology* **58**, 1437-1438.

Webb, L. E. (1970). Infection of potato plants and tubers by *Erwinia atroseptica.* Ph.D. Thesis, University of London.

Wilson, C. L., Steers, D. L. and Smith, G. G. (1970). Fungal lysosomes or spherosomes. *Phytopathology* **60**, 216-227.

DISCUSSION

Professor R. K. S. Wood: Before the discussion starts, I should like to refer to the recent work of Dr Harry Mussell which he has been describing at the Symposium on diseases caused by *Verticillium* spp. held this week at Wye College. He believes that leaf symptoms in cotton plants infected by *Verticillium albo-atrum* may be caused by peroxides and that these are produced following the action on cell walls of chain-splitting pectic enzymes secreted by the pathogen. Very similar symptoms develop in plants treated with peroxides, and the development of symptoms can be mitigated by treatments which will decrease production of peroxides. This is a provocative and stimulating development which is, I think, very relevant in the light of Dr Lund's recent work on ethylene in soft rots caused by bacteria.

Can I now start by asking a question myself, relating to the method, which is used by most people, of estimating cell death by plasmolysis and neutral red. Do we know what we are doing when we use this method, because it interests me that the neutral red accumulates essentially in vacuoles, not necessarily only in the central vacuole, but also in vacuoles within the cytoplasm and these of course are lined by tonoplasts. We tend to assume that when we are experimenting with the permeability of cells we are mainly concerned with the plasmalemma, which is usually examined because it is next to the cell wall and we can see it most easily. In fact, fine structure studies show that the tonoplast is a very different limiting membrane from the plasmalemma. Thus, if the neutral red *is* contained within vacuoles which are limited by tonoplast, we must consider that the tonoplast is a much tougher structure than the plasmalemma. Are we working rather blindly here? Has anyone any views about plasmolysis and the neutral red method as a means of estimating cell death? Any views about the tonoplast and the plasmalemma in this connexion? I remember when Tribe was doing this work many years ago he thought he had isolated protoplasts, but when he looked at them closely they were not protoplasts at all, they were tonoplasts just floating around in a plasmolyticum. The rest of the cytoplasm and the plasmalemma had gone. I was also hoping to provoke some questions on plasmodesmata.

Dr R. J. W. Byrde: In our paper we do vaguely question the neutral red plasmolysis stain. We were wondering whether plasmolysis and the ability to take up neutral red were synonymous. Working with Dr Calonge on protoplasts of cucumber and tomato fruit tissue, we found that we could often keep protoplasts intact but they gradually lost their ability to take up neutral red. This certainly raised a question in our minds, but I can't answer the questions which you pose.

Professor P. W. Brian: The most mysterious part of this cell death business, to my mind, is the fact that you can get a considerable degree of protection by a mild degree of plasmolysis. Now I have no doubt that the cytoplasm and the cell wall are a good deal more intimately connected than we are in the habit of thinking, and so I can believe that the pectic enzyme may kill, as it were under natural conditions, but I don't really see why the slight degree of retraction of the plasmalemma can possibly protect it. Have you any views on this?

Professor Wood: Yes I have—because in the paper published by Mount *et al.* (1970) they suggested ways in which pectic enzymes may act upon some undetermined component in the plasmalemma itself and also when retraction of the protoplast from the cell wall occurs in plasmolysis this susceptible component in the plasmalemma becomes in some way not accessible to the pectic enzymes. I don't find this very convincing and for the reasons you give, i.e. because you only need a very slight retraction of the protoplasm; I have therefore assumed that it is probably some plasmolytic effect. Provided you can keep the membrane contracted so that it is intact in a plasmolyticum then it no longer bursts.

Professor Brian: If you cause a small retraction plasmolytically, and expose the cell to the pectic enzyme, and subsequently if you remove the pectic enzyme will it die?

Professor Wood: If it is in the plasmolyticum, no. But if you remove the pectic enzyme and the plasmolyticum, then it bursts. I think the implication is that the plasmalemma itself is not damaged directly; it only bursts because something within the cell wall has been removed which stops it bursting, but I don't know what this is.

Dr D. Pitt: We have been interested for some time in membranes and their stability, and I am rather interested in the idea that pectic substances may alter permeability in this way. I am also concerned that many other things can do this as well, and I wonder whether you are concerned that your pectic enzyme preparations may contain other things which could be primarily responsible. Would you comment on this because you are working with preparations which are notoriously complex.

Professor Wood: What substances had you in mind?

Dr Pitt: There are many substances, proteins, enzymes, toxic compounds or potentially toxic substances around the molecular weight 50 000-100 000, which might well be either absorbed on to or be within the preparations. Could you comment on the degree of purification of your pectic enzymes.

Dr Josephine Hall: We separated the enzymes on Sephadex after ammonium sulphate precipitation and we did not estimate for anything except pectic enzyme activities and their macerating and permeability-increasing activities on potato disks. This is something for further study.

Professor Wood: There are a whole range of things you can eliminate, phosphatidases, practically any other wall-degrading enzyme, proteases and many things which are not involved. In the work of Mount *et al.* where they have done very careful electro-focusing, I think there is sound evidence that it is this pectate lyase that is responsible.

Dr Josephine Hall: I think so as well, but we obviously weren't necessarily looking for other enzymes—I think we can disregard phosphatidases.

Professor Wood: And it can't have a low molecular weight, it must be thermostable, it must be activated by calcium. The circumstantial evidence is now very good indeed that it is this enzyme that kills cells.

Dr J. A. Sargent: We tend so easily to think of membranes in general, particularly perhaps the plasmalemma, as being static organelles, whereas there is good evidence that this is a membrane which is in a continual state of flux, continually being re-formed. We can see this happening, and see the results of it occurring.

Presumably, under the normal healthy condition, the plasmalemma is being continually dissolved, for want of a better word. Thus any mechanism which interferes with either the process of degradation or rebuilding, will of course affect its permeability.

Professor S. H. Crowdy: Could I come back to this question of plasmolytica, for it seems that in natural circumstances the pectic enzyme outside the cell is producing its own plasmolyticum. What happens to the osmotic pressure? I can quite see that if you wash a cell to get rid of the pectic enzyme you will then have removed any low molecular weight materials from the middle lamella, but if you don't wash the cell the osmotic pressure outside should be getting higher all the time—or shouldn't it? Why does a possible osmotic effect not protect the protoplast?

Professor Wood: Are you suggesting that the enzymes themselves are hydrolysing the polysaccharides within the cell wall to lower molecular weight compounds?

Professor Crowdy: Well isn't this what they are doing, I was under the impression that something like this was going on.

Professor Wood: It is an extraordinarily difficult thing to prove, because you have to try to get the concentration of the low molecular weight compounds at the site of action. Certainly the end product itself, galacturonic acid, or some such derivative, in concentrations well above those which would arise if you completely hydrolysed the cell wall, is without effect. But that does not answer your question about the local concentration at the point. It seems to me to be technically impossible to decide this. Can you answer that, Dr Byrde?

Dr Byrde: No, I certainly can't answer this question, but I think one other thing to bear in mind is that in the healthy cell wall the pectic substances are heavily hydrated in a gel form. It is possible that attack on them may lead to liberation of free water. This might produce protoplast bursting.

Professor Wood: But that would be the other way round.

Dr Byrde: Yes, and this would tend to lead to bursting, which I think is what Margaret Dean observed.

Professor P. H. Williams: Many membrane physiologists consider themselves to be working in what they call 'black-box' chemistry, and although this question may lead us deeper into the blackness, I'm interested in developing some of the thoughts that Dr Sarjeant brought up, i.e. should we consider the membrane as a single unit concept, or rather should we consider the protoplast, the active cytoplasm, as being part of this system. Is there any evidence that the site of killing of PG is associated here with the cytoplasm (which is more responsible for membrane function and integrity than the membrane itself).

Professor Wood: There is little evidence for these pectic substrates within cytoplasm, although I think that Albersheim has claimed to find them by using stains that are fairly specific for pectic substances.

Professor M. A. Stahmann: Some pectic enzymes have very high pH optima, 9-10. I would like to ask two questions, first, do you consider these to be very active *in vivo,* and then secondly, is there a connexion between enzyme activity and oxidases. I ask this because of the observation of Tomiyama that treatment of potato tissue with pectic-hydrolysing enzymes increased peroxidase and polyphenol oxidase activity in the underlying tissues.

Professor Wood: The question you raise about the very high pH values only applies to the pectate and pectin lyases. I don't know what the answer to that is. We are faced with this problem in the *Erwinia* rots of potato tubers, where the evidence would stress that pectate lyase is the most active in these rots, but it has a pH optimum of 9 or above. In fact, we have never found the true optimum pH for this enzyme. Whereas if you take a soft rotted potato tuber, it has a pH of about 6.5 or 7.

Professor Stahmann: Yes, I wonder how important they are *in vivo.*

Dr Hall: We do not know whether maceration at high pH values i.e. pH 9.0 is relevant to rotting *in vivo* because of the technical difficulties in determining pH conditions at the site of enzyme action in potato tissue.

Professor Wood: Regarding your second question, I can only quote the work of Mussell, which in some way raises this point, and also that of Daphne Osborne and Irene Ridge, which clearly indicate that peroxidases are wall-bound enzymes and that if you have a pectic enzyme which is doing something drastic to the structure of the cell wall, then it could well be releasing these peroxidases from the bound state, but I don't know of any work on the direct release, or whether the mere treatment of cell walls with pectic enzymes does lead to a large increase in free peroxidase compared with bound peroxidase.

Professor Stahmann: In my laboratory, when white potato was treated with commercial peroxidase preparations, which may not have been pure, there was a marked increase in both polyphenol oxidase and peroxidase in the underlying layers.

Professor Wood: This is very true, but how are you going to relate peroxidases to cell death?

Professor Stahmann: We have been studying the interaction of the peroxidase system with proteins, and my paper will show how peroxidase can react with the histone group of proteins, e.g. to deaminate; it may disrupt protein structure, and this can upset enzyme action.

Professor J. Friend: You did mention that there was no evidence for polysaccharides being present in the plasmalemma, yet if we look at Dr Northcote's studies, in which he feeds labelled glucose and watches it being transported towards the cell and deposited in the middle lamella, one sees accumulations of radioactivity inside the cell which presumably are either labelled glucose or polymers of glucose or other sugars. Is it not possible that these are the beginning of the pectic molecules which are bound up in membranes inside the cell near the plasmalemma, and therefore there could be some connexion between the plasmalemma and the pectic substances which are not yet fully formed into their large molecular size when they are present in the wall, and could these then be the target for your pectic enzymes.

Professor Wood: Yes, but if you look at both the classical and current pictures of the cell membrane with all its little dots and squares, and the unit membrane structure, I don't recollect seeing a pectic substance attached to any of these. Is this not true, Dr Sargent?

Dr Sargent: It is quite clear that the membrane does dissolve, we must therefore have enzymes doing it, and probably quite a complex set of enzymes is involved. But at the same time we must have enzymes there which are rebuilding it continually. If we interfere with any one of them, and also interfere with any of the reactions involving the dictyosomes–not only the production of packages of wall-building material which pass through the plasmalemma, but also the membrane-building materials themselves–then we will have altered the permeability of that organelle.

Professor Wood: Yes, but I want to know the role of a very highly substrate-specific pectic enzyme in this. Referring to Professor Stahmann's other point, the question one asks fine structure workers concerns the relation between the limiting unit membrane, and the innermost layer of the cell wall. In most pictures the inner membrane abuts the cell wall. Occasionally you get rather more complicated pictures of it going in and out, but what is the relation between these two? This point still seems unresolved. The other point refers to the structure of the cell wall. You've got the middle lamella, you've got the primary cell wall and the secondary cell wall. Again the classical picture shows that the secondary cell wall, which is adjacent to the plasmalemma, contains very little pectic substance, whatever one means by pectic substances. I was hoping to provoke you into some pertinent questions on what is meant by a pectic substance, but that perhaps is too wide a subject, but it is a critical point. Again the classical concept sees maceration as occurring mainly along the line of the middle lamella, which is well removed from the plasmalemma. The secondary cell wall is not supposed to be the main repository of the substrates of these enzymes; it is supposed to be dominated by cellulose and hemi-cellulases. Again there is a remoteness from the site of action.

Professor J. H. Burnett: On this question of localization, why can't you label your enzymes, and then combine autoradiography with the electron microscopy or light microscopy, and see where they end up. Is there any objection to this technique?

Professor Wood: I don't think there is any objection to it.

Professor Burnett: Well this would perhaps give you a more direct answer than some of these more indirect methods.

Professor Wood: No one has yet done that so far as I know. What would be the object? Would you then end up with a labelled pectate lyase?

Professor Burnett: That is right, then apply it to your cells, and then you go through the electron microscopy procedure and look for autoradiography. You've got a labelled enzyme and you are simply looking for the autoradiographic pattern.

Professor Wood: In the hope that you would find out where that enzyme is acting?

Professor Burnett: Well if you can think of any better way, that's fine, but it seems to me that in the state of ignorance that we are all in on this, any method is worth trying, and this is, after all, analogous to the way that Northcote and other people have used to trace the paths of other compounds.

Professor Wood: But they have used labelled substrates.

Professor Burnett: If the enzyme is bound on to plasmalemma, for instance, then it ought to be possible to follow this.

Professor Wood: The number of molecules involved, of course, would be very, very small indeed. This enzyme is active in remarkably low concentrations, and whether you could ever label enough material to get your autoradiographs out, I don't know, but it's worth trying.

Professor C. E. Bracker: In response to what Professor Burnett said, there are, of course, some mammoth technical problems involved in doing the autoradiography, e.g. concerning distances from the source, which would have to be taken into account.

In regard to Harry Mussell's work, he has developed an assay technique for pectic enzymes in which he uses cucumber tissue, and this seems to be a reliable method. He has also now isolated and purified an endopolygalacturonase from *Verticillium.* He can subject cucumber tissue to this enzyme, without any other contaminating materials that might be present in the vascular system of the cotton as a result of the fungus. Can he then tell whether for example these cells die, approximately when they die, and whether the peroxidases he finds in the cotton leaf, are also present in this little model system he has? Do you know?

Professor Wood: Yes, I do. Incidentally, Mussell's system works beautifully. I think that the preparations of *Verticillium* that act in cotton do in fact kill cucumber cells, but I think so far he has been unable to implicate peroxides in the killing of this tissue. I don't think he has succeeded in doing it with potatoes either.

I.2 The Role of Extracellular Enzymes in the Rotting of Fruit Tissue by *Sclerotinia fructigena*

R. J. W. BYRDE, A. H. FIELDING AND S. A. ARCHER

Long Ashton Research Station

AND

ELEANOR DAVIES

Department of Microbiology
University of Bristol, England

INTRODUCTION

The fungus *Sclerotinia fructigena* Aderh. and Ruhl. causes a brown rot disease of apple and related fruits characterized by the comparative firmness of the invaded tissue. The importance of extracellular 'cytolytic' enzymes in the pathogenicity of the genus *Sclerotinia* dates back to the classical paper of de Bary (1886) working with *S. libertiana.* Bruschi (cited by Valleau, 1915) was the first to suggest that extracellular pectolytic enzymes were active in a fruit-rotting species, and much of the subsequent work has been restricted to these enzymes.

The nomenclature of the pectolytic enzymes, at one time confused, was standardized by Demain and Phaff (1957). Bateman and Millar (1966) subsequently proposed enlargements to take account of the newly-recognized transeliminase enzymes; their nomenclature is used in this paper.

The production by *S. fructigena* of extracellular enzymes in culture has received considerable attention. J. S. Cole (1956) who summarized prior work on the subject, demonstrated the secretion of polygalacturonase (PG) and pectin methylesterase (PME) in a synthetic medium with either glucose or pectin as carbon source. In addition, the filtrates would macerate potato disks. Enzyme activities were shown to increase with increasing amounts (up to 2%, w/v) of ammonium tartrate, the nitrogen source used in the medium. These results were confirmed by M. Cole and Wood (1961b).

J. S. Cole (1956) showed that the PG was able to reduce the viscosity of sodium polypectate solutions more rapidly than that of pectin (implying that the enzyme is an endo-PG), and that the pH optimum for the breakdown of the former substrate was about 6.0. Subsequent work (Fielding and Byrde, 1969) confirmed that the enzyme is an endo-PG, though a rather lower pH optimum was found. The enzyme existed in at least two forms, of mol. wt. approx. 77 000 and 38 500, and electrophoresis suggested that these carried a net basic charge which may assist in the adsorption of the enzyme on acidic polyuronides in the host cell wall. By contrast, the PME secreted *in vitro* has not received further study.

The macerating activity mentioned above was shown by Byrde and Fielding (1962) to be distinct from PG, and subsequent work demonstrated the presence of an α-L-arabinofuranosidase (AF) in partially purified enzyme preparations free of PG, yet capable of macerating potato tissue (Byrde and Fielding, 1965). This enzyme was further characterized as an exo-type enzyme, again existing in multiple forms, with a pH optimum of about 4.0 (Fielding and Byrde, 1969). However, by that time the macerating activity had been correlated with a pectin methyl transeliminase (PMTE) also present in culture filtrates: this enzyme was found to exist in at least two forms, with pH optima of 7.3 and 8.3. The latter required activation by an uncharacterized component in potato extract, or by sodium polypectate (Byrde and Fielding, 1968).

While the secretion *in vitro* of β-galactosidase has been recorded, the following extracellular enzymes have not been detected: cellulase, proteases, xylanase, β-D-xylosidase, polygalacturonate transeliminase, and phosphodiesterase (Byrde and Fielding, 1968).

Physiological Effects *In Vivo*

KILLING OF TISSUE

As already mentioned, the rotting of fruit by *S. fructigena* is characterized by the comparatively firm texture of the infected tissue. The infected skin often assumes a chestnut brown colour, and the underlying tissue a lighter shade of brown, due to post-mortem oxidation of polyphenolic compounds (M. Cole, 1958a). The killing of the cells in the region of the advancing hyphae and behind them was demonstrated by use of Tribe's (1955) neutral red plasmolysis method (J. S. Cole, 1956). These results have readily been confirmed by one of us (E. D.) in attempts to delineate the effect more finely both spatially and temporally. Hyphal tips were often seen among the zone of living cells (see Fig. 1); in some cases, there was death of cells apparently in advance of the hyphae (as shown by J. S. Cole, 1956, Fig. 1), but this may have been due to the presence of adjacent hyphae not then visible. Clearly, the effects described could be due either to a slow-acting toxin generally diffusing some distance ahead of the hyphae (which advance at approximately 200 μm/h) or to a more-rapidly-acting compound remaining in the near vicinity of the hyphal tips.

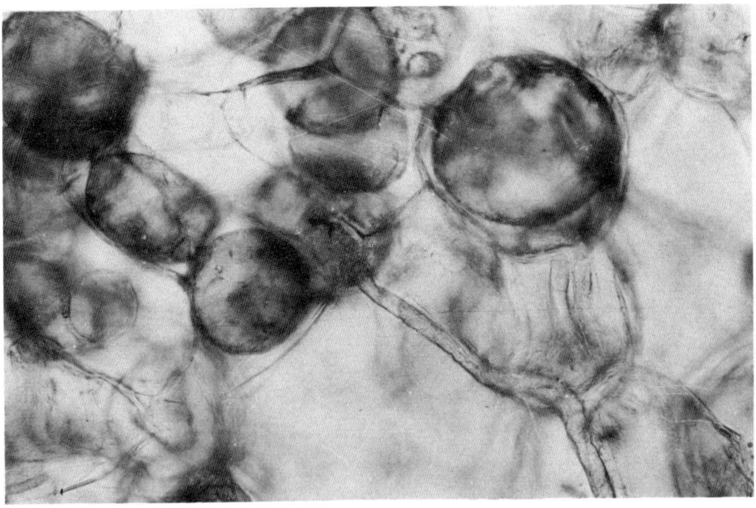

Fig. 1. Photomicrograph of invading hypha of *S. fructigena* adjacent to stained plasmolysed protoplast of apple fruit cell. Stained and plasmolysed with neutral red in buffered 1.7 M KNO_3. ×120.

CELL LEAKAGE

Tribe's method for determining whether cells are living or dead is based on the ability of a living cell to be plasmolysed by a hypertonic solution and of its vacuole to be stained by neutral red. These two characteristics are not necessarily identical, and the physiological basis of the uptake of neutral red is not clear. The permeability characteristics of plant cell membranes, often changed in disease (Wheeler and Hanchey, 1968), can also be examined by determination of ion leakage, either by the use of labelled isotopes, e.g. ^{86}Rb (Mount *et al.*, 1970) or by conductivity measurements (e.g. Hall, 1971). The latter method has proved useful in examining changes in semi-permeability of apple cells during invasion by *S. fructigena*. Some modification was required because of the osmotic fragility of apple cells, already recorded by Burg and Thimann (1960), who found that apple cells actually lost water (and other cell constituents) when placed in water. Experiments were therefore done in 0.4 M-sucrose as stabilizing medium and conductivity was measured directly on the solution in which the disks were immersed, as shown in Fig. 2. Preliminary results using either a conductivity probe on the intact tissue, or a cell containing 20 disks (5 mm dia.) in 0.4 M-sucrose (20 ml), suggested that permeability changes occurred only at the edge of the obviously rotted area. The absence of leakage more than 1 mm in advance of the hyphae was confirmed in triplicate experiments in which finer spatial limits were used (Table I).

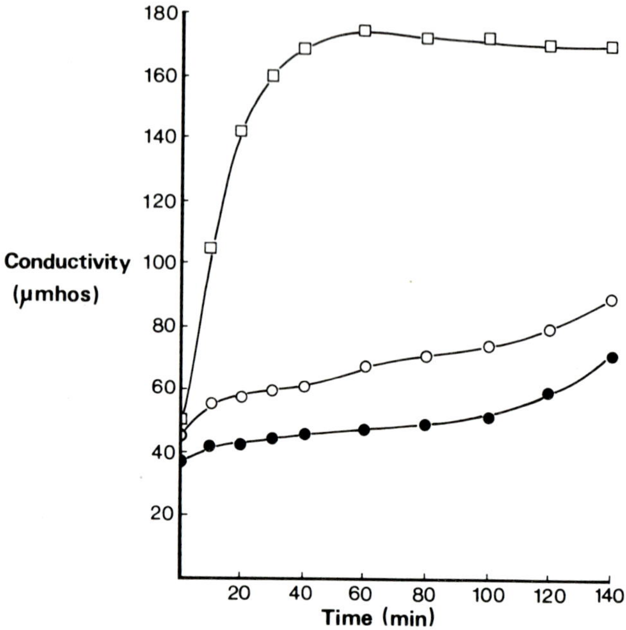

Fig. 2. Comparison of leakage of apple tissue slices immersed in water (□), 0.4 M mannitol (○) and 0.4 M sucrose (●).

Conductivity was read directly on 20 ml liquid containing 10 disks of fruit tissue (1 cm dia., 1 mm thick) of apple, Lord Lambourne, at room temperature.

TABLE I

Electrolyte leakage from apple fruit tissue

Position relative to advancing rot edge[1]	Mean conductivity increase (μmhos)
± 1 mm	34.7
+ 1 to + 3 mm	15.7
+ 3 to + 5 mm	14.0
Healthy tissue	15.0
Least significant difference ($P = 0.05$)	12.9

Equal lengths (*c.* 150 mm) of ribbons of tissue, 1 mm deep including peel, were cut parallel to the advancing edge of the rot, and immersed in 0.4 M-sucrose solution (20 ml). Conductivity increase over the ensuing 15 min was recorded.

[1] Positive measurements signify non-invaded tissue.

Occurrence of Enzymes *In Vivo*

A complicating factor in the detection of extracellular enzymes in apple tissue, whether healthy or diseased, is the susceptibility of these enzymes to inactivation by oxidized host constituents (J. S. Cole, 1956) of which polyphenols have been particularly implicated (M. Cole, 1958*a*; M. Cole and Wood, 1961*b*; Byrde, 1963).

M. Cole and Wood (1961*b*) recorded high levels of PME in extracts of tissue infected by *S. fructigena*, relative to sound tissue, and rather higher than with two other fruit-rotting pathogens. PG was also detected in small quantities, but was lower than with the other two pathogens. Macerating activity was not detected with *S. fructigena*. In later work on the fine structure of infected apple tissue, Calonge *et al.* (1969) confirmed the presence of PME and PG, and demonstrated that AF and a β-galactosidase were present in infected tissue. PMTE was not detected.

Following preliminary experiments by Akinrefon (1967) on the spatial distribution of PG, one of us (E. D.) has examined the enzyme levels in extracts of the tissue in four zones relative to the advancing front, with the results shown in Table II. These confirm the presence of PME in healthy tissue, higher levels in infected tissue, with AF but no PMTE in infected tissue. The increase in PG ahead of the rot, reminiscent of the demonstration by Balasubramani *et al.* (1971) of PG outside *Botrytis* lesions on *Vicia faba* leaves suggests that some

Table II

Enzyme activities extracted from different parts of apples with infections of *S. fructigena*

Sample[1]	PG[2] (U.)		PME[3] (ml 0.01 N NaOH)		AF[4] (ΔE)	PMTE[4] (ΔE_{240})
	Expt 1	Expt 2	Expt 1	Expt 2	Expt 1 only	Expt 1 only
A	6.5	7.3	0.6	0.8	0.05	0.00
B	35.8	36.6	1.1	1.5	0.05	0.00
C	94.9	78.0	3.4	3.6	0.21	0.00
D	220.5	221.5	4.0	3.5	0.27	0.00

Excised tissue was immersed for 3 h in acetone in an ice-salt bath. It was then macerated and washed repeatedly on a Buchner funnel with cold acetone. The residues were dried under reduced pressure and ground to a fine powder. This was extracted with 0.25 M Na_2HPO_4 (20 ml/g) at 0° C for 1 h, and filtered through muslin.

[1] *A*. Healthy tissue; *B*. Healthy tissue 1-2 mm in advance of the hyphae; *C*. Diseased tissue from zone edge; *D*. Well-rotted tissue from body of rot.

[2] Estimated by cup-plate method (Dingle *et al.*, 1953), pH 4.7, 25° C.

[3] Estimated by back-titration after 20 h at 25° C. Substrate mixture was that described by Smith (1958) adjusted to pH 5.0.

[4] For methods, see Byrde and Fielding (1968).

forward diffusion of this enzyme may have occurred. By contrast, PME did not appear to increase greatly until the fungus arrived.

ACTIVITY OF THE ENZYMES *IN VIVO*

In infected tissue, PME is not only present but also acts on its substrate. M. Cole and Wood (1961*a*) showed that in such tissue there was an increase in the amount of pectic substances soluble in dilute alkali, indicating that demethylation had occurred. In our experiments, histochemical examination of infected tissue using the iron-hydroxylamine stain method described by Reeve (1959) also indicated that walls were demethylated. Although it was not easy to see hyphae in tissue when this stain was used, the onset of demethylation appeared to correspond approximately with the arrival of the hyphae.

The liberation of methanol has been confirmed by two methods: permanganate oxidation followed by the use of chromotropic acid reagent, which is specific for formaldehyde (Boos, 1948), and by gas chromatography.

By the first method, healthy apples (Dunn's Seedling), were shown to contain 3.93 mg methanol/100 g of fresh tissue; whereas for rotted tissue the comparable figure was 73.0 mg. For Bramley's Seedling the differences were even more marked, the respective figures being 0.09 and 84.4 mg. This greater difference may reflect the very low levels of host PME known to be present in this cultivar (Pollard and Kieser, 1951). When sections were cut through the advancing front of the rot and methanol was assayed in tissue disks cut serially along the section, high levels were found slightly in advance of the zone of browning corresponding to the arrival of fungal hyphae and demethylation of the cell walls as detected histochemically.

Further evidence for the identity of methanol was provided by gas chromatography. Volatile components from infected apple tissue included ethylene (Hislop *et al.*, 1972), methanol and ethanol, all of which were essentially absent from healthy fruitlets at a similar stage of maturity. A typical chromatogram is shown in Fig. 3. Evidence for the origin of methanol arising from demethylation of pectin was provided by the fact that methanol could be detected after incubating a crude wall preparation overnight with mycelial pellets of *S. fructigena.* Further evidence was obtained by incubating highly purified apple cell walls and sections of apple tissue with fungal PME, essentially free of other pectolytic enzymes, the liberated methanol being detected by gas chromatography in both cases.

The presence, in substantially increased amounts, of both arabinose (Byrde and Fielding, unpublished), and D-galacturonic acid (Cole and Wood, 1961*b*) in extracts of infected tissue indicates that both PG (at least an exo-enzyme) and AF are also active. Electron micrographs, however, suggest that, at least in pear tissue, breakdown of cell walls is largely localized round the hyphae (Calonge *et al.*, 1969).

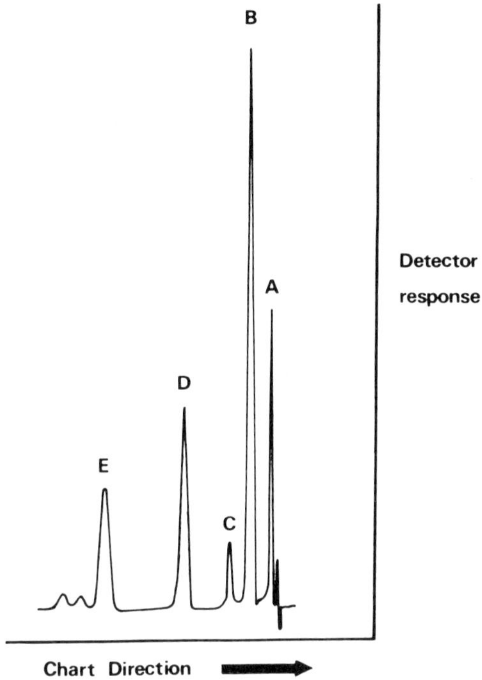

Fig. 3. Gas chromatogram of volatile constituents from apple fruits infected with *S. fructigena.* A, ethylene; B, methanol; C, unknown; D, ethanol; E, unknown.

1 ml gas samples were injected into a Varian Aerograph 205-2B fitted with flame-ionization detector. Glass column 150 cm x 3 mm packed with Porapak Q 100-120 mesh. Injector temp. 110° C. Column Temp. 105° C. Nitrogen carrier gas. Flow rate 20 ml/min.

ORIGIN OF PECTOLYTIC ENZYMES PRESENT *IN VIVO*

What is the origin of the increased levels of PME and PG in infected tissue? Such increases are commonly encountered in other host-pathogen interactions. PG is generally accepted as being of fungal origin (Wood, 1967), although Barash and Khazzam (1970) demonstrated the presence of induced host PG in anthracnose disease of avocado. Increases in PME have often been attributed to activation of host enzymes (e.g. Bateman, 1963) rather than to secretion by the pathogen.

The enzymes in the *S. fructigena*–apple system were examined by iso-electric focusing, which has already proved useful in pectolytic enzyme resolution (Garibaldi and Bateman, 1971). It is seen in Fig. 4 that the host PME had two major components, with pI values of 9.6 and 6.5 and a minor component of pI 2.7. In culture, *S. fructigena* produced PME with a pI value of 4.9. In the

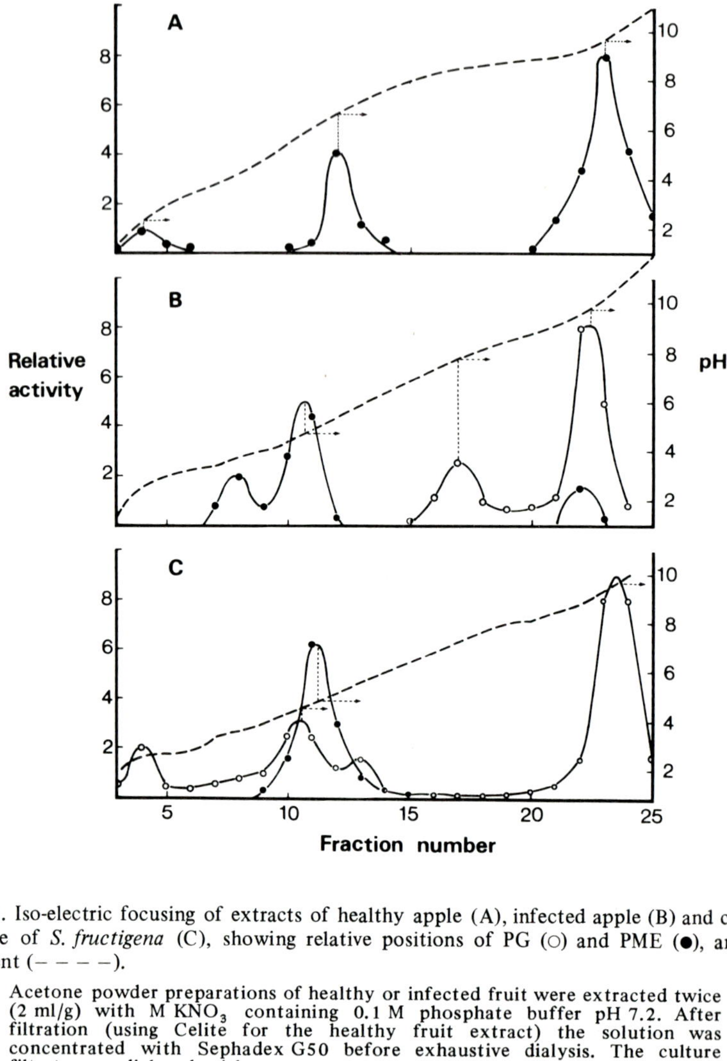

Fig. 4. Iso-electric focusing of extracts of healthy apple (A), infected apple (B) and culture filtrate of *S. fructigena* (C), showing relative positions of PG (○) and PME (●), and pH gradient (– – – –).

Acetone powder preparations of healthy or infected fruit were extracted twice (2 ml/g) with M KNO_3 containing 0.1 M phosphate buffer pH 7.2. After filtration (using Celite for the healthy fruit extract) the solution was concentrated with Sephadex G50 before exhaustive dialysis. The culture filtrate was dialysed without pre-treatment. Iso-electric focusing (Vesterberg and Svensson, 1966) was done at 10° C for 40 h on a 110 ml column with carrier ampholytes at a final concentration of 1% (w/v). The enzyme sample was added to the light component of the sucrose gradient. Voltage 200 V increasing to 500 V. Enzyme assays as in Table II.

extract of rotted apple the major PME component had a pI value of 5.1; a second component was present with pI 4.1, and a small peak at pI 9.6 presumably corresponded to the residual host enzyme. These results indicate that the marked increase in PME was due to the pathogen and not to the host.

This view was strengthened by the pH values found for optimum activity which were: *i.* healthy apple, a broad peak from 5.5 to 7.0; *ii. S. fructigena* (*in vitro*), 5.0; *iii.* rotted apple, 4.5-5.0. Polygalacturonase was absent in healthy tissue; the pI values for the enzyme produced *in vitro* were 9.8 and 4.6. In infected tissue, the main component had a pI value of 9.8 with a minor peak at pI 7.6. AF (not shown in the Figure) was not present in healthy apple; two components (pI values of 6.8 and 3.0) were present *in vitro,* but only the former was detected *in vivo.*

PHYSIOLOGICAL EFFECTS OF ENZYME PREPARATIONS

We have made repeated, but uniformly unsuccessful, attempts by several methods, using extracts of infected tissue to simulate the cell leakage and death which occurs *in vivo.* Such failures may well be associated with a modification of the active agent, possibly as a result of necrotic reactions.

However, a dialysed culture filtrate of *S. fructigena* grown on a polypectate medium (Byrde and Fielding, 1968) rapidly induced cell leakage in apple tissue as seen in Fig. 5. For fractionation, iso-electric focusing was used: this method based, as is ion-exchange chromatography, on separation by net charge of molecules, has two advantages over other methods. Unlike column chromatography, where adsorption can occur, the final fractions include all the initial constituents. Unlike gel filtration, the components are focused and concentrated rather than becoming diffused and hence diluted. Figure 5 shows a clear peak of cell leakage at a pI value of 5.4, which did not correspond exactly with that for any other enzyme activity recorded for the fractions, although nearest to that for PME. When fractions were heated at 100°C for 20 min, they were no longer active. Overnight exposure to fractions inducing leakage led to browning of the tissue and death of the cells, as shown by the plasmolysis/neutral red method of Tribe (1955). These effects on apple tissue could not be simulated by methanol, up to 4% (v/v), a concentration in excess of that which could be expected to occur even locally following PME action. M. Cole (1958*b*) had reached a similar conclusion on the non-involvement of methanol.

Fractions from another iso-electric focusing experiment, corresponding to a pI range of 4.9-5.6 were subjected to gel filtration on Sephadex G100. The phospholipase, PME and PG activities of these fractions, following dialysis, and their ability to bring about conductivity changes are shown in Fig. 6. From this and Fig. 5 it is clear that the ability to induce cell leakage was not associated with PMTE, AF or phospholipase activity: further work is required to clarify the role of PG and PME. A preliminary experiment with disks treated with 30% (v/v) ethanol (Hall, 1971) indicated that a minor proportion of leakage induced by the active fractions was due to ion release from cell walls.

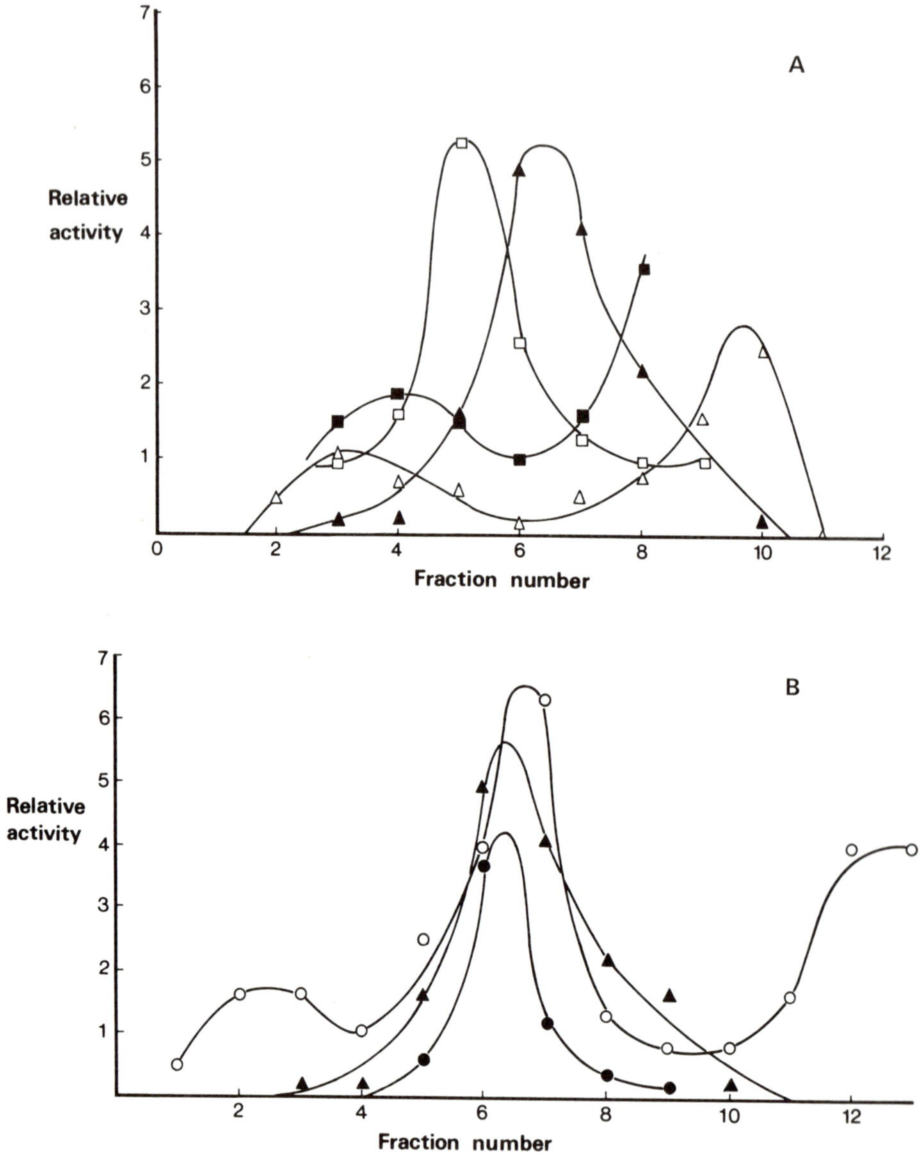

Fig. 5. Cell leakage of apple fruit tissue induced by dialysed fractions from iso-electric focusing (pH 3-10) of a dialysed culture filtrate of *S. fructigena*. Comparison of induced leakage (▲) with: A. PMTE (△), AF (■) and phospholipase (□). B. PG (○) and PME (●).

Iso-electric focusing carried out as for Fig. 3. Phospholipase assayed by method of Doery *et al.* (1965). Other enzymes as for Table II.
Peak of cell leakage corresponded to a pI value of 5.4.

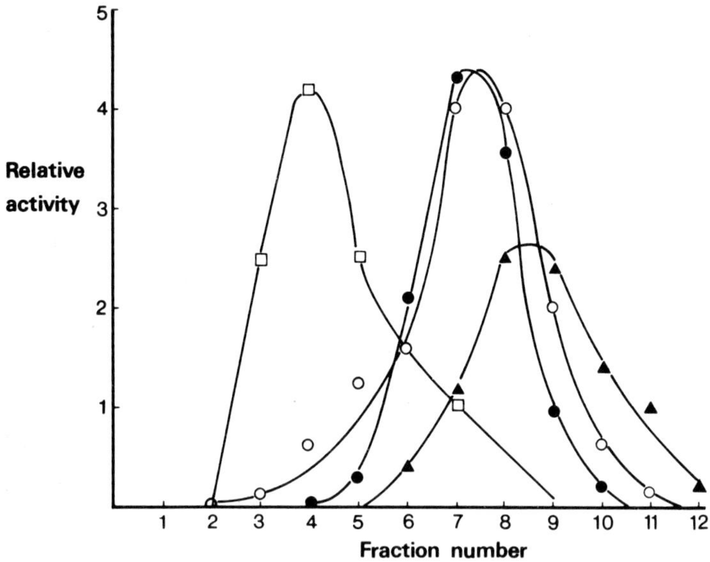

Fig. 6. Gel filtration of leakage-inducing peak from iso-electric focusing, showing further resolution of conductivity increase (▲), PG (○), PME (●) and phospholipase (□).

Gel filtration on Sephadex G100 (35 × 3.5 cm) using 0.05 M phosphate buffer pH 7.3 as eluant. Fractions (14 ml) subsequently dialysed against water. Assays as in Fig. 5.

Conclusions

In culture, *Sclerotinia fructigena* is capable of secreting an array of extracellular enzymes. Most seem to be functional when the fungus invades apple tissue: a notable exception is PMTE, which is often associated with pathogenicity but which has not been detected in extracts of apples infected by *S. fructigena.*

On the arrival of infecting hyphae, marked physiological and structural changes occur in the tissue, but apparently little happens before this stage. These include cell death, associated with loss of membrane semi-permeability, and subsequent polyphenol oxidation leads to browning of the tissue. The pectic substances are also modified, although overall loss is not great: the cellulose component does not appear to be attacked, and the rot remains comparatively firm.

The role of extracellular enzymes in bringing about these changes is still not clear. There is good reason to think that PME is much involved in the changes in the pectic substances, since multiple evidence of demethylation has been obtained.

Extracts of diseased tissue, although rich in PME, have repeatedly failed to induce physiological effects in healthy tissue. However, a crude extracellular enzyme preparation from *S. fructigena* has been shown to cause leakage from apple tissue, and subsequent cell death. Although in preliminary experiments on fractions of this preparation these effects were not well correlated with any single characterized enzyme component, it should now be possible to resolve the identity of the lytic factor.

Acknowledgements

We are grateful to Dr G. V. Hoad for the gas chromatographic analysis, and to Mrs C. H. Perry for technical assistance.

References

Akinrefon, O. A. (1967). Improved extraction of polygalacturonase in apple tissue rotted by *Sclerotinia fructigena* Aderh. and Ruhl. *Rep. Long Ashton Res. Stn for 1966* 168-173.

Balasubramani, K. A., Deverall, B. J. and Murphy, J. V. (1971). Changes in respiratory rate, polyphenoloxidase and polygalacturonase activity in and around lesions caused by *Botrytis* in leaves of *Vicia faba*. *Physiol. Pl. Pathol.* **1**, 105-113.

Barash, I. and Khazzam, S. (1970). The relationship and properties of pectic glycosidases produced by host and pathogen during anthracnose disease of avocado. *Phytochemistry* **9**, 1189-1197.

de Bary, A. (1886). Uber einige Sclerotinien und Sclerotinienkrankheiten. *Bot. Z.* **44**, 377-474.

Bateman, D. F. (1963). Pectolytic activities of culture filtrates of *Rhizoctonia solani* and extracts of *Rhizoctonia* infected tissues of bean. *Phytopathology* **53**, 197-204.

Bateman, D. F. and Millar, R. L. (1966). Pectic enzymes in tissue degradation. *A. Rev. Phytopathol.* **4**, 119-146.

Boos, R. N. (1948). Colorimetric microdetermination of methanol with chromotopic acid reagent. *Anal. Biochem.* **20**, 964-965.

Burg, S. P. and Thimann, K. V. (1960). Studies on the ethylene production of apple tissue. *Pl. Physiol. Lancaster* **35**, 24-35.

Byrde, R. J. W. (1963). Natural inhibitors of fungal enzymes and toxins in disease resistance. *In* 'Perspectives of biochemical plant pathology' (ed. S. Rich). *Conn. agric. Exp. Sta. Bull.* **663**, 31-47.

Byrde, R. J. W. and Fielding, A. H. (1962). Resolution of endopolygalacturonase and a macerating factor in a fungal culture filtrate. *Nature, Lond.* **196**, 1227-1228.

Byrde, R. J. W. and Fielding, A. H. (1965). An extracellular α-L-arabinofuranosidase secreted by *Sclerotinia fructigena*. *Nature, Lond.* **205**, 390-391.

Byrde, R. J. W. and Fielding, A. H. (1968). Pectin methyl-*trans*-eliminase as the maceration factor of *Sclerotinia fructigena* and its significance in brown rot of apple. *J. gen. Microbiol.* **52**, 287-297.

Calonge, F. D., Fielding, A. H., Byrde, R. J. W. and Akinrefon, O. A. (1969). Changes in ultrastructure following fungal invasion and the possible relevance of extracellular enzymes. *J. exp. Bot.* **20**, 350-357.

Cole, J. S. (1956). Studies in the physiology of parasitism. XX. The pathogenicity of *Botrytis cinerea, Sclerotinia fructigena* and *Sclerotinia laxa,* with special reference to the part played by pectolytic enzymes. *Ann. Bot.* **20**, 15-38.

Cole, M. (1958a). Oxidation products of leuco-anthocyanins as inhibitors of fungal polygalacturonase in rotting apple fruit. *Nature, Lond.* **181**, 1596-1597.

Cole, M. (1958b). 'A comparative study of the mechanisms by which certain fungi and bacteria rot apple fruit'. Ph.D. Thesis, University of London.

Cole, M. and Wood, R. K. S. (1961a). Types of rot, rate of rotting, and analysis of pectic substances in apples rotted by fungi. *Ann. Bot.* **25**, 417-434.

Cole, M. and Wood, R. K. S. (1961b). Pectic enzymes and phenolic substances in apples rotted by fungi. *Ann. Bot.* **25**, 435-452.

Demain, A. L. and Phaff, H. J. (1957). Recent advances in the enzymatic hydrolysis of pectic substances. *Wallerstein Lab. Commun.* **20**, 119-140.

Dingle, J., Reid, W. W. and Solomons, G. L. (1953). The enzymic degradation of pectin and other polysaccharides. II. Application of the 'cup-plate' assay to the estimation of enzymes. *J. Sci. Fd Agric.* **4**, 149-155.

Doery, H. M., Magnusson, B. J., Gulasekharam, J. and Pearson, J. E. (1965). The properties of phospholipase enzymes in staphylococcal toxins. *J. gen. Microbiol.* **40**, 283-296.

Fielding, A. H. and Byrde, R. J. W. (1969). The partial purification and properties of endopolygalacturonase and α-L-arabinofuranosidase secreted by *Sclerotinia fructigena. J. gen. Microbiol.* **58**, 73-84.

Garibaldi, A. and Bateman, D. F. (1971). Pectic enzymes produced by *Erwinia chrysanthemi* and their effects on plant tissue. *Physiol. Pl. Path.* **1**, 25-40.

Hall, J. A. (1971). The maceration of tissues and killing of cells by *Erwinia carotovora* and *Corticium praticola.* Ph.D. Thesis, University of London.

Hislop, E. C., Hoad, G. V. and Archer, S. A. (1972). See p. 87-117 of this book.

Mount, M. S., Bateman, D. F. and Basham, H. G. (1970). Induction of electrolyte loss, tissue maceration and cellular death of potato tissue by an endopolygalacturonate *trans*-eliminase. *Phytopathology* **60**, 924-931.

Pollard, A. and Kieser, Margaret E. (1951). The pectase activity of apples. *J. Sci. Fd Agric.* 2, 30-36.

Reeve, R. M. (1959). A specific hydroxylamine ferric chloride reaction for histochemical localization of pectin. *Stain Technol.* **34**, 209-211.

Smith, W. K. (1958). A survey of the production of pectic enzymes by plant pathogenic and other bacteria. *J. gen. Microbiol.* **18**, 33-41.

Tribe, H. T. (1955). Studies in the physiology of parasitism. XIX. On the killing of plant cells by enzymes from *Botrytis cinerea* and *Bacterium aroideae. Ann. Bot.* **19**, 351-368.

Valleau, W. D. (1915). Varietal resistance of plums to brown rot. *J. agric. Res.* **5**, 365-396.

Vesterberg, O. and Svensson, H. (1966). Isoelectric fractionation, analysis and characterization of ampholytes in natural pH gradients. *Acta Chem. Scand.* **20**, 820-834.

Wheeler, H. and Hanchey, P. (1968). Permeability phenomena in plant disease. *A. Rev. Phytopathol.* **6**, 331-350.

Wood, R. K. S. (1967). 'Physiological Plant Pathology.' Blackwell, Oxford and Edinburgh. 570 pp.

DISCUSSION

Professor P. H. Williams: I will make both you and Harry Mussell happy, by referring to the double peak of PG activity, one peak only correlating with the conductivity changes. At the Wye conference Harry Mussell showed us a graph which looked almost identical. He has assayed these, and one of his peaks is an endo-PG and one is an exo-PG, and it is the endo-PG which is the active peak, and the exo-PG has no conductivity effect.

Dr R. J. W. Byrde: Yes, we have obviously got to look at the relative endo and exo activities. Certainly they both show positive in an endo assay, but we have just a little evidence to suggest that perhaps the later peak has a much higher ratio of exo activity than the earlier peak.

S. A. Archer: Both PG peaks possess both exo and endo activity, although most exo activity is associated with the pI 9.75 isoenzyme–mono, di, and trigalacturonic acids are the eventual breakdown products.

Professor R. K. S. Wood: This is a rather puzzling feature which was also raised by Mount and Bateman because they isolated, by the elegant electro focusing technique, a number of different PGs. Although one thinks of a PG as having only one activity, yet some of these PGs kill cells, and cause conductivity changes, and others don't. You have a pectin transeliminase from *Sclerotinia fructigena* which you have implicated in maceration.

Dr Byrde: It will macerate potato.

Professor Wood: And yet basically the effect of this transeliminase is the same as that of an endo PG, and yet you've got quite different activities in terms of conductivity.

Dr Byrde: We are also puzzled as to the relationship between these two PGs. There is always a trail between these two peaks and the PG never goes down to zero. It does suggest that one is constantly being transformed into the other; there is perhaps monomer and dimer, with one migrating across as the focusing is being done. It recalls Swinburne's published results.

Dr T. R. Swinburne: I think the process of iso-electric focusing might avoid many of these difficulties. Much of what happens in the changes in the pectic enzymes during the process of separation is a problem of ion-exchange cellulose, and I think the enzyme tends to associate or dissociate in the presence of this ionic separating medium. I think iso-electric focusing should avoid many of these difficulties, and it might also enable the form which is actually present *in vivo* to be separated.

Dr Byrde: I didn't in fact refer to this in the lecture. The form which we got *in vivo* was the pI 9.75 peak, but we are a bit doubtful whether this is an artefact due to our extraction methods. In culture we get this main peak and another. The ratio in size between these two culture peaks is not constant; we are not sure at the moment why in some experiments one peak is so very much bigger than the other, but sometimes they are almost the same size. But we do get this very characteristic peak, with a high iso-electric point, very similar to an enzyme from *Verticillium* described by Wang and Keen (*Archs Biochem. Biophys.* **141**, 749-757, 1970). There is also another component in rotted tissue, pI 7.8, which doesn't correspond with anything in culture, or of course in healthy tissue where PGs are absent. We haven't looked into this further at this stage but in every assay we have done we always get a trail between the peaks.

Professor C. E. Bracker: Are you saying that there is not a close relationship between phospholipase and the conductivity which signals the leakiness of the cell?

Dr Byrde: Those are the results which we have obtained, and I think this agrees both with Dr Hall's work and with Bateman's.

Professor Bracker: Because that is an enzyme which perhaps would be acting on the membrane since the membrane does consist to a large extent of various phospholipids.

Dr Byrde: When Bateman first demonstrated the presence of this phosphatidase, I thought he had the answer, and I expect he did too!

Professor Bracker: And is the phospholipase produced by the fungus or by the host?

Dr Byrde: It is produced by the fungus. I think Mr Archer would perhaps comment on the phospholipase, because he has done the work on this.

S. A. Archer: We have found in the *Sclerotinia* culture filtrate two phospholipases in fact, with differing iso-electric points, and differing substrate specificities. Only one of them is found in the *in vivo* preparation, and that has a rather high iso-electric point, again in the region of about 9.75-9.8. We have wondered why phospholipases don't attack the membranes, perhaps they are important in a rather later stage of pathogenesis. They may break down some of the internal membranes of the cells, possibly the mitochondrial membrane or something like that which also has a high phospholipid content, but they certainly don't seem to correspond with the killing.

Professor Wood: I think Tribe, in 1955, stressed that a membrane-attacking enzyme might be responsible, but no one did anything about it until Bateman did it. It is rather puzzling why phospholipase doesn't kill. Why doesn't it alter the permeability?

Professor Bracker: Of course, we've still the matter of membrane models, and just how the various membranes of the cell are constructed. This is a matter of great debate in almost any cell biology meeting one goes to. Perhaps the phospholipid or part of the phospholipid is protected within the membrane, and phospholipase could still be acting on the membrane, but perhaps at a later stage, after the phospholipids were exposed by something else acting at the surface of the membrane.

Dr Byrde: Yes, I agree. Pronase gave no maceration effect, but we haven't tried this in this assay, although others have probably done so.

Professor J. Friend: Could I follow up the previous question, by asking what is the specificity of the phospholipase, does it hydrolyse, and which of the fatty acids does it hydrolyse?

S. A. Archer: In our assays for phospholipase we have always used soya bean lecithin; other lecithins, such as are isolated from eggs, are not degraded to anything like the same extent. It would appear that the nature of the fatty acids present in the phospholipid is important in determining the specificity. This work is still actively proceeding, and the phospholipases present aren't fully characterized yet.

Professor Friend: In that case it might be worth while looking at the fatty acid composition of the phospholipids in your host tissue. This might give you some indication of what is going on.

S. A. Archer: Yes, that is something that we are certainly intending to do. In iso-electric focusing patterns, corresponding to the phospholipase we have enzymes present which hydrolyse various *para*nitrophenol derivatives, caprylate, laurate, etc. Whether or not these represent the same enzyme or not I wouldn't know at this stage. It could be that this is the phospholipase 'A' or something like that, which is breaking off the fatty acids from the phospholipids.

Professor K. Verhoeff: I would like to ask you a question about methods, you were talking about PG enzymes. When do you think you have a mixture of endo- and exo-PG and when do you think you have one of the two? You can imagine that after a long time of reaction with endo-PG you can expect mono-galacturonic acid.

Dr Byrde: Yes, I was basing my comment on the exo activity on some reducing group assays which Mr Archer did on one iso-electric focusing run where it seemed that the pI 9.8 peak gave much more reducing-group activity than would be suggested by the endopolygalacturonase assay.

Professor Verhoeff: But after how many minutes of reaction time?

S. A. Archer: 60 minutes.

Dr Byrde: Certainly this is something that we must look at again, now that we have discovered this effect that possibly one of the PG peaks is implicated in causing leakage but not the others. This could be a function of endo versus exo activity, which we have only looked at for the mixed preparation, but not for each of the isoenzymes.

I.3 Control of the Vertical Distribution of Apple Scab Disease on Shoots of the Apple Rootstock MM109

D. S. KIRKHAM AND R. C. HIGNETT

East Malling Research Station, Maidstone, Kent

SUMMARY

A position of maximum susceptibility to *Venturia inaequalis* is usually observed on the shoots of the apple rootstock MM 109. Treatment of inoculated shoots with either kinetin or pigmented metabolites isolated from culture filtrates of *V. inaequalis,* caused a simultaneous stimulation of scab on certain leaves and inhibition on others, leading to alterations in the vertical distribution of disease. Differences were observed between the effects of kinetin, the metabolites and environmental factors.

INTRODUCTION

The development of the apple scab disease is most often seen on young growing leaves, while those approaching the mature state during the infection period tend to be resistant. Factors controlling this onset of mature resistance are obscure. Observations on plants of a very susceptible cultivar showed that some immature leaves developed few or no symptoms of infection (Kirkham and Hignett, 1970). Since it appears to be unlikely that these apparently resistant leaves are genetically different from their diseased neighbours the expression of symptoms may be determined at another metabolic level. One such control would be the availability of substrates suitable for the pathogen. The reorganization of solute transport in the host by *Venturia inaequalis* and some effects of kinetin on the disease have been demonstrated (Hignett and Kirkham, 1967; Kirkham and Hignett, 1970). Interference with host hormone systems by pathogens in other disease systems has frequently been observed (Dekhuijzen and Staples, 1968; Bailiss and Wilson, 1967; Sequeira, 1963).

Although it is known that the apple scab disease requires cool humid conditions in the field, the effects of temperature, humidity and light in the glasshouse have not been thoroughly investigated. Work on other diseases indicates that these factors are very important (Smith and Kennedy, 1970). The present study is concerned with interactions between *V. inaequalis,* the apple rootstock MM 109 and the environment.

METHODS

A single-conidium isolate of *V. inaequalis* (Clone E 1; Kirkham, 1957) was used for infection in the glasshouse experiments. Spore inoculum was raised in artificial culture on filter paper cylinders standing in 10% (w/v) malt extract solution at 18° C (Kirkham, 1956). Pigmented metabolites produced by the pathogen in leaf extract solution were isolated from culture filtrates by ethanol precipitation and dialysis (Hignett and Kirkham, 1967).

Leaf extract was prepared from leaves of the apple cultivar Edward VII, the terminal six leaves on growing tips being harvested during July. Leaves (1-2 kg) were refluxed for a total of 4 h in two changes of methanol. The methanol extract was vacuum dried at 50° C, and the residue suspended in water for 1 h. Insoluble matter was removed and re-extracted with water. The pooled aqueous extracts (300 ml) were allowed to stand overnight at 18° C and any precipitate was again removed. 20 ml ammonia (14 N) was added to the solution which was extracted four times with 250 ml wet *n*-butanol. The aqueous layer was vacuum dried at 50° C, taken up in 300 ml water and 40 ml glacial acetic acid was then added. The butanol extraction was repeated with this solution. Both butanol extracts were dried under vacuum at 50° C and each of the residues suspended in 100 ml water. The suspensions were extracted four times with 100 ml ether, then all aqueous residues were pooled and concentrated to remove volatile substances. The aqueous concentrate was then extracted four times with an equal volume of ethyl acetate, and traces of ester removed under vacuum Three vol. alcohol were added, the precipitate being removed after 4 h at 0° C. The solids were suspended in 2 N HCl, and partially hydrolysed at 100° C for 20 min. Acid was removed under vacuum and the pH of the water soluble residue was adjusted to 6.5 with 2 N NaOH. Three vols. alcohol were then added and the precipitate removed after 4 h at 0° C. The pooled alcohol soluble fractions were taken to dryness and used as a supplement (1% w/v) in basal medium 'NC' (Kirkham, 1956) in which casein digest was replaced by L-asparagine (0.5% w/v).

Rooted shoots of the apple rootstock clone MM 109 grown in pots served as host material. Shoots (with stem thickness 5-6 mm) were selected in the nursery from the stoolbed crop. The potted material was vernalized in stacks without further selection. Plants for an experiment were picked at random from the stacks and single shoots grown in the glasshouse at 15-22° C. Weak and damaged plants were rejected at this stage and the remainder were then selected at random for treatment. Before inoculation, the first fully unrolled and partially expanded leaf below each shoot tip was labelled (for purposes of recording) on the petiole and designated L_0, the two leaves above being +1 and +2 and the two below −1 and −2. The plants were then distributed randomly in the humid (75-85% r.h.) inoculation chambers at 15-22°C, inoculated by spray application of conidial suspensions at the rate of 3 ml to 10 plants, and held for 24 h in moist conditions. Each shoot tip was individually sprayed using compressed air to give a finely atomized mist of inoculum: Experiments with dye indicated that this technique gave a satisfactory distribution of droplets. The amount of dye was greatest on the larger leaves (as expected) i.e. Leaves −1 and −2. It was concluded that the largest leaves on control plants received the greatest number of spores on inoculation. The inoculum density used on each occasion was approximately 50 000 conidia/ml.

The pigmented fungal metabolites and kinetin were applied as sprays at the rate of 3 ml to 10 plants two days after inoculation. The kinetin treatment was repeated on the third day. Kinetin and metabolite solutions were applied at a concentration of 0.06 mg/ml and 5 mg/ml respectively. After treatment, the plants were distributed at random on the bench for the duration of the experiment. The glasshouse was maintained at 15-22°C. Relative humidity normally varied diurnally from 45% (minimum) during the day to 90% (maximum) at night, except where a 70% minimum was imposed.

The incidence of disease was recorded by counting the numbers of sporulating lesions four times during 14 days after their first appearance. Plants having five or more lesions on one leaf and at least one on another were used for the estimation of disease distribution. Other plants were rejected.

Visible light incident upon the plants was measured using photoelectric cells (Jackson and Slater, 1967).

Results

OCCURRENCE OF A PEAK IN DISEASE RESPONSE

A large proportion of the test plants showed a maximum number of lesions at one position (subsequently referred to as the 'peak'), in the sequence of five recorded leaves. 'Peaking' plants are those showing such a peak. The peak could occur at any position but in control sets of plants it was observed most frequently on the first fully unrolled leaf (Leaf 0), rather than on the larger leaves below, which had received more spore inoculum. At each record (Tables I and II) the percentage of the total number of peaks is given for each of the five leaf positions. While shoots often showed minor peaks separated by at least two inter-nodes from the major position, the latter is clearly the chief characteristic of disease distribution.

In any group of plants one or more usually appeared to be immune, others showed a high degree of resistance, while the remainder illustrated the typical peak distribution with variable levels of disease. The cause of inter-plant variation is quite unknown and is not singly correlated with leaf surface microbial populations, inter-stool differences, latent virus, root system size or visible shoot characteristics. When shoots were re-inoculated after further growth the initial disease response was seldom repeated. In most experiments less than 50% of each responding group showed their peaks at the same position (Tables I and II). This may suggest the occurrence of different disease-categories of plants corresponding to the five leaf positions.

VERTICAL DISTRIBUTION OF DISEASE PEAKS

Table I shows that two experiments (at different times) gave similar results despite the high level of inter-plant variation. The differences seen in each experiment between the distribution of disease peaks on untreated and on kinetin treated plants were comparable irrespective of the numbers of lesions involved. Kinetin stimulated disease at Leaf +2 and caused inhibition at Leaf +1 throughout both experiments; the effects on other leaves were minimal. These experiments were done with diurnal variation in humidity (45%-90% r.h.).

Table II shows the effects of fungal metabolites on the development of disease peaks under condition, of controlled humidity (Experiment 3, 70% r.h. min). Stimulation of desease occurred at Leaf +1 simultaneously with inhibition at Leaves 0 and +2. These effects were masked in conditions of variable humidity. In the previous experiments where humidity was controlled, the inhibition by kinetin at Leaf +1 was eliminated and the effects at other leaf positions were erratic and not reproducible.

In an experiment to determine the effect of light on disease developing in conditions of high humidity, it was observed that a reduction in the light received (from 1206 to 911 cal. cm^{-2}) was accompanied by a 30% decrease in total numbers of lesions on control plants. The differences in total numbers of lesions observed between Experiments 1 and 2 could not be ascribed to this effect as the overall light levels were similar (1165 and 1290 cal. cm^{-2} respectively). It seems that the differences in lesion numbers were due either to the intensity of incident light occurring during certain critical short periods after infection or to a combination of these with changes in humidity. Humidity differences between Experiments 2 and 3, which received the same amount of light must account for the higher final total numbers of lesions on control plants in Experiment 3.

DISCUSSION

The results show that a peak of disease occurs on a particular leaf after shoot infection. This happens where favourable metabolic interactions in the disease

TABLE I

Distribution (%) of disease peaks as affected by kinetin and conditions of diurnal variation of humidity

Leaf no.	Expt. no.	Treatment	Record no. 1	2	3	4
+2	1	Control (C)	24	18	12	0
		Kinetin (K)	62	38	44	29
	2	C	33	18	18	18
		K	50	46	31	31
+1	1	C	29	29	29	35
		K	15	19	6	7
	2	C	50	36	27	27
		K	0	9	8	8
L_0	1	C	41	41	35	35
		K	23	38	38	43
	2	C	17	36	46	46
		K	50	36	46	46
−1	1	C	6	12	18	18
		K	0	6	6	14
	2	C	0	9	9	9
		K	0	9	15	15
−2	1	C	0	0	6	12
		K	0	0	6	7
	2	C	0	0	0	0
		K	0	0	0	0

	Expt. no.	Treatment	Final total lesions on peaking plants	Peaking plants at 4th record	Plants inoculated
	1	C	1084	17	17
		K	746	14	17
	2	C	353	11	17
		K	311	13	17

TABLE II

Effects of pigmented fungal metabolites on the development and percentage distribution of disease peaks in conditions of controlled high humidity (Experiment 3)

Leaf no.	Treatment	Record no. 1	2	3	4
+2	Control (C)	29	13	13	7
	Fungal Product (F.P.)	15	6	6	0
+1	C	29	33	27	13
	F.P	62	53	41	41
L_0	C	36	47	47	60
	F.P.	23	35	41	41
−1	C	7	7	13	13
	F.P.	0	6	12	12
−2	C	0	0	0	7
	F.P.	0	0	0	6

	Final total lesions on peaking plants	Peaking plants at 4th record	Plants inoculated
C	744	15	17
F.P.	816	17	17

system are expressed, even though larger leaves on the same shoot receive more spore inoculum. The particular leaf within which this situation occurs will be determined by the host and pathogen and also by the environment. Some degree of disease resistance is observed on other leaves, which indicates the essentially defensive nature of the host plant. The dynamic nature of this situation is demonstrated by the way in which it can be altered by treatments applied after infection.

The effects of kinetin indicate that the disease is under hormonal control. The relative resistance of leaves was disturbed by application of kinetin, which led to changes in the distribution of disease where diurnal variation of humidity was allowed. These effects were suppressed by continuous high humidity and may therefore be connected with transpiration rates and solute transport. In contrast, the effects of fungal metabolites were maximal in conditions of high humidity. In these circumstances stimulation of disease occurred at Leaf +1 where under variable humidity kinetin had caused inhibition.

The effects of fungal metabolites and kinetin at Leaf +2 under constant and variable humidity respectively again were opposed. In addition the fungal products inhibited the disease at Leaf 0. Though the differences between these effects were very considerable they both altered distribution of disease, suggesting that they both ultimately affected the same disease-control systems. The differences occurring between adjacent leaves in a group of plants indicates the difficulty of interpreting experiments involving hormones or pathogens in which leaves are used without regard to their disease potential. The response of the disease to changes of incident visible light and humidity in the post-infection period underline the importance of the environment in the whole question of host-pathogen relations. Successful infection followed by the interplay of the many factors involved determines how the disease will develop. It seems that the whole environment must be controlled to within very fine limits to make possible studies of metabolic interactions in the scab disease and quite possibly in any plant disease.

Acknowledgements

Thanks are due to Miss C. Baker, Mrs J. Town, J. H. Carder, H. Hutchins and A. L. Roberts for technical assistance.

References

Bailiss, K. W. and Wilson, Irene M. (1967). Growth hormones and the Creeping Thistle Rust. *Ann. Bot.* **31**, 195-211.

Dekhuijzen, H. M. and Staples, R. C. (1968). Mobilization factors in Uredospores and bean leaves infected with bean rust fungus. *Contr. Boyce Thompson Inst. Pl. Res.* **24**, 39-51.

Hignett, R. C. and Kirkham, D. S. (1967). The role of extracellular melanoproteins of *Venturia inaequalis* in host susceptibility. *J. gen. Microbiol.* **48**, 269-275.

Jackson, J. E. and Slater, C. H. W. (1967). An integrating photometer for outdoor use particularly in trees. *J. appl. Ecol.* **4**, 421-424.

Kirkham, D. S. (1956). A culture technique for *Venturia* spp. and a turbidimetric method for the estimation of comparative sporulation. *Nature, Lond.* **178**, 550-551.

Kirkham, D. S. (1957). Relationships between cultural characters and pathogenicity in *Venturia inaequalis* and *Venturia pirina*. *J. gen. Microbiol.* **16**, 360-373.

Kirkham, D. S. and Hignett, R. C. (1970). Antagonism between the effects of kinetin and extracellular metabolites of the pathogen in apple scab disease. *Nature, Lond.* **225**, 388.

Sequeira, L. (1963). Growth regulators in plant disease. *A. Rev. Phytopathol.* **1**, 5-30.

Smith, Mark A. and Kennedy, Bill W. (1970). Effect of light on reaction of soybean to *Pseudomonas glycinea. Phytopathology* **60**, 723-725.

DISCUSSION

Dr H. M. Dekhuijzen: The increase or decrease of the symptoms is very interesting; do you think that the disease is under hormonal control? If so, would you expect that other growth hormones, e.g. IAA or gibberellins, would have similar effects? My second question is that as kinetin is not a natural hormone, would it not be better to use zeatin or zeatin riboside, for this kind of experiment?

Dr D. S. Kirkham: Yes, I think kinetin is proving adequate, firstly for indicating that the system is under hormonal control, and it is also very useful in showing what effects a hormone can have on disease distribution. We have also used it to test our control system, and the influence of environmental effects on disease distribution. Kinetin is readily available and easy to use; zeatin is expensive and difficult to handle. Both are apparently inactive *in vitro.*

Dr Dekhuijzen: Both do not inhibit growth?

Dr Kirkham: There is no direct action, therefore it should be all right to use it.

Dr R. C. Hignett: We have studied IAA, but not to any great extent, and the indications were that it could behave similarly and could certainly disturb the growth of the fungus on the plant.

Dr J. P. Blakeman: Could you suggest reasons why the older leaves don't respond to the hormonal treatment, and to treatments with fungal products. Does this imply that the mechanism of resistance of older leaves is rather different from that of younger leaves?

Dr Kirkham: They can respond.

Dr Hignett: The whole thing depends to such an enormous extent on the environment, the amount of visible light received by the plant, the size of the root system, the age of the shoots, almost anything you care to mention, will affect the results you get out of this particular system and will also affect which leaves respond in what manner. We have had enormous response from very large −2-type leaves which presumably should have been showing mature resistance, but under certain conditions we have had enormous stimulation of disease on them. This question of mature resistance is something which has a convenient label but there seems to be fog of ignorance. We can only say, in our system at any rate, that mature resistance is a very variable quantity.

Professor P. H. Williams: Do you have any idea what the relationship of normal leaf microflora might be to infection by *V. inaequalis*? I'm thinking that perhaps the kinetin and leaf age interaction may be due to your sunlight studies, perhaps as kinetin is a bacteriostat, this is affecting natural leaf flora to the point of permitting greater numbers of propagules to penetrate the cuticle.

Dr Kirkham: We have managed to isolate nothing from the leaf surface which had any effect on the pathogen at all, either *in vivo* or *in vitro*. There was no disturbance of disease, but that doesn't mean to say there is no other active factor.

Dr G. E. Russell: Have you looked at the concentrations of sugars in the leaves which have varying disease reaction? In sugar beet, for example, the first four leaves which are produced have quite different disease reactions from the leaves produced subsequently. These first four leaves have markedly lower concentrations of monosaccharides than the older adult leaves. We can alter the disease reactions by spraying with sugars, putting plants in darkness, etc. Have you considered such a possible association between sugar content and susceptibility to apple scab?

Dr Kirkham: No we haven't, but it would obviously be interesting.

Dr E. C. Hislop: You have recorded the visible symptoms of disease, may I ask if you have looked at the effects of your treatments, shall we say, on the germination, penetration and sporulation of the pathogen that you apply in your inoculum. I'd like to know, for example, whether in varying your environmental treatments you've modified perhaps some phytoalexin-type production. Secondly, could I ask what was the time scale of the humidity trace which you showed, was it a 24-h period?

Dr Kirkham: Yes, it was a 24-h period. I'm sure we have a lot of lesions on these leaves which we never see; in other words, they never sporulate. They don't get to that stage. I am pretty sure this happens, we have looked at this to some extent, by stripping cuticle, epidermis, and then staining, by which we see developing mycelium which has never got beyond a certain stage. Again this might be due to qualities of the environment before the time when lesions are due to appear, and we have to look into it.

Dr Hislop: May I suggest, if you require to examine a system where the youngest leaves are normally more resistant than older leaves, that you try *Botrytis fabae* on broad beans, which will give you an answer in 24 h.

Dr Kirkham: Yes, that is a very good idea, because we want to broaden the work, to take in other diseases, and *B. fabae* on beans is a good example. Helminthosporium on tomato would perhaps be another.

Professor P. W. Brian: Did you see any visible effects on leaf senescence as a result of the kinetin or fungal metabolite treatments.

Dr Kirkham: No.

Professor Brian: Is that because the experiments did not go on long enough?

Dr Kirkham: We've never had any effect on the host itself by any of these treatments, none whatsoever, either when done late in the season or early.

R. Copeland: Have you applied kinetin to individual leaves, e.g. to Leaf −2 and no others, and examined the flow of metabolites and susceptibility to *Venturia* under these circumstances.

Dr Hignett: We had a quick look at the reaction of individual leaves, but at that time we had no environmental control, and weren't so aware of its vital importance. Regarding the sugar content, I very much doubt if the sugar content of the cell underneath the developing lesion has much effect on the rate of growth of that lesion because the mycelium is developing at a considerable distance from the cell, and does not penetrate it at all.

Dr G. E. Russell: We have found an effect of sugars on several diseases in sugar beet–rusts, powdery mildews, downy mildews and so on. I am not suggesting that it is necessarily a direct effect of the sugars.

Dr L. J. Littlefield: Have you studied incandescent light versus fluorescent light on this?

Dr Kirkham: Well, not incandescent light.

Dr Littlefield: I ask this because Professor Flor has shown very nicely with flax rust that there is generally a more susceptible reaction or, in quantitative terms, a greater production of uredia under fluorescent light than under incandescent. However, in certain cases, he can show a very drastic qualitative change from a rather highly resistant reaction to a very susceptible reaction, when going from incandescent to fluorescent light.

Dr Kirkham: We are using mercury and Kolor-arc lamps. These Kolor-arc lamps are extremely efficient, they are very bright, with a very wide spectral range, in fact we don't really need our mercury lamps.

Dr Hignett: We have tried some experiments with tungsten-iodine high intensity lighting, but these tests indicated that wide spectrum Kolor-arc lamps are in fact better, particularly in view of the short life of the tungsten-iodine lamps. We also tested high pressure sodium lighting, and again there was an indication that it didn't favour the growth of the disease as effectively as wide spectrum Kolor-arc. I would think that the quality of the light is quite an important factor, and just as important as the overall amount of visible light that the plants receive.

Dr R. J. W. Byrde: Could you remind us of the biochemical nature of the fungal pigmented metabolites? I think these are melano-proteins.

Dr Hignett: We had a great deal of difficulty obtaining these compounds, particularly in persuading the fungus to produce the same materials every time we culture it, and having produced it, we've got to make sure that there are no remnants of the culture medium mixed with the fungal product. We are working on this, it is very tricky, the products depend to a great extent on the substrates offered to the fungus. We have now started some tracer work, which indicates, so far, that the fungal products contain amino acids, carbohydrates, and other compounds which are being resolved.

Professor R. K. S. Wood: May I ask a supplementary question to that? Have you got the melano-proteins out of infected plants?

Dr Hignett: No we haven't attempted this yet, largely because it is difficult to characterize precisely what is produced *in vitro* even, and to go looking for something inside the plant, of which there will be very little indeed is not to be contemplated at present. Sooner or later of course, it would be a good thing to try and get out of the plant whatever the fungus is putting in, and to compare this with what is produced in deep culture.

If I may put a question to the audience, something which has concerned us is this variation, what you might call a symptomless resistance. As all our plant material is clonal, vegetatively propagated, and presumably is genetically identical, each individual plant should be a replica of every other plant. And yet we have this terrible business where in any group of plants with a given inoculum, say in a group of 50 plants, some plants have 50-100 lesions/leaf, and the vast majority have rather less. But there are always two or three which have no lesions whatsoever, and no symptoms. It's just as if you never inoculated them. One knows perfectly well that the inoculum has arrived, but what has happened to it? The secondary question is the problem of shoots, in which, say, a leaf 0 has a considerable number of lesions, and yet a leaf above that (which should not be showing mature resistance) shows no lesions at all. Again quite symptomless—there are no indications whatsoever that anything has happened to such a leaf. This phenomenon must be fairly widespread, and if anybody has any ideas, I shall be very glad to hear.

Dr Hislop: May I ask one possibly irrelevant question. Have you ever tried washing your leaves before inoculating them? In some systems, this will reduce variability?

Dr Kirkham: Yes, but without effect.

Dr R. B. Drysdale: I think it is always a great mistake to regard any two cells as being genetically identical. As soon as you have division the chances of the daughter cells being genetically identical is pretty small. All you can hope is that the genes in which you are particularly interested are the same in the two cells. I think it is a gross over-simplification to think that after a cell division you have two identical cells.

Dr Hignett: Are you suggesting in fact that this symptomless resistance in plants which you know originate vegetatively from a fully susceptible stock are showing a type of resistance which is present in all of that stock, but is only expressed by that particular plant at that particular time? A plant, which has no symptoms whatsoever at a particular time, if allowed to grow on and re-inoculated will then be susceptible to disease in the normal way.

Dr Drysdale: I am not implying that my remark has any real value to your problem, all I'm suggesting is the assumption that cell division produces two identical cells is completely wrong. I would not like to say that this is offering any explanation helpful in solving your problem.

Dr Hignett: It could though.

Professor Wood: I think some of our people working with *Colletotrichum lindemuthianum* on bean leaf would support what you say, Dr Drysdale.

Section II

The Involvement of Ethylene

II . 1 The Effect of Certain Bacteria on Ethylene Production by Plant Tissue

BARBARA M. LUND

A.R.C. Food Research Institute, Norwich, England

INTRODUCTION

An increase in ethylene production following infection of plant tissue with fungi has been reported by many workers (Burg, 1962; Pratt and Goeschl, 1969) and this effect has also been reported for plant tissue infected with viruses (Ross and Williamson, 1951; Balazs *et al.*, 1969; Lockhart and Semancik, 1970; Nakagaki *et al.*, 1970). To the author's knowledge, the only reports of increased ethylene production associated with bacterial infections are those of Freebairn and Buddenhagen (1964) and Lund and Mapson (1970). Many fungi (Ilag and Curtis, 1968) and some bacteria (Swanson, 1971) including *Pseudomonas solanacearum* (Freebairn and Buddenhagen, 1964) produce ethylene when grown *in vitro* on laboratory media; for plant tissue infected with such organisms ethylene may be produced in part by the pathogen and in part by the diseased host. In some instances the pathogen has not been shown to form ethylene *in vitro*, and the evidence suggests that the olefine is produced by the tissues of the host in response to injury by the parasite (Wood, 1967).

Our interest in this subject arose following the observation that *Erwinia carotovora* stimulated ethylene production by cauliflower floret tissue, and that the pectic enzymes of the bacterium appeared to be responsible for this effect (Lund and Mapson, 1970).

MATERIALS AND METHODS

Materials. Cauliflowers (*Brassica oleracea* L., var. *botrytis*) were obtained from a local market and green sprouting calabrese (*Brassica oleracea* var. *italica*) from a local grower.

Sodium polypectate, polygalacturonate and pectin (US National Formulary) were obtained from Sunkist Growers Inc., Ontario, California, USA.

Protease (from *Streptomyces griseus*, 0.8 units/mg), trypsin (11 000 BAEE units/mg), pectinesterase (from tomato) and pectinase (0.8 units/mg) were obtained from the Sigma Chemical Co.

Ethylene production from cauliflower florets. From the head, pieces of floret tissue (about 5 mm dia. and 7 mm long) were separated by cutting the petiole rather than the floret tissue. The florets, in conical flasks, were partially immersed in the appropriate buffer solution, the flasks were then flushed with oxygen, closed, and incubated at 25° C or at 20° C. Duplicate flasks were set up for each experiment.

Ethylene was estimated by gas-liquid chromatography either using a column (275 cm x 6 mm) packed with 30% silicone oil (May and Baker, Ltd.) on Celite (85-100 mesh) or using a stainless steel column (150 cm x 3 mm) packed with Porapak S (80-100 mesh) operated at 65° C, and a flame-ionization detector. Sample volumes ranged from 0.5-2.0 ml. A gas mixture containing 31.6 ppm of ethylene in air was used as a reference standard.

Bacteria-free culture-supernatant of *Erwinia carotovora* was prepared as described by Lund and Mapson.

Enzyme assays for pectate lyase (EC 4.2.99.3), polygalacturonase (EC 3.2.1.15) and pectinesterase (EC 3.1.11) were described by Lund and Mapson. Activities determined by these assays are expressed in units, where a unit of pectate lyase liberates 1 μmol of aldehyde groups/min from polygalacturonic acid at pH 8.6 and 25° C; a unit of polygalacturonase liberates 1 μmol of aldehyde groups/min from polygalacturonic acid at pH 5.2 and 25° C; a unit of pectinesterase releases 1 μmol of carboxyl groups/min from pectin at pH 7 and 25° C. In addition, for screening large numbers of fractions for pectate lyase and polygalacturonase, cup-plate assay methods were devised based on the method of Dingle *et al.* (1953). The cup-plate assays were semi-quantitative, the zone diameter being proportional to the logarithm of the concentration of the enzyme. Enzyme activities based on the cup-plate assays are expressed in arbitrary P-units based on 100 for a 20 mm dia. zone.

Proteolytic enzyme activity was estimated by a cup-plate method using 1% gelatin as substrate and a pH of 6.5. Enzyme activities are expressed in arbitrary units based on 100 for a 20 mm dia. zone.

Protein was estimated by the method of Lowry *et al.* (1951) using bovine serum albumen as a standard or from the extinction at 280 nm and 260 nm (Layne, 1957).

Purification of pectate lyase and polygalacturonase. The crude bacterial enzyme preparation was treated with $(NH_4)_2SO_4$ to give 90% saturation. The precipitate was collected by centrifuging, redissolved in 0.05 M sodium acetate buffer pH 5.2 and dialysed against 0.05 M acetate buffer until the dialysis liquid was free from sulphate ions. The solution was concentrated by ultrafiltration and fractionated on columns of microgranular carboxymethylcellulose (Whatman

CM52 CM-cellulose) using sodium acetate buffer pH 5.2 and gradient elution, following similar methods to those described by Nasuno and Starr (1966) and Moran *et al.* (1968).

RESULTS

ETHYLENE PRODUCTION BY PLANT TISSUE INOCULATED WITH *ERWINIA CAROTOVORA*

In certain experiments with cauliflower florets it was found that rapid production of ethylene from the florets was caused by contamination with *E. carotovora* (Lund and Mapson). Deliberate inoculation of florets with this bacterium resulted in a high rate of ethylene production, and the tissue became water-soaked in appearance due probably to breakdown of the plant tissue by this pectolytic micro-organism (Fig. 1). When florets were inoculated with

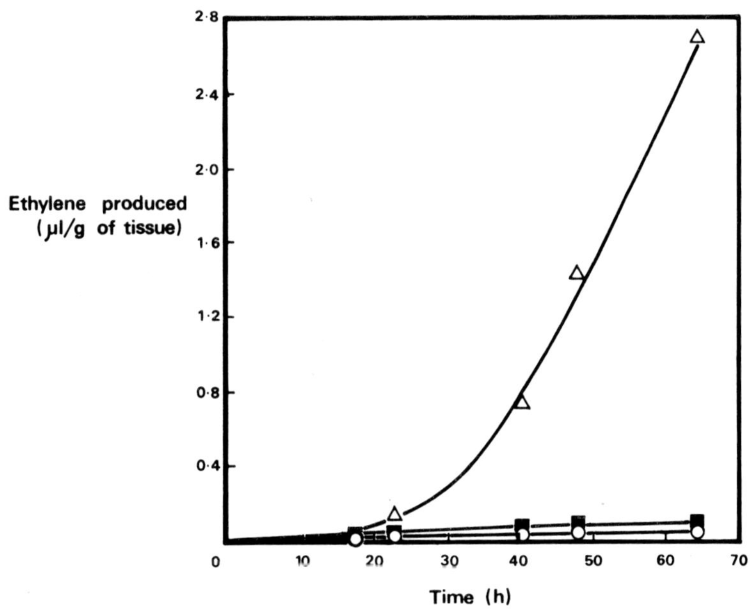

Fig. 1. Ethylene production by cauliflower florets inoculated with bacteria. Samples (12 g) of florets were placed in 250 ml flasks and to each flask was added 20 ml of sucrose (0.4 M) + EDTA (2 mM) solution and 1 ml of the inoculum indicated. After 30 min, excess of liquid was drained from the florets; flasks were flushed with oxygen and incubated on a shaker at 20° C.
○ flask 1, no added inoculum;
△ flask 5, inoculated with 1 ml of suspension of *E. carotovora*;
■ flask 9, inoculated with 1 ml of a mixed suspension of non-pectolytic isolates.
Replicate flasks were set up for viable counts of bacteria.

non-pectolytic bacteria isolated from cauliflower florets, these bacteria multiplied to the same extent as did *E. carotovora,* but no stimulation of ethylene formation occurred. Inoculation of calabrese florets with *E. carotovora* also resulted in an increased rate of ethylene formation. The maximum rates of production of the hydrocarbon by florets inoculated with *E. carotovora* and incubated at 20° C in oxygen were 0.05 μl/g tissue/h and 0.1 μl/g tissue/h for cauliflower and calabrese respectively. Florets inoculated with *Xanthomonas campestris,* another pectolytic bacterium, also showed an increase in ethylene formation.

Whole green tomatoes inoculated with *E. carotovora* produced more ethylene than comparable tomatoes inoculated with sterile water; this was associated with visible rotting of the fruit by the bacterium. The maximum rates of ethylene production in different tomatoes during the first 46 h at 25° C were 0.04-0.10 μl/g tissue/h.

When *E. carotovora* was grown in liquid culture media containing pectate, or containing cauliflower extract + DL-methionine, no synthesis of ethylene could be detected (Lund and Mapson). It therefore seemed possible that when plant tissue was inoculated with the bacterium, the increased amounts of ethylene evolved were not synthesized by the bacterium, but by the damaged plant tissue.

THE MECHANISM OF THE BACTERIAL STIMULATION OF ETHYLENE FORMATION BY FLORETS

E. carotovora was grown in a liquid pectate medium and the bacteria were harvested by centrifugation. The bacteria-free culture-supernatant, containing pectic enzymes, stimulated ethylene production by cauliflower florets; the active principle of the culture-supernatant was heat-labile and ethylene production was also dependent on heat-labile components of the floret tissue (Fig. 2). The bacterial enzymes stimulated ethylene formation by the florets rather than by petiole tissue (Table I). Further studies of the mechanism of stimulation of ethylene production have been made using cauliflower florets. In preliminary fractionations of the culture supernatant, the ability to stimulate ethylene production was retained by fractions with both pectate lyase and polygalacturonase activity (Lund and Mapson).

The demonstration that stimulation of ethylene production was dependent on the action of both bacterial and plant enzymes suggested the possibility that the increased rate of synthesis occurred via the pathway normally occurring in cauliflower florets. There is good evidence that ethylene is formed from methionine in plant tissues (Mapson *et al.,* 1970; Mapson and Hulme, 1970; Baur *et al.,* 1971), and studies involving cell-free extracts of cauliflower florets have led to the formulation of a probable route of ethylene production (Fig. 3) (Mapson and Hulme). This involves (i) transamination of methionine to the oxo

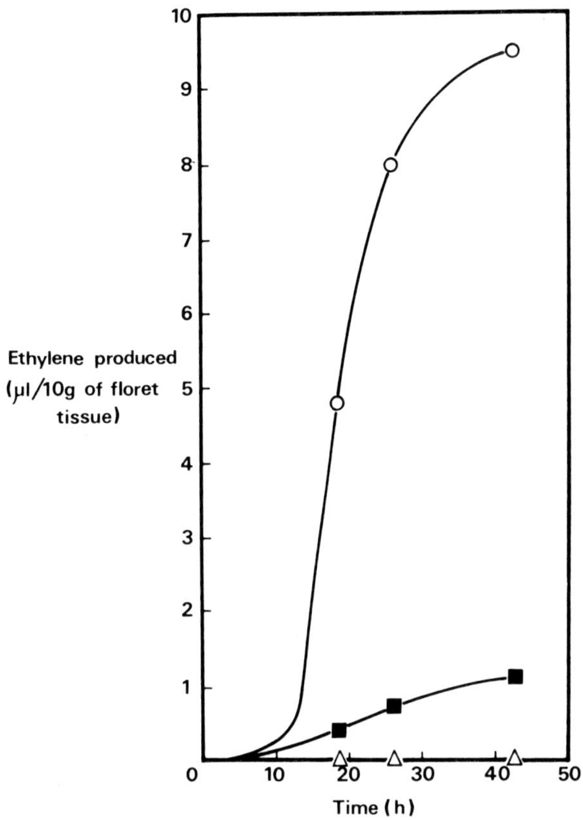

Fig. 2. Stimulation of ethylene production dependent on both plant and bacterial enzymes. Floret tissue (10 g) was incubated in 8 ml of phosphate buffer (0.1 M), pH 6.8, to which the following additions were made:
○, 2 ml of bacterial enzyme preparation;
■, 2 ml of autoclaved bacterial enzyme preparation;
△, 2 ml of bacterial enzyme preparation, but enzymes of floret tissue had been inactivated by heat before addition.

acid 4-methylmercapto-2-oxobutyric acid, (ii) a glucose oxidase generating hydrogen peroxide and (iii) a peroxidase using hydrogen peroxide to catalyse the formation of ethylene from the C-3 and C-4 carbon atoms of the oxo acid. This latter reaction requires the presence of two heat-stable cofactors, a phenolic acid (*p*-coumaric acid) and a sulphinic acid (methane sulphinic acid). The role of the oxo acid as an intermediate in ethylene synthesis from methionine was supported by experiments with apple and tomato tissue (Mapson *et al.*) but has been disputed in the case of cauliflower florets by Lieberman and Kunishi

TABLE I

The effect of a culture-supernatant of *E. carotovora* on ethylene production by cauliflower tissue

Tissue	Culture-supernatant	Ethylene nl/g tissue
floret	+	401
floret	–	14
petiole	+	23
petiole	–	11

Flasks (25 ml) contained 2 g florets; culture-supernatant, 0.4 ml; phosphate buffer 0.1 M pH 6.5 to 2 ml. After flushing with oxygen, flasks were incubated at 25° C for 8 h. Ethylene production is the mean of duplicate flasks.

The culture supernatant added contained the following amounts of enzymes expressed in arbitrary units (*P*-units)/ml: pectate lyase 481, polygalacturonase 438, protease 71.

$$CH_3{-}S{-}CH_2{-}CH_2{-}CH(NH_2){-}COOH + \text{oxo acid (phenyl pyruvic)}$$

$$\text{Transaminase} \rightleftharpoons \text{(pyridoxal phosphate)}$$

$$CH_3{-}S{-}CH_2{-}CH_2{-}CO{-}COOH + \text{amino acid (phenyl alanine)}$$

$$\beta\text{-D-glucose} + O_2 \xrightarrow{\text{Glucose oxidase}} \text{D-glucono-}\delta\text{-lactone} + H_2O_2$$

$$H_2O_2 + CH_3{-}S{-}CH_2{-}CH_2{-}COOH \xrightarrow[\text{Phenolic acid + sulphinic acid}]{\text{Peroxidase}} CH_2{=}CH_2 + \text{other products}$$

Fig. 3. Synthesis of ethylene from methionine in cauliflower florets. (Mapson and Hulme, 1970.)

(1971), while in apple tissue Baur *et al.* concluded that methionine was a closer precursor of ethylene than was the oxo acid.

Culture-supernatants of *E. carotovora* were used in experiments to elucidate the mechanism of the bacterial stimulation of ethylene production by cauliflower florets (Lund and Mapson, 1970). When florets plus culture-supernatant were incubated with 1,2,3,4-^{14}C labelled methionine or

4-methylmercapto-2-oxobutyric acid both ethylene production and incorporation of labelled substrates were greater than in the absence of the culture-supernatant, suggesting that the bacterial enzymes stimulated the normal mechanism of ethylene production occurring in the florets. The percentage increase in incorporation was slightly lower than the percentage increase of ethylene production; the possibility was not excluded, therefore, that the bacterial enzymes also stimulated ethylene formation from substrates other than methionine or the oxo acid, but later work made this appear unlikely.

Ethylene is formed by homogenates of cauliflower florets in the presence of 4-methylmercapto-2-oxobutyric acid, and this reaction in homogenates was also accelerated by the bacterial culture-supernatant (Fig. 4). The stimulatory effect

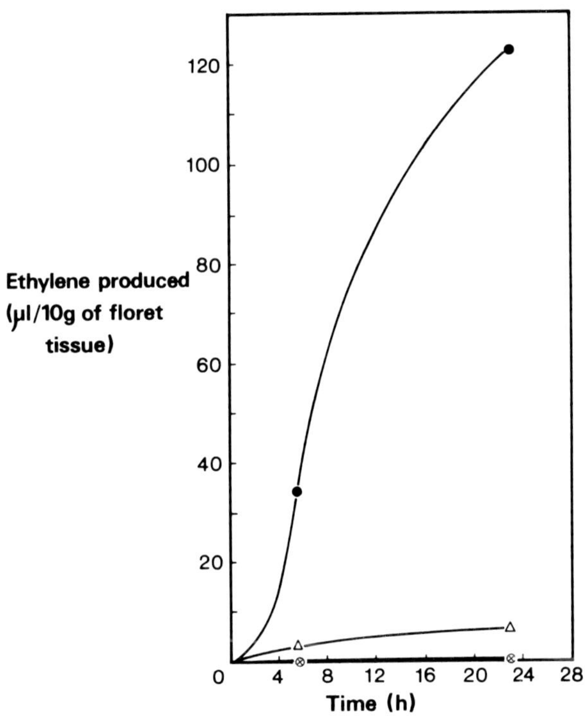

Fig. 4. Stimulation by bacterial enzyme preparation from *E. carotovora* of the synthesis of ethylene from 4-methylmercapto-2-oxobutyric acid by homogenate of cauliflower tissue. Homogenate was prepared from floret tissue (20 g) with 15 ml of a solution containing 0.4 M-sucrose, 2 mM-EDTA and 0.1 M-phosphate buffer, pH 6.5. Homogenate (5 g) was placed in each flask with the following additions:

●, oxo acid (3 mM) and bacterial enzyme preparation (0.5 ml);

△, oxo acid (3 mM);

○, no addition;

x, bacterial enzyme preparation.

of the bacterial enzymes in this system could be reproduced by the addition of small amounts of glucose oxidase, which would result in an increased rate of production of hydrogen peroxide. The bacterial culture-supernatant did not itself contain a glucose oxidase or any other oxidase active on substrates in the cauliflower homogenate. This suggested that the bacterial enzymes might cause an increase in the activity of the glucose oxidase present in cauliflower tissue, and hence stimulate ethylene production from oxo acid. In an attempt to locate the site of action of the bacterial enzymes, separate fractions of floret tissue were prepared containing (i) plant cell wall material, (ii) cell contents. When the cell wall fraction was incubated with oxo-acid no ethylene was formed unless a peroxidase (horseradish peroxidase), cofactors (a phenolic acid and a sulphinic acid) and glucose were added. When these components were added, ethylene production was initiated; pre-treatment of the cell wall fraction with the culture-supernatant for 2 h at 25° C resulted in a greatly increased rate of synthesis of ethylene after the subsequent addition of the peroxidase, cofactors and glucose (Fig. 5). Ethylene production by the cell contents in the presence of added oxo acid was not increased by pre-treatment with the culture-supernatant.

The experiments with the cell-wall fraction suggested that glucose oxidase was present in this fraction, and that the acceleration of ethylene formation brought about by the bacterial enzymes resulted from an increase in activity of this glucose oxidase. Direct evidence of an increase in glucose oxidase activity of cell wall preparations after treatment with the bacterial culture-supernatant was obtained by manometric studies of oxygen uptake following the addition of D-glucose, and it was shown that the increase in activity of glucose oxidase was accompanied by detachment of some of the enzyme from the cell wall with consequent solubilization.

THE EFFECT OF PURIFIED BACTERIAL ENZYMES ON ETHYLENE FORMATION BY FLORETS

Preliminary fractionation of the culture-supernatant (Lund and Mapson, 1970) showed that ability to stimulate ethylene production occurred in fractions containing both pectate lyase and polygalacturonase, these latter two enzymes were not separated. The pectic enzymes of *E. carotovora* which are mainly responsible for tissue maceration appear to be an endopolygalacturonase (Nasuno and Starr, 1966) and an endo-pectate lyase (Moran *et al.*, 1968; Dean and Wood, 1968; Mount *et al.*, 1970). Exo-pectate lyase and exo-polygalacturonase have also been isolated from cells of *E. carotovora* (Okamoto *et al.*, 1963, 1964) but are probably of minor importance in tissue maceration (Bateman and Millar, 1966). In our experiments a typical batch of culture supernatant contained the following enzymes:

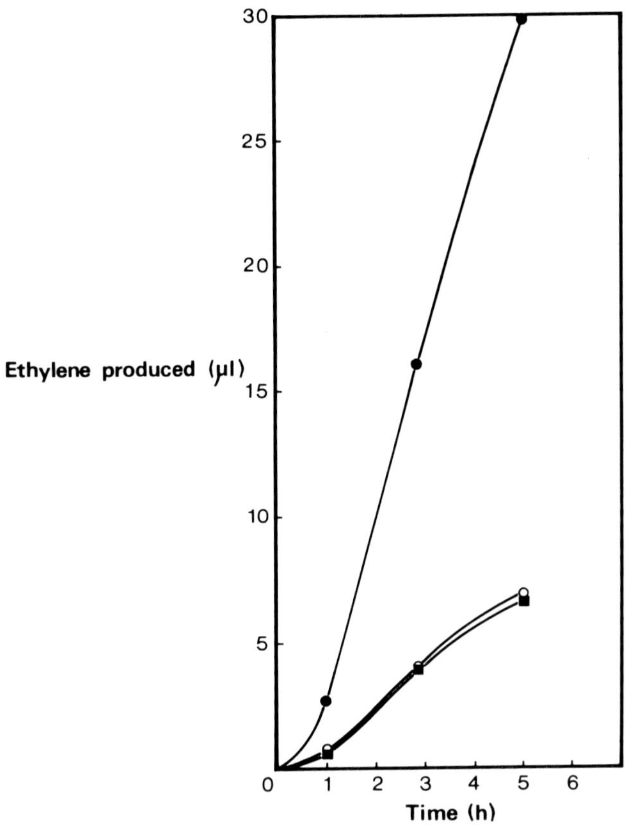

Fig. 5. Stimulation of ethylene production from 4-methylmercapto-2-oxobutyric acid by cell-wall material supplemented with cofactors after pretreatment with bacterial enzyme preparation. Cell-wall material (≡ 5 g of floret tissue in 5 ml of 0.1 M-sodium potassium phosphate buffer, pH 6.5), was treated as follows:
○, not pre-incubated;
■, pre-incubated at 25° C for 2 h;
●, pre-incubated at 25° C for 2 h with bacterial enzyme preparation (0.5 ml).
After pre-incubation oxo acid (1 mM), benzene-sulphinic acid (0.5 mM), *p*-hydroxybenzoate (0.5 mM), D-glucose (0.5 M) and horseradish peroxidase (0.9 purpurogallin unit) was added to each sample. The ethylene formed at 25° C was subsequently determined.

pectate lyase	polygalacturonase	pectinesterase
1.5 units/ml	0.25 units/ml	0.05 units/ml

In the later work it was found that proteolytic enzymes were also present.

By chromatography on CM-cellulose, separation of pectate lyase and polygalacturonase was obtained. From two different experiments fractions were selected which showed 52-fold and 185-fold increases (respectively) in specific activity of pectate lyase compared with the crude culture-supernatants, and which contained only traces of polygalacturonase and protease activity. These fractions stimulated ethylene production by cauliflower florets, the stimulation was equivalent to that obtained with a crude enzyme preparation with similar pectate lyase activity but also containing polygalacturonase (Table II).

TABLE II

The effect of purified pectate lyase on ethylene production by cauliflower florets

Enzyme preparation added	Amount of enzyme added: pectate lyase (units)	Amount of enzyme added: poly-galacturonase (*P*-units)	Ethylene nl/g tissue
Experiment 1. Incubation time 10.25 h			
None	0	0	37
Crude enzyme preparation	3	382	302
Crude enzyme preparation	0.3	38	229
Purified pectate lyase	0.31	trace	244
Experiment 2. Incubation time 5.5 h			
None	0	0	7.5
Crude enzyme preparation	3	382	256
Crude enzyme preparation (1 : 10 diln)	0.3	38	114
Crude enzyme preparation (1 : 100 diln)	0.03	3.8	21
Purified pectate lyase	5	9	237
Purified pectate lyase (1 : 10 diln)	0.5	0.9	133
Purified pectate lyase (1 : 100 diln)	0.05	0.09	11

Flasks (25 ml) contained 2 g florets; enzyme preparation 0.5 ml; phosphate buffer 0.1M pH 6.5 + EDTA 2mM 1.5 ml. After flushing with oxygen, flasks were incubated at 25°C.

Pectate lyase activity expressed in units/ml based on chemical assay.

Polygalacturonase activity expressed in arbitrary units (*P*-units)/ml, based on cup-plate assay.

From these fractionation experiments, bacterial proteolytic enzymes did not appear to be involved in the stimulation of ethylene formation; preparations containing pectic enzymes but lacking proteolytic activity were as effective as those containing both pectic and proteolytic activity (Table III). Commercial proteolytic enzymes were also tested for ability to stimulate ethylene production (Table IV). Using the cup-plate assay (see Methods section) the concentrations of commercial proteases used in this experiment were much greater than the concentrations found in the bacterial enzyme preparations. Neither the *Streptomyces griseus* protease nor trypsin gave any significant stimulation of ethylene production during the incubation time used.

TABLE III

The effect of bacterial enzyme preparations with or without protease activity on ethylene production by cauliflower florets

Enzyme preparation added	*P*-units added pectate lyase	poly-galacturonase	protease	Ethylene nl/g tissue
None	0	0	0	19
Preparation (a) lacking protease	382	382	0	241
Preparation (a) lacking protease	95	95	0	171
Preparation (a) lacking protease	38	38	0	140
Preparation (b) containing protease	664	382	151	171
Preparation (b) containing protease	166	95	38	260
Preparation (b) containing protease	66	38	15	201

Flasks (25 ml) contained 2 g florets; enzyme preparation, 0.5 ml; phosphate buffer 0.1 M pH 6.5, 1.5 ml. After flushing with oxygen, flasks were incubated at 25° C for 5.5 h.
Enzyme activities expressed in arbitrary units (*P*-units).

TABLE IV

The effect of commercial proteolytic enzymes on ethylene production by cauliflower florets

Enzyme preparation added	*P*-units added pectate lyase	poly-galacturonase	protease	Ethylene nl/g tissue
None	0	0	0	19
Bacterial	477	477	0	145
Protease	–	–	3303	19
Protease	–	–	330	25
Trypsin	–	–	5875	23
Trypsin	–	–	587	25

Conditions as in Table III, phosphate buffer (0.1 M, pH 6.5) also contained EDTA, 2mM. Incubation time 6 h.
Enzyme activities expressed in arbitrary units (*P*-units/ml) based on cup-plate assays.
Protease (Sigma) 0.5% solution was equivalent to 6607 *P*-units/ml.
Trypsin (Sigma) 0.1% solution was equivalent to 11 750 *P*-units/ml.

In early experiments, attempts to study the effect of commercial, fungal pectic enzymes were discontinued because of the presence of large amounts of other volatile material, thought to be of fungal origin. Recent experiments have shown that Pectinase (Sigma) will also stimulate ethylene production by cauliflower florets (Table V). This pectinase is produced from a strain of

TABLE V

The effect of Pectinase (Sigma) on ethylene production by cauliflower florets

Tissue	Enzyme preparation added	Ethylene nl/g tissue
floret	none	27.5
floret	bacterial	373.5
floret	Pectinase	548
floret	heated Pectinase	284.5
heated floret	Pectinase	13
none	Pectinase	0

Conditions as Table III, phosphate buffer (0.1 M, pH 6.5) also contained EDTA, 2 mM. Incubation time 5.3 h.

Heated Pectinase and florets were placed, in tubes, in a boiling water bath for 10 min then cooled.

The bacterial enzyme preparation contained the following activities, pectate lyase 7.5 units/ml based on chemical assay, polygalacturonase 995 *P*-units/ml based on cup-plate assay.

The solution of Sigma Pectinase contained 30 mg of the crude enzyme/ml in acetate buffer 0.05 M, pH 5.2.

Aspergillus; data is not available on the nature of the pectic enzymes present, and the product probably contains a number of other enzymes.

DISCUSSION

It was reported by Freebairn and Buddenhagen (1964) that bananas infected with *Pseudomonas solanacearum* produced more ethylene and ripened earlier than uninfected fruit. Many strains of this pathogen formed ethylene when grown in peptone glucose broth, one strain failed to do so when grown *in vitro*, and it was suggested that this strain may accelerate synthesis of the hydrocarbon by host cells—although it was also possible that the bacterium itself produced ethylene in the presence of undetermined substrates within the banana fruit. *Ps. solanacearum* forms pectic enzymes (Husain and Kelman, 1958), the nature of these enzymes is not clear, and it would be interesting to know whether the enzymes can stimulate ethylene production by banana tissue.

In our experiments, synthesis of ethylene by *E. carotovora* growing *in vitro* was not detected, but it is possible that synthesis may occur in different cultural conditions. Whether the bacterium can carry out this synthesis or not, its ability to stimulate formation of ethylene by certain plant tissues is of some interest.

The fact that pectate lyase rather than polygalacturonase appeared to account for the effect of bacterial culture-supernatants is perhaps surprising in view of the pH optima of these enzymes. When assayed against polygalacturonate the pH optimum for *E. carotovora* pectate lyase is about 8.5 (Starr and Moran, 1962) and activity falls to a low level when the pH is lowered to 6.5; the pH optimum for *E. carotovora* polygalacturonase is about 5.2-5.4 (Nasuno and Starr, 1966) and this enzyme shows considerable activity at pH 6.5, which was the pH used in our experiments with cauliflower and calabrese florets. Possibly there is a difference between the pH optima for these enzymes acting on substrates within plant tissue, and the pH optima for assays *in vitro*. Purification of polygalacturonase, in order to test directly whether this enzyme has any effect on ethylene synthesis, is in progress. The observation that proteolytic enzymes alone were ineffective, and did not appear to enhance the effect of the bacterial pectic enzymes may be worth investigating further, as proteolytic enzymes could provide an increased concentration of methionine, as a precursor for ethylene synthesis (Demorest and Stahmann, 1970).

The effect of the bacterial enzymes on ethylene synthesis by cauliflower florets could be accounted for by its effect on the activity of glucose oxidase attached to the plant cell wall tissue. Glucose oxidase had previously been found in the non-particulate fraction of the cytoplasm of cauliflower florets (Mapson and Wardale, 1968). Further study of the mechanism of stimulation of ethylene synthesis may be of interest; the increase in permeability which has been reported when plant tissue is treated with *E. carotovora* pectate lyase (Mount *et al.*, 1970; Hall and Wood, 1970) may also be relevant since there is some evidence, referred to by Mapson (1969), supporting the theory that a change in permeability of cell membranes may play a part in the initiation of rapid ethylene production during ripening of climacteric fruits.

An increase in ethylene formation has also been found when green tomatoes were inoculated with *E. carotovora*. In this tissue the mechanism of ethylene biosynthesis is reported to differ from that in cauliflower florets (Mapson and Wardale, 1971) and further work is required in order to understand the effect of the bacterium on tomato tissue. Pectic enzymes of bacteria and possibly of a fungus have been shown to accelerate ethylene formation by floret tissue, and tissues infected by viruses have been reported to undergo alterations in pectic constituents and show yellowing (Weintraub and Ragetli, 1961). Differences have been demonstrated between the pathways of ethylene synthesis in different plant tissues, and further work is necessary to establish whether pectic enzymes have a general role in triggering formation of this plant hormone in diseased or in normal tissue.

Summary

(1) An increase in ethylene production may occur as a consequence of infection of plant tissues by fungi, bacteria or viruses. In some cases the pathogen is capable of synthesizing ethylene and the relative contribution of host and of pathogen to the total ethylene formed is unknown. The work reported here demonstrates that cauliflower and calabrese florets and tomato fruit infected with *E. carotovora* show an increase in synthesis of this hydrocarbon, and in floret tissue an increase can also be caused by addition of a bacterial culture-supernatant containing pectic enzymes.
(2) In cauliflower florets, bacterial enzyme(s) probably accelerates synthesis of ethylene by the route occurring in normal tissue, this biosynthesis involves methionine as a precursor and is thought to depend on the activities of a transaminase, forming 4-methylmercapto-2-oxobutyric acid, a glucose oxidase, and a peroxidase together with their substrates and cofactors.
(3) The site of action of the bacterial enzyme(s) was on plant cell wall tissue, this contained glucose oxidase the activity of which was increased and solubilized in the presence of bacterial enzyme(s), thus leading to an increase in peroxide available for synthesis of ethylene from the oxo acid.
(4) From culture-supernatants of *E. carotovora,* pectate lyase was purified 180-fold and appeared to account for the ability of the culture-supernatants to stimulate formation of ethylene.

Acknowledgements

I am indebted to the late Professor L. W. Mapson with whose collaboration this work was started and who elucidated the stage at which ethylene biosynthesis in florets was affected by the bacterial enzymes. I wish also to thank Dr A. C. Hulme and Dr M. J. C. Rhodes for helpful discussions, and Mr G. M. Wyatt for valuable technical assistance.

References

Balazs, E., Gaborjányi, R., Tóth, A. and Király, Z. (1969). Ethylene production in Xanthi Tobacco after systemic and local virus infections. *Acta Phytopath. Acad. Sci. Hung.* **4**, 355-358.

Bateman, D. F. and Millar, R. L. (1966). Pectic enzymes in tissue degradation. *A. Rev. Phytopathol.* **4**, 119-146.

Baur, A. H., Yang, S. F., Pratt, H. K. and Biale, J. B. (1971). Ethylene biosynthesis in fruit tissue. *Pl. Physiol., Lancaster* **47**, 696-699.

Burg, S. P. (1962). The physiology of ethylene formation. *A. Rev. Pl. Physiol.* **13**, 265-302.

Dean, M. and Wood, R. K. S. (1968). Cell wall degradation by a pectate transeliminase. *Nature, Lond.* **214**, 408-410.

Demorest, D. M. and Stahmann, M. A. (1970). Ethylene production from peptides and protein containing methionine. *Pl. Physiol., Lancaster* **47**, 450-451.

Dingle J., Reid, W. W. and Solomons, G. L. (1953). The enzymic degradation of pectin and other polysaccharides. II. Application of the 'Cup-plate' assay to the estimation of enzymes. *J. Sci. Fd Agric.* **4**, 149-155.

Freebairn, H. T. and Buddenhagen, I. W. (1964). Ethylene production by *Pseudomonas solanacearum. Nature, Lond.* **202**, 313-314.

Hall, J. A. and Wood, R. K. S. (1970). Plant cells killed by soft rot parasites. *Nature, Lond.* **227**, 1266-1267.

Husain, A. and Kelman, A. (1958). The role of pectic and cellulolytic enzymes in pathogenesis by *Pseudomonas solanacearum. Phytopathology* **48**, 337-386.

Ilag, L. and Curtis, R. W. (1968). Production of ethylene by fungi. *Science, N.Y.* **159**, 1357-1358.

Layne, E. (1957). Spectrophotometric and turbidimetric methods for measuring protein. *In* 'Methods in Enzymology' (eds S. P. Colowick and N. O. Kaplan). Vol. III, 447-454. Academic Press, New York.

Lieberman, M. and Kunishi, A. T. (1971). An evaluation of 4-S-methyl-2-ketobutyric acid as an intermediate in the biosynthesis of ethylene. *Pl. Physiol., Lancaster* **47**, 576-580.

Lockhart, B. E. and Semancik, J. S. (1970). Growth inhibition, peroxidase and 3-indoleacetic acid oxidase activity, and ethylene production in Cowpea mosaic virus-infected Cowpea seedlings. *Phytopathology* **60**, 553-554.

Lowry, O. H., Rosebrough, N. J., Farr, A. J. and Randall, R. J. (1951). Protein measurement with the Folin phenol reagent. *J. biol. Chem.* **193**, 265-275.

Lund, B. M. and Mapson, L. W. (1970). Stimulation by *Erwinia carotovora* of the synthesis of ethylene in cauliflower tissue. *Biochem. J.* **119**, 251-263.

Mapson, L. W. (1969). Biogenesis of ethylene. *Biol. Rev.* **44**, 155-187.

Mapson, L. W. and Hulme, A. C. (1970). The biosynthesis, physiological effects, and mode of action of ethylene. *In* 'Progress in Phytochemistry' (eds L. Rheinhold and Y. Liwschitz). Vol. 2, 343-384. Interscience Publishers, London.

Mapson, L. W., March, J. F., Rhodes, M. J. C. and Wooltorton, L. S. C. (1970). A comparative study of the ability of methionine or linolenic acid to act as precursors of ethylene in plant tissues. *Biochem J.* **117**, 473-479.

Mapson, L. W. and Wardale, D. A. (1968). Biosynthesis of ethylene. Enzymes involved in its formation from methional. *Biochem. J.* **107**, 433-442.

Mapson, L. W. and Wardale, D. A. (1971). Enzymes involved in the synthesis of ethylene from methionine, or its derivatives, in tomatoes. *Phytochemistry* **10**, 29-39.

Moran, F., Nasuno, S. and Starr, M. P. (1968). Extracellular and intracellular polygalacturonic acid trans-eliminases of *Erwinia carotovora. Archs Biochem. Biophys.* **123**, 298-306.

Mount, M. S., Bateman, D. F. and Basham, H. G. (1970). Induction of electrolyte loss, tissue maceration, and cellular death of potato tissue by an endopolygalacturonate trans-eliminase. *Phytopathology* **60**, 924-932.

Nakagaki, Y., Hirai, T. and Stahmann, M. A. (1970). Ethylene production by detached leaves infected with Tobacco Mosaic Virus. *Virology* **40**, 1-9.

Nasuno, S. and Starr, M. P. (1966). Polygalacturonase of *Erwinia carotovora. J. biol. Chem.* **241**, 5298-5306.

Okamoto, K., Hatanaka, C. and Ozawa, J. ,(1963). On the saccharifying pectolytic enzymes of *Erwinia aroideae*. *Agr. Biol. Chem.* 27, 596-597.

Okamoto, K., Hatanaka, C. and Ozawa, J. (1964). Some properties of the saccharifying pectate trans-eliminase of *Erwinia aroideae*. *Ber. Ohara Inst. Landw. Biol.* **12**, 107-114.

Pratt, H. K. and Goeschl, J. D. (1969). Physiological roles of ethylene in plants. *A. Rev. Pl. Physiol.* **20**, 541-584.

Ross, A. F. and Williamson, C. E. (1951). Physiologically active emanations from virus-infected plants. *Phytopathology* **41**, 431-438.

Starr, M. P. and Moran, F. (1962). Eliminative split of pectic substances by phytopathogenic soft-rot bacteria. *Science, N.Y.* **135**, 920-921.

Swanson, B. T. (1971). 'Relationship of ethylene to senescence'. Ph.D. Thesis. University of Minnesota, USA.

Weintraub, M. and Ragetli, H. W. J. (1961). Cell wall composition of leaves with a localized virus infection. *Phytopathology* **51**, 215-219.

Wood, R. K. S. (1967). 'Physiological Plant Pathology'. Blackwell, Oxford and Edinburgh.

DISCUSSION

Dr G. A. Kamerbeck: We know in tulip bulbs, a very heavy gummosis can be caused by small quantities of ethylene, but it may be that the ethylene is produced by *Fusarium oxysporum*, or it may arise from an exogenous source. We also know that infection of *Erwinia carotovora* in hyacinth bulbs can cause heavy gummosis after the infection. It is therefore obvious from your work that the *Erwinia* is producing the ethylene which, as a secondary effect, causes this heavy gummosis. Did you observe any symptoms of gummosis in cauliflower or tomatoes? My second question is perhaps more wild. Do you suppose that your *Erwinia* is not producing ethylene where it is in culture, and can only produce ethylene by help of the host tissue, so that it arises from co-operation between the healthy and damaged parts of the tissue? The cofactors are produced by the affected tissue, and normal healthy tissue is supplying the ethylene-synthesizing system. The same idea can be found in the work of Uritani, and from Stahmann's work with *Ceratocystis*. When an organism (such as *Fusarium oxysporum* f. *tulipae*) that can produce relatively great amounts of ethylene *in vitro* is cultured, ethylene production starts only after a first growth period. Does the speaker give support to the idea that also in this instance there may be a cooperation between the young and older starving mycelium?

Dr Barbara Lund: Let's consider gummosis first. I think our systems were too unlike the systems you are talking about to expect to see this, and with cauliflower, or anything like that, there was only marked water soaking and rotting of the tissue. With tomato, the way inoculation was made meant that the organism was inoculated mainly into the centre of the fruit, and I certainly did not see anything specific as you mention. I think your second question speculates more on the effect of the mycelium. We did deliberately restrict ourselves to looking at the effects of the extracellular enzymes, because this is a particularly manipulable system, and I've no information on ethylene production by *Erwinia* in culture. I've not seen it described at all in the literature, but it may well happen.

Dr R. C. Hignett: If you increase the concentration of ethylene in a disease system, is there any effect on the course of the disease, its rate of development, etc.?

Dr Lund: These are artificial systems, and to say that it affects the course of a disease is supposing a rather more specific interaction than I think is occurring. These soft rots involve rather non-specific types of reaction, and we were working in unnatural systems, while the tomato disease would involve a more natural system.

Professor M. A. Stahmann: You suggested that your culture supernatants increased glucose oxidase, which tends to increase ethylene formation, but did you make any direct measurements on glucose-oxidase activity?

Dr Lund: I did not give you the data, but measurements of glucose oxidase activity have been made by manometric methods, and in addition other carbohydrate substrates were used. The activity was specific to glucose with some effects on 2-deoxy-D-glucose.

Professor Stahmann: Did you ever measure peroxidase activity?

Dr Lund: No we did not. Looking back, we should have done, and it would be interesting to do this. The trend of Mapson's experiments, right through, had been to indicate that peroxidase was not rate-limiting in ethylene production but that glucose oxidase was in fact rate-limiting. This is why it appeared that we looked more particularly at the activation of that system. It could well be that peroxidase was also activated.

R. C. Codner: If you add the reaction products of a pectic enzyme on a pectic substrate does this stimulate ethylene production in your system?

Dr Lund: We have not done that experiment. You are suggesting that some of the degradation products of polygalacturonate would act as substrates for ethylene production. Had this been so, it would have occurred in our heated systems but it did not. You would also have expected it to occur when we grew *Erwinia* on culture medium containing polygalacturonate, but we did not find this.

S. A. Archer: You mention that certain components of your system are heat labile, just how heat labile are they? Did you boil, or heat to a specific temperature?

Dr Lund: When I say heat labile, they were mostly at 100° C for 5-10 min.

S. A. Archer: I ask this because some of the heat-labile components in the apple system are inactivated by treatment at 50° C.

Dr Lund: As regards the high optimum pH to which Professor Stahmann referred, this has always been a stumbling block in some way. All one can say is that the purified material does result in maceration at pH 6.5, presumably acting suboptimally. Also, possibly, we are using a rather unusual artificial assay system, with a certain concentration of calcium ions and particular substrates, and perhaps the assay system we adopt determines to some extent the pH optimum.

D. E. Stead: Have you ever tried this on potatoes to find the release of ethylene from potatoes infected by *E. carotovora*?

Dr Lund: Yes, I have tried it. The results have not been very convincing.

II. 2 The Involvement of Ethylene in Plant Diseases

E. C. HISLOP, G. V. HOAD AND S. A. ARCHER

Long Ashton Research Station, University of Bristol, England

INTRODUCTION

A little over 100 years ago illuminating gas and smokes were shown to cause remarkable growth responses in plants, and seventy years ago the active principle was shown to be the simple unsaturated hydrocarbon ethylene, which was effective at concentrations of less than 0.1 ppm. Ethylene, now known to be a natural product of plant metabolism, is considered increasingly to be an integral part of plant auto-regulation (Osborne, 1968). Typical responses of land plants to ethylene are inhibition of growth, yellowing and premature shedding of leaves, earlier ripening of fruits, fading of flowers, the epinasty of leaves and stems, loss of bending responses to light and gravity, the breaking of dormancy in buds and seeds, enhancement of flowering and stimulation of adventitious roots (Osborne, 1971).

Many plants have been shown to produce increased amounts of ethylene under conditions of stress or injury, and tissues damaged by pathogens are not exceptions to this general rule. Burg (1962) reviewed studies on ethylene production by wounded tissues and concluded that almost all that had been published to that date was purely observational. In their comprehensive review of the physiological roles of ethylene in plants, Pratt and Goeschl (1969) considered that the relations between ethylene production and disease, wound and stress responses deserved further study. The object of this paper is therefore to examine the production of ethylene by diseased plant tissues and to review and speculate upon the implications of this phenomenon.

THE PRODUCTION OF ETHYLENE BY DISEASED TISSUES

The few diseased plants which have been examined have a higher rate of ethylene evolution than similar healthy plants. This appears to be true for viral, bacterial and fungal infections as indicated by the following selected examples covering some of the major groups of pathogens.

One of the earliest reports of increased emanation of volatile materials was from decaying citrus fruits infected with the fungus *Penicillium digitatum* This observation was of particular interest because it was shown that the volatiles could cause epinasty in plants and because it so happened that this was one of the few fungi which, even now, are known to produce large amounts of ethylene *in vitro* (Muller *et al.*, 1940). A few years later, Williamson (1950) examined the capacity of 19 pathogenic fungi on 12 hosts to initiate the triple response of etiolated Alaska pea seedlings. He concluded that certain diseased tissues, particularly rose leaves infected with *Diplocarpon rosae* and Chrysanthemum infected with *Ascochyta chrysanthemi*, showed a marked stimulation of ethylene production, and that it was a response to injury occurring only as long as the infected tissue was alive. Further, of five pathogens grown on potato dextrose agar, only *P. digitatum* produced measurable amounts of ethylene.

The following year Ross and Williamson (1951) examined virus-infected leaves for physiologically active emanations and made the interesting observation that *Physalis floridana* leaves with necrotic lesions caused by potato virus Y elicited a marked response in etiolated pea seedlings, but that systemically-infected symptomless leaves with a higher virus content caused a smaller response. Similar data were obtained for other host–virus interactions, and it was also shown that leaves of *P. floridana* and *Nicotiana tabacum* with necrotic lesions induced by phytotoxic chemicals such as copper sulphate also produced considerable amounts of ethylene. It was concluded from these data that the active emanation, presumably ethylene, was a product of the necrotic cells rather than the cause of the necrosis.

The first report implicating a bacterial pathogen in the increased ethylene production by diseased tissue seems to be that by Freebairn and Buddenhagen (1964). These workers showed that increased ethylene was produced by bananas infected with *Pseudomonas solanacearum* and that several strains of this bacterium produced considerable quantities of ethylene when grown in shake culture in a peptone-glucose medium. Several other bacteria from soil, as secondary organisms associated with banana tissue, and from banana fruits affected by tip rot did not produce ethylene under similar conditions. Unlike earlier reports involving pathogens, Freebairn and Buddenhagen used a gas chromatographic technique for the identification of chemically-adsorbed ethylene. Co-chromatography with known ethylene and a positive epinasty test proved the identity of the gas, a confirmation not always possible in some earlier studies on emanations from infected tissue, although the presumed identity of the active principle on the basis of bioassays was reasonable. Flame-ionization gas chromatography now permits quick, direct, yet highly sensitive and accurate measurements of ethylene.

These examples of greater evolution of ethylene from diseased tissues in comparison with that from healthy tissues raise the following points to be considered in this paper:

(i) Is ethylene produced by the pathogen, the host, or by the host–pathogen interaction?
(ii) To what extent is ethylene responsible for the symptoms of plant disease?
(iii) What is the mechanism of ethylene biosynthesis in diseased tissues?
(iv) Is ethylene involved in interactions between pathogens and their hosts?

IS ETHYLENE PRODUCED BY THE PATHOGEN, THE HOST, OR BY THE HOST–PATHOGEN INTERACTION?

It is now clear that many fungi and some bacteria do produce ethylene *in vitro*. Ilag and Curtis (1968) examined 228 species of fungi and detected and verified ethylene as a metabolic product in 22 of them. Since 58 out of the 228 produced a gas with the same chromatographic retention time it was suggested that ethylene is probably a frequent metabolic product of fungi. However, the production of ethylene was usually very low, since 0.1-0.2 g dry weight of mycelium incubated in a 10 ml syringe produced less than 0.5 ppm (15 nl) during 24 h in 94% of the tests. Notable exceptions to this were *Aspergillus clavatus* (514 ppm), *A. flavus* (12.8), *Ascochyta imperfecta* (9.9), *Cephalosporium gramineum* (12.4), *Penicillium corylophilum* (10.7) and *Thamnidium elegans* (15.5). The situation is complicated by the fact that different strains of the same fungus have been shown to differ in their capacity to produce ethylene (Chalutz and DeVay, 1969).

As already stated, *P. digitatum* is also a prolific producer of ethylene *in vitro* and for this reason has been used in many metabolic studies. Ethylene is produced during active growth of this fungus on a range of carbon sources. Tracer studies indicate that any metabolite that can be incorporated into the methylene carbons of isocitrate can serve as an ethylene precursor.

The production *in vitro* of ethylene from bacterial pathogens is not so well documented. *Erwinia carotovora* did not produce ethylene in culture (Lund and Mapson, 1970) but the work of Freebairn and Buddenhagen (1964) indicates that strains of the same bacterium can behave differently and that nutritional factors may have to be considered. The levels of ethylene produced by *P. solanacearum* were quite high, 350 nl being obtained from 20 ml of bacterial suspension in a 50 ml flask in 5 h.

Production of ethylene by healthy plant tissues is variable but usually very low for all but climacteric fruits, when compared with the levels of production by diseased tissues. It appears that the increased ethylene produced by diseased tissue may be derived from either the damaged host tissues or from the pathogen which has been supplemented with a substrate from the host, or from both sources combined. There is no evidence for or against the supplementation of the pathogen by the host, but there is some evidence that the host is largely responsible for ethylene production. In addition to the work of Ross and Williamson (1951), data from Balázs *et al.* (1969) and Nagagaki *et al.* (1970)

confirm that plants which exhibit local virus lesions produce larger amounts of ethylene than those infected systemically, and that enhanced ethylene production coincides with the appearance of the local lesions.

Moreover, ethylene production is known to be stimulated by conditions of stress other than that of pathogen attack, e.g. gamma radiation (Maxie *et al.*, 1965), chloride damage (Rasmussen *et al.*, 1969) and low temperature stress (Cooper *et al.*, 1969) have all been shown to increase ethylene production by *Citrus* spp. It is also known that the higher concentrations of ethylene found around sliced tissues of apple fruits are not due solely to increased ventilation (Burg, 1962) but also to increased ethylene production.

Evidence that ethylene is produced by tissues damaged by fungi is less clear cut, but still convincing. Williamson (1950) concluded that the response to infection occurs only as long as the infected tissue is alive; and this was also shown to be true for the stimulation of ethylene production by sweet potato tissue injured by chemicals (Imaseki *et al.*, 1968c). Tissue plugs from sweet potato roots infected with *Ceratocystis fimbriata* produced ethylene only if the plugs consisted of both fungus-invaded and non-invaded parts (Imaseki *et al.*, 1968a). Chalutz and DeVay also examined this host–parasite system and found that ethylene production was dependent upon the rate and amount of fungal growth on agar media and in host tissue but there was no consistent relationship between the relative amounts of ethylene produced *in vitro* and *in vivo*.

Hislop and Stahmann (1971) measured ethylene evolution from barley leaves infected with *Erysiphe graminis* f. sp. *hordei* and found a massive stimulation in infected leaves compared with healthy leaves or immune leaves inoculated 36-48 h before examination. However, some inoculated immune leaves produced more ethylene than similarly-treated susceptible leaves for a short period about 16-18 h after inoculation. Microscopic observations of leaves harvested 16 h after inoculation indicated that the fungus had developed in an identical manner on compatible and incompatible hosts. Since the inoculum level on both was the same, it was concluded that this increased ethylene production was a host response to injury perhaps indicating some biochemical lesion which did not occur in the susceptible tissue. Forty-eight hours after inoculation, ethylene production by immune leaves decreased appreciably while that from susceptible leaves increased steadily after inoculation (Fig. 1). Wheat leaves infected for several days with *Puccinia graminis* f. sp. *tritici* also showed an increased production of ethylene compared with infected resistant leaves which produced more than healthy control leaves (Daly *et al.*, 1970).

We have been examining the production of ethylene from apple fruits infected with the brown rot fungus *Sclerotinia fructigena* Aderh. and Ruhl. This fungus produces no ethylene *in vitro* but infected pre-climacteric apples produce very large quantities of this gas compared with similar healthy fruits. When sections of apple parenchyma taken from plugs of tissue (Fig. 2) are incubated in

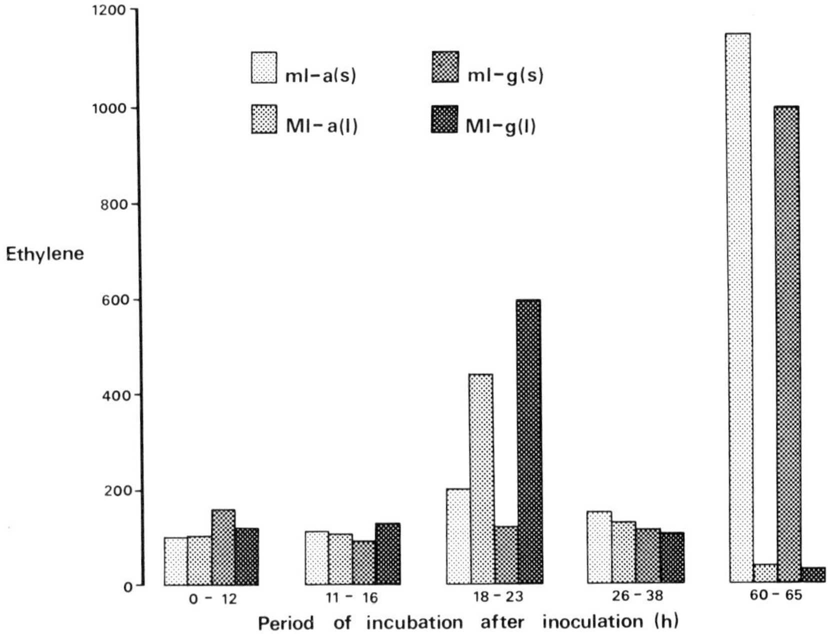

Fig. 1. Ethylene evolution (nl/g/h) from inoculated detached susceptible (S) and immune (I) barley leaves incubated in darkness at 19° C. (Hislop and Stahmann, 1971).

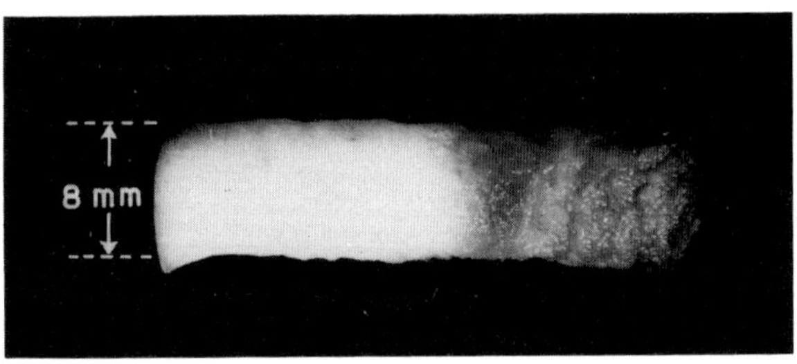

Fig. 2. Plug of apple tissue infected (darker portion at right) with *S. fructigena*. Margin of rot corresponds to disk no. 4 in Fig. 3.

sealed containers, it is obvious that most of the ethylene produced comes from the margin of the rot where hyphae can be seen penetrating apparently healthy tissue (Fig. 3). The bulk of the rot which contains a large amount of viable mycelium contributes little to the production of the ethylene and therefore once again it seems that the gas is produced by the host in response to the presence of the fungus. The data in Table I obtained from disks of apple tissue from

TABLE I

Oxygen uptake and pectic enzyme production by disks (2 mm thick) taken serially from healthy (1-3), partly rotted (4) and wholly rotted (5-7) apple pulp

	Disk No.						
	1	2	3	4	5	6	7
	← Healthy			→←		Rotted →	
QO_2	0.30	0.36	0.49	0.49	0.55	0.41	0.39
PG	0.00	–	–	7.70	–	–	10.20
AF	0.10	–	–	0.17	–	–	0.28
PME	0.15	–	–	2.70	–	–	3.30

Key
QO_2 = μl/mg dry wt./h
PG = Polygalacturonase, arbitrary units
AF = Arabinofuranosidase, arbitrary units
PME = Pectin methyl esterase, arbitrary units
– signifies no test

different areas around a lesion similar to those used to measure ethylene production (Fig. 3) indicate that oxygen uptake by tissues near the margin of the rot is high compared with that from healthy or well rotted tissue and that some pectic enzymes also occur in high amounts in the margin and body of the rot.

The conclusion that the host produces the ethylene is further supported by the fact that infected pre-climacteric fruits heated in a water bath at 50° C for 20 min do not produce large quantities of ethylene even though the rot develops normally. How this treatment inhibits ethylene production is not clear, because the host cells from heated fruits have the same respiration rate and the same conductivity and plasmolysis characteristics as unheated fruits.

TO WHAT EXTENT IS ETHYLENE RESPONSIBLE FOR THE SYMPTOMS OF PLANT DISEASE?

A student of physiological plant pathology can hardly fail to be impressed with the similarity between some of the symptoms of disease in plants and some of the effects of ethylene on plants. Since increased ethylene production is a feature of diseased tissue it seems reasonable to suspect that some of the symptoms of disease are in fact caused by excess ethylene.

Symptoms characteristic of senescence are common in diseases of shoots and leaves, and as Williamson (1950) pointed out, the yellowing and abscission of rose leaves infected with *D. rosae* could be due to the excess ethylene they produce.

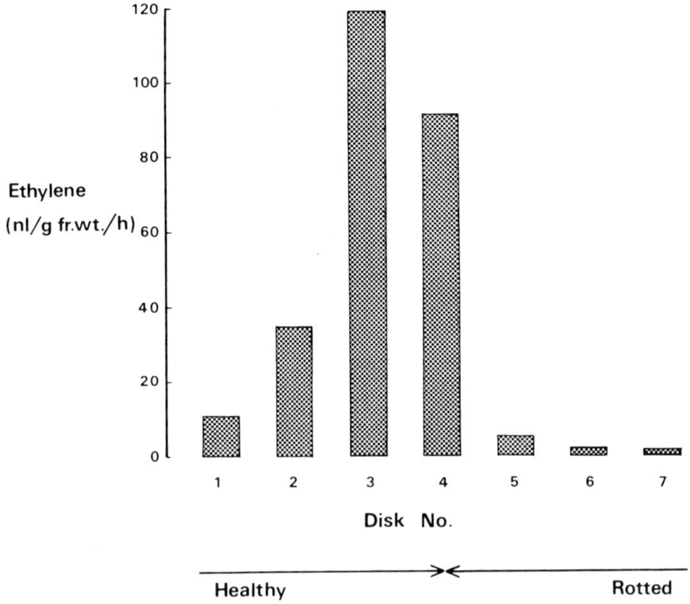

Fig. 3. Ethylene production by disks (2 mm thick) from healthy (1-3), partially rotted (4), and wholly rotted (5-7) apple pulp.

Another common symptom of certain diseases is epinasty of the petioles, and Dimond and Waggoner (1953) concluded that the ethylene produced by tomatoes infected with *Fusarium oxysporum* f. sp. *lycopersici* could be responsible for this symptom of infection. Abscission of tomato leaves, also a symptom of infection by this pathogen, was not however reproduced in their experiments on the effects of ethylene on healthy tomato plants. Another disease characterized by symptoms similar to those induced by ethylene is that caused by *Cercospora personata* on groundnut. Gaseous emanations from infected leaves caused epinasty in a tomato bioassay and the active priciple was presumed, but not proven, to be ethylene (Swamy, 1961).

F. oxysporum f. sp. *tulipae* is a pathogen of tulip bulbs and it is often observed that the normal development of healthy bulbs is altered by the presence of infected bulbs which produce high local concentrations of ethylene in soil. The work of de Munk and de Rooy (1971) has shown that this ethylene may be responsible for the observed symptoms of stunted growth of shoots and roots and blasting of the flower buds. For other crops, damage to healthy plants by ethylene evolved by diseased tissues may also be of some commercial importance. Smith *et al.* (1964) reported increased ethylene production from carnation flowers infected by *Botrytis cinerea* and stated that the levels reached were high enough to damage uninfected flowers in the same pack. Serious damage to dormant apple and pear nursery stock maintained in cold storage has also been reported by Curtis and Rodney (1952) who found that bud damage was evident at 1 ppm of ethylene, a value frequently exceeded in cold stores containing pome fruit.

Recently, evidence has accumulated to suggest that natural leaf-fall is triggered by ethylene production in senescing cells close to abscission zones (Jackson and Osborne, 1970); and it would be tempting to attribute pathogen-induced leaf abscission solely to excess ethylene production. As Wood (1967) points out however, diseases such as that caused by *Sphaceloma rosarum* which has a similar mode of parasitism to *D. rosae,* apparently does not produce excess ethylene. Auxin inactivation has been implicated in the leaf fall of coffee caused by *Omphalia flavida* (Ray, 1958), but although auxin degradation was demonstrated *in vitro,* activity of an IAA oxidase induced by *O. flavida* has never been demonstrated in diseased host tissues. Clearly insufficient information has accumulated to implicate ethylene universally in premature abscission and there is no reason to suppose that its involvement will be the same in every syndrome studied.

Ethylene may also be involved in the injury to various plant species caused by waterlogged soil. Kramer (1951) and Jackson (1956) list leaf yellowing, epinasty and adventitious root formation as occurring in a number of species and noted that greater symptom development occurred in waterlogged soil than in sand or water culture. Jackson (1956) mentioned ethylene as one possible toxin contributing to the observed damage and a recent report by Smith and Scott-Russell (1969) has indicated that levels of ethylene up to 10 ppm may occur in anaerobic soil under waterlogged conditions. A possible connection here is purely speculative but sufficient to warrant further work.

Plants infected with fungi, bacteria or viruses usually show an increased respiratory rate, which Goodman *et al.* (1967) have suggested is one of the most general phenomena in the physiology of diseased plants. As they point out it is not a specific reaction, because respiration, just as ethylene production, may be increased by chemical and mechanical injury. Since ethylene can stimulate respiratory activity, for example in initiating the climacteric of fruits and perhaps even in less conventional systems, e.g. potato tubers (Reid and Pratt, 1970), it could be argued that increased respiration in infected tissues is initiated by ethylene. Goodman *et al.* (1967) suggest that, in general, only plants in an advanced stage of systemic virus infection show an increased respiration rate, while in hosts showing local necrosis there is a marked enhancement of respiration at the time lesions appear, which it will be remembered is exactly the time when enhanced ethylene production is detected. The same authors suggest that the increase in the respiratory rate in incompatible fungal-plant interactions is greater than in compatible interactions: such respiratory changes coincided with the production of ethylene at certain stages in the compatible and incompatible reactions examined by Hislop and Stahmann (1971), as shown in Fig. 1.

It is of course dangerous to generalize about interactions occurring between very different hosts and parasites but since the object of a symposium is to generate discussion we would like to raise again the question—which comes first, the increased ethylene production or increased oxygen uptake; or are these two interrelated, since the production of ethylene by healthy plants is oxygen dependent (Burg, 1962)?

Other symptoms of disease which might be affected by ethylene but about which there is little information, are the initiation of adventitious roots (e.g. Dimond and Waggoner, 1953) and the various degrees of tissue proliferation seen in many diseases. Growth-regulating compounds such as IAA have been implicated in such disease syndromes as tumour formation by *Agrobacterium tumefaciens* (e.g. Braun and Laskaris, 1942; Sequeira, 1964), and hypertrophy of corn infected with *Ustilago zeae* (Turian and Hamilton, 1960). Many results suggest that auxins may modify the effects of ethylene in plants but the interplay between them is extremely complex and beyond the scope of this paper.

WHAT IS THE MECHANISM OF ETHYLENE BIOSYNTHESIS IN DISEASED TISSUES?

Anyone familiar with the literature on ethylene will realize at once that this is a highly presumptuous section heading because relatively little is known about the biochemistry of ethylene production even in healthy tissues. Therefore, our object in this section is to review briefly some of the information available about healthy tissue and then to consider the situation in diseased tissue.

The observation that *P. digitatum* would produce large amounts of ethylene when grown in defined media prompted a considerable amount of research with this system with the object of elucidating the mechanism of biogenesis of the gas. The state of our knowledge about this system was reviewed by Pratt and Goeschl (1969), but they were forced to conclude that although much had been done, none of the tracer feeding experiments carried out to that date conclusively showed ethylene production from specific substrates by specific enzymes. One point of interest in relation to the production of ethylene from higher plant systems compared with *P. digitatum* was the finding that uniformly labelled methionine was not metabolized to ethylene by the fungus (Ketring *et al.*, 1968). It seems likely therefore that the mechanisms of ethylene production in this and possibly other fungi are different from those of higher plants (Pratt and Goeschl, 1969).

A number of model systems have been described in which ethylene is produced non-enzymically from linolenic acid or methionine in the presence of ascorbic acid and copper salts (Lieberman and Mapson, 1964). In one system linolenic acid is first oxidized before ethylene and ethane are produced in approximately equal quantities. Only when C-3 and C-4 of methionine are labelled is the isotope incorporated into ethylene (Lieberman *et al.*, 1966) and this was confirmed when it was found that methional was even more readily converted to ethylene in the same system. In a second model system methionine was converted to ethylene by flavine compounds in the light (Yang *et al.*, 1966).

Since both methionine and linolenic acid occur commonly in plants these model systems were considered as prototypes for the process *in vivo* which was thought in all probability to be an enzymic one. Lieberman *et al.* (1966) showed that methionine can induce more than a 100% increase in ethylene production by tissue slices from post-climacteric apples, and suggested that a copper-containing enzyme might be involved. Reports on the enzymic formation of ethylene from methional by extracts of cauliflower (Mapson and Wardale, 1967) and by extracts from pea seedlings (Ku *et al.*, 1967) soon followed, while Yang (1967) characterized a system for the aerobic production of ethylene from methional in the presence of horseradish peroxidase with Mn^{2+}, sulphite and a monophenol as cofactors. Methionine is inactive as a precursor of ethylene in such a system but α-keto-γ-methylthiobutyric acid is as active as methional (Yang, 1969). Free methional does not occur in plants but an important step in the elucidation of the process whereby ethylene may be produced from methionine was the demonstration that the keto acid can be produced from methionine by the action of a transaminase present in cauliflower plant tissue (Mapson *et al.*, 1969). This keto acid was then degraded by a peroxidase which utilizes hydrogen peroxide generated by the oxidation of glucose by glucose oxidase.

Methionine and its derivatives are precursors of ethylene in apple, tomato and cauliflower tissue, but linolenic acid is inactive (Mapson *et al.*, 1970). However, linolenate and an enzyme with lipoxygenase activity, as well as a transaminase and a peroxidase, were involved in the synthesis of ethylene from methionine in tomatoes (Mapson and Wardale, 1971). The failure to convert labelled linolenic acid to ethylene was not due to poor uptake, since it was effectively converted to carbon dioxide (Baur and Yang, 1969). These authors further found that the keto acid was converted inefficiently to ethylene by apple tissue compared with methionine, contrasting with the finding of Mapson *et al.* (1969) who used cauliflower tissue. An explanation for this discrepancy has been given by Lieberman and Kunishi (1971) who showed that cauliflower tissue leaks peroxidase and cofactors into a buffer medium which can then degrade the keto acid to ethylene. On the other hand, apple tissue does not leak peroxidase and consequently does not respond to the presence of the keto acid. The whole question of the nature of the enzymes and substrates involved in ethylene biosynthesis was therefore confused by their conclusion that the keto acid probably was not an intermediate in the pathway between methionine and ethylene, and that peroxidase may not be involved in the biosynthesis of the gas; this despite the fact that Takeo and Lieberman (1969) had isolated, purified and characterized an enzyme from apple tissue which was a peroxidase catalysing the formation of ethylene from methional in a system which required *p*-coumaric acid as the phenolic cofactor. Peroxidase also leaked from tomato tissue in the experiments of Lieberman and Kunishi (1971). Ku *et al.* (1969) have isolated a peroxidase-like enzyme from this tissue which produced ethylene from the keto acid, but not from methionine. In all cases, the peroxidase-like enzymes from apple, cauliflower or tomato require essentially the same cofactors as used in Yang's (1967) model system. Circumstantial evidence that a peroxidase may be involved in the formation of ethylene by intact tissues was provided by Ku *et al.* (1970) who showed that both the activity of peroxidase, and ethylene production increased as tomato fruits ripened.

Further evidence that it is methionine and not its α-keto analogue which acts as a precursor of ethylene in higher plant systems has been obtained from studies on the inhibition of ethylene production by rhizobitoxine (Owens *et al.*, 1971). Rhizobitoxine, a phytotoxin produced by certain strains of *Rhizobium japonicum,* inhibits greening of new leaf tissue of many plants and inhibits β-cystathionase in the methionine biosynthetic pathway in *Salmonella typhimurium* (Owens *et al.*, 1968) and in spinach (Giovanelli *et al.*, 1971). A surprise finding was that rhizobitoxine appears to inhibit ethylene production not by inhibiting methionine synthesis but by either directly or indirectly preventing the conversion of methionine to ethylene. Rhizobitoxine did not inhibit ethylene production by *P. digitatum,* providing further evidence that in this case methionine is not a precursor of ethylene.

Peptides containing a C-terminal methionine residue, but not N-terminal or internal residues, also serve as precursors of ethylene in model systems (Ku and Leopold, 1970b; Demorest and Stahmann, 1971). Free methionine occurs only in very small quantities in apple fruits (L. F. Burroughs, private communication) and if this is a natural precursor of ethylene its level could be limiting. We have shown that acetone-dried powders made from apple tissue rotted by *S. fructigena* and acetone-dried powders made from the margins of the rot contain proteolytic activity which is not present in acetone dried powders of healthy tissue. Similar results were shown for other pathogens of apple both *in vitro* and *in vivo* where the enzymes were apparently endopeptidases (Kuć and Williams, 1962). Demorest and Stahmann (1971) suggested that precursors of ethylene could be produced by the proteolysis of tissues during disease, a factor of possible importance since Ku and Leopold (1970b) pointed out that while methionine acts optimally as a precursor only at unphysiological pH values the optima for the peptides are much nearer to those common to plant cells.

The present status of linolenate as a substrate is somewhat ambiguous because although a label from this substrate was incorporated into ethylene in the work of Galliard *et al.* (1968a) it was not incorporated in later work (Mapson *et al.*, 1970). It was found that the incorporation of label from linolenate was some 20 times less frequent than from methionine and in many respects the system used resembled the copper/ascorbate model system (Mapson, 1970). The production of ethylene by whole apple fruits, tissue slices and cell-free extracts prepared from the fruit supplied with linolenic acid increased simultaneously during the development of the respiration climacteric, whilst as the climacteric peak is reached the ability of the extracts and disks of peel to produce ethylene declines (Rhodes *et al.*, 1970). It is known that lipoxidase activity appears at the onset of the climacteric in apples (Wooltorton *et al.*, 1965; Meigh *et al.*, 1967) and it seems probable that the stimulation of ethylene production when linolenic acid is fed to apple tissue, or extracts of tissue, may be due to a secondary role of this substrate, namely, the replacement of the glucose oxidase system for generating hydrogen peroxide. Similarly, Galliard *et al.* (1968b) were able to show a stimulation of ethylene production by aged apple peel disks by peroxidation products of linolenate.

A free radical mechanism was proposed for the generation of ethylene by the copper/ascorbate system (Lieberman and Hochstein, 1966) and for the Yang system (Yang, 1967) as well as for the radiation effects studied by Shah and Maxie (1965). Beauchamp and Fridovich (1970) have produced evidence that it is the hydroxyl radical produced by xanthine oxidase in the presence of its substrate and oxygen, rather than the superoxide anion radical or hydrogen peroxide which is involved in the production of ethylene from methional. Beauchamp and Fridovich concluded that xanthine oxidase generates O_2^- and H_2O_2 as the primary products of the reduction of oxygen and generates $\cdot OH$ as the secondary consequence of the interaction of O_2^- and H_2O_2. Schemes for the enzymic production of ethylene from methional in cauliflower tissue and for a suggested free radical mechanism for the reaction as summarized by Mapson (1970) are reproduced in Figs 4 and 5 respectively.

Sakai *et al.* (1970) used sweet potato tissue instead of the popular apple, tomato or cauliflower tissues and attempted to examine, for the first time, the biosynthesis of ethylene in healthy and fungal-infected tissues. As a result of experiments in which glucose U-^{14}C, acetate-1-^{14}C, acetate-2-^{14}C, and pyruvate-3-^{14}C were fed to healthy or *Ceratocystis fimbriata*-infected tissue disks, Sakai and co-workers concluded that since the two carbon atoms of acetate appeared to enter ethylene without splitting in healthy tissue, non-involvement of the TCA cycle was indicated, agreeing with the conclusions of Gibson and Young (1966). However, in diseased tissue where ethylene was mainly derived from acetate-2-^{14}C, the TCA cycle must be involved in the metabolism of the acetate. Further, a striking increase in ethylene production by diseased tissue 6 h after inoculation, which did not reflect incorporation of label from glucose-U-^{14}C, suggested that ethylene was produced from some unknown cellular component not easily synthesized from glucose.

Enzymes	Particulate (mitochondria)	Transaminase. Catalyst for conversion of methionine to 4-methylmercapto 2-oxo butyric acid $CH_3-S-CH_2-CH_2-CH(NH_2)-COOH \rightarrow CH_3-S-CH_2-CH_2-CO-COOH$
	Glucose oxidase	Produces H_2O_2 in the oxidation of β-D-glucose
	Peroxidase	Uses H_2O_2 to produce ethylene from $CH_3-S-CH_2-CH_2-CO-COOH$ in the presence of two cofactors Methional can substitute for the oxo acid
Cofactors	Phenolic	Esters of *p*-coumaric acid Other phenols having $-OH$ group in *para* position and conjugated system can substitute
	Sulphinic acid	Methane sulphinic acid $CH_3-S(OH)=O$ Benzene sulphinic acid can substitute. Also sulphite, but latter less effective

Fig. 4. Enzymic formation of ethylene from methionine (cauliflower tissue). (Mapson, 1970.)

(a) From $CH_3{-}S{-}CH_2{-}CH_2{-}CHO$

$$\text{Phenolic} + H_2O_2 \xrightarrow{\text{peroxidase}} \text{phenoxy free radical}$$

$$\text{phenoxy radical} + \text{sulphinic acid} \rightarrow \text{phenolic} + \text{sulphinic free radical}$$

O_2 + sulphinic free radical → stepwise reduction of O_2 with production of free radicals $O_2^{\dot{+}}$, $HO_2^{\cdot}$, $OH^{\cdot}$, etc.

(b) $$CH_3{-}S{-}CH_2{-}CH_2{-}CHO + HO_2^{\cdot} \rightarrow CH_3{-}\overset{+}{\dot{S}}{-}CH_2{-}CH_2{-}CHO + HO_2{-}$$

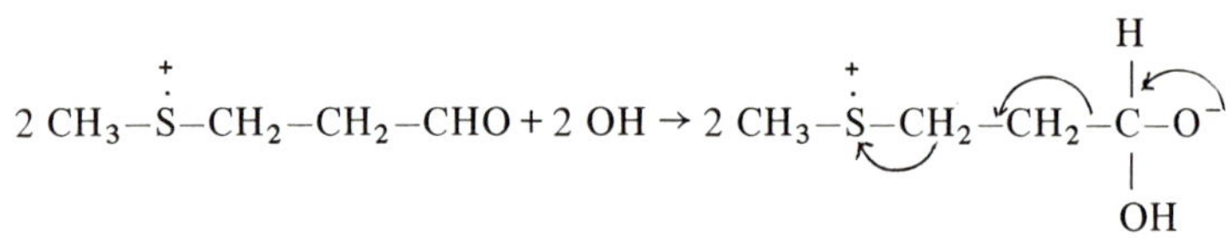

$$\rightarrow CH_3{-}S{-}S{-}CH_3 + 2\ CH_2 = CH_2 + 2\ HCOOH$$

Fig. 5. Suggested free radical mechanism for formation of ethylene from methional. (Mapson, 1970.)

The interpretation of these studies is not easy, especially as the literature on the incorporation of ^{14}C-labelled respiratory intermediates and related compounds into ethylene in healthy tissue is considerable and sometimes contradictory. A useful review of this topic is given by McGlasson (1970).

In our own experiments we have attempted to obtain information on the nature of the ethylene-generating system by supplementing fruit and pulp disks from pre-climacteric apples infected by *S. fructigena* with likely precursors of the gas. Results indicate that methional and linolenic acid alone and in combination with several cofactors do not give a significant and repeatable boost to ethylene production, and methionine gives only a marginal increase. Some data from these experiments are summarized in Table II, where disks of peel were suspended in 0.1 M phosphate buffer, pH 6.5, containing 0.4 M mannitol and 1% soluble polyvinylpyrrolidone.

Perhaps the enzymic processes involved in the production of ethylene in climacteric apples and other fruits are not directly responsible for the increased production of ethylene in the infected apple tissue. For example, we have been unable to demonstrate any increase in peroxidase or lipoxidase activity in the bulk of the rot or the margin of the rot compared with the healthy tissue. In fact, in pre-climacteric apples we cannot find peroxidase activity in a variety of preparations which have been shown to be non-inhibitory to peroxidase in a model system and not to contain high amounts of catalase which might compete for the added hydrogen peroxide. We obtained a stimulation of ethylene

TABLE II

Effect of potential substrates on ethylene production by infected apple peel disks

Additives (2 mM)	Ethylene (μl/kg/h)	% of Control
Control	17.0	100
DL-Methionine	27.5	165
Acetate	8.5	50
Pyruvate	17.5	105
Propionate	7.5	45
Glucose	20.0	120
Homocysteine	23.0	140
Methional	20.0	120
Linolenate	8.5	50
+Ascorbate (50 mM) +Cu^{2+}(0.4 mM)	51.0	300
	L.S.D. (P = 0.05) = 4.7	
	L.S.D. (P = 0.01) = 6.4	

production from infected peel disks and peel extracts compared with healthy disks and extracts, incubated in a medium containing copper/ascorbate and linolenate as reported by Galliard *et al.* (1968a), but heated peel disks behaved similarly, suggesting that the stimulation may have been elicited by a system different from that active *in vivo*.

Our attempts to implicate the phenolase activity of the fruit disks or tissue extracts directly in the production of ethylene have also been negative and at the moment our only possible explanation of increased ethylene production in diseased tissue would involve a theoretical modification of the phenolic content of the tissues by phenolase enzymes either to remove inhibitors or to provide cofactors (e.g. Yang, 1967; Mapson and Wardale, 1968; Hislop and Stahmann, 1971). Either host or pathogen derived enzyme systems could be responsible for this conversion, as *S. fructigena* is known to synthesize several monophenolic acids from chlorogenic acid, one of the main phenolics of healthy apple tissue (Fawcett and Spencer, 1968).

We have been able to stimulate the production of ethylene from cauliflower tissue supplied with methionine and incubated in a crude culture filtrate of *S. fructigena* containing several pectic enzymes, in the manner described by Lund and Mapson (1970), but we were unable to obtain a similar stimulation when apple disks were substituted for cauliflower tissue. Negative results were also obtained when apple fruit disks were incubated in selected pectic enzyme fractions of the crude culture filtrate separated on an iso-electric focusing column. Extracts of fungal mycelium obtained from liquid cultures and extracts of rotten apple pulp also failed to stimulate the production of ethylene from disks of healthy pre-climacteric apples.

In another experiment, pre-climacteric apple fruitlets pre-incubated in approx. 0, 1, 10 or 100 ppm ethylene were inoculated with a wild strain of *S. fructigena* and with two single spore variants isolated following mutagen treatment (kindly supplied by Hazel Howell). A strain producing unusually high pectic enzyme levels (769), and the wild type fungus, produced lesions which were not significantly different in size or ethylene-producing capacity, whilst a slow growing isolate (684) producing low enzyme levels gave smaller lesions and less ethylene (Table III). While not statistically significant there was a tendency

TABLE III

Production of ethylene by apples pre-incubated in a range of ethylene/air mixtures, and then inoculated with three isolates of *S. fructigena*. Measurements were made after 24 h incubation, commencing three days after inoculation

	Fungal Isolate					
	Wild type		769		684	
Pre-incubation ethylene (ppm)	Ethylene (ppm)	Lesion increase (mm)	Ethylene (ppm)	Lesion increase (mm)	Ethylene (ppm)	Lesion increase (mm)
0	85	11.8	92	11.0	71	6.3
1	77	14.7	93	11.3	19	2.3
10	64	11.0	79	10.6	11	2.0
100	68	12.2	76	11.6	<1	0.3

for the 769 isolate to produce rather more ethylene from somewhat less rapidly spreading lesions. Also for a given isolate of the fungus, lesion size decreased with increasing pre-incubation concentrations of ethylene, a factor which was re-examined in a second experiment reported in the next section. Our experiments also confirmed that ethylene production from diseased fruits was inhibited in anaerobic conditions and that infection did not raise the level of ethylene produced by climacteric apples. In fact, the amount of ethylene produced by infected climacteric apples fell rapidly as tissue was killed by the advancing fungus. Ethylene production by disks of peel from healthy and infected pre-climacteric and climacteric apple fruits is shown in Table IV where it is evident that normal ethylene production from climacteric peel was again reduced by infection.

A further point of difference between the pathogen-induced and climacteric systems is their sensitivity to heat inactivation. Ethylene production by

TABLE IV

Ethylene production (nl/g dry wt./h) by pre-climacteric and climacteric apple peel and pulp tissue

State of tissue	Pre-climacteric Peel	Pre-climacteric Pulp	Climacteric Peel	Climacteric Pulp
Healthy	25	11	100	10
Half infected	300	350	50	0
Rotted	0	5	0	0

climacteric fruit is known to be inhibited by high temperatures (see Burg, 1962) but synthesis of the hydrocarbon is resumed at a high rate within hours of restoration to room temperature, at least for the apple cultivar 'Emneth Early'. However, as mentioned earlier, the same heat treatment (50° C for 20 min) totally inhibited the pathogen-induced system for 24 h and production comparable with unheated, infected controls was not obtained until seven days after heating, although after this time considerably more ethylene was produced by the heated apples than the unheated controls (Fig. 6). Clearly, at least one factor in the pathogen-induced biosynthetic pathway is heat labile and only slowly re-synthesized.

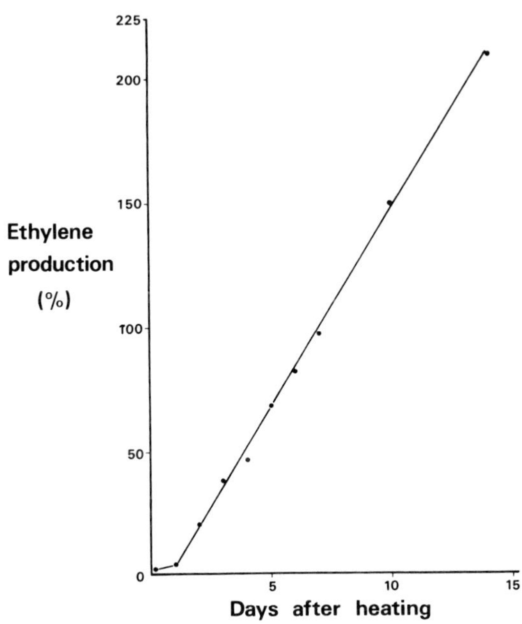

Fig. 6. Ethylene production by heat-treated inoculated apples as a percentage of unheated inoculated controls.

We are thus ignorant of the mechanism of ethylene production in diseased or stressed tissues; in the absence of definite information we must be prepared to consider mechanisms which are different from those operative in healthy tissue. Further, it is possible that in both healthy and diseased tissue, ethylene may be produced by more than one system. In fact, McGlasson (1970) has suggested that for healthy tissues both enzymic and non-enzymic systems might be involved.

IS ETHYLENE INVOLVED IN INTERACTIONS BETWEEN PATHOGENS AND THEIR HOSTS?

The object of this section is to consider the implications of the possible involvement of ethylene in altering the development of plant diseases rather than the symptoms of disease as previously considered.

Studies with labelled ethylene indicate that this gas does not normally react with cell constituents (McGlasson, 1970), although other data indicate that it may apparently be incorporated into RNA (Shimokawa and Kasai, 1968), and may increase incorporation of ^{32}P into RNA (Holm and Abeles, 1967). The effects of ethylene on protein synthesis are of considerable interest to plant pathologists, since there is much evidence indicating changed enzyme levels in diseased tissues compared with healthy tissues, and there is speculation on the role of enzymes in the regulation of disease resistance and host–pathogen specificity (Stahmann *et al.*, 1968). It had previously been shown (Stahmann *et al.*, 1966) that exposure to ethylene of tissue from susceptible sweet potato induced resistance to infection by *Ceratocystis fimbriata,* and increased the activity of peroxidase and polyphenol oxidase in the tissue. Other results have shown (Weber and Stahmann, 1964) that similar changes in these enzymes and in the susceptibility of the tissue could be induced by prior inoculation with a non-pathogenic strain of *C. fimbriata* or by exposing the tissues to volatile materials from infected tissue, implicating the involvement of ethylene. Stahmann *et al.* (1968) were able to demonstrate an increase in polyphenol oxidase but not peroxidase in slices of potato tuber treated with ethylene, but there was no change in the levels of either of these enzymes in the storage tissues of carrot, radish or turnip. In subsequent studies with sweet potato tissue, Imaseki *et al.* (1968b) also showed that ethylene stimulated phenylalanine ammonia-lyase. Chalutz and Stahmann (1969) demonstrated the induction of pisatin formation in peas; the induction of isocoumarin formation in carrot tissue exposed to the gas was shown by Carlton *et al.* (1961) and also by Chalutz *et al.* (1969). Riov *et al.* (1969) also demonstrated the induction of phenylalanine ammonia-lyase by ethylene in citrus fruit peel, and Hyodo and Yang (1971) have shown enhanced activities of this enzyme and cinnamic acid-4-hydroxylase in etiolated pea seedlings following ethylene treatment.

However, when Chalutz and De Vay (1969) examined the effect of ethylene on sweet potato tuber tissue semi-resistant to *C. fimbriata* in which penetration was already limited, they were unable to demonstrate that penetration was further reduced by treatment with the gas. This may partly be explained by differences in the experimental techniques for whereas Stahmann *et al.* (1966) incubated sliced tissue in large closed containers, these authors incubated whole tubers in a continuous airstream.

Abeles *et al.* (1971) were able to show enhanced activities of β-1,3-glucanase and chitinase in extracts from *Phaseolus vulgaris* leaves treated with 10 μl/litre ethylene for three days, compared with extracts from control plants not exposed to the gas. These enzymes have uncertain functions in higher plants, and the authors suggested that they may represent an endogenous protective mechanism against micro-organisms.

On the basis of work with black-rot-infected sweet potatoes, Stahmann *et al.* (1966, 1968) have suggested that in some host–pathogen interactions, ethylene might act as a trigger which regulates the amount or activity of specific enzymes which could be involved in resistance or immunity mechanisms. It was not suggested that this was the only mechanism involved, but the hypothesis has gained some backing from the fact that enzymes such as phenylalanine ammonia-lyase can be activated by ethylene, and that in some cases this can be correlated with phytoalexin production in tissues infected with fungi or treated with chemical compounds which can stimulate ethylene production (Hadwiger *et al.*, 1970). However, for the present, the importance of ethylene-induced pisatin production in peas must be questioned, since the level found was much less than that induced by fungi (Chalutz and Stahmann, 1969). Bearing in mind the effects of ethylene on respiration and metabolism in fruits, McGlasson (1969) was prompted to suggest that ethylene may play a role in the recovery of wounded tissues by temporarily stimulating the mobilization of reserves to provide energy for repair processes.

Peroxidase is one of the enzymes commonly stimulated by the presence of ethylene and there is now considerable evidence to suggest that it is the synthesis of the enzyme, rather than its activation, which is responsible for the increased amounts found in some tissues (Gahagan *et al.*, 1968; Ridge and Osborne, 1970). Using etiolated pea seedlings supplied with ^{14}C-leucine, Ridge and Osborne showed that after electrophoresis, peaks of radioactivity were associated with the main peroxidase bands, while experiments with actinomycin D indicated that some RNA synthesis is necessary for the increase in peroxidase activity to occur. *De novo* synthesis of peroxidase was also indicated following ethylene treatment of sweet potato tissue by Shannon *et al.* (1971), while RNA and protein synthesis were demonstrated in apple fruit tissue by Hulme *et al.* (1971).

Although peroxidase is a common enzyme in plants, little is known about its biological function. On the basis of evidence presented earlier, it would seem that it may be involved in the *in vivo* production of ethylene and there are reports indicating positive correlations between peroxidase levels and resistance to pathogens in plants (e.g. Clare *et al.*, 1966; Fehrman and Dimond, 1967; Simons and Ross, 1970). Polyphenol oxidase is another enzyme sometimes stimulated by ethylene and which has been implicated in disease resistance, as reviewed by Kosuge (1969). It must be stressed that disease resistance is not an absolute or static state but depends on many factors which are adequate to prevent disease development under particular conditions (Kuć, 1966, 1968). Peroxidase and/or polyphenol oxidase activity is not always stimulated by ethylene (Stahmann *et al.*, 1968; Hislop and Stahmann, 1971; Nakagaki *et al.*, 1970); ethylene production by infected resistant tissues may be inversely related to their peroxidase levels, while endogenous ethylene may not be involved in either the susceptible or resistant reactions (Daly *et al.*, 1970; Hislop and Stahmann, 1971).

The importance of phenolases in ethylene production is not clear, but as suggested by a number of workers they could have a very important indirect role in regulating ethylene synthesis by modifying the levels of phenolic materials which have been shown to be essential in model systems. Mapson and Wardale (1968) and Takeo and Lieberman (1969) demonstrated a specific requirement for *p*-coumaric acid in their systems, while catechol and resorcinol were strong inhibitors. However, the Yang (1967) model system utilized resorcinol but was inhibited by catechol. To confuse the situation further, Fuchs (1970) has demonstrated a stimulation of ethylene production by citrus peel supplemented with catechol or methyl-catechol while resorcinol, guaiacol and *p*-coumaric acid were ineffective. Of particular interest in this study was the observation that stimulation by catechol could be reversed by a specific competitive inhibitor of phenolase. At the moment there is no evidence for or against the involvement of the pectic enzymes of *S. fructigena* in the production of ethylene by infected pre-climacteric apples, but it may be pertinent to recall that pectic enzymes have been implicated in the activation of latent phenolase (Deverall and Wood, 1961).

We have been unable to show an effect of ethylene on the peroxidase content of apples, but have obtained some indication that pre-treatment of apples with ethylene reduces the speed at which lesions of *S. fructigena* develop. Similar results were obtained in experiments with fruitlets where pre-treatment with ethylene did not induce endogenous ethylene evolution, and with older pre-climacteric apples where the ethylene pre-treatments induced the climacteric. When isolates of *S. fructigena* were grown in various ethylene–air mixtures there was no significant effect of increasing ethylene concentrations on colony diameter, colony appearance or the synthesis of pectic enzymes. Some of these results are summarized in Table V which shows values for the mean colony diameter of each of three isolates of the fungus and the mean diameters of the rots measured at the same time.

TABLE V

Growth *in vitro* (mm) of *S. fructigena* in various concentrations of ethylene and the development of lesions (mm) in apples pre-incubated in the same concentrations of the gas. Measured 4 days after inoculation

Ethylene concentration (ppm)	Fungal Isolate Wild type *in vitro*	*in vivo*	769 *in vitro*	*in vivo*	684 *in vitro*	*in vivo*
0	31.5	42.8	28.0	40.2	10.8	14.0
1	29.4	41.4	25.6	38.8	11.8	8.4
10	29.8	40.8	30.0	36.8	10.2	7.6
100	29.5	33.2	32.0	32.6	9.5	4.8

This result was a little unexpected, since in many cases susceptibility of fruits to infection increases as they ripen (e.g. Sitterly and Shay, 1960); although Lockhart *et al.* (1968) have shown that ethylene levels considerably higher than ours reduced rot development by *Gloeosporium album* in McIntosh apples but had no effect on growth of the fungus *in vitro.*

Just as increased respiration and ethylene production are common phenomena in diseased or wounded tissue, so apparently is altered permeability (Wheeler and Hanchey, 1968). It is tempting to suggest that there is a common trigger for all these processes, although there is at present no justification for such an assumption. Kuć (1966) suggested that enzyme induction and repression could be such a trigger, but one is tempted to query what it is that triggers enzyme synthesis or activation. Wheeler and Hanchey (1968) suggest that altered permeability which occurs as a result of almost any stimulus is another attractive candidate for the trigger. Could ethylene be a third candidate? Ethylene is produced by many stimuli, and has profound effects at very low concentrations. This gas can affect enzyme synthesis, as has been discussed, and has frequently been implicated in altered permeability (McGlasson, 1970). A considerable number of workers (e.g. Sacher, 1962; Lyons and Pratt, 1964; Bain and Mercer, 1964) have postulated that ethylene may evoke a response in tissues by directly altering membrane permeability. For example, mitochondria swell in the presence of ethylene (Lyons and Pratt, 1964) and ADP-induced volume changes in active mitochondria occur more quickly in the presence of the gas (Olson and Spencer, 1968). However, recent work (Mehard and Lyons, 1970; Ku and Leopold, 1970a) has shown that the swelling response of mitochondria is not specific to ethylene, nor does the gas exert any specific influence on oxidative activity. It would seem therefore that mitochondria may not be the site of ethylene regulation of plant response to pathogens. Abeles *et al.* (1971) obtained some indication that ethylene may increase membrane permeability in an extremely specific and well regulated manner, since the synthesis and release or secretion of cellulase is regulated by the gas. In our own work we did not find an effect of ethylene on the secretion of extra-cellular pectolytic enzymes by *S. fructigena* growing in liquid culture.

The mechanism of action and importance of ethylene in pathogenesis are clearly topics about which we know very little at present, but which should provide great scope for further study.

References

Abeles, F. B., Bosshart, R. P., Forrence, L. E. and Habig, W. H. (1971). Preparation and purification of glucanase and chitinase from bean leaves. *Pl. Physiol., Lancaster* **47**, 129-134.

Abeles, F. B., Leather, G. R., Forrence, L. E. and Craker, L. E. (1971). Abscission: regulation of senescence, protein synthesis, and enzyme secretion by ethylene. *HortSci.* **6**, 371-376.

Bain, J. M. and Mercer, F. V. (1964). Organisation resistance and the respiration climacteric. *Aust. J. biol. Sci.* **17**, 78-85.

Balázs, E., Gáborjányi, R., Tóth, A. and Király, Z. (1969). Ethylene production in Xanthi tobacco after systemic and local virus infections. *Acta Phytopath. Acad. Sci. Hung.* **4**, 355-358.

Baur, A. H. and Yang, S. F. (1969). Precursors of ethylene. *Pl. Physiol., Lancaster* **44**, 1347-1349.

Beauchamp, C. and Fridovich, I. (1970). A mechanism for the production of ethylene from methional. *J. biol. Chem.* **245**, 4641-4646.

Braun, A. C. and Laskaris, T. (1942). Tumor formation by attenuated crown gall bacteria in the presence of growth-promoting substances. *Proc. natn. Acad. Sci. U.S.A.* **28**, 468-477.

Burg, S. P. (1962). The physiology of ethylene formation. *A. Rev. Pl. Physiol.* **13**, 265-302.

Carlton, B. C., Peterson, C. E. and Tolbert, N. E. (1961). Effects of ethylene and oxygen production of a bitter compound by carrot roots. *Pl. Physiol., Lancaster* **36**, 550-552.

Chalutz, E. and De Vay, J. E. (1969). Production of ethylene *in vitro* and *in vivo* by *Ceratocystis fimbriata* in relation to disease development. *Phytopathology* **59**, 750-755.

Chalutz, E., De Vay, J. E. and Maxie, E. C. (1969). Ethylene-induced isocoumarin formation in carrot root tissue. *Pl. Physiol., Lancaster* **44**, 235-241.

Chalutz, E. and Stahmann, M. A. (1969). Induction of pisatin by ethylene. *Phytopathology* **59**, 1972-1973.

Clare, B. G., Weber, D. J. and Stahmann, M. A. (1966). Peroxidase and resistance to *Ceratocystis* in sweet potato increased by volatile materials. *Science, N.Y.* **153**, 62-63.

Cooper, W. C., Rasmussen, G. K. and Waldon, E. S. (1969). Ethylene evolution stimulated by chilling in *Citrus* and *Persea* sp. *Pl. Physiol., Lancaster* **44**, 1194-1196.

Curtis, O. F., Jr. and Rodney, D. R. (1952). Ethylene injury to nursery trees in cold storage. *Proc. Am. Soc. hort. Sci.* **60**, 104-108.

Daly, J. M., Seevers, P. M. and Ludden, P. (1970). Studies on wheat stem rust resistance controlled at the S-6 locus. III. Ethylene and disease reaction. *Phytopathology* **60**, 1648-1652.

Demorest, D. M. and Stahmann, M. A. (1971). Ethylene production from peptides and protein containing methionine. *Pl. Physiol., Lancaster* **47**, 450-451.

Deverall, B. J. and Wood, R. K. S. (1961). Chocolate spot of beans (*Vicia faba* L.)–interactions between phenolase of host and pectic enzymes of the pathogen. *Ann. appl. Biol.* **49**, 473-487.

Dimond, A. E. and Waggoner, P. E. (1953). The cause of epinastic symptoms in Fusarium wilt of tomatoes. *Phytopathology* **43**, 663-669.

Fawcett, C. H. and Spencer, D. M. (1968). *Sclerotinia fructigena* infection and chlorogenic acid content in relation to anti-fungal compounds in apple fruits. *Ann. appl. Biol.* **61**, 245-253.

Fehrman, H. and Dimond, A. E. (1967). Peroxidase activity and Phytophthora resistance in different organs of the potato plant. *Phytopathology* **57**, 69-72.

Freebairn, H. T. and Buddenhagen, I. W. (1964). Ethylene production by *Pseudomonas solanacearum. Nature, Lond.* **202**, 313-314.

Fuchs, Y. (1970). Ethylene production by citrus fruit peel. Stimulation by phenol derivatives. *Pl. Physiol., Lancaster* **45**, 533-534.

Gahagan, H. E., Holm, R. E. and Abeles, F. B. (1968). Effect of ethylene on peroxidase activity. *Physiologia Pl.* **21**, 1270-1279.

Galliard, T., Hulme, A. C., Rhodes, M. J. C. and Wooltorton, L. S. C. (1968a). Enzymic conversion of linolenic acid to ethylene by extracts of apple fruits. *FEBS Letters* **1**, 283-286.

Galliard, T., Rhodes, M. J. C., Wooltorton, L. S. C. and Hulme A. C. (1968b). Metabolic changes in excised fruit tissue. III. The development of ethylene biosynthesis during the ageing of disks of apple peel. *Phytochemistry* **7**, 1465-1470.

Gibson, M. S. and Young, R. E. (1966). Acetate and other carboxylic acids as precursors of ethylene. *Nature, Lond.* **210**, 529-530.

Giovanelli, J., Owens, L. D. and Mudd, S. H. (1971). Mechanism of inhibition of spinach β-cystathionase by rhizobitoxine. *Biochim. biophys. Acta* **227**, 671-684.

Goodman, R. N., Kiraly, Z. and Zaitlin, M. (1967). 'The biochemistry and physiology of infectious plant disease.' D. Van Nostrand Company Inc., New York, 354 pp.

Hadwiger, L. A., Hess, S. L. and Sharon von Broembsen (1970). Stimulation of phenylalanine ammonia-lyase activity and phytoalexin production. *Phytopathology* **60**, 332-336.

Hislop, E. C. and Stahmann, M. A. (1971). Peroxidase and ethylene production by barley leaves infected with *Erysiphe graminis* f. sp. *hordei. Physiol. Pl. Pathol.* **1**, 297-312.

Holm, R. E. and Abeles, F. B. (1967). Abscission: the role of RNA synthesis. *Pl. Physiol., Lancaster* **42**, 1094-1102.

Hulme, A. C., Rhodes, M. J. C. and Wooltorton, L. S. C. (1971). The relationship between ethylene and the synthesis of RNA and protein in ripening apples. *Phytochemistry* **10**, 749-756.

Hyodo, H. and Yang, S. F. (1971). Ethylene-enhanced formation of cinnamic acid-4-hydroxylase in excised pea epicotyl tissue. *Archs Biochem. Biophys.* **143**, 338-339.

Ilag, Lina and Curtis, R. W. (1968). Production of ethylene by fungi. *Science, N.Y.* **159**, 1357-1358.

Imaseki, H., Teranishi, T. and Uritani, I. (1968a). Production of ethylene by sweet potato roots infected by black rot fungus. *Pl. Cell Physiol., Tokyo* **9**, 769-781.

Imaseki, H., Uchiyama, M. and Uritani, I. (1968b). Effect of ethylene on the inductive increase in metabolic activities in sliced sweet potato roots. *Agr. biol. Chem., Japan* **32**, 387-389.

Imaseki, H., Uritani, I. and Stahmann, M. A. (1968c). Production of ethylene by injured sweet potato root tissue. *Pl. Cell Physiol., Tokyo* **9**, 757-768.

Jackson, M. B. and Osborne, D. J. (1970). Ethylene, the natural regulator of leaf abscission. *Nature, Lond.* **225**, 1019-1022.

Jackson, W. T. (1956). The relative importance of factors causing injury to shoots of flooded tomato plants. *Am. J. Bot.* **43**, 637-639.

Ketring, D. L., Young, R. E. and Biale, J. B. (1968). Effects of mono-fluoroacetate on *Penicillium digitatum. Pl. Cell. Physiol., Tokyo* **9**, 617-631.

Kosuge, T. (1969). The role of phenolics in host response to infection. *A. Rev. Phytopathol.* **7**, 195-222.

Kramer, P. J. (1951). Cause of injury to plants resulting from flooding of the soil. *Pl. Physiol., Lancaster* **26**, 722-736.

Ku, H. S. and Leopold, A. C. (1970a). Mitochondrial responses to ethylene and other hydrocarbons. *Pl. Physiol., Lancaster* **46**, 842-844.

Ku, H. S. and Leopold, A. C. (1970b). Ethylene formation from peptides of methionine. *Biochem. biophys. Res. Commun.* **41**, 1155-1160.

Ku, H. S., Yang, S. F. and Pratt, H. K. (1967). Enzymic evolution of ethylene from methional by a pea seedling extract. *Archs Biochem Biophys.* **118**, 756-758.

Ku, H. S., Yang, S. F. and Pratt, H. K. (1969). Ethylene formation from α-keto-γ methyl thiobutyrate by tomato fruit extracts. *Phytochemistry* **8**, 567-573.

Ku, H. S., Yang, S. F. and Pratt, H. K. (1970). Ethylene production and peroxidase activity during tomato fruit ripening. *Pl. Cell Physiol., Tokyo* **11**, 241-246.

Kuć, J. (1966). Resistance of plants to infectious agents. *A. Rev. Microbiol.* **20**, 337-370.

Kuć, J. (1968). Biochemical control of disease resistance in plants. *Wld Rev. Pest Contr.* **7**, 42-55.

Kuć, J. and Williams, E. B. (1962). Production of proteolytic enzymes by four pathogens of apple fruit. Abstr. in *Phytopathology* **52**, 739.

Lieberman, M. and Hochstein, P. (1966). Ethylene formation in rat liver microsomes. *Science, N.Y.* **152**, 213-214.

Lieberman, M. and Kunishi, A. T. (1971). An evaluation of 4-S-methyl-2-keto-butyric acid as an intermediate in the biosynthesis of ethylene. *Pl. Physiol., Lancaster* **47**, 576-580.

Lieberman, M., Kunishi, A., Mapson, L. W. and Wardale, D. A. (1966). Stimulation of ethylene production in apple tissue slices by methionine. *Pl. Physiol., Lancaster* **41**, 376-382.

Lieberman, M. and Mapson, L. W. (1964). Genesis and biogenesis of ethylene. *Nature, Lond.* **204**, 343-345.

Lockhart, C. L., Forsyth, F. R. and Eaves, C. A. (1968). Effect of ethylene on development of *Gloeosporium album* in apple and on growth of the fungus in culture. *Can. J. Pl. Sci.* **48**, 557-559.

Lund, Barbara M. and Mapson, L. W. (1970). Stimulation by *Erwinia carotovora* of the synthesis of ethylene in cauliflower tissue. *Biochem. J.* **119**, 251-263.

Lyons, J. M. and Pratt, H. K. (1964). An effect of ethylene on swelling of isolated mitochondria. *Archs Biochem. Biophys.* **104**, 318-324.

McGlasson, W. B. (1969). Ethylene production by slices of green banana fruit and potato tuber tissue during the development of induced respiration. *Aust. J. biol. Sci.* **22**, 489-491.

McGlasson, W. B. (1970). The ethylene factor. *In* 'The biochemistry of fruits and their products' (ed. A. C. Hulme). Vol. 1, p. 475. Academic Press, London and New York.

Mapson, L. W. (1970). Biosynthesis of ethylene and the ripening of fruit. *Endeavour* **19**, 29-33.

Mapson, L. W., March, J. F., Rhodes, M. J. C. and Wooltorton, L. S. C. (1970). A comparative study of the ability of methionine or linolenic acid to act as precursors of ethylene in plant tissues. *Biochem J.* **117**, 473-479.

Mapson, L. W., March, J. F. and Wardale, D. A. (1969). Biosynthesis of ethylene. 4-methyl-mercapto-2-oxybutyric acid, an intermediate in the formation from methionine. *Biochem. J.* **115**, 653-661.

Mapson, L. W. and Wardale, D. A. (1967). Biosynthesis of ethylene. Formation of ethylene from methional by a cell-free enzyme system from cauliflower plants. *Biochem. J.* **102**, 574-585.

Mapson, L. W. and Wardale, D. A. (1968). Biosynthesis of ethylene. Enzymes involved in its formation from methional. *Biochem. J.* **107**, 433-442.

Mapson, L. W. and Wardale, D. A. (1971). Enzymes involved in the synthesis of ethylene from methionine, or its derivatives, in tomatoes. *Phytochemistry* **10**, 29-39.

Maxie, E. C., Eaks, I. L., Sommer, N. F., Rae, H. L. and El-Batal, S. (1965). Effects of gamma radiation on rate of ethylene and carbon dioxide evolution by lemon fruit. *Pl. Physiol., Lancaster* **40**, 407-409.

Mehard, C. W. and Lyons, J. M. (1970). A lack of specificity for ethylene-induced mitochondrial changes. *Pl. Physiol., Lancaster* **46**, 36-39.

Meigh, D. F., Jones, J. D. and Hulme, A. C. (1967). The respiration climacteric in the apple. Production of ethylene and fatty acids in fruit attached to and detached from the tree. *Phytochemistry* **6**, 1507-1515.

Muller, E. V., Winston, J. R. and Fisher, D. F. (1940). Production of epinasty by emanations from normal and decaying citrus fruits and from *Penicillium digitatum*. *J. agric. Res.* **60**, 269-277.

de Munk, W. J. and de Rooy, M. (1971). The influence of ethylene on the development of 5°C precooled 'Apeldoorn' tulips during forcing. *HortSci.* **6**, 40-41.

Nakagaki, Y., Hirai, T. and Stahmann, M. A. (1970). Ethylene production by detached leaves infected with tobacco mosaic virus. *Virology* **40**, 1-9.

Olson, A. O. and Spencer, M. (1968). Studies on the mechanism of action of ethylene. I. The effects of ethylene on mitochondria prepared from bean cotyledons. *Can. J. Biochem.* **46**, 277-282.

Osborne, Daphne J. (1968). Ethylene as a plant hormone. *Soc. Chem. Ind. Monograph* **31**, 236-249.

Osborne, Daphne J. (1971). Ethylene as a plant growth regulator. *New Scientist* **50**, 511-512.

Owens, L. D., Guggenheim, S. and Hilton, J. (1968). Rhizobium synthesised phytotoxin: an inhibitor of β-cystathionase in *Salmonella typhimurium*. *Biochim. biophys. Acta* **158**, 219-225.

Owens, L. D., Lieberman, M. and Kunishi, A. (1971). Inhibition of ethylene production by Rhizobitoxine. *Pl. Physiol., Lancaster* **48**, 1-4.

Pratt, H. K. and Goeschl, J. D. (1969). Physiological roles of ethylene in plants. *A. Rev. Pl. Physiol.* **20**, 541-584.

Rasmussen, G. K., Furr, J. R. and Cooper, W. C. (1969). Ethylene production by citrus leaves from trees grown in artificially salinized plots. *J. Amer. Soc. Hort. Sci.* **94**, 640-641.

Ray, P. M. (1958). Destruction of auxin. *A. Rev. Pl. Physiol.* **9**, 81-118.

Reid, M. S. and Pratt, H. K. (1970). Ethylene and the respiration climacteric. *Nature, Lond.* **226**, 976-977.

Rhodes, M. J. C., Wooltorton, L. S. C., Galliard, T. and Hulme, A. C. (1970). The production of ethylene by whole apple fruits and by tissue slices and cell-free extracts prepared from the fruit. *J. exp. Bot.* **21**, 40-48.

Ridge, Irene and Osborne, Daphne J. (1970). Regulation of peroxidase activity by ethylene in *Pisum sativum:* Requirements for protein and RNA synthesis. *J. exp. Bot.* **21**, 720-734.

Riov, J., Monselise, S. P. and Kahan, R. S. (1969). Ethylene-controlled induction of phenylalanine ammonia lyase in citrus fruit peel. *Pl. Physiol., Lancaster* **44**, 631-635.

Ross, A. F. and Williamson, C. E. (1951). Physiologically active emanations from virus-infected plants. *Phytopathology* **41**, 431-438.

Sacher, J. A. (1962). Relations between changes in membrane permeability and the climacteric in banana and avocado. *Nature, Lond.* **195**, 577-578.

Sakai, S., Imaseki, H. and Uritani, I. (1970). Biosynthesis of ethylene in sweet potato root tissue. *Pl. Cell Physiol., Tokyo* **11**, 737-745.

Sequeira, L. (1964). Inhibition of indoleacetic acid oxidase in tobacco plants infected by *Pseudomonas solanacearum. Phytopathology* **54**, 1078-1083.

Shah, J. and Maxie, E. C. (1965). Ethylene formation in pea epicotyl tissues following irradiation with γ-rays from ^{60}Co. *Physiologia Pl.* **18**, 1115-1120.

Shannon, L. M., Uritani, I. and Imaseki, H. (1971). *De novo* synthesis of peroxidase isozymes in sweet potato slices. *Pl. Physiol., Lancaster* **47**, 493-498.

Shimokawa, K. and Kasai, Z. (1968). A possible incorporation of ethylene into RNA in Japanese Morning Glory (*Pharbitis nil*) seedlings. *Agric. biol. Chem. Japan* **32**, 680-682.

Simons, T. J. and Ross, A. F. (1970). Enhanced peroxidase activity associated with induction of resistance to tobacco mosaic virus in hypersensitive tobacco. *Phytopathology* **60**, 383-384.

Sitterly, W. R. and Shay, J. R. (1960). Physiological factors affecting the onset of susceptibility of apple fruit to rotting by fungus pathogens. *Phytopathology* **50**, 91-93.

Smith, W. H., Meigh, D. F. and Parker, J. C. (1964). Effect of damage and fungal infection on the production of ethylene by carnations. *Nature, Lond.* **204**, 92-93.

Smith, K. A. and Scott Russell, R. (1969). Occurrence of ethylene, and its significance, in anaerobic soil. *Nature, Lond.* **222**, 769-771.

Stahmann, M. A., Clare, B. G. and Woodbury, W. (1966). Increased disease resistance and enzyme activity induced by ethylene and ethylene production by black rot infected sweet potato tissue. *Pl. Physiol., Lancaster* **41**, 1505-1512.

Stahmann, M. A., Woodbury, W., Lovrekovich, L. and Macko, V. (1968). The role of enzymes in the regulation of disease resistance and host-pathogen specificity. *In* 'Biochemical regulation in diseased plants or injury', pp. 263-274. The Phytopathological Society of Japan.

Swamy, R. N. (1961). Gaseous emanation from groundnut infected by *Cercospora personata* (Berk et Curt) Ell. et Everh. *Phytopath. Z.* **40**, 245-247.

Takeo, T. and Lieberman, M. (1969). 3-Methyl-thiopropionaldehyde peroxidase from apples: an ethylene-forming enzyme. *Biochim. biophys. Acta* **178**, 235-247.

Turian, G. and Hamilton, R. H. (1960). Chemical detection of 3-indoleacetic acid in *Ustilago zeae* tumors. *Biochim. biophys. Acta* **41**, 148-150.

Weber, D. J. and Stahmann, M. A. (1964). *Ceratocystis* infection in sweet potato: its effect on proteins, isozymes and acquired immunity. *Science, N.Y.* **146**, 929-931.

Wheeler, H. and Hanchey, Penelope (1968). Permeability phenomena in plant disease. *A. Rev. Phytopathol.* **6**, 331-350.

Williamson, C. E. (1950). Ethylene, a metabolic product of diseased or injured plants. *Phytopathology* **40**, 205-208.

Wood, R. K. S. (1967). 'Physiological plant pathology.' Blackwell Scientific Publications, Oxford and Edinburgh. 570 pp.

Wooltorton, L. S. C., Jones, J. D. and Hulme, A. C. (1965). Genesis of ethylene in apples. *Nature, Lond.* **207**, 999-1000.

Yang, S. F. (1967). Biosynthesis of ethylene. Ethylene formation from methional by horse-radish peroxidase. *Archs Biochem. Biophys.* **122**, 481-487.

Yang, S. F. (1969). Further studies on ethylene formation from α-keto-γ-methylthiobutyric acid or β-methylthiopropionaldehyde by peroxidase in the presence of sulphite and oxygen. *J. biol. Chem.* **244**, 4360-4365.

Yang, S. F., Ku, H. S. and Pratt, H. K. (1966). Ethylene production from methionine as mediated by flavine mononucleotide and light. *Biochem. biophys. Res. Commun.* **24**, 739-743.

DISCUSSION

Professor P. W. Brian: In my experience there is very little literature on the effects of ethylene on the growth of fungi. Is there anything relevant in the literature that you have found?

Dr E. C. Hislop: Yes, it has been shown by Lockhart that *Gloeosporium* infections in apples can be reduced by ethylene but he used concentrations a good deal higher than we have done, up to 10 000 ppm. On the other hand, much information about the development of rots in store suggests that many apples increase their susceptibility as they reach their climacteric and, of course, storing apples in ethylene will induce the climacteric. We were rather surprised to see this result in the lesion development. It was repeated in two experiments, the first using immature apples which were not induced into their respiration climacteric by the ethylene treatment, and the second experiment where they were induced into climacteric, and we got essentially the same result in both.

Professor Brian: What I am particularly interested in are direct results on fungi. Is there any other information on this?

Dr Hislop: Yes, the only work I know of is that involving *Gloeosporium* where there was no effect of ethylene *in vitro.*

Professor M. A. Stahmann: I am very much impressed to see the increased interest in ethylene. I think ethylene is now recognized as a volatile hormone, and I wonder what its function could be. It might be worth considering it as a hormone that could be produced at sites of injury or infection, whose function might be to diffuse very rapidly to cells adjacent to the infected area, and there to trigger off other events. It is now known that four or five enzymes are induced by treatment with ethylene; one function of these enzymes might be to protect these adjacent cells from invasion by the fungus. This seems to be possible in some plants, but not in others. I think we are going to learn a great deal more as we continue to study the effect of ethylene on infection and its relationship to resistance or susceptibility. It also appears that there are several methods by which ethylene may be produced. I think all these have in common the possible production of free radicals from peroxidase, polyphenoloxidase and glucose oxidase, which act on substrates. These substrates may be different, but derivatives of methionine seem to be involved; not just methionine, but methional and methionine peptides all give rise to ethylene, so that there may be several sources for ethylene in healthy or infected plants.

Dr Hislop: Methional does not, I think, occur *in vivo,* but we are interested in testing some of the peptides of methionine, as examined by yourself and Mr Demorest. I would not like to hazard a guess as to the importance of ethylene, but I think it is now looked upon as a plant hormone.

Dr J. Beyersbergen: In tulips there is possibly a barrier which prevents *Fusarium oxysporum* from penetrating. We have found that this barrier is synthesized as soon as the bulbs are lifted, but when they are placed in air, with 1 or 2 vpm ethylene synthesis of this fungitoxic substance (tulipalin) is completely inhibited, and then the fungus can very easily penetrate. So this contrasts with what Professor Stahmann stated. We have found in tulips that ethylene is produced *in vitro* at a very high level by *Fusarium* on different media, and we believe that *Fusarium* possibly uses ethylene to penetrate into the bulb.

Dr Hislop: This is a most interesting observation, and one of which I was not aware. This is the first instance I have ever come across of this type of pathogenicity.

Professor R. K. S. Wood: There was a paper by De Vay published recently about the possible involvement of ethylene in the *Verticillium* wilt of cotton. He rather regarded this as an after-effect.

Dr Hislop: I think his work, and also that of Daly on wheat rust, came to the same conclusion; that ethylene itself is not primarily involved, but it may be involved as a secondary factor. Likewise in the work that I did on barley and barley mildew, ethylene could not be implicated as a primary factor. It did not seem to be involved in peroxidase or phenylalanine ammonia lyase synthesis, and it was not involved in resistance. So, in these respects I would be inclined to agree with Drs De Vay and Daly.

Dr J. A. Kavanagh: To what extent is *Sclerotinia* rot accompanied by a halo effect immediately surrounding the lesions?

Dr Hislop: No halos are visible externally although we have certainly noticed them internally, as I think you can see on the slide.

Dr Kavanagh: Obviously this degradation effect is accompanied by some changes in the organelles within the cells immediately adjacent. Have you looked at this?

Dr Hislop: Dr Pitt has had a look at the structure of organelles in tissues infected with fungi but I believe he failed to reproduce similar changes in organelles with fungal enzymes. We have not yet looked at the tissues adjacent to the rot, although now that we have managed to purify, in fairly large quantities, some of the pectic enzymes produced by the pathogen, we intend to examine the effects of these on tissues, protoplasts and membranes.

Dr I. M. Smith: As a healthy apple is ripening, at some point it begins to produce ethylene in larger quantities, and at some point it also begins to soften. Do these points coincide?

Dr Hislop: I won't pretend to be an expert on the physiology of fruit ripening, but generally speaking, although they do not precisely coincide, there is a fairly close agreement between the onset of increased ethylene production, increased respiration, and those changes recognized as ripening.

Dr Smith: I was interested in the possibility that the degradation of walls by pectic enzymes might stimulate ethylene production. How does ethylene production in ripening apples relate in time to softening and the presumably related cell wall changes?

S. A. Archer: The peak of ethylene evolution usually slightly precedes the respiration climacteric and the peak of the respiration climacteric usually corresponds with the changes in ripening.

Dr Smith: What actually induces the sudden increase in ethylene production? Some substrate or some essential metabolism must be changing.

Dr Hislop: We have been totally inhibited in our work by being unable to find any treatment that would stimulate the production of ethylene by healthy tissue. We have tried supplementing tissues with various substrates and with glucose oxidase, but we failed completely to get any stimulated production of ethylene comparable to that produced by diseased tissues. It may be, that in our system the pathogen must be present, but we would like to try some of Dr Lund's enzyme preparations to see whether these would stimulate ethylene production.

Professor Wood: I wonder if I could make a quick comment on the tendency of all of us to assume because what we call a healthy tissue does not contain any of these degradative enzymes, that the host tissue when it is affected by the pathogen may contain them. I would refer to the work of Tani, which indicated quite clearly the involvement of wall-degrading enzymes of host origin. Do you think this might happen?

Dr Hislop: I would not like to commit myself. We have been very worried because we cannot extract any enzyme with peroxidase-type activity from our apple tissues. I don't know whether anyone else has ever tried? We have even been led to wonder whether, in fact, it is another enzyme which can generate free radicals, such as polyphenol oxidase, which we do know to be there in large quantities, and to be, shall we say, de-compartmentalized in infected cells. We wondered whether that is an important process.

Dr J. A. Sargent: I would like to ask one probably rather naïve question. Almost any higher plant cell when it is damaged, e.g. by stroking a brush across the surface, will produce ethylene. In a similar way, could not the pathogen hyphae travelling through a tissue (thereby mechanically disturbing those cells, although not killing them) be the basic cause of the production of ethylene?

Dr Hislop: It could be, I suppose. On the other hand we have instances where cell-free systems will stimulate the production of ethylene, and therefore it seemed to us reasonable to consider this. I do not know how to answer your question, but you are right to ask it. There are examples where alteration of the tropism of a plant, just by laying it on its side, will stimulate it to produce ethylene you do not even have to touch it. So almost any stimulus could perhaps produce ethylene. Are there fundamental implications in this?

Dr D. Pitt: I would like to ask Dr Hislop about the substrates he used for his peroxidase determinations, because some of these are highly specific.

Dr Hislop: We have only tried three substrates, catechol, *o*-dianisidine and guaiacol.

Dr Pitt: Did you use benzidine?

Dr Hislop: Not recently, but earlier I used benzidine without effect.

Dr Pitt: You also mentioned the localization of polyphenols. In what sort of sub-cellular organelle do you think that these might be located?

Dr Hislop: Presumably they are compartmentalized somewhere, because they are apparently inactive in healthy tissue, and when the tissue is damaged they are released. One would like to know how and why. As you know we have been attempting to further some of the work that you did on this topic, but so far with no success.

Professor S. H. Crowdy: I was wondering if you had treated your tissues with any of the Ethrel-type chemicals which are thought to release ethylene inside the tissue.

Dr Hislop: We have not done so with apples. But I think Ethrel usually works by breakdown on the surface. Although there has been one reference to the possible stimulation of the natural production of ethylene, in most instances it seems to rely on the straightforward breakdown of the compound. I do not think it stimulates ethylene production by the host. In my work with barley I did find that some treatments such as maleic hydrazide and CCC would stimulate peroxidase, but not ethylene production.

S. A. Archer: With apples, Ethrel may be rather ineffective in view of the acidity of the tissues.

Professor Wood: I would like to finish with a comment which was made by a rather cynical colleague of mine, who pointed out in the first place that the great interest in peroxidases may be connected with the fact that they are enzymes the activity of which is extremely easy to measure; and secondly, the tremendous increase in current interest in ethylene coincides rather remarkably with the widespread introduction of the use of g.l.c., which has provided a quick and direct means by which this gas can be measured. We should be rather careful–there may be lots of other systems involved that we cannot yet measure quite so readily as we can the peroxidases and ethylene.

Section III
Obligate Parasitism

III . 1 The Study of Obligate Parasites *in vitro*

D. S. INGRAM AND INEZ C. TOMMERUP

A.R.C. Unit of Developmental Botany, Cambridge, England

INTRODUCTION

The term obligate parasite was applied by Brian (1967) to those fungi which could grow and achieve full development only in association with a suitable living host plant. The obligate parasites were then divided into two categories, ecologically obligate and physiologically obligate. Members of the latter category, which are considered here, were said to be unable to survive saprophytically in pure culture, even on the most complex media so far tested. A large range of fungi were considered to be physiologically obligate, including certain plasmodial parasites such as *Plasmodiophora brassicae*, members of the Peronosporaceae (downy mildews), the Albuginaceae (white blisters), the Erysiphales (powdery mildews), and the Uredinales (rusts). Brian suggested that techniques for the growth of obligate parasites in host-tissue cultures might be further developed for studies *in vitro* of host–parasite interactions, and recognized that some of the obligate parasites might eventually be grown in true axenic culture, once suitable media had been devised. In fact, axenic culture of certain rust fungi (Uredinales) is already an established procedure (Scott and Maclean, 1969).

GROWTH OF OBLIGATE PARASITES IN TISSUE CULTURE

It is surprising that tissue cultures have not been used more widely in studies of plant diseases caused by fungi because it is more than twenty years since Morel (1944, 1948) realized the possible advantages of their use as tools in plant pathology, particularly for studies of physiologically obligate parasites. The potential advantages of the dual culture system as envisaged by Morel seem obvious; obligate parasites, which would otherwise need to be grown on whole plants, can be cultured on an apparently simplified host in a controlled physical and nutritional environment, and in the absence of contaminant micro-organisms. In practice, however, there may be many problems.

THE ESTABLISHMENT OF DUAL CULTURES OF OBLIGATE PARASITES AND THEIR HOSTS

The downy mildew fungus of sugar beet, *Peronospora farinosa* f. sp. *betae,* provides an example of this technique. It is a pathogen of young plants of sugar beet (*Beta vulgaris*) whose leaves become thickened and distorted as a result of infection. The infected leaves may be killed, but most plants eventually recover from the disease (Russell, 1969a). Callus tissue cultures were grown from the surface-sterilized laminae and petioles of the first and second seedling leaves of the commercial sugar beet cultivars Maris Vanguard and Sharpe's Klein E on a basal medium supplemented with 2,4-dichlorophenoxyacetic acid (2,4-D, 6.0 mg/litre), 1-naphthalene acetic acid (NAA, 0.1 mg/litre) and coconut milk (150 ml/litre) or on a defined medium containing the basal medium of Murashige and Skoog (1962) supplemented with kinetin (1.5 mg/litre) and NAA (1.0 mg/litre) or 2,4-D (6.0 mg/litre) (Ingram and Joachim, 1971). It is frequently difficult to obtain contaminant-free inoculum of obligate parasites in order to infect established host calluses (Brian, 1967). With *P. farinosa,* Ingram and Joachim overcame this problem by using a surface sterilization procedure. Detached seven-day-old pairs of susceptible sugar beet cotyledons were inoculated with non-sterile conidia of *P. farinosa,* incubated at 15°C on moist filter paper in the light for 72 h, and then surface sterilized and placed on a salt + sucrose + agar medium and incubated further.

Many of the cotyledons remained free of contaminants and *P. farinosa* sporulated on them freely after seven days of incubation. Contaminant free cotyledons bearing conidia were placed in contact with the established sugar beet calluses, which then became infected. A similar technique has been used to infect Brassica calluses with *Peronospora parasitica* (Ingram 1969c).

After infection *Peronospora farinosa* readily became established in the sugar beet calluses, forming a dense weft of aerial mycelium (Fig. 1). When incubated in the light at 15°C the dual cultures continued to grow well, and although the infection was heavy, the callus tissues were not killed. Indeed, infected calluses grew at about the same rate as non-infected calluses and host and parasite appeared to be in complete balance. New infected cultures were established by transferring small pieces of infected callus to fresh medium, where they continued to grow. By histological investigations of the dual cultures, Ingram and Joachim revealed that the *P. farinosa* mycelium was largely aerial, and that within the infected tissues the hyphae were sparse and largely intercellular, causing little tissue damage. Superficially normal digitate haustoria were present and frequently closely associated with intact host nuclei (see Ingram and Joachim, 1971, Plate 2, Figs 6 and 7). Normal viable conidia were produced in culture on branched conidiophores. It is important that obligate parasites grown *in vitro* should be shown to retain their pathogenicity to intact hosts, and with

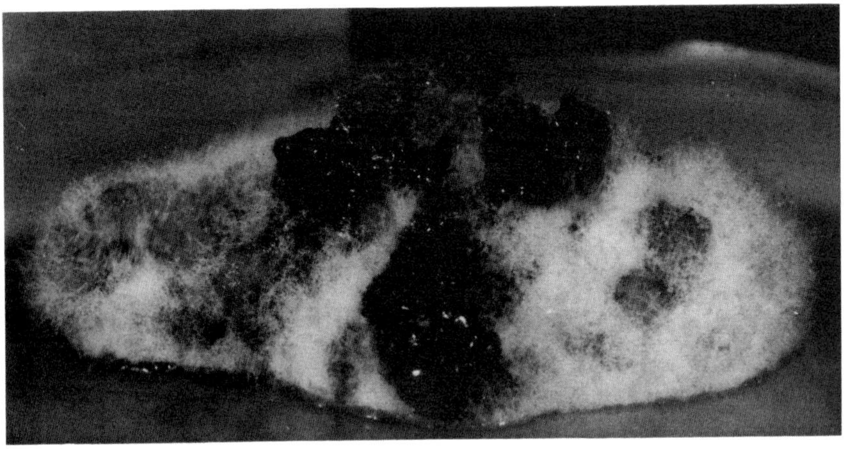

Fig. 1. A sugar beet callus infected with mycelium of *P. farinosa* f. sp. *betae*.

P. farinosa this was demonstrated at intervals during a period of two years after the initiation of dual cultures. Sporulation occurred on sugar beet cotyledons nine days after they had been inoculated with callus-produced conidia or with small pieces of infected callus tissue (see Ingram and Joachim, 1971, Plate 1, Fig. 4); the fungus also became established in seedlings of beet (Maris Vanguard) when these were inoculated with callus-produced conidia.

The initiation of dual cultures of *Peronospora farinosa* and its host was quite straightforward, but this is not the case with all host–parasite combinations and there may be many obstacles to be overcome before dual cultures can be produced. It may be difficult to infect some host callus tissues because certain fungi are unable to establish infections in the absence of a cuticle, epidermis or other differentiated tissue (Brian, 1967). Moreover, callus tissues of many plant species are known to produce abnormal metabolites which are fungitoxic. Maheshwari *et al.* (1967) could not infect Antirrhinum callus with uredospores of *Puccinia antirrhini* because the tissues produced an abnormal extracellular inhibitor of uredospore germination. Similarly P. A. Mason (personal communication) was unable to establish *Bremia lactucae* in callus tissues derived from the leaves of a susceptible lettuce cultivar. The fungus penetrated the callus cells, but a post-infection reaction then occurred to limit its spread to a small area around the point of inoculation. An abnormal, post-infection fungitoxic compound was apparently involved and could be extracted from the inoculated tissues.

A further problem that may be encountered in growing dual cultures of obligate parasites and their hosts is that of maintaining a balance between the growth rate of the selected fungus and the growth rate of the host callus tissues. Under natural conditions there is usually a high degree of balance existing between obligate parasites and their hosts, so that diseased organs are killed very slowly. This balance may be reflected in culture, as with *Peronospora farinosa* and sugar beet callus and *Plasmodiophora brassicae* and Brassica callus (Ingram 1969a). Indeed, unlike calluses derived from healthy Brassica plants, Brassica callus tissues that are systemically infected with secondary plasmodia of *P. brassicae* have been shown to be independent of certain exogenous growth factors (Ingram, 1969b; Williams *et al.*, 1969; Dekhuijzen and Overeem, 1971). In contrast to these balanced situations, a slow-growing obligate parasite may, under certain circumstances, be quickly outgrown by a rapidly enlarging callus; Turel and Ledingham (1957) found that the rust fungus *Melampsora lini* was often outgrown by the flax callus on which it was being cultured. The reverse situation may also apply as, for example, with *Peronospora parasitica* (Ingram, 1969c). When susceptible cabbage leaf calluses were inoculated with this fungus they were killed within 7-14 days.

THE VALIDITY OF THE DUAL CULTURE SYSTEM

Despite the many technical problems associated with growing obligate parasites in host callus tissue cultures a number of successful dual cultures suitable for experimental study have now been established. It is, therefore, important to consider whether the results obtained from experiments where dual cultures are used can be interpreted in terms of the intact diseased plant. Tissue cultures are quite different metabolically from the plants from which they were derived: they often lack chlorophyll, are usually in a state of constant meristematic activity, may be undifferentiated and may show abnormalities of secondary metabolite production. It is likely that many of the differences between intact and cultured plant tissues are due to permanent genetic changes such as the loss or addition of chromosomes and the development of mutations. The populations of some such altered cells might be expected to increase rapidly as a result of artifical selection for fast growing, or other types of tissue at the times of transfer of cultures to fresh media. Our studies with sugar beet showed such an example of chromosomal change when there was a dramatic increase in the ploidy levels of cells during a period of culture *in vitro.* The increases were not constant from cell to cell, so that most cultures became chromosome mosaics (Table I). Callus tissues were initiated from segments of the first seedling leaves of the experimental sugar beet Lines F and G on five different culture media. In each case the basal medium was that of Murashige and Skoog (1962) and this was supplemented with auxin and kinetin or coconut milk as indicated in Table I. Samples of the seedling leaves and seedling root tips were fixed in Newcomer's fixative (Newcomer, 1953) at the time of callus initiation, and samples of callus tissue were fixed after six transfers at monthly intervals on the test media. Chromosome counts were obtained from tissue squashes after hydrolysis and staining with propionic orcein. Diploid counts of 18 chromosomes only were always obtained from the nuclei in squashes of the first seedling leaves and root tips of Line F and G plants, but in six-month-old calluses diploid counts were obtained only in some of the Line G nuclei. Polyploidy had developed in all of the Line F callus nuclei counted, and in many of the Line G callus nuclei grown on three out of the five test media. It has not yet been possible to regenerate whole plants from sugar beet callus, but Heinz and Mee (1971) have shown recently that plants differentiated from callus of *Saccharum* species hybrids are morphologically, cytogenically and enzymatically different from the parent plants from which the calluses were derived.

Little is known about the differences between tissue cultures and intact plants in their interactions with fungal parasites. Williams and Yukawa (1967) found no ultrastructural differences between secondary plasmodia of *Plasmodiophora brassicae* in naturally-infected clubroot tissues and those in infected callus cultures, and Dekhuijzen and Overeem (1971) demonstrated certain correlations between the auxin and cytokinin content of natural clubroot tissues and the behaviour in culture of callus tissue infected with secondary plasmodia. Tommerup and Ingram (1971) and Ingram and Tommerup (1972) showed that the cytological development of the primary phase of the life cycle of *P. brassicae* was not the same in callus tissue cultures as in intact *Brassica* plants, although the secondary phase was normal. Some comparative studies have also been carried out on the expression of resistance and susceptibility by cultured tissues to infection by fungal pathogens. Experiments with *Phytophthora infestans* have suggested that with the potato cultivar Orion there may be good correlation between intact plants and callus cultures derived from them in the expression of the R1 major gene for resistance (Ingram and Robertson, 1965; Ingram, 1967; Robertson *et al.*, 1968), although recent work by Professor Friend (personal communication) suggests that the biochemical mechanism of resistance expression operating in Orion tissue cultures may not be the same as that operating in the intact Orion plant. Warren and Routley (1970) have shown that a major gene for resistance to *P. infestans* may be expressed in tomato callus culture. Bailey (1970) has demonstrated that pea calluses produce the phytoalexin pisatin, but calluses which had been established for over 18 months showed a marked reduction in their ability to produce the compound when compared with newly established cultures. Further differences between intact plants and callus cultures in the expression of resistance and susceptibility have also been found in experiments with *Peronospora parasitica* (Ingram, 1969c). The susceptibility of different *Brassica* callus clones and root organ cultures to *P. parasitica* was not constant and results obtained with callus were frequently at variance with results obtained using intact *Brassica* plant parts. Host–parasite specificity was apparently not lost in tissue culture, however, for *P. parasitica* would not infect callus cultures derived from cultivars

TABLE I

The ranges of chromosome counts obtained from the dividing nuclei of calluses of sugar beet Lines F and G after six transfers (at monthly intervals) on five test media (about 50 dividing nuclei were counted in each treatment). Counts of 18 chromosomes were always obtained from dividing nuclei of Lines F and G first seedling leaves and root tips fixed at the time of callus initiation

Supplements to the basal medium (1 litre) (Murashige and Skoog, 1962)	Range of chromosome numbers in nuclei of: Line F	Line G
2,4-D (5.0 mg) + kinetin (1.5 mg)	36 to 108	18 only
NAA (1.0 mg) + kinetin (1.5 mg)	36 to 108	18 only
Benazolin[1] (5.0 mg) + kinetin (1.5 mg)	36 to 200 approx.	18 to 108
IAA (5.0 mg)[2] + kinetin (1.5 mg)	54 to 200 approx.	18 to 54
2,4-D (6.0 mg) + NAA (0.1 mg) + coconut milk (150 ml)	36 to 200 approx.	18 to 108

[1] Benazolin = 4-chloro-2-oxobenzothiazolin-3-ylacetic acid.
[2] IAA = Indolyl-3-acetic acid.

of the non-hosts oat, wheat, potato, tomato, lettuce and sugar beet (D. S. Ingram, unpublished data). In contrast, Harvey and Grasham (1971) have shown that the rust *Cronartium ribicola* will infect calluses derived from the non-host species *Pseudotsuga menziesii* as readily as it will infect calluses from its normal host, *Pinus monticola.* Further abnormalities of resistance expression in tissue culture have been reported by Saad and Boone (1964) for the combination of *Venturia inaequalis* with apple callus and by Maheshwari *et al.* (1967) for the *Puccinia antirrhini* and Antirrhinum callus combination.

In recent studies of two inbred lines of sugar beet, differences between callus cultures and intact plants in their behaviour to *Peronospora farinosa* f. sp. *betae* have been demonstrated. Leaves of the sugar beet Line G, a homozygous diploid, were very susceptible to attack by *P. farinosa* while leaves of Line F were highly resistant through the operation of a single dominant gene which led to a hypersensitive reaction of the host cells upon infection (Russell, 1968, 1969a and b). The six-month-old callus cultures of Lines F and G initiated on the five test media described in Table I were used for comparison: at the time when sample callus tissues were fixed for cytological examination, other replicate samples of tissue were laid out on their respective media in petri dishes. These calluses were then inoculated with *P. farinosa* by placing a small piece of the sugar beet (Maris Vanguard) callus tissue, permeated with fungal mycelium, in contact with each test callus. The results of the experiment, which were assessed after one month of incubation at 15°C in the light, are summarized in Table II. Most replicates of the Line F ('resistant') calluses initiated on three of the test media were readily invaded by mycelium of *P. farinosa.* On two of the media, mycelial growth was poor on some of the callus replicates and did not occur at all on others. Some of the Line G ('susceptible') callus replicates supported only poor fungal growth on all of the test media while others were immune. Complete susceptibility of Line G callus occurred in only some of the replicates on four out of the five test media. Further differences between calluses and intact sugar beet plants in the expression of the major gene for resistance have been recorded elsewhere (Ingram and Joachim, 1971). Many more comparative studies are necessary, but the findings so far suggest that tissue cultures may in some cases be quite different from the plants from which they were derived in their interactions with pathogens; data on host–parasite interaction obtained from tissue culture studies should, therefore, be interpreted with extreme caution until more information on the nature and extent of the differences is available.

Growth of Obligate Parasites in Axenic Culture

Dual cultures offer a possible means of studying host-obligate parasite interaction under controlled conditions, but it is logical that attempts should also be made to culture obligate parasites independently of their host tissues so

TABLE II

The range of resistance and susceptibility to infection by *P. farinosa* in 18 replicates each of Line F or Line G sugar beet tissue cultures after six transfers (at monthly intervals) on five test media.
Susceptible (S)—profuse mycelial growth on the test calluses;
Resistant (R)—poor fungal growth;
Immune (I)—no fungal growth.

Supplements to the basal medium (Murashige and Skoog, 1962)	No. of susceptible, resistant or immune calluses Line F			Line G		
	S	R	I	S	R	I
2,4-D (5.0 mg) + kinetin (1.5 mg)	17	1	0	4	6	8
NAA (1.0 mg) + kinetin (1.5 mg)	13	5	0	5[1]	2	1
Benazolin (5.0 mg) + kinetin (1.5 mg)	15	3	0	10	8	0
IAA (5.0 mg) + kinetin (1.5 mg)	2	11	5	0	6	12
2,4-D (6.0 mg) + NAA (0.1 mg) + coconut milk (150 ml)	0	5	13	1[2]	1	10

[1] Eight replicates only.
[2] Twelve replicates only.

that the metabolism and genetics of the parasite may be studied in isolation. Many of the attempts to grow obligate parasites in host tissue cultures have been made with a view to obtaining contaminant-free mycelium or spores for axenic culture studies.

THE PERONOSPORACEAE (DOWNY MILDEW FUNGI) AND ALBUGINACEAE (WHITE BLISTER FUNGI)

Little progress in the culture of downy mildew fungi in the absence of host tissue has yet been reported, but it has been observed that certain members of this group are sufficiently independent of host metabolism to grow for short distances away from host callus tissue cultures on the surface of their culture media. Such a phenomenon was observed by Griffin and Coley-Smith (1968) in their experiments with *Pseudoperonospora humuli.* Similarly, mycelium of *Peronospora farinosa* grew for distances of 1.5-2.0 cm away from infected sugar beet calluses on the surface of the Murashige and Skoog (1962) basal medium supplemented with kinetin and 2,4-D, NAA or benazolin (Ingram and Joachim, 1972). In some instances peninsulas of mycelium with conidiophores and conidia (Fig. 2) were formed. Many of these peninsulas were connected to the parent callus by only a few hyphal strands or, in some instances, by a single hypha (Fig. 3). However, when connections with the parent callus were severed

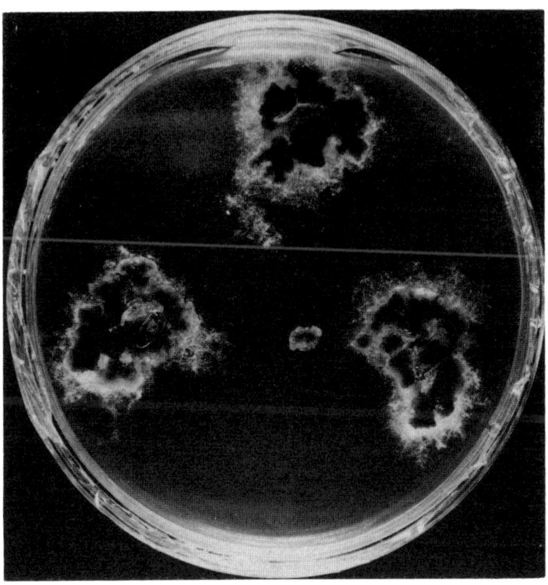

Fig. 2. Mycelial growth of *P. farinosa* away from parent calluses on the surface of a chemically defined culture medium (petri dish photographed from the underside).

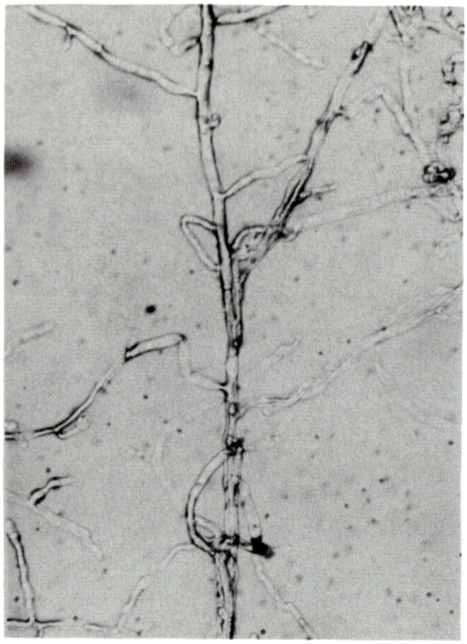

Fig. 3. Enlarged view of the hyphal connection between a peninsula of mycelium of *P. farinosa* and the infected parent callus on a chemically defined tissue culture medium.

the isolated mycelium did not survive. There is a report by Guttenburg and Schmoller (1958) that limited vegetative growth and sporulation of *Peronospora brassicae* was obtained on a beer wort–phosphate agar medium, and more recently Tiwari and Arya (1969) obtained sporulation and axenic growth of *Sclerospora graminicola* mycelium arising from host callus. This survived for two transfers in the absence of living host tissues.

THE ERYSIPHALES (POWDERY MILDEW FUNGI) AND THE UREDINALES (RUST FUNGI)

Although axenic cultures of powdery mildew fungi have not yet been obtained, considerable success has been achieved in attempts to culture the rust fungi. It is now 20 years since Hotson and Cutter (1951) claimed that in some instances mycelium of *Gymnosporangium juniperi-virginianae* grew out from dual cultures of this fungus and *Juniperus* species callus and became established on the culture medium. The saprophytic mycelium was maintained in axenic culture over a very long period and was, under some conditions, capable of re-infecting living host plants (Cutter, 1951, 1959). It was later reported (Cutter, 1960) that saprophytic mycelium of *Uromyces ari-triphylli* had been obtained in a similar way. Unfortunately other workers were unable to repeat the findings of

Hotson and Cutter, and their work remained the subject of controversy (see Brian, 1967) until Williams *et al.* (1966) obtained vegetative colonies of a strain of *Puccinia graminis* f. sp. *tritici* from contaminant-free uredospores on a simple medium supplemented with yeast extract. The saprophytic mycelium of *P. graminis* could be transferred, and was later shown to be capable of sporulation and pathogenicity when the culture medium was further supplemented with Evans's peptone (Williams *et al.*, 1967). Further experiments showed that the complex extracts in the culture medium could sometimes be replaced by aspartic acid and sulphur amino acids such as cysteine (Kuhl *et al.*, 1971). The variation of *P. graminis* in culture has been discussed recently by Maclean and Scott (1970) and by Maclean *et al.* (1971), and the suitability of axenic cultures for genetical studies has been pointed out. Several other strains of *P. graminis* have now been cultured (Bushnell, 1968; Coffey *et al.*, 1969; Bushnell and Stewart, 1971), and cultures have also been obtained from spores of *Melampsora lini* (Turel, 1969a and b; Coffey *et al.*, 1970), *P. graminis* f. sp. *avenae* (Scott and Maclean, 1969), *P. graminis* f. sp. *secalis* and *P. coronata* f. sp. *avenae* (Kuhl *et al.*, 1971) and *P. recondita* (Singleton and Young, 1968; Kuhl *et al.*, 1971). Harvey and Grasham (1970a and b) have grown mycelium of *Cronartium ribicola* on a membrane separating it physically from a host callus culture, and also in isolation on a medium pre-conditioned by host callus tissues. Recently attempts have been made to obtain saprophytic mycelium of certain British rusts, but these have met with only limited success.

In one series of experiments the culture of *Puccinia punctiformis* (thistle rust), *P. coronata* f. sp. *avenae* Race 8 (crown rust of Oat cv. Blenda), *P. recondita* f. sp. *tritici* (brown rust of wheat cv. Wilhelmina) and *P. striiformis* f. sp. *tritici* Race 1B (yellow rust of wheat cv. Maris Ranger) was attempted using contaminant-free uredospores. Infected seedling leaves of the appropriate hosts were surface-sterilized in a calcium hypochlorite solution immediately prior to the opening of the uredosori and, after washing in sterile distilled water, were laid out in petri dishes on a medium containing 10.0 g glucose and 10.0 g agar in 1 litre of distilled water. Incubation was at 15° C in alternating periods of 16 h low-intensity white light and 8 h darkness. When the rust pustules opened, uredospores were transferred to the test media in petri dishes with the tip of a sterile scalpel. Various test media with complex additives were used, but the one that gave best growth of all species tested consisted of Czapek's salts supplemented (/ litre) with glucose (10.0 g), Evans's peptone (5.0 g), Difco casamino acids (2.0 g), Difco lactalbumin hydrolysate (1.0 g) and agar (7.0 g) at pH 6.4-6.8. Incubation was always at 15° C in alternating periods of 16 h low-intensity white light and 8 h darkness. Under these conditions macroscopic colonies (2.0-4.0 mm dia.) of *P. punctiformis, P. coronata* and *P. recondita* were formed from a dense inoculum of uredospores (Fig. 4). However, these colonies staled, becoming brown after about six weeks, and

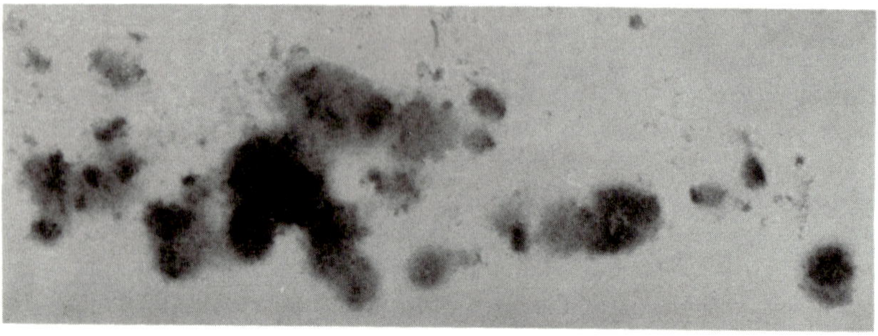

Fig. 4. Macroscopic colonies, consisting of vegetative mycelium of *P. punctiformis*, growing from a heavy inoculum of uredospores on a salts + glucose medium containing agar, peptone, casamino acids and lactalbumin. The isolated colonies are of dia. 0.5-4.0 mm.

could not be subcultured, although their survival in culture was sometimes improved by the addition of washed powdered charcoal (2.0 g/litre) to the medium. Sporulation did not take place in culture. Colony formation only occurred when dense uredospore inocula were used; when uredospores were sown thinly, highly branched germ tubes developed (Fig. 5), but did not grow into colonies, suggesting that developing spores and sporelings stimulate each other in the culture medium. Mycelial growth of *P. striiformis* could not be obtained on any of the media tested.

In another series of experiments, seedling leaves from appropriate hosts were infected with *Puccinia coronata* f. sp. *avenae* Race 8 or *P. recondita* f. sp. *tritici* or *P. striiformis* f. sp. *tritici* and were surface sterilized immediately prior to the opening of the uredospore pustules. They were then laid out in petri dishes on the surface of a medium containing distilled water, Noble agar (10.0 g/litre) and glucose (10.0 g/litre) only, and were incubated for 10 days in the cooled and lighted incubator described above. At the end of this time the leaves, which had senesced and turned yellow, were removed. With all three rust species tested macroscopic colonies had formed from the detached uredospores on the culture medium (Fig. 6). The colonies survived for six weeks before staling, but could not be subcultured, even to more complex culture media. Sporulation did not take place. Fungal colonies were not formed on the agar-glucose medium in the absence of a host leaf and it must be assumed that saprophytic growth was supported by substances which had diffused from the senescing leaves.

In a third series of experiments, seedling leaves of the oat cultivar Blenda infected with *Puccinia coronata* f. sp. *avenae* Race 8 and of the wheat cultivars Maris Ranger infected with *P. striiformis* f. sp. *tritici* and Wilhelmina infected with *P. recondita* f. sp. *tritici* were surface sterilized immediately prior to the opening of the uredospore pustules. Segments of infected leaf (1.5 cm long) were then laid out on the surface of a medium containing Czapek's salts, sodium citrate (3.0 g/litre), glucose (40.0 g/litre), Evans's peptone (10.0 g/litre) and agar (15.0 g/litre) at pH 6.0 and incubated at 15°C in alternating periods of 16 h low-

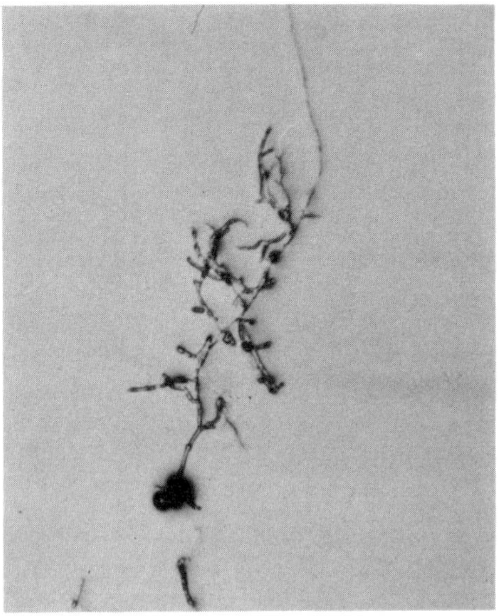

Fig. 5. A much-branched germ tube growing from an isolated uredospore of *P. recondita* f. sp. *tritici* on a salts + glucose medium containing agar, peptone, casamino acids and lactalbumin.

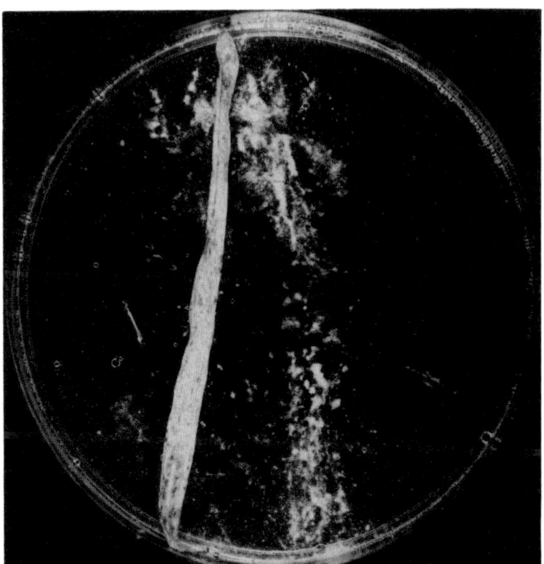

Fig. 6. Vegetative mycelium of *P. recondita,* which arose after an infected wheat leaf had been allowed to senesce, with uredosori facing downwards, on the surface of a water + agar + glucose medium for 10 days. The senescent leaf was moved aside, and the photograph was then taken after a further 10 days of incubation.

intensity white light and 8 h darkness. The leaf segments usually senesced and became yellow within 7 days and were apparently dead after 14 days. Aerial mycelium of *P. coronata, P. striiformis* or *P. recondita* was formed on the surface of the appropriate dead leaf tissues after about 21 days and persisted for several weeks, although mycelium did not spread on to the culture medium. Later, after about two months of incubation, large fungal stromata (0.5-1.0 cm across) with uredospores and sometimes teleutospores were formed on the dead leaves. Clearly the combination of dead host tissues and the culture medium was providing a more suitable chemical and physical environment for saprophytic growth and sporulation of the three rusts tested than the culture medium alone.

Although considerable effort has recently been directed towards obtaining axenic growth of rusts, little is yet known concerning the nature and significance of the specialized conditions required for saprophytic growth. It is clear that both the nutritional and the physical conditions required vary considerably between different species and even between different strains of the same species, and it is impossible to make generalizations. Cutter believed that his axenically-cultured rusts were mutants and that an observed loss of ability to grow saprophytically, associated with re-inoculation into host tissue, was the result of a mutation in the opposite direction. However, with regard to their work with *Puccinia graminis* Scott and his collaborators (Scott and Maclean, 1969; Kuhl *et al.*, 1971) have suggested that a change in the expression of the rust genome, leading to a reorientation of metabolism, occurs between germ tube elongation and the establishment of saprophytic mycelium. The fact that only a small number of sporelings survive to form macroscopic colonies is attributed to variation in the extent to which developing hyphae are able to adapt their metabolism to the saprophytic rather than the parasitic environment. They go on to suggest that further progress in the culture of rust fungi (and presumably other obligate parasites) will be facilitated by investigation of the nature of this metabolic transition between the germ tube and the initiation of saprophytic hyphae, and of the importance of leakage of metabolites during the development of both sporelings and colonies.

Acknowledgements

We wish to thank Dr Gordon Russell for advice and for generous gifts of sugar beet seed and inoculum of *Peronospora farinosa,* Professor P. W Brian and Dr K. J. Scott for discussion, the International Federation of University Women, the South Australian Women Graduates' Association and the University of Cambridge for the support of one of us (I. C. T.) and Boots Pure Drug Co. Ltd. for the sample of Benazolin.

REFERENCES

Bailey, J. A. (1970). Pisatin production by tissue cultures of *Pisum sativum* L. *J. gen. Microbiol.* **61**, 409-415.

Brian, P. W. (1967). Obligate parasitism in fungi. *Proc. R. Soc. B.* **168**, 101-118.

Bushnell, W. R. (1968). *In vitro* development of an Australian isolate of *Puccinia graminis* f. sp. *tritici. Phytopathology* **58**, 526-527.

Bushnell, W. R. and Stewart, D. M. (1971). Development of American isolates of *Puccinia graminis* f. sp. *tritici* on an artificial medium. *Phytopathology* **61**, 376-379.

Coffey, M. D., Bose, A. and Shaw, M. (1969). *In vitro* growth of gelatin suspensions of uredospores of *Puccinia graminis* f. sp. *tritici. Can. J. Bot.* **47**, 1291-1293.

Coffey, M. D., Bose, A. and Shaw, M. (1970). *In vitro* culture of the flax rust, *Melampsora lini. Can. J. Bot.* **48**, 773-776.

Cutter, V. M., Jr. (1951). The isolation of plant rusts upon artificial media and some speculations on the metabolism of obligate plant parasites. *Trans. N.Y. Acad. Sci.* **14**, 103-108.

Cutter, V. M., Jr. (1959). Studies on the isolation and growth of plant rusts in host tissue cultures and upon synthetic media. I. *Gymnosporangium. Mycologia* **51**, 248-295.

Cutter, V. M. Jr. (1960). Studies on the isolation and growth of plant rusts in host tissue cultures and upon synthetic media. II. *Uromyces ari-triphylli. Mycologia* **52**, 726-742.

Dekhuijzen, H. M. and Overeem, J. C. (1971). The role of cytokinins in clubroot formation. *Physiol. Pl. Path.* **1**, 151-161.

Griffin, M. J. and Coley-Smith, J. R. (1968). The establishment of hop tissue cultures and their infection by downy mildew *Pseudoperonospora humuli* (Miy. & Tak.) Wilson under aseptic conditions. *J. gen. Microbiol.* **53**, 231-236.

Guttenburg, H. von and Schmoller, H. (1958). Kulterversuche mit *Peronospora brassicae* Gaum. *Arch. Mikrobiol.* **30**, 268-279.

Harvey, A. E. and Grasham, J. L. (1970a). Growth of *Cronartium ribicola* in the absence of physical contact with its host. *Can. J. Bot.* **48**, 71-73.

Harvey, A. E. and Grasham, J. L. (1970b). Survival of *Cronartium ribicola* on a medium containing host tissue culture diffusates. *Mycopath. Mycol. appl.* **40**, 245-248.

Harvey, A. E. and Grasham, J. L. (1971). Inoculation of a non host tissue culture with *Cronartium ribicola. Can. J. Bot.* **49**, 881-882.

Heinz, D. J. and Mee, Grace W. P. (1971). Morphological, cytogenetic and enzymatic variation in *Saccharum* species hybrid clones derived from callus tissue. *Am. J. Bot.* **58**, 257-262.

Hotson, H. H. and Cutter, V. M. Jr. (1951). The isolation and culture of *Gymnosporangium juniperi-virginianae.* Schw. *Proc. natn. Acad. Sci. U.S.A.* 37, 400-403.

Ingram, D. S. (1967). The expression of R-gene resistance to *Phytophthora infestans* in tissue cultures of *Solanum tuberosum J. gen. Microbiol.* **49**, 99-108.

Ingram, D. S. (1969a). Growth of *Plasmodiophora brassicae* in host callus. *J. gen. Microbiol.* **55**, 9-18.

Ingram, D. S. (1969b). Abnormal growth of tissues infected with *Plasmodiophora brassicae. J. gen. Microbiol.* **56**, 55-67.

Ingram, D. S. (1969c). The susceptibility of Brassica callus to infection by *Peronospora parasitica. J. gen. Microbiol.* **58**, 391-401.

Ingram, D. S. and Joachim, Irene (1971). The growth of *Peronospora farinosa* (Fr.) Fr. f. sp. *betae* and sugar beet callus tissues in dual culture. *J. gen. Microbiol.* **69**, 211-220.

Ingram, D. S. and Robertson, N. F. (1965). Interaction between *Phytophthora infestans* and tissue cultures of *Solanum tuberosum. J. gen. Microbiol.* **40**, 431-437.

Ingram, D. S. and Tommerup, I. C. (1972). The life history of *Plasmodiophora brassicae* Woron. *Proc. Roy. Soc. B.* **180**, 103-112.

Kuhl, Joy L., Maclean, D. J., Scott, K. J. and Williams, P. G. (1971). The axenic culture of Puccinia species from uredospores: experiments on nutrition and variation. *Can. J. Bot.* **49**, 201-209.

Maclean, D. J. and Scott, K. J. (1970). Variant forms of saprophytic mycelium grown from uredospores of *Puccinia graminis* f. sp. *tritici. J. gen. Microbiol.* **64**, 19-27.

Maclean, D. J., Scott, K. J. and Tommerup, I. C. (1971). A uninucleate wheat infecting strain of the stem rust fungus isolated from axenic cultures. *J. gen. Microbiol.* **65**, 339-342.

Maheshwari, R., Hildebrandt, A. C. and Allen, P. J. (1967). Factors affecting the growth of rust fungi on host tissue cultures. *Bot. Gaz.* **128**, 153-159.

Morel, G. (1944). Le développment du mildiou sur les tissus de Vigne cultives *in vitro. C.r.hebd. Séanc. Acad. Sci., Paris* **218**, 50-52.

Morel, G. (1948). Recherches sur la culture associée de parasites obligatoires et de tissus végétaux. *Ann. Epiphyt. Sér. Path. Vég.* **14**, 1-112.

Murashige, T. and Skoog, F. (1962). A revised medium for rapid growth and bio-assays with tobacco tissue cultures. *Physiolo. Pl.* **15**, 473-497.

Newcomer, E. H. (1953). A new cytological and histological fixing fluid. *Science, N.Y.* **118**, 161.

Robertson, N. F., Friend, J., Aveyard, M., Brown, J., Huffee, M. and Homans, A. L. (1968). The accumulation of phenolic acids in tissue culture pathogen combinations of *Solanum tuberosum* and *Phytophthora infestans. J. gen. Microbiol.* **54**, 261-268.

Russell, G. E. (1968). Experiments in selecting for resistance to downy mildew in sugar beet. *J. agric. Sci., Camb.* **71**, 251-256.

Russell, G. E. (1969a). Resistance to fungal diseases of sugar beet leaves. *Br. Sug. Beet Rev.* **38**, 27-35.

Russell, G. E. (1969b). Recent work on breeding for resistance to downy mildew (*Peronospora farinosa*) in sugar beet. *J. Inst. Sug. Beet Res.* (I.I.R.B.) **4**, 1-10.

Saad, A. T. and Boone, D. M. (1964). Growth of *Venturia inaequalis* in apple callus tissue *in vitro* in relation to pathogenicity. *Phytopathology* **54**, 905 (abstr.).

Scott, K. J. and Maclean, D. J. (1969). Culturing of rust fungi. *A. Rev. Phytopathol.* **7**, 123-146.

Singleton, L. L. and Young, H. C. (1968). The *in vitro* culture of *Puccinia recondita* f. sp. *tritici. Phytopathology* **58**, 1068 (abstr.).

Tiwari, M. M. and Arya, H. C. (1969). *Sclerospora graminicola* in axenic culture. *Science, N.Y.* **163**, 291-293.

Tommerup, I. C. and Ingram, D. S. (1971). The life-cycle of *Plasmodiophora brassicae* Woron. in Brassica tissue cultures and in intact roots. *New Phytol.* **70**, 327-332.

Turel, F. L. M. (1969a). Saprophytic development of the flax rust *Melampsora lini*, race No. 3. *Can. J. Bot.* **47**, 821-823.

Turel, F. L. M. (1969b). Low temperature requirement for saprophytic flax rust cultures. *Can. J. Bot.* **47**, 1637-1638.

Turel, F. L. M. and Ledingham, G. A. (1957). Production of aerial mycelium and uredospores by *Melampsora lini* (Pers.) Lév. on flax leaves in tissue culture. *Can. J. Microbiol.* **3**, 813-819.

Warren, K. S. and Routley, D. G. (1970). The use of tissue culture in the study of single gene resistance of tomato to *Phytophthora infestans. Proc. Am. Soc. hort. Sci.* **95**, 266-269.

Williams, P. G., Scott, K. J. and Kuhl, Joy L. (1966). Vegetative growth of *Puccinia graminis* f. sp. *tritici in vitro. Phytopathology* **56**, 1418-1419.

Williams, P. G., Scott, K. J., Kuhl, Joy L. and Maclean, D. J. (1967). Sporulation and pathogenicity of *Puccinia graminis* f. sp. *tritici* grown on an artificial medium. *Phytopathology* **57**, 326-327.

Williams, P. H., Reddy, M. N. and Strandberg, J. C. (1969). Growth of non-infected and *Plasmodiophora brassicae* infected cabbage callus in culture. *Can. J. Bot.* **47**, 1217-1220.

Williams, P. H. and Yukawa, Y. B. (1967). Ultrastructural studies on the host-parasite relations of *Plasmodiophora brassicae. Phytopathology* **57**, 682-687.

DISCUSSION

Dr D. S. Ingram: Before the discussion begins may I comment that I am no expert on axenic culture, but I have included this in the hope that the audience will discuss it and give their own ideas and views.

Dr H. M. Dekhuijzen: Your results show clearly that after many transfers, your tissue culture has changed. Does the fungus also change? So, let us suppose you start the culture with one physiological race of fungus, how many races have you after, say, 15 transfers?

Dr Ingram: Do you mean in tissue culture?

Dr Dekhuijzen: Yes, growth of an obligate parasite in a tissue culture.

Dr Ingram: I do not know, but I imagine that you get as many changes in obligate parasites cultured in tissue cultures as in any fungal parasite cultured axenically. In other words, organisms such as *Phytophthora infestans* grown in culture on bean medium certainly change; for example, they lose pathogenicity. I imagine the same kind of changes might well occur in pathogens cultured on host tissues.

Dr Dekjuijzen: But what happens when you assay the races obtained from tissue culture on living plants?

Dr Ingram: All that I know from our work on *Peronospora farinosa*, is that in the short time we have had it in culture, it does not seem to have changed appreciably in its reaction with Line F and Line G, but we have yet to do more tests to check this.

Dr G. E. Russell: Obviously the hypersensitive reaction of Line F to *Peronospora farinosa* does not work in tissue culture, but I would be very interested to know if other kinds of resistance, collectively known as non-specific resistance, work in tissue culture.

Dr Ingram: As far as resistance is concerned, tissue cultures are so different from the whole plant that behaviour might be different or it might be the same, and it is almost a matter of chance. I have grown calluses from Sharpe's Klein E which has a fairly high level of non-specific resistance. Some calluses are apparently immune, some are susceptible, and there is no consistent pattern that one can see.

Professor N. F. Robertson: Is there any correlation between the ability to invade a meristem, and ability to grow in culture? My impression is that meristems in general are not easily invaded by fungi, but I imagine *Peronospora farinosa* may well be invading the meristem.

Dr Ingram: Yes, meristems are invaded, and there may be a correlation here, but I really have very little evidence to say either yes or no. Perhaps John Coley-Smith can tell us about *Pseudoperonospora humuli* entering meristems and growing in culture.

Dr J. R. Coley-Smith: I have always thought that it did go into the apical meristem, but David Royle (who is sitting next to me) seems to think that it doesn't quite get into the meristem, so perhaps I had better get him to answer the question.

Dr D. J. Royle: I do not think that *Pseudoperonospora humuli* gets into the apical dome of hop. The first 5-6 cell layers of shoot apex are not invaded intercellularly, although the fungus will colonize other non-vacuolate cell regions.

Dr Ingram: And yet it grows well in culture.

Dr Coley-Smith: I do not think it grows as well as your *Peronospora farinosa.*

Dr Ingram: Is this partly because the hop tissue grows very slowly?

Dr Coley-Smith: It could well be. The hop tissue certainly does not grow very well in artifical cultures.

Dr Ingram: It might be that fungi grow better on a tissue that grows well, but I do not think much evidence is available, although our work with sugar-beet tends to support this. There is one other point, we have tried unsuccessfully to get thistle rust (*Puccinia punctiformis*) into thistle tissue cultures. This is a meristem invader, so for this system this is no correlation.

Professor R. K. S. Wood: A point of information. Is it right that callus tissue does not contain plasmodesmata?

Dr Ingram: There are some who say not, but plasmodesmata have been seen in callus tissue.

Professor Wood: I ask this question because in considering the killing of plant cells by pectic enzymes, we have speculated on the possible role of plasmodesmata. If there are none in the callus, then these cells might be killed far less rapidly by these enzymes.

Dr Ingram: It is possible that they are present, but not very probable, especially where there is a friable tissue, because we may presume that cells are continually moving about during growth.

Professor Wood: That would make it very interesting, from my point of view, to try callus tissue with these pectic enzymes.

Dr Ingram: Yes, it would definitely be worth trying. Actually, Dr Heale, at Queen Elizabeth's College, is infecting carrot calluses with various rotting fungi.

Dr I. M. Smith: Can the immunity of sugar beet calluses derived from both the resistant and susceptible cultivars be related to any other attribute which would explain it?

Dr Ingram: I have no explanation for it, except to say that with lettuce callus we can get a new reaction to *Bremia lactucae* which gives rise to a post infection toxin. On calluses infected with *Bremia lactucae* spores, there is initial penetration, after which a post infection toxin is produced. There is then no further growth of the fungus, thus giving an apparent immunity.

Hazel Howell: I wondered if with the changes you have been getting (in your Lines) towards a more immune or a more susceptible reaction, you have noticed any correlation with the ploidy of the callus cells.

Dr Ingram: No, we have not done enough counts, but I don't think there is any correlation.

Hazel Howell: The numbers you quoted are by no means even multiples of 18 and if, as this implies, there are unbalanced chromosome sets dominance could be upset.

Dr Ingram: Yes. As far as I can see there are no correlations, but we would need many more counts to check this.

Dr R. Johnson: Might there be changes in ploidy in the pathogen as well as in the callus tissue? This might have some effect.

Dr Ingram: We have been looking at chromosomes of *Plasmodiophora* and *Peronospora*, but have found no changes.

P. W. Wilkins: There are some recorded instances of doubling the complement (i.e. diploid to tetraploid) with the result that plant resistance is increased, as occurs with the resistance of tetraploid red clover (*Trifolium pratense*) to *Sclerotinia trifoliorum.*

Dr Ingram: That is very interesting indeed, although in the example I quoted, some of the polyploid calluses from the same sugar beet leaf were susceptible, but others were immune.

Dr Inez Tommerup: With reference to the question by Roy Johnson, we have examined the behaviour of the nuclei of *Plasmodiophora brassicae* during all phases of its life cycle in callus cultures of turnips and compared these findings with the behaviour of the fungal nuclei during its life cycle in turnip plants. We found no difference in ploidy levels of the fungus *P. brassicae,* even though the callus culture cells had extremely high ploidy levels. In very preliminary studies of *Peronospora farinosa,* the numbers of chromosomes in fungus callus cultures appears to be the same as that of the fungus growing in sugar beet leaves.

Dr Ingram: This work is far from complete.

Dr R. C. Hignett: I wondered if you could enlarge on the resistant reaction that you get in the tissue cultures that were initially susceptible. Can you say any more about what happens?

Dr Ingram: With Line G tissue cultures (which is a susceptible line), we can establish calluses on a whole series of media. We can then test their resistance or susceptibility either by applying spores or a mass inoculum of fungal mycelium, growing on another piece of callus. In some instances we get invasion of the tissues very rapidly, and fluffy mycelial growth ensues. In others, only a very slow growth of fungus occurs on the tissues, but in still other cultures from the same clone there is good growth of the fungus. In a third reaction we might get absolutely no growth of the fungus on the callus we are trying to infect. I have not seen any evidence that any fungitoxic metabolites may be diffusing from the callus to prevent growth of the fungus on the tissue we are using as inoculum.

Dr Hignett: There is no kind of collapse of the tissue culture?

Dr Ingram: We have not yet looked at the cytology and histology of this particular reaction.

III . 2 Host–Parasite Relations in Cabbage Clubroot

P. H. WILLIAMS, J. R. AIST AND P. K. BHATTACHARYA

Department of Plant Pathology, University of Wisconsin, Madison, U.S.A.

INTRODUCTION

The selection of a system and design of experiments to gain deeper insight into obligate parasitism between fungi and higher plants requires a number of basic considerations. The first step in the establishment of a host–parasite relationship normally involves an exchange of information between one or both of the partners. The nature of this exchanged information, the environment in which it is exchanged, the genetic make-up of the host and the parasite and the ontogenetic state of the particular partners may all be important in determining the events which lead to a parasitic relationship. Although no system of host and parasite may yet be considered ideal for the study of obligate host–parasite relations, the combination of *Plasmodiophora brassicae* Wor. on various crucifers has been useful for the examination of certain aspects of obligate parasitism (Williams *et al.*, 1971). By growing seedlings of cabbage (*Brassica oleracea* var. *capitata*) in solution culture and exposing their root hair cells to suspensions of *P. brassicae* zoospores, the events leading to the establishment of a host–parasite relationship may be followed at the cellular level (Williams *et al.*, 1971).

Under phase-contrast and interference-contrast optics the processes of encystment and penetration may be examined on living root hair cells, and at desired times these stages may be fixed and observed under the electron microscope (Aist and Williams, 1971). Following penetration, the growth of the plasmodium of *P. brassicae* may be observed throughout its life in the hair cell, and at appropriate times various cytological and cytochemical measurements may be made (Bhattacharya and Williams, 1971). The seedling root growing in liquid culture produces a linear array of hair cells ranging in age from those only a few hours old to those several days old. Thus, an exposure of the seedling root to a suspension of *P. brassicae* zoospores provides the opportunity for observing the parasite in host cells of varying ages. The linearity of the hair cell usually results in microscopic views of the host nucleus unobstructed by the parasite. Thus, growth of the parasite and various responses of the host can be observed within the same cell.

Methods and Results

INOCULUM

Inoculum of *P. brassicae* usually consisted of a suspension of resting sporangia extracted from clubroot gall tissue (Williams *et al.*, 1971). Resting sporangia are replete with mitochondria, free and bound ribosomes, endoplasmic reticulum and large lipid bodies. They are uninucleate, without a nucleolus, and have a golgi complex (Williams and McNabola, 1967). After 26-30 h, resting sporangia were layered on to the bottom of a vial in which three or four cabbage seedlings were growing in dilute salts solution; a high concentration of primary zoospores could be found swimming in the solution (Macfarlane, 1958).

ENCYSTMENT

When cabbage seedlings (Jersey Queen) germinated on moist filter paper and grown for 24 h in dilute salts were placed for 30-60 min in a suspension of *P. brassicae* primary zoospores, and then returned to a solution free of zoospores, a relatively synchronous 'pulse' of infections occurred in the root hair cells (Williams *et al.*, 1971). Zoospores usually collided with root hairs several times before becoming finally attached to one. Attachment occurred on the side of the spore opposite the point of flagellar insertion. After attachment, the flagellae coiled around the zoospore and were retracted in less than 1 min. Following retraction of the flagellar axonemes the attached spore rounded up and became encysted 2-3 min later (Aist and Williams, 1971). The encysted zoospore remained apparently quiescent for about 3 h. However, during this time the penetration apparatus consisting of the Stachel, the Schlauch, and the Rohr (Keskin and Fuchs, 1969) was formed within the cyst (Figs 1, 2).

PENETRATION

Root hair penetration was examined by exposing seedlings to zoospores for a 30-min pulse, then 2 h after the beginning of inoculation two seedlings were observed every 30 min and the percentage of full cysts, half full cysts and empty cysts determined (Fig. 6). The development of papillae on the inside of the hair cell wall at the point of cyst attachment was also recorded. About 15 min prior to penetration, a vacuole within the cyst enlarged to fill about half the cyst volume. Many of the lipid bodies within the cyst were closely adpressed to this vacuole. At the beginning of penetration, the Rohr evaginated in the period of about 1 min to produce the bulb-shaped adhesorium which was firmly adpressed to the cell wall (Figs 3, 4, 5, 7). From within the adhesorium the Stachel was forced through the hair cell wall and, in about 1 s, the parasite was injected into the host cytoplasm of the cell. Simultaneously, the cyst vacuole expanded to fill the volume of the cyst and the adhesorium shrank slightly (Fig. 5). The young amoeba remained attached to the adhesorium by a short strand, presumably the Schlauch, for a few seconds before being swept away by cyclosis. Lipid bodies within the encysted zoospore did not pass into the host, but remained in the empty cyst and in the adhesorium as a coagulated droplet (Fig. 5).

ESTABLISHMENT AND GROWTH OF THE PLASMODIUM

Young amoebae within the hair cell cytoplasm contained all types of organelles found in the resting sporangium with the exception of lipid bodies (Fig. 8). Upon entry the amoebae were without nucleoli. The young amoeba was bounded by a seven-layered envelope similar to that observed in the infected clubroot galls (Williams and McNabola, 1970). Often the outer unit membrane of the plasmodial envelope appeared to be part of a membrane bounding large flattened vacuoles situated between the parasite and the host cytoplasm (Aist and Williams, 1971).

Several parameters were used to determine the growth of *P. brassicae* in cabbage root hairs. Since it was known that nuclear division in each plasmodium was synchronous (Williams *et al.*, 1971), growth could be expressed as the function $N = 2^n$, where N was the number of nuclei in a given plasmodium and n was the number of nuclear divisions undergone by the plasmodium Following a 1-h pulse inoculation, the percentage of nuclei $N = 2^0$ to 2^6 appearing at 3-h intervals was plotted. From these data it was determined that *P. brassicae* remained uninucleate for 21 h (Fig. 9). After the first division, nuclei divided synchronously at about 4-h intervals until sporulation at 72-96 h.

Under the light microscope, the first measurable growth responses of the parasite were increases in size of the plasmodium and the reappearance of a nucleolus (Table I). Between 2 h and 4 h after penetration, the parasite quadrupled in volume, then grew at a more linear rate. Nucleoli also first became visible between 2 and 4 h; however, the first small lipid bodies did not appear until 4-6 h after penetration.

RESPONSES OF THE HOST TO PENETRATION AND PARASITE ESTABLISHMENT

Penetration by *P. brassicae* resulted in measurable changes in the metabolism of the hair cell nucleus. Within 4 h after penetration the volume of the host cell nucleolus had begun to increase and by 6 h it had doubled (Table I). Nucleolar enlargement continued for about 24 h. Cytofluorometric measurements of nuclear protein, histone and RNA indicated that increased nucleolar volume was accompanied by increased nuclear RNA and protein (Bhattacharya and Williams, 1971). Although the total protein content of the nucleus increased considerably, the histones decreased slightly (Table II). Within the histones, the lysine-rich

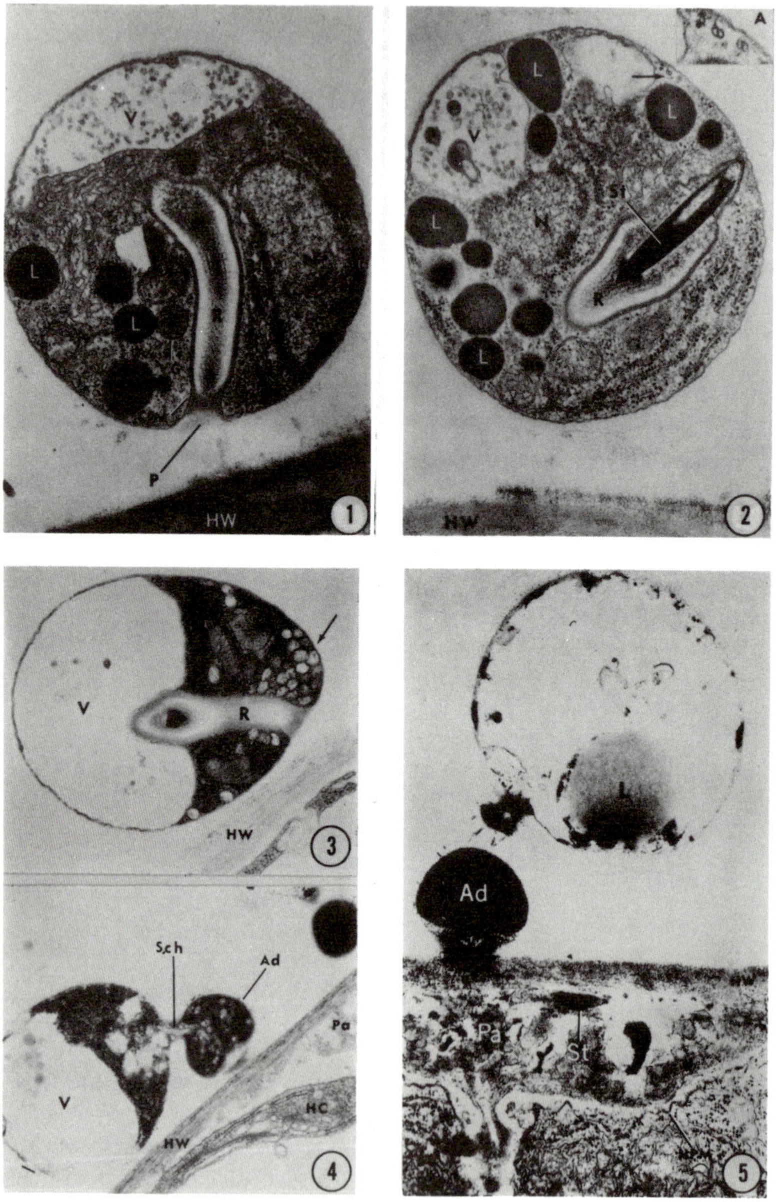
V
L
R
P
HW
1
A
N
St
2
3
Sch
Ad
Pa
HC
4
5

fraction decreased by 25% whereas the arginine-rich fraction remained unaltered (Table III). Regardless of its age at the time it became infected, or the number of parasite plasmodia within it, the hair cell nucleolus never increased in size beyond a 1.5-3.0 μm diameter. No changes in the levels of host DNA occurred as the result of infection.

In addition to the chemical changes taking place in the nucleus of the parasitized host cell, the morphology of the hair cell was often affected by the parasite. Instead of the normal linear extension of the root hair, the tip became enlarged and clubshaped or branched. Frequently, thick deposits of PAS-positive material (Jensen, 1962) occurred in these clubbed tips of the parasitized cell. The swelling of the hair cell tip could be detected within 4-6 h after the parasite had entered the cell, and though not all parasitized cells had swollen tips, as

---

Fig. 1. Primary cyst showing orientation of Rohr toward the host wall. The Rohr is lined by the cyst plasma membrane and is occluded by a plug. Fixation–Embedding Schedule D. (See Aist and Williams, 1971.) x36 700.

Fig. 2, 2A. Primary cyst showing location of Stachel within the Rohr. Fig. 2A shows the doublets at arrow in Fig. 2 at higher magnification. These are the only remaining doublets of an axoneme, and the doublet at the right appears to be breaking down. Fixation–Embedding Schedule D. Fig. 2–x36 700; Fig. 2A–x82 500.

Fig. 3. Electron micrograph of primary cyst just prior to adhesorium formation. The cyst vacuole has enlarged to fill about half the cyst volume. Golgi vesicles (arrow) are concentrated near the Rohr plug. Fixation–Embedding Schedule D. x25 700.

Fig. 4. Primary cyst which has produced an adhesorium. The adhesorium appears to be fastened to the host wall by a fibrillar adhesive material. Part of the Schlauch can be seen in the neck of the adhesorium. Fixation–Embedding Schedule D. x17 200.

Fig. 5. A penetration site after penetration, in which the cyst is seen to retain a large lipid body. Fixation–Embedding Schedule C. x23 500.

ABBREVIATIONS IN FIGURES

Ad	adhesorium	N	nucleus
AV	vacuole between amoebal envelope and host cytoplasm	NP	nuclear pore
		P	Rohr plug
CH	chromatin	Pa	Papilla
CW	cyst wall	PC	parasite cytoplasm
E	amoeba envelope	Pl	plastid
ER	endoplasmic reticulum	R	Rohr
FAM	fibrillar adhesive material	RW	Rohr wall
G	Golgi body	Sch	Schlauch
HC	host cytoplasm	St	Stachel
HPM	host plasma membrane	UIB	unidentified inclusion body
HW	host wall	V	cyst vacuole
L	lipid body	VG	vesicle with granular matrix
M	mitochondrion		

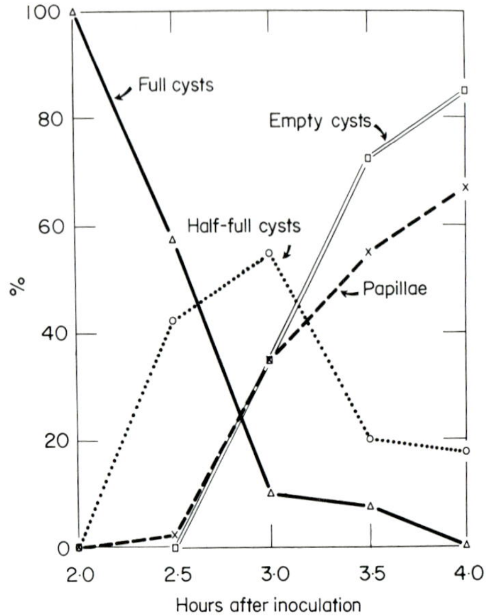

Fig. 6. The time course of cabbage root hair penetration by *P. brassicae.* Seedlings were exposed to zoospores for 30 min (pulse inoculation), then 2 h after beginning of inoculation, two seedlings were observed every 30 min and the percentage of cysts in each stage of development was determined. Ten cysts were observed per root. Most penetrations, indicated by appearance of empty cysts, occurred 2.5-3.5 h after the beginning of the pulse inoculation. Development of papillae was closely related in time to penetration. The difference at 4 h between the percentage of empty cysts and the percentage of penetration sites with papillae probably represents the percentage of cysts which forced most of their contents into the adhesoria without achieving host penetration.

many as 97% showed the response (Table I). We have observed that the younger a cell was at the time of infection, the greater was the distortion (Williams *et al.*, 1971).

The most rapid response to infection we have observed in the hair cell while the parasite was present has been the deposition of materials to form a papilla at the penetration site. Within 2-4 min after penetration a swelling, visible under the light microscope, appeared at the root hair wall just beneath the adhesorium. This swelling contained callose as indicated by a bright yellow-green fluorescence under u.v. illumination after staining with aniline blue (Jensen, 1962). In electron micrographs, the papilla was seen located between the host plasma membrane and the cell wall. It was composed primarily of irregularly-shaped light and moderately dark staining areas. The moderately dark staining areas resembled the host wall in texture and staining properties, but a parallel orientation of microfibrils was not apparent in papillae. Occasionally, the

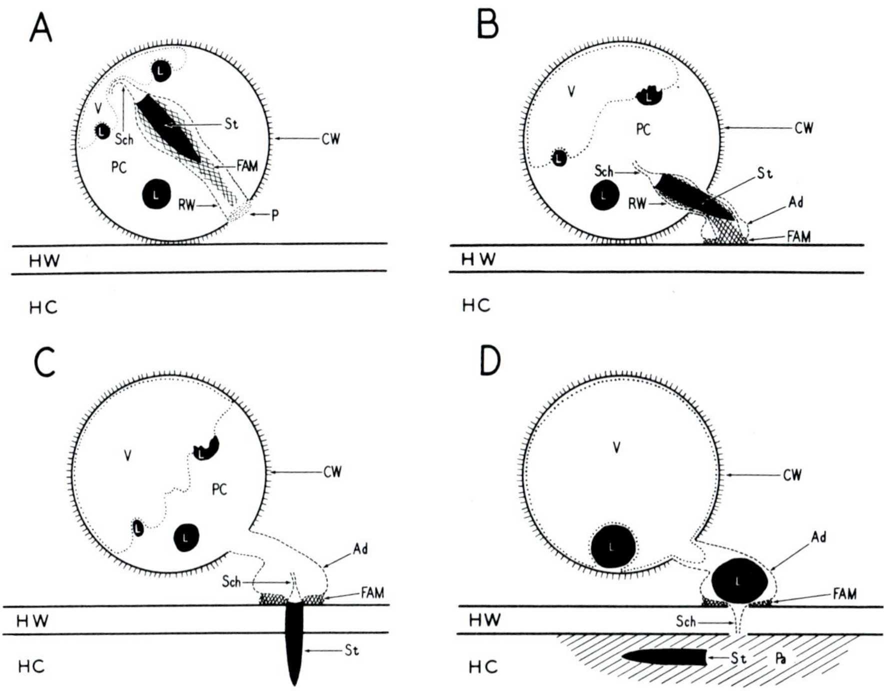

Fig. 7. Diagrammatic summary of penetration process. (A) Cyst vacuole has not yet enlarged; (B) vacuole enlarges and small adhesorium appears; (C) Stachel punctures host wall; (D) penetration has occurred and host protoplast has deposited a papilla at the penetration site.

papillae contained numerous moderately dense staining bodies with light staining borders. Vesicles with contents resembling these spherical bodies were found in areas of host cytoplasm adjacent to the papillae, suggesting that the contents of these vesicles may have been extruded through the host plasma membrane into the papilla. Several dense-staining bodies which were usually membrane-bounded were also found in papillae. The Stachel which was pushed aside when the parasite entered the host was also commonly found embedded in the papilla.

Discussion

The processes of encystment and penetration of cabbage root hairs by *P. brassicae* are remarkably similar to that described by Keskin and Fuchs (1969) for *Polymyxa betae* Keskin on beet roots. The terms for the infection structures are those used by Keskin and Fuchs with the exception of the 'adhesorium'

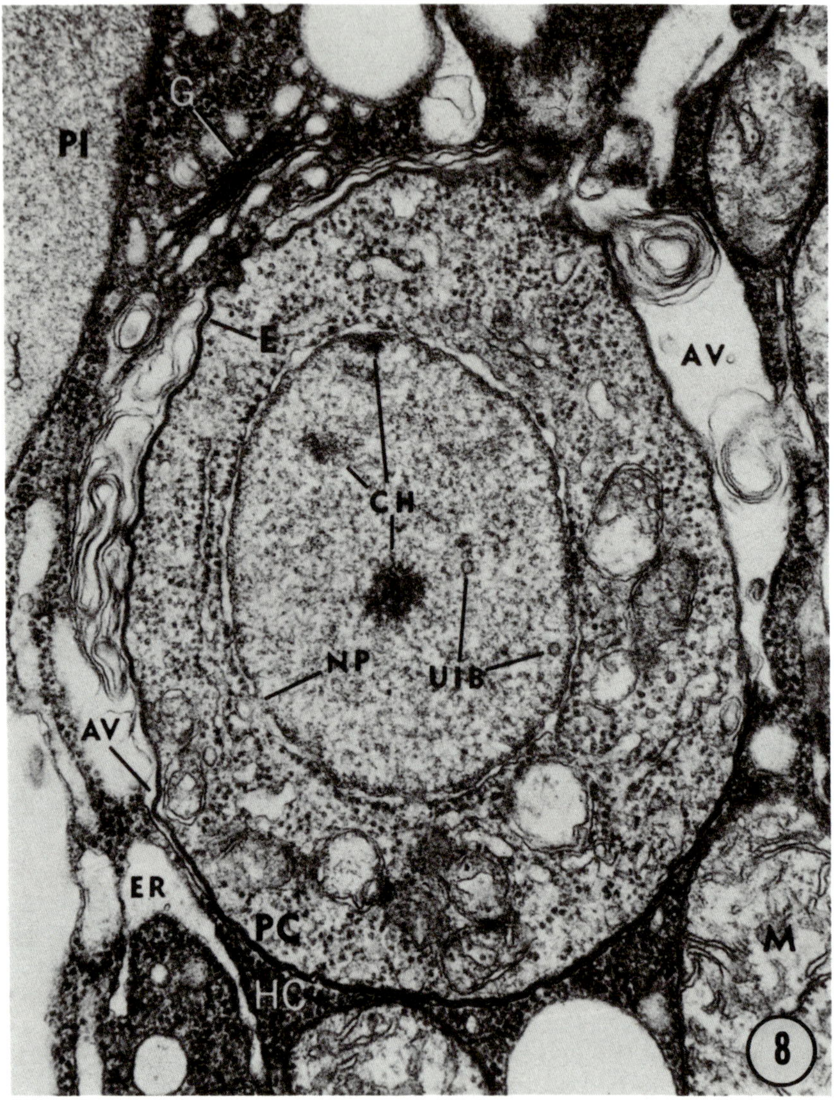

Fig. 8. A young amoeba in a root hair, surrounded by various host organelles. Over much of its surface the parasite envelope is separated from host cytoplasm by a large flattened vacuole, AV. Fixation–Embedding Schedule D. ×32,300.

which we have coined to replace more appropriately their term 'Stillet'. Penetration appears to be primarily a mechanical process without any conspicuous alterations in host wall texture or staining properties as occurs in the penetration by powdery mildews (McKeen *et al.*, 1969). The absence of

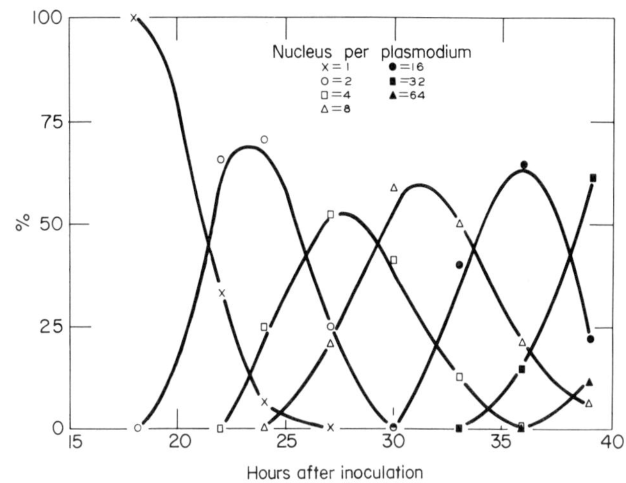

Fig. 9. The percentage of *Plasmodiophora brassicae* plasmodia containing 1, 2, 4, 8, 16, 32, or 64 nuclei per plasmodium recorded at 3 h intervals after a 1 h exposure of cabbage seedling root hair cells to zoospores of *P. brassicae.* At least 40 plasmodia were measured at each time.

stress signs in the wall microfibrils is probably due to the sharpness of the Stachel and the speed with which it is thrust through the wall. Though the nature and source of the forces involved in the penetration process are unknown, it is possible that adhesorium production and injection of the parasite result from pressure created within the cyst vacuole. Injection of the parasite may also be aided by contraction of the adhesorium which appears to be somewhat elastic.

Although the root hair stages of *P. brassicae* provide a measure of precision for the timing and observation of the infection process, those stages within the root hair represent only a short part of the life cycle of the parasite (Karling, 1968). The major portion of the life cycle of *P. brassicae* occurs within the cortical and stelar tissue of crucifer roots and involves the alteration of normal host cell differentiation into actively proliferating galls. Recently, Tommerup and Ingram (1971) have illustrated *P. brassicae* undergoing fusion of protoplasts from primary sporangia, mitosis within the multinucleate plasmodium and subsequent cleavage of the plasmodium into zoosporangia, all within dead cells of *Brassica napus* callus growing in tissue culture. Such stages, although appearing similar to those occurring in the root hairs, are not strictly analogous. In the dead callus cells, *P. brassicae* presumably did not undergo the net increase in volume observed when the plasmodia were actively growing within the cytoplasm of the living hair cell. The mitotic divisions preceding cleavage into zoosporangia in the dead callus cells resembled more closely the later stages of

TABLE I

The growth of uninucleate plasmodia of *Plasmodiophora brassicae* in cabbage root hair cells and the influence of the parasite on hair cell tip distortion and nucleolar size

Age of infection (h)	Condition of hair cell	Dia. of amoeba (μm)	% Amoebae with nucleoli	Dia. of hair cell nucleolus (μm)	% Hair cells distorted
0	noninfected	–	–	1.17 ± 0.01	10
	infected	0.85[1]	0	1.20 ± 0.04	13
2	noninfected	–	–	1.19 ± 0.02	7
	infected	0.85	0	1.21 ± 0.04	13
4	noninfected	–	–	1.04 ± 0.03	10
	infected	1.33	30	1.25 ± 0.05	20
6	noninfected	–	–	1.06 ± 0.04	13
	infected	1.54	77	1.43 ± 0.05	73
9	noninfected	–	–	1.11 ± 0.02	7
	infected	1.92	97	1.82 ± 0.03	87
15	noninfected	–	–	1.17 ± 0.01	10
	infected	2.43	100	1.93 ± 0.03	97
21	noninfected	–	–	1.18 ± 0.01	13
	infected	2.63	100	2.13 ± 0.03	90

[1] Figures represent averages of 30 cells. Root hairs were 20-24 h old. Roots were fixed in formalin-acetic acid-alcohol (Jensen, 1962) for 1 h following 1 h of pulse inoculation with zoospores. Small amoebae were detected under u.v. illumination after staining with acridine orange. Measurements were made under phase contrast optics.

TABLE II

The effect of *P. brassicae* infection on cabbage root hair cells, nuclear DNA, total protein, histone and non-histone protein

Cell condition	DNA	Histone	Total protein	Non-histone protein	DNA / histone	DNA / non-histone protein
Noninfected[1]	11.1 ± 0.36	10.2 ± 0.40	17.3 ± 0.92	7.1	1.08	1.56
Infected[2]	11.4 ± 0.19	8.8 ± 0.37	23.3 ± 1.0	14.5	1.35	0.77

[1] Figures represent arbitrary units of fluorescence from acridine yellow-Schiff (for DNA), geranine G, pH 8.1 (for histone), and geranine G, pH 2.8 (for total protein), corrected for background. Non-histone protein figures are obtained by subtracting histone from total protein values. Averages and standard errors are derived from 16-20 nuclear measurements.

[2] Infected cells were 42 h old and contained 1-5 plasmodia with 2-4 nuclei/plasmodium. (After Bhattacharya and Williams, 1971.)

TABLE III

The effect of *P. brassicae* infection on cabbage root hair cells, nuclear DNA, RNA and protein-bound lysine and arginine

Cell condition	DNA + RNA	DNA	RNA	Lysine	Arginine	DNA / lysine	DNA / arginine	Lysine / arginine
Noninfected[1]	28.3 ± 0.65	16.3 ± 0.32	12.0	7.2 ± 0.20	8.1 ± 0.27	2.26	2.0	0.88
Infected[2]	38.4 ± 1.04	17.0 ± 0.42	21.4	5.4 ± 0.09	8.0 ± 0.52	3.14	2.1	0.67

[1] Figures represent arbitrary units of fluorescence from berberine sulphate (for DNA + RNA and for DNA after RNA extraction), dansylchloride (for lysine) and ninhydrin (for arginine) corrected for background fluorescence. The values for RNA were obtained by subtracting DNA values from the combined DNA + RNA values. Averages and standard errors are for 20-30 nuclear measurements.

[2] Infected cells were 42 h old and contained 1-5 plasmodia with 2-4 nuclei/plasmodium. (After Bhattacharya and Williams, 1971.)

plasmodial growth and cleavage in the dead root hair cells. An electron microscope examination of the envelope surrounding the plasmodium in dead callus would provide important insight into the nature of the host–parasite interface. Both in our study and previously (Williams and McNabola, 1970), we have observed that during active vegetative growth the plasmodium was surrounded by a distinct seven-layered envelope, the outer part of which was thought to have been contributed by the host. In infected clubroot gall cells as cleavage into sporangia began the outer membrane of the envelope disintegrated, concomitantly with the death of the host cell, leaving the plasmodium bounded by a single unit membrane (Williams and McNabola, 1967).

Even though *P. brassicae* may be capable of existing saprophytically for periods of time in the absence of a living host, the need for a compatible nutritional relationship with the host is essential for growth of the young uninucleate amoeba. If it is assumed that the abundant supply of lipid within the resting sporangium and the zoospore serves as a primary source of carbon and energy, it appears that formation of the plasmodium by fusion of the zoospores would not deprive the parasite of a nutritional base for survival. Yet, the single zoospore upon penetration of the root hair is left without any lipid reserves and must rapidly establish a nutritional relationship with the host, if it is to survive.

Within the parasite, the reappearance of a nucleolus and lipid bodies was taken as an indication of the establishment of a compatible relationship between the host and the parasite. Nucleoli were first visible under the light microscope 4 h after penetration, suggesting that the events leading to the establishment of the parasite occur within this time. The accumulation of lipid droplets in the young plasmodium implied that the parasite was growing sufficiently well within the host to be undergoing net lipid synthesis.

During the first 4 h after penetration, the host also was undergoing profound changes in response to the parasite. In addition to the rapid deposition of material to form papillae at the puncture sites, the enhanced level of nuclear metabolism attested to an influence of the parasite on the host's genetic machinery. The decrease in the lysine-rich portion of the histone together with concomitant increases in nucleolar size, RNA, and non-histone protein suggests that the parasite may be altering the normal transcriptional processes of the nucleus. Higher levels of messenger RNA may require additional ribosomes to affect their expression in enhanced protein synthesis (Harris, 1968).

Though the nature of the regulatory information from the parasite remains unknown, the role of cytokinins and auxins in the clubroot gall formation has been investigated by a number of workers (Katsura *et al.*, 1966; Matsubara and Nakahira, 1968; Ingram, 1969a, b; Kavanagh *et al.*, 1969; Reddy and Williams, 1970; Dekhuijzen and Overeem, 1971). Auxins and cytokinins have both been implicated in the hypertrophy and hyperplasia of infected tissues. Whether *P. brassicae* is the source of these growth regulators or whether the parasite is stimulating the host to synthesize abnormal amounts of them is unknown (Ingram, 1969b). The restriction of host nuclear and nucleolar enlargement to infected cells in the clubroot gall (Williams, 1966) implicates regulatory compounds which are not transported, rather than auxins and cytokinins, beyond the parasitized cell.

The limited responses in nuclear metabolism of the root hair cell to infection by *P. brassicae* were in contrast to the clubroot gall cells. In the gall cells nuclear RNA, DNA, and histone were correlated positively with the number of parasite nuclei within the cell (Williams, 1966). Thus, in cells containing large plasmodia the nucleolar volumes were increased 30-fold and the DNA contents 16-fold compared with non-infected cells. In the root hair cell, although increasing numbers of plasmodia resulted in greater amounts of nucleolar RNA and protein, the lateral growth of the hair cell nucleolus was always less than 3 μm and nuclear DNA never increased. As we have suggested previously (Bhattacharya and Williams, 1971), perhaps the time at which the regulatory information of the parasite is received influences the host's subsequent development. In gall cells the parasite is within each cell and daughter cell from the time of its inception, whereas the hair cell is at least 6 h old before it is infected. The failure of host DNA to increase upon infection of the hair cell suggests that either the parasite is unable to stimulate host DNA synthesis or that the necessary receptors in the root hair for stimulation of DNA synthesis have been blocked or lost. The active DNA, RNA and protein synthesis accompanying plasmodial growth in the gall cells suggests that either the regulatory information from the parasite in the gall differs from that in the root hair, or that the information is being received by cells capable of responding differently from the root hairs.

The events determining the success of a compatible host–parasite relationship undoubtedly occur very soon after penetration. Perhaps an examination of interactions of the host with the parasite in the first few moments after penetration will provide a deeper understanding of this parasitic relationship.

SUMMARY

Penetration of cabbage root hairs by *Plasmodiophora brassicae* occurs by the injection of the parasite through a puncture in the host cell wall. This puncture is produced when a bullet-shaped 'Stachel' is forced from within the encysted zoospore through the hair cell wall. Penetration occurs in about one second, and once inside the host cytoplasm the young amoeba is swept away from the point of entry by cyclosis. Immediately following penetration, the host deposits a callose-rich papilla around the entry point. Shortly thereafter, the tip of the hair cell may swell and become club-shaped. The young uninucleate amoeba is surrounded by a multilayered envelope and has no nucleolus or lipid bodies.

Within 4 h after penetration, the growing amoeba acquires a nucleolus and begins to accumulate lipid bodies. After about 20 h in the hair cell, the amoeba undergoes nuclear division. Thereafter, synchronous divisions occur at about 4 h intervals up to about 48 h at which time the plasmodium sporulates and the hair cell dies. By 2 h after penetration, the nucleolus of the host cell has begun to enlarge, and by 20 h it has increased 6-fold in volume compared to nucleoli in non-infected cells. This increase in host nucleolar volume is accompanied by increases in nuclear RNA and non-histone protein content. Within the histone, the lysine-rich fraction declines whereas the arginine-rich fraction remains unchanged. Host nuclear DNA content also does not change with infection.

Acknowledgements

This research was supported by the College of Agricultural and Life Sciences, University of Wisconsin, Madison; by the National Kraut Packers Association; by Public Health Service Grant AI 4149; and by National Science Foundation Predoctoral Fellowships to J. R. Aist, Wisconsin Agricultural Experiment Station Project 118.

References

Aist, J. R. and Williams, P. H. (1971). The cytology and kinetics of cabbage root hair penetration by *Plasmodiophora brassicae* Wor. *Can. J. Bot.* **49**, 2023-2034.

Bhattacharya, P. K. and Williams, P. H. (1971). Microfluorometric quantitation of nuclear proteins and nucleic acids in cabbage root hair cells infected by *Plasmodiophora brassicae. Physiol. Pl. Pathol.* **1**, 167-175.

Dekhuijzen, H. M. and Overeem, J. C. (1971). The role of cytokinins in clubroot formation. *Physiol. Pl. Pathol.* **1**, 151-162.

Harris, H. (1968). 'Nucleus and cytoplasm'. The Clarendon Press, Oxford.

Ingram, D. S. (1969a). Growth of *Plasmodiophora brassicae* in host callus. *J. gen. Microbiol.* **55**, 9-18.

Ingram, D. ,S. (1969b). Abnormal growth of tissues infected with *Plasmodiophora brassicae. J. gen. Microbiol.* **56**, 55-67.

Jensen, W. A. (1962). 'Botanical histochemistry.' W. H. Freeman and Co., San Francisco and London.

Karling, J. S. (1968). 'The Plasmodiophorales,' 2nd edn. Hafner Publishing Company, New York and London.

Katsura, K., Egawa, H., Toki, T. and Ishii, S. (1966). On the plant hormones in the healthy and *Plasmodiophora* infected roots of *Brassica rapa* var. Neosuguki Kitam. I. *Ann. Phytopath. Soc. Japan* **32**, 123-129.

Kavanagh, J. A., Reddy, M. N. and Williams, P. H. (1969). Growth regulators in clubroot of cabbage. *Phytopathology* **59**, 1035.

Keskin, B. and Fuchs, W. H. (1969). Der infektionsvorgang bei Polymyxa betae. *Arch. Mikrobiol.* **68**, 218-226.

Macfarlane, I. (1958). A solution-culture technique for obtaining root-hair or primary infection by *Plasmodiophora brassicae*. *J. gen. Microbiol.* **18**, 720-732.

McKeen, W. E., Smith, R. and Bhattacharya, P. K. (1969). Alterations of the host wall surrounding the infection peg of powdery mildew fungi. *Can. J. Bot.* **47**, 701-706.

Matsubara, S. and Nakahira, R. (1968). Cytokinin activity in an extract from the gall of *Plasmodiophora*-infected root of *Brassica rapa* L. *Bot. Mag.* (*Tokyo*) **80**, 373-374.

Reddy, M. N. and Williams, P. H. (1970). Cytokinin activity in *Plasmodiophora brassicae*-infected cabbage tissue cultures. *Phytopathology* **60**, 1463-1465.

Tommerup, I. C. and Ingram, D. S. (1971). The life-cycle of *Plasmodiophora brassicae* Woron. in Brassica tissue cultures and in intact roots. *New Phytol.* **70**, 327-332.

Williams, P. H. (1966). A cytochemical study of hypertrophy in clubroot of cabbage. *Phytopathology* **56**, 521-524.

Williams, P. H. and McNabola, S. S. (1967). Fine structure of *Plasmodiophora brassicae* in sporogenesis. *Can. J. Bot.* **45**, 1665-1669.

Williams, P. H. and McNabola, S. S. (1970). Fine structure of the host-parasite interface of *Plasmodiophora brassicae* in cabbage. *Phytopathology* **60**, 1557-1561.

Williams, P. H., Aist, S. J. and Aist, J. R. (1971). Response of cabbage root hairs to infection by *Plasmodiophora brassicae*. *Can. J. Bot.* **49**, 41-47.

DISCUSSION

Dr D. S. Ingram: Would you like to speculate on the function of the papilla?

Professor P. H. Williams: I would not like to speculate on the function, but the papilla is a relatively non-specific response to mechanical injury of all sorts that may be commonly found in many types of cells. Material resembling the papilla develops around haustoria in resistant reactions and in some susceptible reactions of many of the obligate parasites. I suspect that this is almost a ubiquitous type of response to some form of wound in plant material. I do not know about algae, but it occurs in higher plants. Whether it is plugging the hole or not, I do not know.

Professor C. E. Bracker: I was interested to note that the older root hairs that you had worked with showed a very high percentage of clubbing, 90-97% on one of the slides that you showed. Were such root hairs elongating at the time that they were infected by *Plasmodiophora,* or had they ceased elongation?

Professor Williams: On that particular slide, all of the root hairs measured were within the same age range, about 20 h old. What you were looking at were root hairs that were now older, because they had been in contact with the parasite. At the time they were inoculated all the cells measured in that slide were less than two hours old, and were in a stage of elongation.

Professor Bracker: Do you know about root hairs that have ceased elongating? Do they club also?

Professor Williams: A general observation has shown that in the younger root hairs there is a much higher percentage of clubbing than occurs in the older ones that have slowed down or stopped elongating.

Professor Bracker: These root hair cells elongate at their tips, and have apical cytoplasmic apparatus very much like that of pollen tubes and fungal hyphae which also grow by tip growth. This apparatus consists of secretory vesicles that apparently participate in apical growth. Have you observed any disruption, alteration or any sort of change in the infected cells that undergo clubbing that would explain the different morphological manifestation of growth pattern at the apex of the clubbed root hair?

Professor Williams: The answer is no, but it is something that is begging to be done. You saw the deposition, that great blob of cell wall-like material, right there on the tip.

Professor Bracker: What is it? Does it look like the papilla?

Professor Williams: I should not say cell wall material, but it is PAS positive, it has a carbohydrate nature, it is not callose though, it is not wound type material, it does not fluoresce, so I suspect that it may be a product of disorganized secretion at the tip.

Professor Bracker: Once the clubbing occurs, does elongation of the hair cell continue or is growth shifted to the radical expansion in the production of the distorted club?

Professor Williams: They elongate a little, and sometimes they will even fork, but they lose their orientation. The ones I showed are quite distorted.

Professor M. A. Stahmann: You showed a very beautiful picture of the penetration of the Stachel through the cell wall and you thought it was mechanical penetration because there was no distortion of the cell wall. I would like to point out that if you drive a nail into a piece of wood you get considerable distortion of the fibres, and that the lack of distortion may suggest that this is not merely mechanical penetration. May I suggest that the penetration could be caused by insoluble enzymes coupled to the surface of the Stachel that hydrolyze the cell-wall constituents as they come into contact with the Stachel. This will give the same effect as drilling a very clean hole with a bit through a piece of wood. The pieces chipped out are chewed up or dispersed, but there is no effect beyond that. Recently, ways have been developed for linking enzymes to insoluble supports, and these insolubilized enzymes are often more stable than enzymes in solution. They are still active and they could act on the surface. So if I were a fungus and I wanted to drill through a cell wall in the most economical way, I would bind my hydrolytic enzymes to the surface which contacts with the cell wall. They then could drill a clean hole that would show no distortion. As plant pathologists, we should give serious consideration to a possible function for insoluble enzymes on the tip of a penetrating hypha, or on the tip of a penetrating Stachel, because this would be a very economical way for the fungus to hold on to its enzymes, and to penetrate with the least possible expenditure of enzymes or protein.

Professor Williams: Perhaps I did not make it clear that the actual time taken by the Stachel to pass through the wall is less than a second. I think this is a very interesting suggestion, but have you any ideas as to how we could study this problem?

Professor Stahmann: People do tend to study enzymes in solution, but I think that a high percentage of enzymes in cells are not in solution, and yet they are still active. We should search for enzyme activity in insoluble cell fractions. Contact between insoluble enzymes and the host surface may allow hydrolysis in a limited area. A localized hydrolysis by insoluble enzymes of the Stachel might give the appearance of mechanical penetration for there may be no visible change until the Stachel breaks through the wall.

Dr H. M. Dekhuijzen: Do you get the development of plasmodia in the root hairs in resistant cultivars?

Professor Williams: Yes we do. Resistance does not seem to be manifest at the root hair level as far as I know.

Dr Dekhuijzen: Then it is probably in the next stage of development?

Professor Williams: Probably.

Dr D. Pitt: I think the suggestion by Professor Stahmann of penetration of zoospores by insolubilized enzymes or packages of soluble enzymes, is very similar to the way in which certain penetrations of ova may be achieved by sperm acrosomes. This work of A. C. Allison and M. R. Young was reported some time ago, so it is not quite so farfetched as one might believe. (See 'Lysomes in Biology and Pathology' (ed. J. T. Dingle and H. B. Fell) Vol. 2, pp. 600-628. North-Holland Publishing Co., Amsterdam)

Dr J. A. Kavanagh: To what extent will you be able to adapt your techniques to detect metabolites or auxins, cytokinins or other hormones within the root hair?

Professor Williams: I do not think we have a hope of achieving this.

Dr Kavanagh: What are your views on the relationship of the plasmodium, zoosporangia etc., in the life cycle of *P. brassicae* and when does conjugation of the amoebae emerging from the infected root occur (or does it occur?).

Professor Williams: I would not say this is the beginning of the life cycle, but it is that phase of the life cycle that we have illustrated. If you can recall the life cycle it is interesting to see that the plasmodium grows rapidly, and you saw a fairly large one (towards the end of my talk) stained with acridine orange; then it rounds up, cleaves and produces a zoosporangium, in which there are zoospores. These zoospores, let us call them secondary zoospores, germinate from the zoosporangia and swim around in the root hair. They then leave the root hair by the same mechanism using a Stachel, as they got in. After they get out of the root hair and fuse, as Dr Ingram and Dr Tommerup have shown, the zoospore gets back into the host to finally cause the clubroot gall, but how this occurs is something we do not yet know.

Dr Ingram: Am I right in assuming the clubbing of the root hairs is not a response specific to *Plasmodiophora brassicae,* but is fairly common in occurrence?

Professor Williams: The clubbing response is common to a wide range of things that are probably injurious or at least which alter the orientation of the cell extension apparatus. We know that if we apply auxin, the hairs club, and this occurs with many other toxins and bacteria, although the concentration of contaminating bacteria may itself produce auxin. There are many things that may cause this clubbing response. I think this is a pretty non-specific type of response to a parasite.

Dr E. C. Hislop: Did I understand rightly that the papilla is only formed after penetration?

Professor Williams: Yes, we get no papilla throughout the process of penetration, or prior to it.

Dr Hislop: Following some interference pictures that you showed, may I ask if there is any indication of a host reaction to the presence of the encysted zoospore prior to penetration such as occurs in hosts inoculated with powdery mildews?

Professor Williams: What you saw in the interference pictures was cytoplasm streaming past the penetration point. As it streams it forms into blobs and all sorts of shapes, which often look like a papilla.

III.3 Structural Concepts of Host–Pathogen Interfaces*

C. E. BRACKER

Department of Botany and Plant Pathology, Purdue University, Lafayette, Indiana, U.S.A.

and

L. J. LITTLEFIELD

Plant Pathology Department, North Dakota State University, Fargo, North Dakota, U.S.A.

Introduction, Objectives and Scope

When a fungus invades a plant and establishes a parasitic relationship, it is entering into an association which obviously is not the same as when the fungus is cultured on artificial media in a laboratory. The fungus must confront the host. The host is alive; it has highly organized cells and barriers which must be breached if the fungus is to gain a foothold. The host acts, reacts, and interacts. As a result it may exclude the fungus, prevent it from developing, or even kill it. Or the host may provide the conditions that are conducive and necessary to the development of the fungus, but often at great expense to itself. Although interfaces occur at tissue, cellular, subcellular, and molecular levels, we limit our discussion mainly to cellular and subcellular interfaces.

The host-pathogen interface is one of the most significant, yet elusive, regions of a diseased organism for understanding how a disease is initiated and maintained. It is important because it is the region of direct interaction between a host and pathogen and thus is the zone through which materials that elicit responses in either partner are exchanged. It is elusive because it is so difficult to define or to delimit. Where are the boundaries of the host-pathogen interface, what does it consist of, and how can it be recognized? What is its real significance? We can even ask, what is the concept of the host-pathogen interface, and is it a useful concept to employ in considering disease phenomena?

First, it is necessary to establish the scope of this chapter:

(1) At the Long Ashton Symposium we presented information on the ultrastructure of two host-parasite systems: powdery mildews and rusts. But in

* A table of contents appears after this paper, on p. 318.

our written contribution, we consider it far more valuable to consider a broad spectrum of host–pathogen combinations rather than merely repeating the specific information that we have published elsewhere (Bracker, 1967, 1968; Littlefield, 1972; Littlefield and Bracker, 1970, 1972). Thus, we are concerned with host–pathogen interfaces generally in plant diseases, and we have gone beyond the associations between fungi and higher plants to include information from other systems that contributes to wider concepts of host–pathogen or host–symbiont interfaces. However, we emphasize associations in which at least one of the partners is a plant, with only brief mention of systems that do not involve plants. The terms *host–symbiont, host–pathogen*, and *host–parasite* are considered nearly equivalent for this discussion and are sometimes used interchangeably (see section on Terminology). Therefore, several non-pathogenic, symbiotic relationships are included because of the striking similarities among interface types in highly diverse kinds of associations. We are struck by the large number of organisms that live on or within other organisms. When this work was originally conceived, we did not appreciate thoroughly either the uniformity of interface types over a broad taxonomic range of symbiotic partners, or the large number of different interface types related especially to different developmental stages of a single host–pathogen association. However, such an appreciation did develop during the preparation of the chapter, and we hope this will be conveyed to the reader. We are not providing a comprehensive bibliography or list of host–pathogen associations. Rather, we have selected examples which illustrate important similarities and differences among interface types, demonstrate developmental sequences, and contribute to an overall concept of interfaces.

(2) The scope of a discourse is determined by the type of information the authors choose to include in their discussion. We realize that interfaces may be considered from biochemical, structural, and other standpoints. We are chiefly concerned with structural aspects of host–pathogen interfaces, and most of our considerations are based on our knowledge and interpretation of the ultrastructure of interfaces. The histology of host–parasite relations has been reviewed previously (Akai, 1959; Rice, 1927; Suzuki, 1965) and will not be repeated here. Our analysis of ultrastructure will draw on studies based on light microscopy when they contribute to our understanding of ultrastructural phenomena. We realize that there are also biochemical interfaces which may or may not be linked with cellular structures, but we leave the discussion of biochemical interactions to those better qualified to explain disease phenomena in biochemical terms. Obviously, a fully-integrated concept of any disease situation requires biochemical as well as morphological explanations. But it is still too soon to achieve the reconciliation of many cytological and biochemical studies. This remains as an important goal for ever more sophisticated cell biological research.

(3) The reader's and our own interests are served by identifying areas of contention and conflict as well as those issues which are known as uncontested fact and those which have not yet been approached. One of the obvious matters of continuing controversy is the terminology used to refer to structures at host–pathogen interfaces. We recognize the problems of terminology, but we have decided not to develop a full discourse on terminology in this paper. That is a lengthy and separate task. Instead, we will identify and explain the terminology we use (see section on Terminology, p. 165). Ultimately a unified terminology, backed by definitions of terms, must emerge to accommodate intelligent discussion of the facts and problems concerning host–parasite interactions.

Our goal is to provide a conceptual framework into which the various kinds of structural relationships may be placed. We hope that this clarification and categorization will provide a degree of order in an otherwise chaotic segment of biology. The many and diverse studies of host-parasite interactions have provided a wealth of information, and it is now possible to start integrating this information into a coherent framework. Hopefully, the conceptual analysis of the morphological aspects of host-symbiont relations can eventually be coupled with comparable analyses of the physiological bases of symbiotic associations (e.g. Smith *et al.*, 1969) to provide a unified and more complete understanding of the host–symbiont association.

We begin with the necessary premise of our review: the concept of the host-pathogen (host-symbiont) interface. We will then discuss the various types of interfacial situations associated with a variety of host–pathogen and host–symbiont combinations, emphasizing intracellular relationships. Near the end of the chapter is a section illustrating diagrammatically the different combinations of components that comprise host–symbiont interfaces and how these may differ in space and time as a developmental sequence is followed.

The Concept of Interfaces as Applied to Host–Pathogen Associations

Interface is defined as 'a surface forming a common boundary of two bodies, spaces, or phases' (Webster's Seventh New Collegiate Dictionary). Taken literally, this definition is too narrow to be meaningful or accurate in discussions of symbiotic or pathogenic interactions because it presupposes a two-dimensional boundary or surface that constitutes the single interface between two interacting organisms. The concept of host–pathogen interfaces is more complicated and does not yet lend itself to a rigid definition. Perhaps **interfacial zone** better describes the three-dimensional multi-component region that usually comprises the region between interacting protoplasts in a symbiotic/pathogenic relationship.

A **concept** represents an integration of all the individual components included. In contrast, a **definition** specifies only the distinguishing characteristics of a concept and need not identify explicitly each specific example included under the concept. Because a concept refers to all of the attributes of its units, we think it is desirable to develop the interface concept first by describing its scope and the problems of definition and then by discussing concrete examples of interfaces as they exist in plant disease and in several non-pathogenic symbiotic associations. In this section, we will develop our understanding of what constitutes a host-symbiont or host-pathogen interface. The full concept, however, will emerge as a result of the descriptions and interpretations of host-symbiont interactions, their similarities and differences, the structures involved, the development of structures and relationships, and the terminology that applies to these systems.

The interface must be thought of in the broadest terms possible. To illustrate this point, consider the following questions. Are the components of the interface different depending on whether one is considering inter- or intra-cellular parasites within a host? Furthermore, is the interface variable in space and in time, as demonstrated by considering different regions of a haustorium or different stages during its development? Can the limits of the interface be set with precision? Does the interface consist only of structures of the respective organisms that are in direct contact, or does it also include cell components that are closely associated but not in contact? How is the interface defined when a pathogen secretes toxins having drastic effects upon cells and organelles that are distant from the pathogen? Is such a biochemical interface also to be considered under the concept of host–pathogen interfaces? Must a cell component be a functional part of the interaction between host and parasite in order to be considered part of the interface? These are the kinds of questions that must be considered when establishing a framework in which to fit the many host–parasite relationships that have been and will continue to be described.

Cytologically, we consider the host–pathogen interface to consist of those structures and materials occurring at sites of host–pathogen interaction. We specify **structures** (plural) because the interface is actually a three-dimensional zone or region and not a single line or boundary. It is difficult to limit the interface to a single boundary or component because the interactions which do occur may be distributed across several structures, and it is not always clear to which partner a specific component belongs. Moreover, the concept of the host–pathogen interface must include structures in either the host or pathogen which are *specifically* associated with the interaction at or around the site of interaction. Inadvertent or chance associations of cell components may also contribute to a functional interfacial zone, but without some evidence of specific association it is difficult to know whether to include these structures as part of the interface.

Structures at the host-pathogen interface may change during the development of a disease, and may differ from one part of the pathogen or host to another. Thus, the interface covers a region in time as well as space, and the components of the interface at one stage of development may be different from the components at another stage. For example, consider the interacting cell components of an intercellular hypha in a plant leaf. Then consider which components would interact as the fungus contacts a host cell, forms a haustorial mother cell, and begins to penetrate the host cell wall. Then consider the growth and development of a haustorium within the host cell. Finally, consider the cell components of both host and parasite at a time when the host cell has changed drastically, is becoming disrupted, and is approaching death. An example of such a sequence is shown in Fig. 83. For every host-pathogen association, the interfaces involved must be considered over the entire time course of the development of the relationship. No other approach can characterize fully the interfaces or illuminate symbiosis or parasitic disease as a *process*.

What then are the limits of the host–pathogen interface? We hope the reader will appreciate that it is nearly impossible at this stage of understanding to set rigid limits on the components of the interface. We will show examples of what certainly are parts of the interface, but undoubtedly new knowledge will alter our perspective and add new information to expand the list of components that can be considered part of the interfacial region. At any one time or place the interface may consist of any or all of the following:

(i) Normal host cell components (i.e. those in a form and functional state characteristic of a healthy or non-invaded cell).
(ii) Normal components of the pathogen (symbiont) cell.
(iii) Structures of host or pathogen that are modified as a result of the interaction.
(iv) Intimate combinations or mixtures of material or structures derived from both host and pathogen.
(v) Newly formed structures or materials that are not normally present in either host or pathogen when either organism is grown separately.

As a starting point for locating the host–pathogen interface more specifically, we consider that if two closely associated cells are interacting in a parasitic relationship, the boundaries of the living protoplasts should be included in the definition of the interfacial zone. Thus, all structures and materials between the plasma membranes of the respective participants should be considered components of the interface, whether or not they play an active role in disease development or the dynamic interactions between the two organisms. Our premise is that the plasma membrane of a cell is the limit of the protoplasm, and it is mainly the protoplasm that acts and reacts in an interaction. Cell walls and surface coats are often important and even critical in cell–cell interactions. But it is the surface membrane of the protoplasm that would be the first limit of the protoplasmic interaction. In all probability the interface does not end at the plasma membrane. Structures within the cytoplasm of host and/or pathogen (symbiont) should also be included. Several examples discussed in this paper will illustrate this point. Of course there are exceptions to the generalization that plasma membranes of both participants are parts of the interfacial region. The most notable example is with non-cellular pathogens such as plant viruses which have no membrane of their own, but other exceptions also exist in which the plasma membrane of one or the other partner is absent or degenerate.

The concept of the host–pathogen interface is further complicated by the fact that at any given time in one interfacial region there may be many interfaces, depending on what entity is used as a criterion. We noted that there may be biochemical interfaces which are not represented by discrete structures detectable by microscopy. Different molecular constituents may be in contact at different sites in a zone of interaction, and so we must not be deluded into thinking that a single line or even a zone represents the entire interface with respect to all interacting entities. In other words, there may be many sub-interfaces within a single interfacial zone.

If it is recognized that the host–pathogen (symbiont) interface is a three-dimensional multi-component system, we can then proceed to identify the major specific components that comprise the interfacial zone. Any or all of the following may be considered interface components depending on whether or not they are present:– cell walls or other surface coats of host and pathogen (symbiont) host cuticle, wall-like apposition layers on the inner face of the wall of either host or pathogen, matrix materials (amorphous, gel liquid, etc.) which may coat the walls of the host and/or pathogen and intervene between the protoplasts of the two organisms, plasma membranes, and cytoplasmic components of each partner (including moribund protoplasm in some instances).

Based on the presence or absence of the various interface components, we have identified a range of categories of interface types (IT) and presented them diagrammatically (pp. 232-241). Each interface type is assigned a number (IT 1, IT 2, IT 3, etc.), and many of these are cited in the text where they are applicable to a particular example under discussion. We hope this will help the reader to link the descriptive accounts, the pertinent electron micrographs, and the diagrammatic spatial arrangement of components within the respective interfaces.

The type of interface between a host and pathogen is determined in part by the type of interaction. For infections by facultative parasites, in which the host is killed in advance of the fungus, the host–pathogen interface extends over a long distance–from the fungal cell to the place where fungal products are interacting with living host cells. The dead and degenerate host cells in between may be part of that interfacial region, but the interface cannot be assigned to a single site in that region because living host cells at the edge of the lesion are also being influenced by the pathogen, albeit at a considerable distance from the pathogen. On the other hand, in interactions of parasites which form intracellular haustoria, e.g. a living haustorial cell within a living host cell, the host–parasite interface is more localized and perhaps more important conceptually because the interaction is more direct if for no other reason than physical closeness of the two living protoplasts. Thus, most of our considerations of interfaces relate to those systems in which living cells of both host and pathogen exist in intimate association. Surprisingly, there are also many different types of functional interactions characterized by remarkably similar cytological interface types. Thus, it will become obvious that some interface types are widespread, whereas others pertain only to restricted specific examples.

Not all interactions (consequently interfaces) between cells of different organisms result in disease. Good examples include mutual symbiotic relationships such as those encountered with root nodule bacteria, mycorrhizae, lichens, and endosymbionts in lower organisms. Furthermore, an organism may interact with itself in ways that mimic parasitic associations. Examples include the attempted infection of hyphae of *Erysiphe polygoni* by itself (Leong *et al.*, 1970), and penetration of sclerotial cells of *Verticillium albo-atrum* by its own cells (Nadakavukaren, 1963). Normal development processes in fungi also parallel some of the interactions that often characterize host–pathogen interactions (e.g. hyphal anastomosis, sexual unions, formation of intrahyphal hyphae). Thus, cell–cell interfaces exist even without parasitic or symbiotic associations. They deserve brief mention here, but hereafter we shall consider only interfaces between interacting organisms of different types.

In summary, we emphasize the flexibility of interpretation encompassed by the concept of the host–pathogen interface. It is necessarily a broad concept, and we caution against defining it in a way that limits its usefulness. The interface is a three-dimensional zone, which may change in time and space, and the specific components of that zone must be defined and identified for each specific example of host–pathogen interaction. Upon that basis, we can draw generalizations and categorize interfacial types by integrating fundamental similarities and by differentiating them according to objective criteria.

Terminology

Controversies over the terminology used for structures at host–pathogen interfaces still exist (e.g. Bracker, 1968; Bushnell, 1972; Ehrlich and Ehrlich, 1971a; Hardwick *et al.*, 1971; Littlefield and Bracker, 1972), and it is necessary to select some terminology in order to refer to the entities under discussion. We favour a terminology that is broadly applicable and with a hierarchy of terms to match the hierarchy of concepts and structures we are dealing with. We will use terms consistent with those used and explained in our previous studies (Bracker, 1968; Littlefield and Bracker, 1972) but with some minor modifications.

We have found dictionary definitions useful in clarifying the meaning of some terms, but it must be recognized that the terminology used here is contextual, i.e. used in the context of host–pathogen associations. Thus, a generic term such as **sheath** that has wide application over a spectrum of disciplines acquires a specific meaning when used contextually and when used with an appropriate adjective to clarify the meaning, i.e. **haustorial sheath, hyphal sheath**, etc. The specific adjective is part of the complete term, but it may be omitted when the term is repeatedly used, in proper context, and where the meaning of the generic term has been established and is clear.

Hanchey and Wheeler (1971) used the term **wall lesion** to refer to wall-like deposits or elaborations derived from a host cell and laid down on a host wall or around an invading parasitic cell. Wall lesion is a good term but implies a broader meaning than just wall deposits, since *lesion* means a localized abnormal structural change, injury, or impairment (usually induced by some inciting factor). Thus, a wall lesion would include localized degradation or ruptures of the wall as well as abnormally induced swellings or growths or deposits on the wall.

Wall apposition describes the kind of wall lesion characterized by an increase in the wall mass by addition to the surface of the wall. **Apposition** is the act or product of things placed side by side, in contact, or together. Thus, an apposition may occur by deposition upon an existing wall or by appositional growth onto the surface of an existing wall. Therefore, a wall apposition would, by definition, include wall or 'wall-like' growths or deposits upon the cell wall. There may be many types of appositions consisting of various materials and consistencies but with some sort of recognized structure (not merely a solution) which is continuous with the cell wall. Appositions include wall-like materials that appear texturally different from the wall proper as well as those that are indistinguishable from the texture of the wall by electron microscopy. There are several types of wall appositions, viz.:

(i) A **papilla** (Bracker, 1968; Smith, 1900) is characterized by a mound or nipple-shaped lump of material deposited or grown onto the cell wall. The demarcation between the papilla and the wall proper may or may not be clearly evident.

(ii) A **collar** (Bracker, 1968; Littlefield and Bracker, 1972) is a ring or collar-like wall apposition, a flange or perforated disk that surrounds the proximal extremity of a haustorium or other penetrating organ. A collar may result from penetration of a papilla, or by a process of apposition after host penetration.

(iii) An **encasement** (Littlefield and Bracker, 1972) extends over a haustorium or other penetrating organ in such a way that the part of the parasite inserted into the host cell is partially or completely enclosed. This term is distinguished from collar by a matter of degree and requires judgement to distinguish borderline cases.

Intracellular invaders are often surrounded by a **matrix** or **sheath** that is distinct from the wall-like appositions just described, although at our present state of understanding there may be some examples in which it is difficult to distinguish between a wall apposition and a matrix or sheath. We use the terms sheath and matrix interchangeably with suitable adjectives to specify the particular kind involved. The sheath includes the whole of the matrix surrounding an invading cell, but excluding the bounding membrane, if there is one, as well as excluding what can clearly be shown to be the wall of the host and/or parasite, and any intact form of wall apposition. A sheath may vary in thickness and size, may consist of different regions and phases (sol, gel, solutions, colloids, layers, etc.), and is not restricted to any particular biochemical characterization or to a single or specific origin (i.e. is not necessarily host-derived or symbiont-derived). Since a sheath is actually an extracellular matrix, this is consistent with what Bushnell (1972) refers to as the extrahaustorial matrix, a descriptive and useful term that has the same meaning as **haustorial sheath** in our terminology. A matrix which consists only of a solution (no mucilage, fibres, colloids, etc.) would still be a kind of sheath.

The reader will note that we have used the terms **host–symbiont**, **host–pathogen**, and **host–parasite** almost interchangeably in referring to interactions and interfaces between dissimilar organisms. For many situations, the three terms can be used interchangeably. We consider host–symbiont to be more general than the other two, and where parasite or pathogen are accurately applicable, we use them.

For this discussion we consider the term **symbiosis** as defined in its broadest aspect in Webster's Third New International Dictionary: '1a: the living together in more or less intimate association or even close union of two dissimilar organisms (as in parasitism, mutualism, or commensalism) . . .' Henry (1966) traces the term symbiosis to DeBary and notes that the relationship must be constant, intimate, and between dissimilar species. But he points out that the term has been misused to indicate mutualism when in fact **mutualism** and **parasitism** are more aptly considered two of the several types of symbiosis. Consequently, we regard diseases of plants which result from microbial, viral or phanerogamic infections to be a type of symbiosis.

The term **symbiont** is used for a pathogenic as well as a non-pathogenic organism, as long as it is the smaller partner (exceptions in the case of equal-sized mycoparasites and hosts), and resides close to, on, or at least in part within, the **host**, the larger partner. This terminology is consistent with that established by the Committee on Terminology of the American Society of

Parasitologists (Hertig *et al.*, 1937). According to this concept, host–symbiont interface, host–parasite interface, and host–pathogen interface may, for all practical purposes, be used interchangeably since they do not differ in any distinct, consistent, morphological manner, except that some symbionts are not pathogens. Whether associations such as those involving wood-decay fungi or invasion of dead host cells following death caused by toxins of the pathogen are truly symbiotic associations since one of the partners is dead (at least on a cellular level), is open to question. However, to compile a list of host–symbiont interfaces we have included these examples of wood-decay fungi and others in which the pathogen is in contact with a non-living host cell. Likewise, we include a section on predatory relationships as illustrated by nematode-trapping fungi and microbial ingestion by predatory cells. Although these relationships are not truly symbiotic, information concerning their respective interfaces contributes to the understanding of interface types and their interaction in the symbiotic associations.

Other terms used in this paper are defined as they arise or are used as applied by the original authors. Hopefully, the day will come when explanations of terminology in reviews such as this will not be necessary.

Intercellular Relationships

By definition, intercellular symbionts or pathogens are those that grow between or among cells of a host. Consequently, the most intimate interface between two such organisms would be cell wall to cell wall of the respective partners. Some intercellular pathogens may also invade dead or moribund host cells, and we include these post-penetration stages in the section on intracellular relationships (p. 176). Although intercellular pathogens contact host cells, the nature of the association and the regions of mutual influence of the respective organisms upon one another are quite diverse. The actions of diffusible enzymes, toxins, or other materials can effect drastic changes in host cells far removed from the pathogen. Thus, although morphologically distinct interfaces may exist, the functional boundaries of such interfaces are extremely difficult to identify.

Separation of Host and Pathogen

Intercellular hyphae may be in direct contact with cell walls of the host (IT 8, IT 9) (Figs 2 and 4), or the walls of the two organisms may be slightly separated by an extracellular matrix surrounding the hypha (IT 13, IT 14) (Fig. 6). This material forms a sheath-like covering over the hyphae (IT 46) and can be amorphous, granular, fibrillar, gelatinous, or slimy (Horino and Akai, 1968a; Liese and Schmid, 1963; Reichle, 1965; Schmid, 1966; Schmid and Balderman, 1967; Schmid and Liese, 1965; 1968). Electron microscopic cytochemistry has shown the extracellular coating in some species to contain acid mucopolysaccharides (Schmid and Balderman, 1967; Schmid and Liese, 1968). These materials, as well as enzymes or other metabolites of the fungus involved in interactions with the host cells might occur initially in cytoplasmic vesicles near the hyphal tips and then be transferred to the cell surface by exocytosis. Secretory vesicles are known to be involved in hyphal tip growth (Grove and Bracker, 1970) as well as penetration of host cells by some parasites (Lesemann and Fuchs, 1970a) and a variety of secretory processes in eukaryotes (Morré and Mollenhauer, 1972).

SUBCUTICULAR HABIT

Some fungal pathogens, most notably the apple scab fungus, *Venturia inaequalis*, inhabit the subcuticular stratum of epidermal cell walls of plant hosts (Figs 2, 9 and 10). The interface between cells of the host and the hypha in such instances would be IT 8 and IT 13. However, other interfaces exist as well, but not in apposition with the host (e.g. IT 37, IT 39, IT 42). Another example of subcuticular growth of a pathogen occurs in *Helminthosporium oryzae* infections of rice (Horino and Akai, 1968a). For a short time following penetration of the cuticle, and before invasion of the internal tissues of the leaf, the hyphae grow parallel to the leaf surface between the upper limit of the epidermal cell wall and the overlying cuticle. The interface types prior to mesophyll penetration would be equivalent to those occurring with *Venturia* infections. Prior to cuticular penetration by *V. inaequalis,* the host–pathogen interface consists of the two respective cell walls, separated by host cuticle as well as by an amorphous matrix surrounding the appressorium (IT 38). In the appressorium, at the time of cuticular penetration, the contents of a membrane-limited 'infection sac' are contiguous with a thin region of the appressorial wall immediately adjacent to the site of cuticle degradation (Fig. 8) (Maeda, 1970). The association of the infection sac with cuticular penetration makes the sac a component of the interface, and its position in relation to cuticular breakdown suggests that it may function in the penetration process. Nicholson *et al.* (1972) used histochemical methods to demonstrate the presence of esterase activity in the appressoria of *V. inaequalis*, and they suggested an association of the enzyme with cuticular penetration. It remains to determine definitively whether the infection sac is the site of enzymes necessary for cuticle breakdown, but the combined evidence of Maeda (1970) and Nicholson *et al.* (1972) strongly indicates that the cuticle is breached by biochemical breakdown. In contrast, Mercer *et al.* (1971) showed ultrastructural evidence that appressoria of an intracellular pathogen, *Colletotrichum lindemuthianum*, could penetrate cured epoxy resin to a depth twice that of host cuticle, and they concluded that this fungus could probably push a penetration peg mechanically through a cuticle (see also pp. 199-203 for information on cuticular penetration by haustorial pathogens).

ALTERATION OF HOST CELL WALLS

As pathogens grow between host cells, cell walls may separate along the middle lamella (Fig. 4) (Akai *et al.*, 1971; Chilvers, 1968; Foster and Marks, 1966; Heath and Wood, 1969; Horino and Akai, 1968b; von Hofsten, 1969) or be degraded, dissolved, or otherwise altered (e.g. Calonge, 1969). Hyphae of *Ascochyta pisi* split the host wall and grow within the layers of the wall (Fig. 3) (Heath and Wood, 1969). *Venturia inaequalis* causes limited but distinct erosion of the outer epidermal wall just beneath the cuticle (Fig. 10) and in some tissues even causes extensive wall degradation as it grows between and among host cells (Maeda, 1970).

The various patterns of cell wall disintegration at the interface between the walls of host cells and the fungi causing wood decay have been reviewed by Liese (1970) and Cowling (1965). These patterns of disintegration vary from localized bore holes associated with growth of blue stain fungi (Liese, 1970) and the closely related Dutch elm disease pathogen (MacDonald and McNabb, 1970) (Fig. 7) to extensive dissolution of the wall by basidiomycetes which exude enzymes over a long period of time and from regions of hyphae other than the tips (Liese, 1970).

Host cell walls may be inordinately thickened (Heath and Wood, 1969), or extensive dark-staining wall-like or membranous deposits may form on the inner side of the host cell wall adjacent to the plasma membrane (IT 11) (Bird, 1961; Huang and Maggenti, 1969; Luke *et al.*, 1966; Paulson and Webster, 1969). Cell wall elaborations also form on the inner side of host epidermal cell walls underneath subcuticular stromata of *Venturia inaequalis* in tissues exhibiting various host reactions (Maeda, 1970). Wall appositions even occur in cells of bean tissue beneath points of contact with intercellular hyphae of *Uromyces phaseoli* var. *vignae*, a nonpathogen of that plant (IT 11 or IT 16) (Heath, 1972) (see also Fig. 54). A similar response of a nonhost plant to rust mycelium was also shown by light microscopy (Leath and Rowell, 1969).

In some lichens there appear to be no ultrastructural changes in the wall of the phycobiont (IT 8) compared to free-living cells (Chervin *et al.*, 1968; Durrell, 1967; Peat, 1968), whereas in other species the algal wall is thicker in the region of contact with the mycobiont (Galun *et al.*, 1970b). In contrast, the fungal wall is thinned out at points of contact with algal cells in other lichens (Chervin *et al.*, 1968). The cell wall of the intercellular, parasitic green alga *Cephaleuros virescens* is thickened where it contacts the host cuticle (Joubert and Rijkenberg, 1971). Difficulty in establishing a rigid concept of the host–symbiont interface in lichens results from the great range of growth habit from purely intercellular hyphae to distinct haustoria, depending partly on the phylogenetic position of the lichen (Galun *et al.*, 1970a, 1971a), the environment in which a particular species is grown (Ben-Shaul *et al.*, 1969; Galun *et al.*, 1970c), and the stage of maturity of the thallus (Galun *et al.*, 1970a). Chervin *et al.* (1968), has suggested that the degree of penetration of the alga by the fungus (consequently altering the components of the interface) may be an expression of the degree of parasitism exerted by the fungus.

The significance of host cell walls in the interactions between hosts and parasites was discussed in detail by Albersheim *et al.* (1969), although a consideration of ultrastructure was not included. Their hypothesis is that the host cell wall determines the pathogen's ability to produce enzymes capable of degrading the host's cell wall. The production of these enzymes determines whether or not a successful infection will be initiated. The dynamic and variable nature of this wall-wall interface is enhanced by changes in chemical composition of the host wall during normal growth and differentiation as well as by changes resulting from parasitic infections.

ALTERATION OF HOST CELL MEMBRANES

Effects of intercellular pathogens upon the integrity of host cell membranes may result from diffusible substances produced by the pathogen or to deleterious reaction products of the host cells stimulated by materials from the intercellular pathogen. The effects of several bacterial and fungal toxins upon host cells have been reviewed recently in Wood *et al.* (1972). Victorin, the pathotoxin produced by *Helminthosporium victoriae,* causes, among other responses, extensive disruption of the internal membrane systems of susceptible host cells (Luke *et al.*, 1966). Damage to the host plasma membrane is regarded as the major cause of altered permeability and subsequent plasmolysis of cells of susceptible oat tissue treated with victorin (Hanchey *et al.*, 1968; Hanchey and Wheeler, 1969). Recent studies by Keck and Hodges (1973) showed marked changes in permeability of the host cell tonoplast as well as the plasma membrane when oat roots were treated with victorin toxin. Similarly diffusible toxins or enzymes originating from intercellular hyphae of *Sclerotinia fructigena* and *Phytophthora palmivora* (Calonge, 1969; Calonge *et al.*, 1969), *Pyrenochaeta terrestris* (Hess, 1969), *Fusarium solani* f sp. *phaseoli* (Reichle, 1965), *Mycosphaerella pinodes* (Heath and Wood, 1969), *Helminthosporium sacchari* (Strobel *et al.*, 1972), or intercellular cells of the bacteria *Corynebacterium sepedonicum* (Hess and Strobel, 1970; Strobel and Hess, 1968), *Pseudomonas tabaci* (Durbin, 1971), and *Erwinia amylovora* (Goodman and Burkowicz, 1970) result in the disintegration of membrane systems in cells of their respective hosts that may be located a distance of several cells from the nearest cells of the pathogen. The hypersensitive response of tobacco (a nonhost) to *E. amylovora* and *P. pisi* has been shown ultrastructurally to involve widespread damage to membranes, ribosomes, ground cytoplasm, and other cellular components (Goodman and Plurad, 1971). In contrast to bacterial infections which structurally disrupt host membrane integrity, bacterial (*P. glycinea*) induced toxemia shows no ultrastructural disruptions, and diseased cells resemble very young, healthy mesophyll cells. The main effect of the pathogen is a delay in mesophyll maturation (Dueck *et al.*, 1972).

It has been suggested recently that for *Pseudomonas tabaci*, one pathogenic principle is probably a cell wall protein (Hoitink and Bradfute, 1971). Isolated protoplasts were incapable of producing symptoms, whereas isolated cell walls produced water-soaking symptoms when injected into the plant, but the activity was destroyed by heating to 60° C or by pronase, a protein-degrading enzyme. This is the first evidence that a mechanism for the pathogenicity of a bacterial plant pathogen is located in the cell wall.

TRANSFER OF NUTRIENTS TO INTERCELLULAR SYMBIONTS

There is very little information to connect specific interface components with intercellular transport processes, but nevertheless the interfacial zone must be considered the region through which materials are exchanged. Several authors have considered nutrient transfer between host and symbiont to be promoted by structural specializations in the regions of contact between cells of the two organisms. For example, elaborations of the fungal plasma membrane to form 'microvilli' (Brown and Wilson, 1968) or similar structures (Peveling, 1969a, b) increase the surface area of interfacial membrane components and may facilitate the flow of nutrients from phycobiont to mycobiont in lichens. Recent information linking plant plasma membranes with enzymes involved in ion transport (Hodges *et al.*, 1972 and references cited) calls attention to the plasma membrane as an important mediator of exchange and has additional implications in host–symbiont relationships.

Direct connections between adjacent cells are also suspect as routes for intercellular transport. Plasmodesma-like channels, possibly connecting the protoplasts between lichen symbionts, have also been reported (Walker, 1968), but Jacobs and Ahmadjian (1969) did not accept this interpretation. Although plasmodesma-like connections have been demonstrated ultrastructurally between the dwarf mistletoe and its host (Tainter, 1971), definitive work on a wide range of phanerogamic parasites is yet to be done. By light microscopy it has been shown in some examples of parasitism by *Cuscuta* sp. that plasmodesma-like connections occur between the parasite and cortical parenchyma cells of the host (Bennett, 1944) or that the cell walls of the parasite seem to disappear and the protoplasm applies itself directly to the wall of the host's sieve tubes directly over a lateral sieve plate or a sieve field (Thoday, 1911).

Ultrastructurally, numerous 'plasmatic filaments' have been shown to extend through the wall of the apical region of a *Cuscuta* hypha that protrudes into a host cell, 'directly connecting the protoplast of the parasite with that of the host cell' (Dorr, 1969). Later in development these connections are plugged by wall appositions that form in the host adjacent to the hypha. Although the nature of cytoplasmic connections between hosts and phanerogamic parasites is not well understood, the extensive documentation of virus transmission by *Cuscuta* sp. (Hosford, 1967) clearly indicates that some kind of cytoplasmic continuity, albeit separated perhaps by membranes but probably not wall barriers, exists between the host and its *Cuscuta* parasite.

Predatory Relationships

Two kinds of predatory relationships are of interest here: one in which a cell of the predator takes up a cell of the smaller prey by phagocytosis and digests it, the other in which the smaller predator captures and immobilizes the larger prey organism and then grows into the prey and digests it. In such instances it would hardly be appropriate to regard the larger partner as a host, or even as a partner, since the relationship seems to be purely predatory and not symbiotic.

PHAGOCYTOSIS OF PREY

Examples of the first type of predator–prey relationship include the phagocytic uptake of bacteria or other microbial cells by plasmodia and myxamoebae of slime molds and cellular slime molds (Gray and Alexopoulos, 1968; Hohl, 1965). Amoebae of protostelids are sometimes cannibalistic and ingest cysts of the same species (Furtado and Olive, 1970). When a microbial cell is phagocytized, the plasma membrane of the predator is invaginated and forms an envelope around the prey (similar to IT 24). Thus, the prey resides for a time inside a vacuole, termed a 'food vacuole', in a relationship that has the ultrastructural appearance of *Rhizobium* cells inside a legume root nodule cell (Dart and Mercer, 1966). With time, the cells of the prey are lysed and digested inside the food vacuole, and at least parts of the prey are then assimilated by the predator. As in many relationships between intimately associated organisms, a derivative of the plasma membrane of the predator (comparable to the host organism insofar as it is the larger 'partner') serves as a prominent component of the interface between the two organisms. In this type of predatory relationship the plasma membrane even plays an active role in capturing the prey via phagocytosis.

NEMATODE-TRAPPING FUNGI

The second example of predatory relationships involves nematode-trapping fungi which have specialized cells adapted for capturing and subsequently penetrating the nematodes. Only one study has provided an ultrastructural explanation for the mode of action of these biological traps and the formation of functional interfaces between trap cells of fungi and the nematode prey

(Heintz and Pramer, 1972; C. E. Heintz, personal communction). Cell components in these trap cells comprise interface systems which are functionally unique.

Traps are basically of two types: (i) those coated with an adhesive substance that sticks to the nematode on contact and thus secures the nematode to the fungus, and (ii) constricting mechanical traps consisting of rings of fungal cells. In the latter type, when a nematode enters the trap lumen and triggers the trap, the ring cells instantly swell to three times their normal volume and constrict the nematode so that it cannot escape. Both of these trapping mechanisms seem to involve specific secretory systems in the fungus that function in the capture of the nematode and in establishing the interface between fungus and nematode.

It is the sticky material on the surface of adhesive traps that establishes the first permanent interface between the fungus and the nematode (similar to IT 13). These cells are distinguished by membrane-bounded inclusions in the cytoplasm, especially near the surface of the protoplast. The contents of the inclusions resemble the material coating the trap surface and may represent sites of adhesive localization prior to secretion (Heintz and Pramer 1972). In the same sense that vesicle-mediated secretion contributes to specialized cell coatings in eukaryotes generally (Morré and Mollenhauer, 1973), the peripheral vesicles in adhesive traps are also related to a modified cell surface—in this instance a surface which is necessary to ensure a predatory relationship and to provide the vital adhesive component of the interface between the fungus and the nematode.

In at least one example of a fungus with adhesive traps C. E. Heintz (personal communication) has shown that soon after the fungus penetrates the cuticle of the trapped nematode, the invading fungal cell invaginates the plasma membrane of the relatively intact protoplast of the nematode (IT 24). The images resemble those of haustoria and intracellular hyphae of plant endosymbionts (e.g. Figs 14, 57, 66), but no wall appositions or structured layers were present around the invading fungal cell within the nematode.

By far the most dynamic interface occurs in the constricting rings of nematode-trapping fungi. Moreover, the ultrastructure of a constricting ring differs before and after closure of the trap. Before closure, membrane-bounded inclusions with electron-dense contents are clustered beneath the fungal plasma membrane on the inner (luminal) side of the ring only. The inclusions are capable of fusing with the plasma membrane in this region to form a labyrinthine apparatus. The contents of the inclusions are expelled from the protoplast, and the surface area of the plasma membrane is greatly increased in the part of the cell that will later expand rapidly to entrap a nematode. In the open rings, there is an additional electron-lucent region between the plasma membrane and the cell wall on the luminal side of the ring. Thus, prior to triggering and closure, these traps have a specialized ultrastructure on the luminal side of the trap which includes a concentration of secretory components 'poised' for the trap closure. This represents a transitory interface which will later function in the trapping process when properly triggered.

Constriction of a trapping ring occurs within 0.1 second as cells of the ring expand on the luminal side of the ring only (Heintz and Pramer, 1972). The outer layer of the ring cell wall ruptures in the luminal region of the trap, and instantaneous cell expansion occurs to trap the nematode. After trap closure, the expanded protoplast is surrounded only by the inner wall layer in the luminal region of the trap. The membrane-bounded inclusions and labyrinthine apparatus are no longer evident, and the electron-lucent space between the plasma membrane and the wall is also lacking. Thus, within a fraction of a second, there is a drastic change in the interface components as the trap constricts. These cytological changes accommodate the rapidly enlarged cell surface, and the authors (Heintz and Pramer, 1972) suggest that the need for additional wall and membrane may be met by the secretory material held in reserve just before the trap closure. Heintz and Pramer's study provides evidence for involvement of specialized membrane-mediated secretory systems in host–pathogen (predator–prey) interfaces and in localized cell expansion. Other examples may not be as dramatic as this, but the relationship between structured secretory systems and sites of host–pathogen/host–symbiont interaction is being documented in a sufficient number of diverse systems that it must be regarded as a highly significant aspect of predatory, parasitic, pathogenic, and mutual symbiotic interactions.

Intracellular Relationships–Non-haustorial

Intracellular associations encompass a wide variety of interface types and a broad range of host and symbiont types. Although we emphasize fungal symbionts or pathogens (see also Ehrlich and Ehrlich, 1971a), the information on algal and prokaryotic symbionts is particularly relevant to the concept of interfaces in symbiotic associations, and viruses provide still another variant worth considering.

Two generalizations can be made with respect to intracellular symbionts. The first is that when a living cell invades another living cell, the invader (symbiont) is surrounded by an additional membrane that is not its own plasma membrane. This membrane has been shown in many examples to be the modified or invaginated host plasma membrane. Thus, the symbiont occupies a compartment within the confines of the host cell but is separated from the host cytoplasm by the host plasma membrane. The plasma membrane of the host is a nearly universal component of the host–symbiont interface and must be regarded as a significant functional interface. There are exceptions of course, as with some endosymbiotic bacteria (Jenkins, 1970; Leedale, 1969), infections by *Olpidium brassicae* (Lesemann and Fuchs, 1970b; Temmink and Campbell, 1968), and mycoplasmas (Bowyer and Atherton, 1971), but these occur infrequently. The second generalization is that apart from the foregoing statement there is no single specialized infection structure or unique cytological distinction to characterize the relationship between a symbiont and its host cell. No general cytological peculiarities distinguish symbiotic phases from free-living or intercellular forms of symbiotic organisms. Individual examples may display characteristic structural features, but one cannot generalize across a broad range of symbionts.

INTRACELLULAR HYPHAE OF FUNGI

Much of the ultrastructural work on intracellular hyphae has dealt with pathogens that kill host cells in advance of penetration or cause severe disruption of invaded cells. Far fewer studies have explored relationships in which intracellular hyphae confront intact protoplasts of living host cells.

When intercellular pathogens invade dead or moribund host cells, the pathogen is usually not surrounded by the invaginated host plasma membrane as is common with haustorial pathogens and those that do not kill in advance. Invading hyphae are surrounded by disrupted cytoplasm or a mixture consisting of breakdown products of the host protoplasm and vacuole (IT 19) (e.g. Calonge, 1969; Heath and Wood, 1969; Hess, 1969). Often intracellular hyphae in disrupted host cells are surrounded by a sheath-like matrix that appears to be a fungal secretion separating the fungal wall from the degenerate host cell (IT 26). Hyphae of *Fusarium solani* f. sp. *phaseoli* are coated by a layer of densely-staining material (Fig. 5) (Reichle, 1965). This material is not present around the hyphae where they penetrate the host wall, but occurs around intercellular hyphae or around intracellular hyphae after penetration.

Moribund cells, which are sometimes capable of responding to infection, may react by forming a papilla on the inner face of the cell wall (Hashioka and Fukita, 1969; Hashioka *et al.*, 1967; Hess, 1969; Reichle, 1965). If the fungus is successful in penetrating this papilla, then the latter appears as a collar surrounding the hypha near the cell wall. Such papillae may prevent host cell penetration in certain host cultivars or strains (Griffiths, 1971; Leong *et al.*, 1970; Nadakavukaren, 1963) (Fig. 55) (IT 21, IT 23, IT 27, IT 28). Similar wall appositions containing lignin or the wound polysaccharide callose (lignitubers, callosities, etc.) have been examined extensively by light microscopy, but such studies (Akai, 1959) are beyond the scope of this paper. Recent studies by electron microscopy (Holland and Fulcher, 1971) revealed lignitubers in wheat root cells penetrated by *Ophiobolus graminis*, but were unable to verify whether the host plasma membrane was penetrated or was continuous around the localized extension of wall material. However, Kolk (1930) suggested that the host plasma membrane was invaginated around the funnel-shaped wall thickening rather than being penetrated by it (see Plate 27, Fig. 5 of Kolk, 1930).

Wall degradation is of particular interest in relation to host penetration even when host cells have been killed in advance of penetration. Penetration by *Pyrenochaeta terrestris* is accompanied by dissolution of the host cell wall only at the point of penetration (Hess, 1969), whereas a general breakdown of host wall structure accompanies infection by other pathogens (Akai *et al.*, 1971; Bird, 1961; Calonge, 1969; Calonge *et al.*, 1969; Gipson *et al.*, 1971; Heath and Wood, 1969; Mercer *et al.*, 1971; Reichle, 1965). Commonly, at the site of host wall penetration the fungal hypha is constricted, and the fungal wall is in contact with the wall of the host (IT 7) (Figs 1, 5, 7, and 11) (Hashioka and Fukita, 1969; Hess, 1969; Horino and Akai, 1968b; MacDonald and McNabb, 1970; Mason, 1970; Mercer *et al.*, 1971; Reichle, 1965). Differences in the staining of host walls around some penetration sites attest to the biochemical effects of pathogens at the crucial interfaces between fungi and host walls during penetration (Fig. 7) (e.g. Hess, 1969; MacDonald and McNabb, 1970). The host cell wall is altered chemically over a rather large halo-shaped area around penetrations by *Ophiobolus graminis*, although the physical integrity of the area is not altered noticeably (Holland and Fulcher, 1971). Chou and Levi's (1971) studies on wood decay indicate that extensive cell wall dissolution by the brown rot fungus, *Poria vaillantii*, results from enzyme secretion from hyphae in the bore holes and not from hyphae in the cell lumen as has been generally concluded. In addition to localized enzyme secretion, some species of wood-inhabiting fungi possess 'transappressoria' at their hyphal tips which facilitate penetration of cell walls (Liese, 1970; Liese and Schmid, 1964). Some of these fungi grow from cell to cell through pits (Fig. 1) as well as through bore holes (MacDonald and McNabb, 1970; Sachs *et al.*, 1970).

Gibberidea heliopsidis attacking *Helianthus strumosus* is one of the few examples of an intracellular fungal pathogen in which hyphae penetrate cells of a plant organ without killing the host cell in advance or inciting protoplasmic destruction (Mason, 1970) The hyphae of this nonhaustorial pathogen grow through the host walls and invaginate the host plasma membrane. They thus reside outside the protoplast but within the confines of the cell lumen. The wall of an invading fungal cell is separated from the invaginated host plasma membrane by a thin encasement layer which is continuous with an apposition on the host wall (IT 21) (Fig. 11). Some hyphae are encased by a thicker layer of material continuous with the host wall in what could be considered a walling-off phenomenon (Fig. 12). Overall, the host–parasite interface around this intracellular parasite is similar to that around some haustoria (see Fig. 66), and is what would be expected when a living cell penetrates another living cell, at least as far as the invaginated host plasma membrane is concerned.

Systemic smut fungi studied by Fullerton (1970) showed several types of interfaces. Hyphae penetrated host cells directly and sometimes grew from cell to cell, without forming any specialized infection structures such as appressoria or penetration pegs. The host plasma membrane was invaginated and surrounded the invading hyphae. At the hyphal apices, the host plasma membrane was close to the fungal wall (similar to IT 18), whereas the membrane was separated from the hyphal wall by a matrix layer (IT 24) in the subapical regions. A collar-like wall apposition formed around hyphae near the host wall (IT 21), and similar material was subsequently deposited within the matrix surrounding the hyphae (IT 29) until this region was filled and the hyphae were encased (IT 21). Fullerton (1970) also found cytoplasmic vesicles around the invading hyphae in association with encasement formation, an observation which suggests that host secretory vesicles participate in the development of the interface. Encased hyphae eventually degenerated.

Not all intracellular hyphae are surrounded by encasements or wall appositions, however. Infection of the marine alga *Porphyra marinum* by *Pythium marinum* is an example of a short-lived intracellular relationship in which there is a rapid change in the nature of the host–pathogen interface (Kazama and Fuller, 1970). There is little evidence of cytological alteration of the host during penetration, and this is an instance in which the pathogen is not constricted where it penetrates the host wall. Soon after host cells are penetrated, they contract, and organelles are destroyed, but there is a brief time when the host protoplast is intact. A similar situation exists in susceptible bean leaves infected by *Colletotrichum lindemuthianum*, but the period during which host cytoplasm remains intact is about 100 h, whereupon invaded and adjacent cells suddenly break down (Mercer *et al.*, 1971). Evidence presented in the same paper suggests invagination of the host plasma membrane by the fungus and an interface resembling either IT 18 or IT 24. Although Kazama and Fuller (1970) indicated that a sheath matrix did not develop around the invading *Pythium* hyphae, and that a 'sheath membrane' was absent, the evidence of their micrographs is sufficient to illustrate that the pathogen was in fact surrounded by a membrane which was the invaginated host plasma membrane (equivalent to a 'sheath membrane') during the early stages of infection. Furthermore, the membrane was closely appressed to the fungal wall over much of its surface (IT 18). This transitory interface, in which the fungal cell is in intimate contact with the surface of the host protoplast, is lost as the host cell reacts, shrinks, and disintegrates, leaving behind necrotic cytoplasm and masses of fibrillar material interpreted as partially degraded host wall.

Carbonell (1970) has recently reviewed the ultrastructure of human pathogenic fungi and their mycoses. Although information on host–parasite interfaces is scanty, several examples show that the cells (yeast-like) of intracellular pathogens are enclosed in a membrane-bounded compartment within the host cytoplasm and that a matrix (termed a zonal ring) separates the fungal wall from the host membrane (IT 24). Cell wall fibrils of fungi such as *Paracoccidioides brasiliensis* are also found free in host cytoplasm or enclosed in vacuoles. Since cell walls of some human pathogens have antigenic properties, these walls—whether intact or disrupted—may participate directly in the functional interactions between host and pathogen.

Other ultrastructural examples of endophytic fungal hyphae in an intact host protoplast include the symbiotic associations of orchid mycorrhizae (Dorr and Kollmann, 1969; Hadley *et al.*, 1971). Although developmental studies are lacking, it is clear that the hyphae are surrounded by a membrane that is either close to the fungal wall (Fig. 14) (Hadley *et al.*, 1971) or separated from it by a sheath-like separation layer (termed a vacuole by Dorr and Kollmann, 1969). Sites of penetration were not shown, so it is not clear whether any wall appositions occurred on the host wall around penetration sites (cf. Meyer, 1966). The membranous envelope around the hyphae has not been traced to continuity with the host plasma membrane, but it is safe to assume that the membrane is of host origin, since its staining properties resemble those of the plasma membrane, and it constitutes the boundary of the host protoplast in relation to the fungal cells (Dorr and Kollmann, 1969; Hadley *et al.*, 1971). Hadley *et al.* (1971) included freeze-etching of host–symbiont interfaces in their study, and they noted that the fungal walls had hemispherical protuberances that could increase the area of the contact surface between host and symbiont by 15%. In Dorr and Kollmann's (1969) study, the invaded host cells were distinguished from non-invaded cells by a differently organized protoplasm which included cytoplasmic strands aggregated in the centre of the cell. The fungus was found within the plasmic strands where unusual proliferations of endoplasmic reticulum occurred which the authors suggested to be a response to the symbiont. During development, the host cells remained intact, but the fungus degenerated, and the host protoplasts retained residues of digested hyphae, IT 25 (Dorr and Kollmann, 1969; Hadley *et al.*, 1971; Meyer, 1966). This is a rare instance of a mutual symbiotic relationship in which the host cell (large partner) survives, and the symbiont (small partner) is at least partly destroyed. It resembles more the predator–prey relationship than the known examples of parasitic or mutual symbiotic relationships.

Unlike the presumed relationship between obligate parasitic fungi and their hosts, the transfer of metabolites in mycorrhizae is principally from fungus to host, and the eventual degradation of the fungal cells may signify substantial necrotrophic assimilation of nutrients by the host cytoplasm (Hadley *et al.*, 1971). The interfacial zone through which the interactions between living cells are mediated in orchid mycorrhizae (IT 24) appears structurally similar to some parasitic, mutual symbiotic, and predatory relationships. This fact exemplifies the danger in assuming a particular kind of functional relationship from a morphological type of interface. It serves to emphasize the caution necessary in interpreting function as well as the need for documenting the information that will permit a functional evaluation of an interfacial zone.

PLASMODIOPHORA BRASSICAE

An intimate and unique interfacial relationship exists between parasitic cells (plasmodia or amoebae) of *Plasmodiophora brassicae* and cells of cruciferous hosts. One of the most elegant current studies of the physiology and cytology of host–parasite relations has been done on this organism by Williams and his coworkers. Other details of this relationship appear in the symposium contribution of Williams *et al.* (see p. 141) and in articles by Williams and McNabola (1967, 1970), Williams and Yukawa (1967), Williams *et al.* (1971), and Aist and Williams (1971, and references cited).

Plasmodia of *P. brassicae* are entirely intracellular and lack specialized feeding structures such as haustoria. The host–parasite interface consists of a plasmodial envelope, 23–24 nm thick. There is no plasmodial wall and no extracellular layers or matrices that are comparable to the sheaths or appositions surrounding invading cells of bacterial and algal endosymbionts or haustorial and hyphal fungal symbionts.

The plasmodial envelope, seen in thin section (Fig. 16), consists of seven layers (four dark and three light), as if two closely appressed membranes formed a common envelope around the parasitic cell. The envelope is so stable that Williams and McNabola (1970) were able to isolate it intact from host tissue. When components of the plasmodial envelope were measured, subjected to extraction and electron staining procedures, they appeared similar to plasma membrane and unlike endoplasmic reticulum, mitochondrial or other cytomembranes of host or parasite. Williams and McNabola's studies (1967, 1970) convincingly demonstrated that the plasmodial envelope consisted of two intimately associated membranes (IT 4). They suggested that the inner membrane was the plasma membrane of the plasmodium and that the outer membrane was host-derived, probably from the host plasma membrane which was invaginated at the time of penetration.

A compound double membrane consisting of parts derived from both host and parasite would provide an interface that brings the protoplast surfaces of host and parasite into direct contact and would require that two membranes from different organisms must function together to ensure the survival and reproduction of the parasite. This interface is distinct from the single membrane boundary (IT 1) between plasmodia of *Olpidium brassicae* and host cells (Lesemann and Fuchs, 1970b; Temmink and Campbell, 1968) or the 'compound membrane' (IT 3) between *Aphelidium* and its algal host cell (Schnepf, 1972; Schnepf *et al.*, 1971b). The envelope is the only visible boundary separating the cytoplasm of the host from the cytoplasm of the plasmodium, which in turn continues to grow and reproduce. Thus, as with *Rhizobium* cells in root nodules (see p. 191), the envelope around plasmodia must keep pace with the reproduction and growth of the symbiont, although no part of the envelope is continuous with the host plasma membrane next to the host cell wall. At least the outer membrane of the plasmodial envelope can be regarded as part of the surface of the host protoplast, albeit detached from the rest of the plasma membrane. Thus, growth of the parasite would require biosynthesis of new host plasma membrane at a site other than the normal protoplasmic surface adjacent to the cell wall.

Toward the end of vegetative growth of plasmodia, the interface components change (Williams and McNabola, 1967). In the transition from vegetative growth to sporogenesis, the outer membrane of the plasmodial envelope separates from the inner membrane and eventually leaves each plasmodium bounded by a single plasma membrane (similar to IT 1 or IT 2). At the stage where plasmodia are surrounded by only a single membrane, Williams and McNabola (1967) obtained evidence that the parasite ingested portions of the host protoplast through a phagocytic process that had not been observed at earlier stages. When the outer membrane of the plasmodial envelope disintegrated, the host cytoplasm became disrupted, IT 2. Concurrent breakdown of the outer membrane and some of the host cytoplasm led the authors to suggest that the integrity of the membrane was under host control. This also supports the interpretation that the outer membrane is host-derived.

Nuclear division in the plasmodia resulted in multinucleate cells of *P. brassicae* which later divided to form resting sporangia. Following cell division, the young sporangia developed spines on their surfaces, and sporangial wall was subsequently laid down between the spines and the sporangial plasma membrane. An intersporangial matrix surrounded the sporangia. Thus, in the transition from vegetative to reproductive development and sporangial maturation, a transition in the host-parasite interface also occurred which involved the elimination of one membrane, the disruption of host cytoplasm, the formation of sporangial walls, and the accumulation of an intersporangial matrix. From a developmental standpoint, the *Plasmodiophora* system provides a good example of the transitional and ephemeral nature of interfaces.

The same system has also been used as a model for demonstrating the dynamics of host-parasite interactions at a much earlier stage of development, during penetration of host cells and establishment of plasmodia (Aist and Williams, 1971; Williams *et al.*; p. 141, this book). Aist and Williams' study is a classic example of the value of correlating light and electron microscopy in the study of developmental processes. The nature of the interface changes in time and space throughout the sequence leading from a free-living zoospore to an intracellular amoeba or plasmodium.

Before penetration, zoospores of *P. brassicae* collide with the wall of a cabbage root hair and attach to it on the side of the zoospore opposite the place of flagellar insertion (IT 34). Pseudopodial extensions of the attached zoospore are continually extended and withdrawn and then the flagella are retracted, and the zoospores encyst (IT 13 and IT 35). Secretory vesicles in the attached parasite cell fuse with the plasma membrane during encystment and contribute to the surface coating of the cyst. (For details see Williams *et al.*, p. 141, this book.)

Penetration of *P. brassicae* into the root hair is similar to that described by Keskin and Fuchs (1969) for *Polymyxa betae* (Aist and Williams, 1971). After such penetration, the interfaces between the amoebae and the host cytoplasm are of two types. One is a seven-layered envelope (i.e. two apposed membranes) similar to the plasmodial envelope in clubroot galls (Fig. 16). The other type is also seven-layered, but the outer membrane is thought to be continuous with flattened vacuoles that lie between the parasite envelope and the host cytoplasm (Aist and Williams, 1971).

Within a few minutes after host penetration, a callose-containing papilla is laid down just beneath the penetration site. It represents a wound-healing procedure that occurs at the site of prior host–parasite interaction and can be regarded as a tardy interface component. Aist and Williams (1971) provide evidence that the papilla is formed at least in part from secretory vesicles in the host cytoplasm. But this is an example of papilla formation occurring after penetration, in contrast to other host–parasite systems in which papillae are formed before penetration and then must be breached by the invading parasite (e.g. Edwards and Allen, 1970; Temmink and Campbell, 1969).

ENDOPHYTIC CHYTRIDS

Ultrastructural studies have shown that several endophytic chytrids have specialized relationships with host cells which result in different interfaces from those usually associated with parasitism by higher fungi. Some chytrids form haustoria (e.g. Karling, 1932; Schnepf *et al.*, 1971a) and will be discussed in the section on haustoria. But the examples described here are those that release an entire protoplast or thallus into the host cell.

Olpidium brassicae is the notable eukaryotic example of a living cell that enters the protoplast of another living cell but is not surrounded by an additional (host-derived) membrane (Lesemann and Fuchs, 1970b; Temmink and Campbell, 1968). The plasma membrane of the intracellular plasmodium is in direct contact with ground cytoplasm of the host cell (IT 1). This plasma membrane-cytoplasm interface has also been demonstrated for mycoplasmas in plant tissue (Bowyer and Atherton, 1971; Granett and Gilmer, 1971; Igwegbe and Calavan, 1970; Kaloostian *et al.*, 1971; Sinha and Paliwal, 1969) as well as in cells of their insect vectors (Fig. 25) (Bowyer and Atherton, 1971; Hibino *et al.*, 1971; Sinha and Paliwal, 1970).

With *Olpidium*, the interface between host and parasite is established when a zoospore settles on host root cells, encysts on the root surface, and secretes an adhesive material which binds it to the cell wall of the root. The first interface is between fungal membrane and host wall (IT 34), although not firmly attached. During encystment a wall–wall interface is formed (Fig. 19) (IT 8), and Temmink and Campbell's (1969) micrographs show an intervening layer of adhesive substance of varying thickness between the cyst wall and the host wall (IT 13). During encystment, the host cell responds by producing a wall apposition in the form of a papilla on the inner surface of the host wall opposite the attached *Olpidium* cell (IT 16) (Temmink, 1971; Temmink and Campbell, 1969). Significantly, this host response occurs before the fungus begins to penetrate the host. During penetration, additional structures occur in the fungal cell which are associated with entry of the cyst protoplast into the host and are thus related to the interface if not being actual parts of it. Next to the host wall, the cyst cytoplasm is populated by numerous cytoplasmic vesicles, but distal to the attachment site a vacuole develops in the *Olpidium* cyst (Lesemann and Fuchs, 1970a; Temmink and Campbell, 1969). Held (1972) also shows a distal vacuole and cytoplasmic vesicles in cysts of the mycoparasite *Rozella* attacking hyphae of *Allomyces*, as well as wall appositions (papillae) forming beneath the point of fungal attachment to the host cell.

In many ways the structural interfaces in early stages of infection by *Olpidium* and *Rozella* are similar. But the variation in the host-wall apposition is striking and deserves emphasis here to illustrate the conceptual equivalence of wall appositions generally, and yet to recognize that different types of wall appositions exist among different hosts and even within the same host attacked by the same parasite. The papillae in lettuce roots consist mainly of matrix materials with embedded vesicles and irregular heterogeneously staining regions (Temmink and Campbell, 1969). In kohlrabi (Lesemann and Fuchs, 1970b), two types of wall appositions were formed depending on the type of host cell. In calyptra cells with little protoplasm, a thin osmiophilic tube was attached to the host wall and surrounded the penetrating fungus, but in plasma-rich cells the wall apposition consisted of a massive irregular papilla-like structure having a spongy appearance in which trapped membranous structures were embedded in a matrix (similar to Fig. 54). The evidence strongly suggests that this type of wall apposition is formed by fusion of cytoplasmic vesicles with the host plasma membrane, and that some host cytoplasm is trapped in the papilla during its formation, resulting in the membranous units that give the papilla a foamy appearance. In *Allomyces* the wall appositions have two morphological components. Adjacent to the host wall beneath the fungal cell is a papilla through which the penetration tube of the fungus grows. An extension of the inner layer of the host wall covers the papilla. Held (1972) also found membranous elaborations (lomasomes by his terminology) attached to some papillae and immediately beneath some cysts that had recently become attached, but had not yet germinated and had not induced papilla formation. These lomasomal elaborations of membrane (as well as secretory vesicles) cannot be ruled out as components of the host–parasite interface in this and other host–parasite combinations, but the function or significance of such contorted membranes in the host cell is obscure. Held (1972) found wall appositions to be the usual phenomenon at sites of host penetration (he reported only one exception) and did not find papillae where penetration was not attempted. The parasite failed to penetrate previously infected hyphae of the host and neither did it induce wall appositions. Thus, wall appositions, which are secretory products of the host cell, form a prominent component of the host–parasite interface before penetration of the host cell. The immediate cytological precursors of the appositions (possibly secretory vesicles) may also be considered part of the interfacial zone. But when host and parasite are so intimately associated, secretion can work both ways, and the parasite in turn can secrete materials that will alter or form new components of the interface (see discussion of secretory vesicles in the parasite later in this section).

Penetration phenomena by chytrids strikingly illustrate the changing host–parasite interfaces, the ephemeral nature of some interface components, and how the interfaces can change drastically over a very short time. In *Rozella*, before host penetration, a germ tube is formed from the cyst, and small vesicles (secretory vesicles) similar to those in hyphal tips of fungi (Grove and Bracker, 1970) occur at the point of attachment of the germ tube to the cyst. At that point the vesicles become a temporary part of the host–parasite interface. For successful penetrations, a hole must then be formed in the host wall. Then a vacuole in the cyst begins to swell to fill the cyst, and in the process it forces the cyst contents through the germ tube and into the host cell.

In *Olpidium*, as a vacuole begins to form in the part of the cyst distal to the host cell, cytoplasmic vesicles (secretory vesicles) derived from the Golgi apparatus accumulate near the cyst wall next to the host cell (Lesemann and Fuchs, 1970a; see also Fig. 6 of Temmink and Campbell, 1969), and lomasome-like membrane configurations are sometimes continuous with the cyst plasma membrane at that site (Fig. 19). These organelles associated with the cell surface near the point of potential penetration become temporary components of the host–parasite interface. As the vacuole in the cyst grows, a hole appears in the cyst wall, and the host wall is penetrated. Part of the wall remains continuous with a wall-like tube protruding through the host wall part way into the host cell, which suggests that some localized cyst growth has occurred at the penetration site in the process of initiating host penetration. As the cyst vacuole continues to grow, the plasmodium enters the host cell through a channel in the papilla in a process which takes about 10 min (Temmink and Campbell, 1969). A wall continuous with the cyst wall partially surrounds the penetrating cyst plasmodium. Thus, the protoplast is forcibly extruded into the host cell lumen where it must breach the host plasma membrane and detach from the cyst, because thereafter much of the fungal protoplast resides in the host cytoplasm as a plasmodium surrounded by no other membrane than its own plasma membrane (IT 1). During the time of host penetration there are several interfaces at various sites of host-parasite interaction. They include wall-wall (IT 8 and IT 13), wall-papilla (IT 21), membrane-membrane (IT 4 assumed at the site of entry of *Olpidium* into the host protoplast just before entry), and membrane-hyaloplasm (IT 1) interfaces at regions of immediate contact or contiguity. Just how the plasmodium passes through the host plasma membrane is not yet known.

We noted above that much of the fungal protoplast moved into the host cell. A small part of it remains back in the evacuated cyst with the vacuole, and is still surrounded by plasma membrane. This means that a net assembly of new plasma membrane in the fungal cell must occur at the time of host penetration to account for the rapidly increased surface area of the fungal protoplast (consisting of the plasma membrane of the plasmodium and plasma membrane remaining in the cyst). Significantly, the accumulations of secretory vesicles or lomasomal configurations that had been near the host-parasite interface prior to penetration were not present in intracellular plasmodia. The implication is that they were used up during penetration. Secretory vesicles and lomasomes could both provide a ready source of new plasma membrane for the fungus during penetration. Moreover, the possible significance of the secretory vesicle contents should not be discounted in thinking about the host-parasite interaction. Materials contained within the vesicles and released during penetration could facilitate penetration by influencing properties of the fungal and host wall or the papilla, all of which are penetration barriers, or by contributing to the fungal wall that extends from the cyst as a penetration tube. That secretory vesicles derived from the endomembrane system should become transient components of the host-parasite interface further emphasizes the ephemeral nature of the interface and the two-way involvements of secretory systems from different partners in the host-parasite interactions.

Once inside the host protoplast, plasmodia of *Olpidium* do not show striking associations with host cell components, except in plasma-rich cells of kohlrabi roots where Lesemann and Fuchs (1970b) showed that small vacuoles surrounded the plasmodium and were so closely associated with the plasmodial plasma membrane that the tonoplasts were nearly in contact with the plasmodial surface. In host cells with little cytoplasm the plasmodia in the peripheral cytoplasm protruded into the vacuole so that the tonoplast of the host central vacuole was closely appressed to the plasmodial plasma membrane (Fig. 20). Thus, the host tonoplast becomes a candidate for an interface component on a purely morphological basis although the functional significance of the close tonoplast is not clear and can only be estimated.

Further development of the intracellular plasmodium of *Olpidium* leads to the formation of a wall around the cell of the parasite and the pursuit of either of two developmental pathways: formation of a resting spore or formation of a zoosporangium followed by zoosporogenesis and discharge of the spores through an exit tube in the sporangial wall (Temmink and Campbell, 1968). When the naked plasmodium forms a wall, an additional component is interposed into the host–parasite interface, and the host protoplast changes so that there is little host cytoplasm left in the host cell around the parasite.

At least two chytrids (*Chytridium* and *Aphelidium*) are parasitic on the alga *Scenedesmus*. Each has a distinct relationship with the host cell and consequently, a different sort of interfacial region (Schnepf, 1972; Schnepf *et al.*, 1971a, b). *Chytridium* is described in the section on haustoria. Encysted zoospores of *Aphelidium* penetrate the *Scenedesmus* wall and release a plasmodium into the host cell. The host responds to penetration by producing extra wall deposit which forms a collar around the wall of the penetration tube of *Aphelidium*. When *Aphelidium* releases an endophytic amoeboid protoplast into the *Scenedesmus* cell, the host plasma membrane is first invaginated around the invading plasmodium to form a double membrane envelope consisting of the adjacent plasma membranes of host and parasite (IT 4). Host and parasite plasma membranes come in contact and become integrated in places to form what Schnepf (1972) and Schnepf *et al.* (1971b) refer to as a 'compound membrane' surrounding the parasite (Fig. 15) (IT 3). The wall-less parasite phagocytizes parts of the host protoplasm in one of the rare instances of demonstrated mass uptake of material from host to parasite (see also Williams and McNabola, 1967). Phagocytosis is also a common nutritional mechanism for many free-living protistan organisms, but such phagocytosis does not usually involve any mutualistic or parasitic interaction. It is more a predator–prey relationship.

ENDOBIOTIC ALGAE

Several species of green, blue-green, and dinoflagellate algae occur as intracellular endosymbionts of protists or invertebrates, or they live between the cells of other invertebrates. The algae are in communication with cells of their hosts across an interface consisting of various components, depending on the system studied and sometimes on the stage of development of the endosymbiont in the host. A variety of interface components is found in both inter- and intracellular associations. Much research using light microscopy has been devoted to the subject of microbial symbiosis and has been thoroughly reviewed elsewhere (Ahmadjian, 1967; Buchner, 1965; Henry, 1966).

A relatively simple plasma membrane–plasma membrane interface (IT 4) separates the cells of *Convoluta* flatworms from their intercellular green-algal symbionts (Oschman, 1966; Oschman and Gray, 1965; Parke and Manton, 1967; Pedersen, 1964; Sarfatti and Bedini, 1965). This condition, however, is typical of the relationship only in the mature flatworm host. The ova and young

Convolluta do not contain algae, and each generation must be reinfected. During development of the symbiotic relationship the alga loses its flagella and wall (Oschman, 1966). Consequently, the structural components of the host-symbiont interface are not constant, but vary with time following infection.

The simplest type of intracellular interface in terms of the number of components involved, is found in the relationship between *Glaucocystis* sp. (Echlin, 1967; Hall and Claus, 1967) or *Cyanophora* sp. (Hall and Claus, 1963) and their respective blue-green algal symbionts. In all of these associations two membranes, slightly separated in space, separate the symbiont from the host cytoplasm. No intervening wall is present. However, the exact nature of the membranes separating the two organisms is not clear. For example, in *Glaucocystis* sp. Echlin (1967) interprets the two membranes to be a part of the endosymbiont, whereas Hall and Claus (1967) regard the innermost membrane to be the plasma membrane of the symbiont, but consider the outer membrane, i.e. the 'interface membrane', to be a component of the host cell. Likewise, in *Cyanophora* sp. the inner membrane is interpreted as the limiting membrane of the host (Hall and Claus, 1963).

In other examples of intracellular associations, the host-symbiont interface also contains the plasma membrane of the symbiont and a membrane of the host, but with the cell wall of the symbiont separating the two membranes. Although the term *vacuolar membrane* is used for the membrane of host origin is probably equivalent to and derived from the plasma membrane of the host cell. This relationship is characteristic of *Chlorella* (green alga) cells which individually occupy 'perialgal vacuoles' in *Paramecium bursaria* (Fig. 13) (Karakashian *et al.,* 1968). The thickness of the algal wall increases with age. When the algal cells divide, a new cell wall is formed to enclose the daughter cells prior to the rupture and peeling off of the mother cell wall. A similar relationship (IT 18 and IT 24) was described by Drum and Pankratz (1965) (although not including information on wall development) for what they interpreted as possibly a modified coccoid blue-green alga in two species of the diatom *Rhopalodia*. A variant of this kind of interface, i.e. symbiont plasma membrane-symbiont wall-host plasma membrane (IT 18), occurs in the interface separating cells of a green algal symbiont from its host, *Chlorohydra* sp. Although a wall surrounds each algal cell, many algal cells may occupy a single vacuole within a cell of the host (Park *et al.,* 1967). In this association, a precise interface between the host and the symbiont is impossible to identify since some but not all of the algal cells are in contact with the vacuolar membrane of *Chlorohydra.* Cells of *Nostoc* sp. (blue-green alga) exist as endocyanelles in the phycomycetous organism, *Geosiphon pyriforme*. The host plasma membrane surrounding each algal cell is separated from the latter by a wall-like slime coating (Fig. 17) (Schnepf, 1964; Schnepf and Brown, 1971). Although Schnepf

(1964) referred to the association between *Geosiphon* and *Nostoc* as a phycomycetous lichen, this designation is equivocal because of the differences in interpretation of the fungal or algal affinities of *Geosiphon* (Scagel *et al.*, 1966).

The most complex type of interface separating intracellular algae from their hosts occurs around the zooxanthallae (Dinoflagellates) which are symbionts in various marine invertebrates. Although *Symbiodinium microadriaticum* has been reported as an intercellular symbiont in the jelly fish *Casseopeia* (Kevin *et al.*, 1966), it generally occurs as an intracellular symbiont in this host as well as in the anemone, *Condylactis* (Kevin *et al.*, 1969). The algal cells are separated from the host cytoplasm by a complex 'periplast' consisting of several membrane layers and a type of cell wall (Fig. 18). The periplast, described in a centrifugal sequence, consists of the algal plasma membrane, a highly convoluted aggregation of membranes, two more membranes between which is sandwiched an amorphous wall-like layer, and finally an outer membrane surrounding the entire structure. Taylor (1968) has described a similar host–symbiont interface separating yellow-brown algal symbionts from cytoplasm of *Anemonia sulcata*, and he showed clearly that the nature of the complex interface was related to the age of the algal cells. As the cells aged, the components of the interface separating them from their host cells were markedly changed. The exact nature or origin of most of the components is not clearly understood.

Several workers have concluded that the zooxanthallae contribute little to the nutrition of the anemone host, but function primarily in the removal of wastes and in the addition of oxygen (see Taylor, 1968, for discussion). However, later work by Taylor (1969) clearly showed that over 60% of the carbon fixed by photosynthesis in the symbiont was transferred to the host under the conditions employed. This material, so derived from the symbiont, provided only secondary nutritional benefits to the host, however, and could not replace those provided by the animal's normal feeding habits (Taylor, 1969). The transfer of carbohydrates between symbionts has been thoroughly reviewed by Smith *et al.* (1969), who discuss the ecological significance and possible mechanisms of such transfer.

ENDOSYMBIOTIC BACTERIA

Bacterial pathogens in higher plants are usually located in the intercellular spaces between host cells (Goodman *et al.*, 1967) or within non-living cells of vascular tissue. Contrasted to this, in many mutualistic and other non-pathogenic associations bacteria occur within living host cells and exhibit a variety of interface types.

One of the best documented examples of an intracellular bacterial association is that of *Rhizobium* infection in roots of leguminous plants. Infection of roots by cells of *Rhizobium* spp. results in a symbiotic relationship that is not necessarily a disease but nonetheless induces abnormal root growths or nodules. These nodules contain the bacteria (bacteroids) and are effective in nitrogen fixation. There are striking cytological parallels between this bacterium-host relationship and that of many fungus-host associations. The general principle concerning intracellular parasites holds true for *Rhizobium*—that is, when a living cell invades a living cell, the invader is surrounded by an additional membrane peripheral to its own cell surface. Physiological and cytological studies have provided information that illustrates our earlier concept of host–parasite interfaces and the time–space changes that occur with development of the host–symbiont relationship.

The extent of a root nodule is indicated by Bergersen's (1968) estimate that the average soybean nodule contains 35 000 tissue cells. Each cell has up to 10^5 membrane-enclosed units containing 4–6 bacteroids each.

Vincent (1966) summarized the main steps in the establishment of an effective root nodule, each of which involves a different sort of interface between the bacterial symbiont and its plant host. The main stages are: (i) occurrence and proliferation of the bacteria near the host root, (ii) entry of the bacterium, (iii) establishment and advance of the infection thread, (iv) nodule differentiation induced by encounter between infection thread and tetraploid host cells, (v) release of bacteria from infection thread with formation of membrane envelope, (vi) multiplication of released bacteria, (vii) conversion of bacteria to bacteroids, and (viii) establishment and maintenance of functional symbiosis.

The interface between *Rhizobium* cells and the host plant begins in the rhizosphere when soil-borne bacterial cells approach or contact cells of legume roots (IT 8 or 13). The bacteria gain access to the host through any of several sites: root hairs, ordinary epidermal cells, or points of lateral root initiation (Dixon, 1969; Sahlman and Fahraeus, 1963; Vincent, 1967). The bacteria initiate an infection thread in an altered and often contorted root hair. The elongation and deformation of root hairs has been linked to the 'influence of indoleacetic acid, IAA, excreted by rhizobia and formed from tryptophan excreted by the plant' (Dixon, 1969). Thus, prior to infection, secretions by both host and symbiont constitute an important part of the host-symbiont interface. Subsequent passage of the bacteria into the plant is facilitated by enzymes and hormones that may lead to cell-wall softening at the time of infection (Dixon, 1969). The infection thread stimulates cell division in the root cortex, and nodules begin to form.

The infection thread is a cellulose tube, continuous with host walls, which contains the bacteria in a zoogleal matrix. As the infection thread grows through cells, the host plasma membrane extends with the developing infection thread and is the limiting membrane between the thread and the host cytoplasm (IT 13 or IT 27, depending on whether the infection thread wall is considered host wall *per se* or a form of wall apposition) (Dart and Mercer, 1964). The tip of the thread may extend completely through a host cell and fuse with the host wall opposite the point of entry (Jordan *et al.*, 1963) or even thrust into neighboring cells (Goodchild and Bergersen, 1966). According to Dart and Mercer (1964), when an infection thread penetrates a host cell, the wall around the zoogleal matrix becomes thinner toward the tip. The thickness of the infection thread wall also varies along its length which makes the interface between the thread and the host cytoplasm appear irregular. Growth of the infection thread is related to the position of the host nucleus (Dixon, 1969).

Infection threads may also extend through intercellular spaces or along the middle lamella of adjacent cells. Thus, the bacterial membrane and wall, as well as the zoogleal matrix and the host wall (infection thread wall) and plasma membrane, are all components of the host-symbiont interface. The position and extent of the infection thread at any given time will determine the nature of the interface at this stage—prior to entry of the bacteria into the host cells.

Infection threads are not always present, however. In some lupins the bacteria are present in intercellular spaces, without an infection thread (Jordan and Grinyer, 1965), and they pass between the walls of adjacent host cells in a naked zoogleal strand. This infection route differs from the widespread infection threads and alters the interface somewhat because special host wall elaborations (infection thread wall) are not produced. Jordan and Grinyer (1965) thought that in the absence of infection threads the bacteria were able to degrade or rupture host cell walls locally to gain access to the host protoplast. In some nodules that are initiated by infection threads, the bacteria break free from the thread and inhabit the intercellular spaces of the host (Dixon, 1969).

Infection by *Rhizobium* is facilitated by cell wall softening and apparent induction of pectic and cell wall-degrading enzymes in the host plant. Dixon (1969) reviewed evidence showing that *Rhizobium* induces some hosts to produce pectic enzymes and that a polysaccharide coat is part of the host-symbiont interface and apparently exerts a controlling effect upon the host.

Bacteria are released into the host protoplasm when a portion of the infection thread wall breaks down or develops a discontinuity so that the zoogleal mass contacts the host cytoplasm, with the host plasma membrane intervening (IT 24) (Dart and Mercer, 1964; Dixon, 1969). In Goodchild and Bergersen's (1966) study, the release of the bacteria was preceded by a bulge on the infection thread to form a cellulose-free extension bounded by the host plasma membrane.

Bacteria enter the host cytoplasm by endocytosis (Dixon, 1967, 1969), and the zoogleal matrix is left behind. During endocytosis the bacteria invaginate the host plasma membrane and enter the cell lumen surrounded by a membrane derived from the host plasma membrane (=phagocytosis) (Fig. 21).

For the intracellular bacteria, the host-symbiont interface is different from that in the infection thread. The cellulosic wall and the zoogleal matrix are no longer present. The recognizable components of the interface include the bacterial plasma membrane, the bacterial wall, the membrane envelope (=host plasma membrane), and a space or matrix of variable dimensions between the bacterial wall and the membrane envelope (IT 24). This matrix subsequently proves to be a significant part of the interface.

Bacterial cell division occurs after the bacteria enter the host cell. Sometimes each bacterial cell division is accompanied by division of the membrane envelope, whereas in other instances the divisions of bacteria and envelopes are not coordinated, and some membrane envelopes then enclose many bacterial cells. Kidby and Goodchild's (1966) experiments using a single strain of *Rhizobium* on different hosts suggested that the division of membrane envelopes was under host control and either did or did not coincide with bacterial divisions, depending on the host used. In either case, increase in the area of the membrane was required, and it is this membrane that is the apparent boundary of the host-symbiont interface on the host side.

Bacteria in root nodule cells are eventually transformed into bacteroids (Bergersen, 1968; Dixon, 1964, 1969). The transformation involves morphological and biochemical changes resulting in organisms quite different from those in the free-living state. Some bacteria become greatly enlarged, up to 40-fold increase in volume (Dixon, 1964), but some are only slightly changed morphologically (Bergersen, 1968). Bacteroids often lose the ability to grow in culture free from the host plant. Some of the physiological changes experienced by bacteroids have been summarized by Dixon (1969). The morphology of the host-symbiont interface remains similar in the bacterial and the bacteroid state. The bacteroid still has a plasma membrane and a membranous wall and is surrounded by the membrane envelope (Fig. 22). The membrane envelope is frequently separated from the bacteroid by a considerable distance, however, and a prominent sheath or matrix surrounds the bacteroid cell.

A significant physiological transformation accompanies the bacteroid transformation—namely the production of enzymes for nitrogen fixation and the formation of the haem protein, leghaemoglobin. Leghaemoglobin is associated with nodules that are effective in nitrogen fixation (Dixon, 1969), and there is a correlation between the amount of leghaemoglobin and the amount of nitrogen fixed. Although several functions for this protein have been advanced (Dilworth and Kidby, 1968; Dixon, 1969), its specific function is still a matter of conjecture. What is significant about leghaemoglobin in this discussion is its location. It is found within the membrane envelope surrounding the bacteroids (Dilworth and Kidby, 1968; Dixon, 1969) and is not in the protoplasm of the plant or the bacteroids. Furthermore, neither host nor symbiont synthesizes leghaemoglobin without the symbiotic association. Dilworth and Kidby (1968) concluded on the basis of electron-microscopic autoradiography that leghaemoglobin occurs between the bacteroid wall and the membrane envelope. In other words, this vital protein is present in the sheath-like region of the interfacial zone.

The fact that leghaemoglobin is located in the host–symbiont interfaces does not explain which organism produces the protein or which organism controls or specifies its synthesis. Dilworth (1969) discussed evidence indicating that the host plant synthesized at least part of the leghemoglobin molecule but pointed out that because genetic material of both plant and bacteroid are present within the same plant cell, 'the location of the gene and its product may not necessarily be one and the same'. By inoculating dissimilar legumes with the same strain of *Rhizobium lupini* and then inoculating the same legume with different strains of the bacterium and analyzing the resulting leghaemoglobins, Dilworth (1969) concluded that genetic specification of leghaemoglobin in the root nodules was a property of the plant.

The work done with *Rhizobium* root nodules is particularly significant for those interested in host–parasite interfaces because of the many parallels between the components of the *Rhizobium* system and those in parasitic relationships (i.e. the components of IT 24). Dixon (1969) also noted comparisons between legume root nodules and crown gall induced by *Agrobacterium tumefaciens,* a bacterium closely related to *Rhizobium.* But the fact that membranes and matrices occur at the host–symbiont interface in so many symbiotic relationships portends even greater significance as we consider fungus–host interactions and the respective roles of host and parasite in establishing, maintaining, and transforming the interface.

An endosymbiotic relationship in which the symbiont is not surrounded by a host-derived membrane was described by Leedale (1969) for an endonuclear bacterium present in some euglenoid flagellates. These bacteria, which inhabit the nucleoplasm, are surrounded by a gelatinous sheath layer that has an amorphous electron-transparent appearance, but the sheath is not bounded by a membrane; it is in direct contact with the euglenoid nucleoplasm (Fig. 24) (similar to IT 24 but without the host membrane). The bacterial cell itself is surrounded by a double-membraned periplast consisting of the bacterial plasma membrane and an outer coating or wall. The bacteria are found throughout the nucleus, but in some nuclei there is a close association between the bacterial cells and the ribosome-rich 'endosome' of the euglenoid nucleus. Thus, within the nucleus there are several possibilities for interfacial interactions, but in each instance, the bacterial sheath intervenes between the bacterial periplast and any component of the host cell.

Some of the bacteria in euglenoid flagellates occur not only in the nucleus but also within the host cytoplasm. Leedale (1969) reported one euglenoid strain that had intracytoplasmic but not intranuclear bacteria. The intracytoplasmic bacteria have the same structure and interfacial components as the intranuclear bacteria except that their sheaths form interfaces with cytoplasm rather than nucleoplasm.

The functional interaction resulting from the peculiar interface of the endonuclear bacteria is not clear, but it does reflect a highly specific and obligate relationship. Also, it is obvious that the bacteria must derive their nutrition from the host. The bacteria multiply to keep pace with host-cell proliferation (the host nuclear envelope does not break down during mitosis, and so the bacteria may be secured either inside or outside the nucleus by the limits of the nuclear envelope). Leedale was unable to isolate internal bacteria into pure culture and could not transfer the bacteria to uninfected strains of the host. 'Infected' strains of the euglenoid organisms were difficult or impossible to culture axenically. Neither host nor symbiont seemed adversely affected by the relationship, and Leedale (1969) considered the possibility that this relationship could exemplify an aspect of the frequently advocated endosymbiont theory of eukaryotic evolution (Margulis, 1970). In any event, the result of the relationship could reflect a euglenoid cell that is 'physiologically dependent on the bacteria', and the bacteria would thus become permanent and essential parts of the host through successfully integrated multiplications of both cell types.

The endosymbiotic bacteria of *Paramecium* spp. were initially considered to be distinct cytoplasmic genetic entities that were passed from generation to generation of *Paramecium* (Sonneborn, 1938, 1943). Known as kappa particles, these structures were described by Preer in 1950. Subsequent studies revealed that kappa particles as well as several similar inclusions are actually Gram-negative bacteria which live as symbionts within the *Paramecium* cells. Ultrastructure of eight such intracellular particles has been reviewed by Beale *et al.* (1969), and a ninth type has recently been described by Jenkins (1970). Seven of the particle types are located in the host cytoplasm, and two are restricted to the nucleus. Among the nine types described, at least seven have different interfacial components separating the host and the symbiont. Kappa and mu particles are free in the host cytoplasm, and their outer boundaries consist of two distinct membranes (bacterial plasma membrane and wall). Delta particles are similar, but have a distinctive electron-dense material surrounding them which separates the outer of the two membranes from the host cytoplasm. Gamma particles are also free in the host cytoplasm, but are surrounded by three membranes. The outermost of the three membranes has ribosome-like particles attached and also extends for some distance into the host cytoplasm where it has the appearance of endoplasmic reticulum. Lambda and sigma particles are very similar to each other and are located in cytoplasmic vacuoles rather than occurring free in the cytoplasm. One to several particles may occupy a vacuole.

Both of these bacterial forms are peritrichous and have flagella which fill much of the vacuolar space. Nu particles are also located within cytoplasm, embedded in capsules, but little is known about their ultrastructure.

The two endonuclear symbionts of *Paramecium* are alpha and epsilon. Alpha particles lie free in the nucleoplasm of the macronucleus but are not found in the micronucleus. The symbiont is surrounded by a single membrane, but with an additional inner membrane in some regions; thus the host-symbiont interface varies within a single symbiont cell (Preer, 1969). A most intriguing interface separates the epsilon particle from the host nucleus (Jenkins, 1970). Epsilon particles are enclosed by two membranes, and exist only within loculi formed by localized bulbous extensions of the outer membrane of the nuclear envelope (Fig. 23).

VIRUSES

Without dwelling on the extensive literature of virus-host relationships, we call attention to several examples of subcellular localization of plant viruses. Although viruses are intracellular, the particular localization often depends on the type and strain of virus and on the stage of pathogenesis. Many animal and insect viruses, and some plant viruses, are surrounded by a membranous envelope, but the capsids of most plant viruses are not enclosed by an envelope (Luria and Darnell, 1967; Matthews, 1970).

Viruses occur most commonly within the cytoplasm of the host, and some are found within or attached to organelles, or even in non-living cells of vascular tissue (Esau, 1968). Viruses in ground cytoplasm occur as individual dispersed virions or as aggregates (Figs 29 and 30) (Esau, 1968; Esau and Gill, 1969). Virus particles and aggregates of virus particles are often embedded in a protoplasmic 'zone of exclusion'; that is, a zone of cytoplasm appearing clear in electron micrographs and from which ribosomes and other particulate or membranous materials are excluded (Figs 28 and 29) (Esau, 1968). Virions are found within organelles such as nuclei and less frequently in plastids (TMV) (Fig. 28) (Esau, 1968; Esau and Cronshaw, 1967) and in the lumina between membranes of endoplasmic reticulum (Esau, 1968) or nuclear envelope (Figs 26 and 27) (MacLeod *et al.,* 1966). Esau and Gill (1969) described the mixing of scattered virions and aggregates of TMV particles with nuclear material of *Nicotiana* during mitosis when the nuclear envelope broke down. The particles occurred among the chromosomes until the late stages of mitosis when most of the virions were segregated outside nuclei during reformation of the nuclear envelopes. Clusters of intranuclear virions of beet yellows virus were also shown in older leaves of *Tetragonia* by Esau and Hoefert (1971) who discussed other examples of virus localization in nuclei.

Some viruses are located in membrane-limited compartments. There is evidence to support the occurrence of virions in host vacuoles (Esau, 1968; Honda and Matsui, 1972; Russo *et al.*, 1968), a position which interposes an additional zone (vacuolar sap) and a membrane (tonoplast) between the virions and host cytoplasm. However, Esau (1968) cautioned that accidental disruption of the tonoplast during specimen preparation could result in virus particles being spilled into the vacuole, and thus the natural occurrence of viruses in plant vacuoles in some micrographs is controversial. Hirumi *et al.* (1967) showed linear arrays of wound tumor virus particles enclosed by long membranous tubes in infected cells of an insect vector (Fig. 32). A similar configuration occurs with radish mosaic virus (Honda and Matsui, 1972) where the virions are found within long tubular protrusions of the host tonoplast which project from the vacuole into the cytoplasm. Kim and Fulton (1971) have also shown virus-like particles inside membrane-limited tubules in cells infected by bean pod mottle virus. In a local lesion host (Pinto bean) the tubules were found between the plasma membrane and the cell wall, but in a systemic host they were embedded within localized thickenings of the host cell wall. As with other types of pathogens, viruses have been shown to induce thickenings on the inner surface of host cell walls, particularly in host cells in the region of local lesions (Tu and Hiruki, 1971).

Virions may contact or be adsorbed onto various cellular membranes. Plant virus particles have been demonstrated within plasmodesmata linking adjacent host cells (Esau, 1968; Kitajima and Lauritis, 1969), presumably passing from one host cell to the next. There, they contact the plasma membrane lining the plasmodesmata. Harrison and Roberts (1968) have shown particles of tobacco rattle virus specifically attached at their ends to outer mitochondrial membranes (Fig. 31). Although the precise mechanism of tobacco necrosis virus transmission by *Olpidium brassicae* is not known, Temmink *et al.* (1970) showed that during acquisition *in vitro* of the virus by zoospores of the fungus, the virions were tightly adsorbed onto the plasma membrane. The failure of some fungal isolates to transmit the virus was correlated with inability to adsorb virus particles *in vitro*. The well-known bacteriophage-bacterium association is a classic example of specific virus-host adsorption aided by specialized structures on the virus. Simon and Anderson (1967) showed stages of attachment of T2 and T4 bacteriophages to the membranous cell wall of *Escherichia coli*. Binding involves two separate phage components–long tail fibres for initial attachment and short tail fibres for subsequent attachment. They also illustrated the virus configurations as the wall was pierced by a needle-like structure and the DNA component of the virus was injected into the bacterial cells (i.e. through the perforation in the cell wall). See p. 231 for examples.

The recent emphasis on fungal viruses has demonstrated that viral infections of fungi are widespread (Hollings and Stone, 1971). Border's (1971) work on a virus infecting *Penicillium stoloniferum* is outstanding because it shows not only the localization of the virus particles but also the developmental progression of the host-virus relationship. No particles are found in the apical 50–100 μm of a hypha. Thus, the growing region of the cell appears to be free of virus. Basipetal to that apical zone is a region in which virus particles, mainly in clusters, are embedded in host cytoplasm much like clusters of virions in a plant cell. But farther back in the hypha the clusters of virus particles become enveloped by a membrane so that ultimately they reside in a vacuole (Figs 33 and 34). The membrane disappears in older cells towards the centre of the colonies, and the virus particles then become enveloped in a membrane having the ultrastructural appearance of the plasma membrane (D. J. Border, personal communication). Clearly, the relationship between virus and host changes with development, and a membrane is added as a new component of the host–pathogen interface after the clusters of virions are established.

Intracellular Relationships–Haustorial

Haustoria are distinctive fungal organs which deserve special attention because they represent the only intracellular portions of a number of important and highly specialized pathogens. Thus, they have more intimate interfacial relationships with the host than any other part of the fungal thallus, and they have been extensively investigated for clues about their 'unique' properties. Bushnell (1972) has provided a superb discussion of the biology of haustoria, and Ehrlich and Ehrlich (1971a) focused considerable attention on structural aspects of haustoria.

Haustoria seem to be uniquely parasitic structures. But apart from this implicit assumption and information on their occurrence, morphology, and relation to thallus development or certain resistance mechanisms (Bushnell, 1972), there is little firm information to document a direct and unique functional role. Ecologically, haustorial pathogens are mostly obligate parasites, and they rarely form haustoria on artificial substrates (Bushnell, 1972). Bushnell noted comparisons between intercellular biotrophic associations and haustorial counterparts and observed that we still '. . . do not know if the haustorium facilitates biochemical interactions between host and parasite that are not possible when the association is of the wall-to-wall, extracellular type.' Further, '. . . there is neither structural nor physiological evidence to indicate that haustoria of obligate parasites differ from those of fungi with greater natural saprophytic capabilities.' Although haustoria are metabolically active, specialized functional capabilities have not yet been discovered that would distinguish haustoria from other fungal cells.

Ultrastructurally, haustoria have protoplasmic organization typical of eukaryotic cells and are not cytologically distinct from nonhaustorial cells. Haustorial morphology and ultrastructure have been extensively documented (e.g. Allen, 1923a, b, 1927, 1928; Berlin and Bowen, 1964; Blackwell, 1953; Bracker, 1967, 1968; Bushnell, 1972; Coffey *et al.*, 1972; Ehrlich and Ehrlich, 1971a; Fraymouth, 1956; Littlefield and Bracker, 1972; Peyton and Bowen, 1963; Rice, 1927; Smith, 1900). In spite of a great deal of ultrastructural study, surprisingly little is known about the development, significance, and role of interface components, although structural details of the interface are now well known. The early expectations that electron microscopy would reveal the unique features of haustoria and explain their role in disease have not materialized. In fact, there are surprising cytological parallels between the interfaces around haustoria and those around intracellular hyphae of non-haustorial symbionts (see pp. 176-179); they are often indistinguishable by electron microscopy. What, then, are haustoria, and how do they differ from other parasitic structures?

DEFINITION, OCCURRENCE, AND GENERAL CHARACTERISTICS OF HAUSTORIA

The concept of the haustorium includes physiological as well as anatomical considerations. The word *haustorium* comes from a Latin term meaning 'to drink' (Snell and Dick, 1971). According to Rice (1927), credit for the first description of what now is called a haustorium belongs to Visiani, who in 1851 described the structure in grape mildew. Although DeBary included appressoria in his concept of haustoria, he correctly regarded the haustorium as a specialized organ that maintained interrelations between parasite and host (Rice, 1927). The idea that haustoria function as organs of absorption is universally accepted, although it has still not been proven experimentally.

The fungal haustorium is a determinate structure. Bushnell (1972) defines it as '. . . a specialized organ which is formed inside a living host cell as a branch of an extracellular (or intercellular) hypha or thallus, which terminates in that host cell, and which probably has a role in the interchange of substances between host and fungus.' A haustorium must be attached to a cell or thallus outside the host cell and is thus distinct from amoebae or plasmodia of *Plasmodiophora* or *Olpidium* which are wholly intracellular thalli. Haustoria are distinct from intracellular hyphae which may continue to grow for some time after penetration and extend from cell to cell. Haustoria are known to assume a variety of forms (e.g. club-shaped, lobed, elongated, branched etc.). A haustorium cannot properly be considered a single cell, since the intracellular portion may represent only part of a cell (rusts, downy mildews) or may consist of one cell plus part of another cell (powdery mildews). Conceivably, a haustorium could be multicellular if it met other criteria. Implicit in the concept of haustoria is their ability to coexist with the invaded cell for a while after penetration. Karling (1932) regarded haustoria as '. . . feeding organs . . . which do not immediately injure or kill the host cell, but live in a somewhat balanced relationship with it.' The duration of the compatibility period is extremely variable.

Haustoria are formed by fungi which cause rust diseases, powdery mildews, downy mildews, white rust (*Albugo candida*), and some smuts, as well as a few other fungal diseases of higher plants. Some species of *Phytophthora* also produce haustoria as do some chytrids, mycoparasites, and lichen mycobionts (Bushnell, 1972). The intracellular structures of endotrophic mycorrhizae are sometimes considered as haustoria (Bushnell, 1972; Meyer, 1966), but in the two examples mentioned on p. 179 (Dorr and Kollman, 1969; Hadley *et al.*, 1971) the original authors referred to the intracellular organs as hyphae. The hyphae of some endotrophic mycorrhizae are capable of growing from one host cell to the next (Harley, 1968). Admittedly, these are examples for which it is difficult to decide whether the invading structures are haustoria.

The main bulk of a haustorium is termed the **haustorial body**, especially if it forms a globose or club-shaped structure. Haustoria may also have appendages called **haustorial lobes**. The haustorium is connected via a slender tube, the **haustorial neck**, to an **appressorium** or **haustorial mother cell** which lies outside the host cell attached to the surface. The haustorium is surrounded by a membrane (the **extrahaustorial membrane** or **invaginated host plasma membrane**) at the boundary of the host protoplast and a sheath or **extrahaustorial matrix** usually separates the membrane from the **haustorial wall**. Various wall appositions in the form of **collars** or **encasements** may also be associated with haustoria. All of these associated host and fungal structures, including the membrane surrounding the haustorium, are referred to collectively as the **haustorial apparatus** (Bracker, 1968; Bushnell, 1972).

There are some inconsistencies in the terminology applied to the cells from which haustoria arise. *Appressorium* is commonly used to denote a swelling on a germ tube or hypha that functions as an organ of attachment, especially in the early stages of infection (Ainsworth, 1971; Burnett, 1968; Gaumann and Dodge, 1928; Snell and Dick, 1971). Ordinarily, an appressorium forms on the external surface of a host prior to penetration.

In powdery mildews, the haustorium typically develops from a superficial appressorium (Bushnell, 1972; Smith, 1900), except in rare instances where haustoria develop from 'intercellular appressoria' which are specialized hyphae within the host tissue, e.g. *Phyllactinia suffulta* (Smith, 1900). Likewise, appressorium has been used for the structure from which haustoria are derived in the smut fungus, *Entyloma nympheae* (Lutman, 1910).

In rust fungi, an appressorium on the host surface typically does not give rise to a haustorium, but rather to a **substomatal vesicle** or **infection hypha**. The haustorium is subsequently formed from a specialized cell of the intercellular mycelium called a haustorial (or haustorium) mother cell (Allen, 1923a;

Bushnell, 1972; Ehrlich and Ehrlich, 1971a; Rice, 1927). Despite the unfortunate differences in terminology, appressoria of powdery mildews and haustorial mother cells of rust fungi are basically the same with respect to their function and relationship to host-cell penetration.

INTERFACE COMPONENTS DURING HOST PENETRATION

When a fungal cell contacts a host cell prior to penetration, an amorphous electron-dense layer is often found between the walls of host and pathogen (Figs 45, 47, and 54) (IT 13, IT 38) and occupies part of the angle of contact between cells. This material is probably a fungal secretion and probably aids the adhesion of the haustorial mother cell to the host cell. Similar layers of interstitial material have been shown for a variety of haustorial plant pathogens (Berlin and Bowen, 1964; Coffey *et al.*, 1972; Ehrlich *et al.*, 1968; Hardwick *et al.*, 1971; Heath, 1972; Kajiwara, 1971; Littlefield and Bracker, 1972; Olah *et al.*, 1971; Peyton and Bowen, 1963; Schnepf *et al.*, 1971a; Van Dyke and Hooker, 1969). Sometimes cell walls are in direct contact (IT 8, IT 11) and adhesive materials, if any, do not show up as extracellular coats in electron micrographs. The shredded appearance of walls of extracellular hyphae and appressoria of powdery mildew fungi (Bracker, 1968; Edwards and Allen, 1970; Watene, 1968) additionally indicate strong adhesion between walls of the respective organisms that is sufficient to resist the displacement of the external fungal cells during specimen preparation.

The interface before and during penetration sometimes includes wall appositions secreted by the host and laid down between the plasma membrane and the wall adjacent to the fungal cell (IT 11, IT 16). Such appositions, formed in advance of penetration, are not common in rust infections, but have occasionally been observed adjacent to intercellular hyphae of rusts (Ehrlich *et al.*, 1968; Heath, 1972; Heath and Heath, 1971). Sometimes small, lumpy wall deposits form adjacent to penetration sites (Littlefield and Bracker, 1972). With powdery mildews, papilla formation at penetration sites is almost universal (Figs 56, 67-70, 81, and 82) (Bracker, 1968; Bushnell, 1972; Edwards and Allen, 1970; Smith, 1900; Stanbridge *et al.*, 1971), and this seems also be a common phenomenon with *Phytophthora* (Ehrlich and Ehrlich, 1966; Hanchey and Wheeler, 1971) and some downy mildews (Chou, 1970). Where papillae and other appositions are formed they constitute a barrier beyond the host wall which must be penetrated, or less frequently (e.g. *Phytophthora* infections) they remain and form a permanent layer separating the haustorial wall from the host plasma membrane (Fig. 66) (IT 21) (Ehrlich and Ehrlich, 1966; Hanchey and Wheeler, 1971). Information on the nature of wall appositions is included later in this section.

Components of host cytoplasm cannot be excluded from the prepenetration interface. A flurry of cytoplasmic activity was described by Bushnell (1971) at the site of host penetration by *Erysiphe graminis*. Electron microscopy has also shown host organelles collected around penetration sites (Edwards and Allen, 1970; Stanbridge *et al.*, 1971). This suggests that host organelles are involved at the interface during penetration, undoubtedly in response to the pathogen and perhaps with roles in forming the wall apposition (papilla), providing additional surface membrane, or secreting materials that either combat or aid the fungus in its attempt at penetration.

After attachment of an appressorium or haustorial mother cell to a host cell wall, the fungal wall may thicken over the area of contact by the addition of new wall layers in the region where penetration will later take place (Figs 44, 45, and 56) (Coffey *et al.*, 1972; Hardwick *et al.*, 1971; Heath and Heath, 1971; Littlefield and Bracker, 1972). Then, as penetration begins, localized growth of the fungus toward the host cell involves the extension of one or more layers of the fungal wall and gradual erosion of the host wall in contact with the emerging penetration peg (Figs 46, 67, and 74) (Edwards and Allen, 1970; Littlefield and Bracker, 1972) (IT 8, IT 11). The apex of the penetration peg may contain cytoplasmic vesicles or other membrane configurations (Figs 46 and 74) similar to those found in growing hyphal tips of fungi (Grove and Bracker, 1970). It is likely that these apical vesicles will be found with increasing frequency as more study is devoted to penetration and as cell preservation procedures become more sophisticated and reliable. The presence of secretory vesicles at the penetration site could be very important in effecting the localized degradation of host components in advance of the penetrating pathogen.

The diameter of the penetration site in a host wall is variable, from less than 0.5 μm (Littlefield and Bracker, 1972) to 2 μm or more (Chou, 1970). This represents the area of host wall actually removed by the action of the penetrating fungus, and there is so little evidence of displacement or physical disruption of wall components that it is difficult to imagine purely mechanical penetration. An exception is in lichens (Peveling, 1968; Roskin, 1970) where the algal wall is clearly displaced around the penetrating haustorium (hypha), but this still does not rule out some biochemical degradation of the wall as well. Significantly, wall dissolution is limited to the immediate penetration area so that intact host wall (albeit perhaps modified) is in direct contact with the wall of the fungal penetration peg. Therefore, as detailed by Stahmann (p. 156), such enzyme activity as is involved in host wall penetration must be extremely limited and perhaps even bound to the surface of the invading penetration peg.

Because of the difficulty in obtaining thin sections through penetration sites, there is very little ultrastructural information on the penetration process (Edwards and Allen, 1970; Littlefield and Bracker, 1972). Much has been assumed about penetration, however, from observing post-penetration stages.

Ultrastructural evidence suggests that penetration involves a combination of enzymatic degradation of host walls and the exertion of physical force. In some studies there is evidence of altered staining (hence biochemical alteration) of the host wall around penetration pegs (Figs 67 and 74) (Edwards and Allen, 1970; McKeen *et al.*, 1969; Stanbridge *et al.*, 1971), whereas in others the wall retains its normal stainability at the penetration site (Figs 47 and 48) (Coffey *et al.*, 1972; Hanchey and Wheeler, 1971; Heath and Heath, 1971; Littlefield and Bracker, 1972; Peyton and Bowen, 1963). Host wall fibrils end abruptly adjacent to the penetration peg and do not appear distorted or displaced as might be expected if the fungus penetrated purely by mechanical force (Edwards and Allen, 1970; Stanbridge *et al.*, 1971). However, when *Erysiphe graminis* penetrates the host epidermal wall, the host cuticle is displaced and is pushed partway into the penetration hole adjacent to the fungal wall (Figs 74, 75, and 76) (Stanbridge *et al.*, 1971). This configuration can only arise by application of mechanical force. The surface of the host wall is sometimes depressed around the penetration site (Figs 44, 66, 74, 75, 76, and 82). Likewise, we have found that the outermost layers of host wall fibrils are partly displaced adjacent to penetration pegs of *E. graminis* (Figs 75 and 76). The wall fibrils appear crushed by physical force but they are also clearly discontinuous and in a densely staining matrix around the penetration sites, indicating that they had been biochemically degraded in this region.

Edwards and Allen (1970) have shown the degradation of host wall fibrils without any signs of stress during primary haustorium formation by *E. graminis*. They concluded that host penetration was a two stage process. Wall penetration was considered basically a biochemical process, but papilla penetration by the same fungus was thought to be principally mechanical, based on apparent lines of stress in the papilla. In our studies of *E. graminis* (not primary haustoria) on wheat, we found differential staining of the papilla in advance of the penetration peg (Figs 67 and 74). Also, the papilla shows successive layering (Fig. 67) in a manner that would have suggested physical displacement if it were not for the fact that the penetration peg had not even reached the papilla and therefore could not have exerted any mechanical force on it. As the stage at which papillae and collars stop growing in powdery mildew infections is not known, it cannot really be decided whether profiles which suggest mechanical displacement of the papilla are due to the force exerted by the penetrating fungus or to the continued addition of papilla material during and after penetration. However, if the papilla is in a gel or liquid state during penetration (Chou, 1970; Bushnell, 1972) then mechanical force may be a major factor in papilla penetration.

Although figures here (Figs 45, 46, and 74) and by other authors (e.g. Edwards and Allen, 1970) have shown the penetration peg in direct contact with the host wall or papilla (IT 8, IT 11, IT 21), the fungal wall may also be surrounded by an additional layer during penetration. Chou's (1970) study of *Peronospora parasitica* shows a reservoir of densely-staining matrix material around incipient haustoria still within the papillae at penetration sites (IT 27). This material is obviously the result of a biochemical interaction or a fungal secretion and not the result of mechanical penetration.

The fungal wall in the penetration area is usually much thinner than elsewhere in the inter- or intracellular portions of the thallus. With one possible exception (Berlin and Bowen, 1964), the fungal wall is continuous from the intercellular hyphae, through the penetration site, and completely around the haustorium. Claims to the contrary are not substantiated by reliable ultrastructural evidence, but in the study of Hardwick *et al.* (1971) the fungal wall was so thin at the penetration site as to appear absent in some micrographs. With rusts, the wall of the haustorial neck is continuous with the innermost layers of the haustorial mother cell wall (Coffey *et al.*, 1972; Littlefield and Bracker, 1972), whereas the outer layer of the mother cell wall is discontinuous at the penetration site. The amorphous or mucilaginous cell coating that occupies the angle of contact between the intercellular walls of host and pathogen (Figs 45 and 47) (Coffey *et al.*, 1972; Hardwick *et al.*, 1971; Littlefield and Bracker, 1972) usually does not continue through the penetration site and is not present at the wall-wall interface in the penetration hole (Figs 47 and 48). One exception to this is with *Albugo candida* where a layer of electron-dense material surrounds the fungal wall in the penetration hole, and Berlin and Bowen (1964) view this layer as being continuous with the coating around the haustoria.

With some pathogens there is a clear delineation of the fungal wall where it passes through the host wall (Berlin and Bowen, 1964; Bracker, 1968; Peyton and Bowen, 1963). This is especially clear with powdery mildews where there is a sharp boundary between the apposed fungal and host walls (IT 7) (Figs 75 and 82). But with rust infections the host and fungal walls merge with such an obscure boundary that it is difficult to tell where one ends and the other begins (Figs 47 and 48) (Coffey *et al.*, 1972; Hardwick *et al.*, 1971; Littlefield and Bracker, 1972). These diffuse regions of integrated host and fungal walls signify sites at which the walls of the two organisms may have grown together.

The notion that fungal wall is absent at the apex of a penetration peg or that haustorial development proceeds by a blowout process (Calonge, 1969; Ehrlich and Ehrlich, 1963a, 1971a) has not been borne out by studies showing cell detail during the penetration process (Edwards and Allen, 1970; Littlefield, 1972; Littlefield and Bracker, 1972) (Figs 35–42, 46, and 74). In a study on lichens (Galun *et al.*, 1971b), a nonstaining layer around young haustoria was taken as evidence that the wall was absent. But failure to stain does not necessarily mean wall material was lacking. There is no reason to suppose that a penetration peg or incipient haustorium should lack a cell wall any more than it would be valid to assume that germ tubes or apices of growing hyphae lack walls (Grove and Bracker, 1970). Kajiwara (1971) thought that *Puccinia* spp. first formed an 'incipient haustorium' surrounded by a structure he called a *primary encapsulation* which had the appearance of a wall apposition. But we are unable to verify that the micrographs of rust infections (Figs 22 and 28 of Kajiwara, 1971) are actually penetration stages. Kajiwara proposed that the fungus then grew through the primary encapsulation and rapidly formed a haustorial body. The incipient haustorium remained as the haustorial neck. Littlefield's studies (1972) by light microscopy show that after host penetration the slender penetration peg of *Melampsora lini* grows several microns into the host cell with no evidence of a surrounding collar or other wall apposition and then begins to swell at the apex to form the haustorial body (Figs 35–42). The neck ring is formed before the body develops, and taken with electron microscopic studies neither the 'blowout' nor 'breakthrough' contention (Kajiwara, 1971) holds for *M. lini.* Evidence in other studies on rusts (Hardwick *et al.*, 1971; Coffey *et al.*, 1972; Heath and Heath, 1971) supports the developmental sequence indicated by Littlefield's (1972) study. The changing interfaces for an idealized rust infection are shown diagrammatically in Fig. 83.

HAUSTORIAL COMPONENTS OF THE HOST-PATHOGEN INTERFACE

Except for the universal occurrence of the haustorial plasma membrane, there are no consistent protoplasmic features of haustorium-host interfaces. Unlike the invaginated host plasma membrane around haustoria (see later this section), the haustorial plasma membrane does not appear to have any specialized ultrastructural properties that distinguish it from the plasma membrane in other parts of the fungal thallus. Haustoria contain organelles and membranes typical of the fungal group to which they belong. Some are especially rich in mitochondria (Berlin and Bowen, 1964), and most are rich in protoplasm. Nuclei are absent from small capitate haustoria (Fig. 66) (Berlin and Bowen, 1964; Ehrlich and Ehrlich, 1966; Hanchey and Wheeler, 1971), but they migrate through the narrow haustorial necks and enter haustoria of rusts, powdery mildews, downy mildews, and other fungi with large haustoria (Bracker, 1968; Littlefield and Bracker, 1972; Peyton and Bowen, 1963). In the apices of lobes of young *E. graminis* haustoria we find vesicles (Fig. 77) similar to those in apices of growing germ tubes and hyphae of fungi. Lomasomes have been identified in haustoria (e.g. Berlin and Bowen, 1964; Kajiwara, 1971; Peyton and Bowen, 1963) and proposed as interface components that function in uptake of nutrients. However, because of their sporadic occurrence in haustoria, we do not conclude that lomasomes have consistent or significant roles at the host-pathogen interface.

The haustorial wall is an extension of and continuous with the wall of the haustorial mother cell or appressorium. The wall is usually thinner around the haustorium than around inter- or extracellular hyphae or appressoria. Whereas fungal walls are generally thickest just around the penetration site where the appressorium or haustorial mother cell contacts the host cell, only part of that wall is continuous through the hole in the host wall as was noted in the discussion of interface components during penetration. The fungal wall is thinnest where it passes through the host wall (Figs 48, 68, and 75) (e.g. Hardwick *et al.*, 1971).

In almost every example of haustoria studied, the haustorial wall forms a continuous coating around the entire haustorial protoplast. Thus, the most common interface types around haustoria are IT 18 and IT 24, depending on whether a haustorial sheath is present or not. In some lichens, where the host wall is invaginated to form a partial or complete coating around the haustoria of mycobionts (Galun *et al.*, 1970a, c, 1971b), the addition of the host wall to the interface would result in IT 8. But if the host wall is only invaginated and not breached by the mycobiont, there is some question about whether the invading organ should be called a haustorium in the strict sense (Bushnell, 1972).

Plasmodesma-like connections that bridge the haustorial wall and link the haustorial protoplast with the haustorial sheath or the host protoplast were described by Calonge (1969) and Ehrlich and Ehrlich (1963a, 1971a, b). The clearest evidence of such a bridge was shown by Ehrlich and Ehrlich (1971a), but at best such images appear obscure and occur only sporadically, unlike the clear connections linking protoplasts of *Cuscuta* hyphae with host cells (Dorr, 1969). Attempts by many investigators to locate these structures in rust haustoria have failed consistently. Calonge's (1969) claims of host–pathogen continuity cannot be accepted as valid conclusions from electron micrographs. Obscure images (Figs 5, 9, and 13 of Calonge, 1969), obvious artefact (Fig. 13 of Calonge, 1969), and interpretations of continuity between haustorial endoplasmic reticulum and host protoplasm (Fig. 5 of Calonge, 1969) transcend the limits of reasonable interpretation of ultrastructure. We seriously question the existence of any such physical host–pathogen connections based on the evidence presented so far. Caution is essential in this matter because the possibility of direct links between the protoplasts of host and pathogen could be important to our understanding of the nature of interfaces. It is such an important concept that, if it has any validity at all it deserves to be documented by only the most reliable ultrastructural evidence.

The haustorial necks subtending capitate haustoria of *Albugo candida* (Berlin and Bowen, 1964) have unique structure because one-half to two-thirds of the neck lacks any structure that stains comparably to the haustorial wall or intercellular hyphal wall. Between the plasma membranes of host and fungus in the neck region is a layer of amorphous material resembling sheath matrix. If the wall is lacking, the haustorial necks would interact with host cells through IT 5, but it is also possible that a wall is present which stains differently from other regions of the fungal wall. Hardwick *et al.* (1971) also reported a small discontinuous region in the distal portion of the haustorial neck of *Uromyces appendiculatus*, but they interpreted this hiatus to be a localized weak spot or dissolution which occurred during fixation.

There is some evidence to indicate that haustorial walls have a different structure from walls of other cells because of differences in staining or layering Berlin and Bowen, 1964; Hardwick *et al.*, 1971; Littlefield and Bracker, 1972; Van Dyke and Hooker, 1969). The coating of fibrils radiating from haustorial walls of *E. graminis* (Fig. 78) may be part of the haustorial wall rather than part of the sheath, although it is likely that material from the sheath matrix permeates this loosely organized layer. Some of these examples refer only to localized or regional differences of the haustorial wall. For example, in *M. lini* and other rusts the wall of the mother cell–haustorium complex can be divided into several distinct regions. The wall of the haustorial mother cell consists of moderately electron-dense material, but an additional layer of exceptionally electron-dense substance occurs in the thickened region of the wall where it is in contact with the host cell. This layer is continuous through the penetration pore in the host wall and extends along the proximal one-third to one-half of the haustorial neck. There it ends abruptly at the proximal limit of the neck ring in this and other rust fungi (Coffey *et al.*, 1972; Hardwick *et al.*, 1971; Heath and Heath, 1971; Littlefield and Bracker, 1972). The neck ring (see below) then intervenes, and beyond the neck ring the wall of the haustorium stains uniformly with moderate electron density.

The **neck ring**, sometimes referred to as a neck band (Ehrlich and Ehrlich, 1971a; Heath and Heath, 1971; Coffey *et al.*, 1972), is a specialized region of the wall of the haustorial neck in rust fungi. It usually occurs in the mid-region of the neck and stains intensely with osmium tetroxide (Figs 48 and 49) (Coffey *et al.*, 1972; Heath, 1972; Hardwick *et al.*, 1971; Heath and Heath, 1971; Littlefield and Bracker, 1972; Van Dyke and Hooker, 1969) and potassium permanganate (Ehrlich and Ehrlich, 1971a; Hardwick *et al.*, 1971). The neck ring is preferentially removed by periodic acid (Littlefield and Bracker, 1972), but it stains intensely with Giemsa stain (Dr Incz Tommerup, personal communication). This structure is detectable by light microscopy, and was reported as early as 1927 by Rice but went almost unnoticed until its rediscovery by electron microscopy in the early 1970s. Littlefield (1972) showed that in *M. lini* the neck ring formed during the elongation of the penetration peg before the haustorial body was formed. The neck ring, which is marked by extremely close association of host and fungal plasma membrane (IT 18), also denotes the abrupt transition from the wall of the penetration peg to the wall of the haustorium (Littlefield and Bracker, 1972).

HAUSTORIAL SHEATH

By the terminology used here, a **haustorial sheath** is equivalent to the encapsulation shown by Heath (1972), Heath and Heath (1971), Ehrlich and

Ehrlich (1963a; 1971a, b), Calonge (1969), Berlin and Bowen (1964), Shaw and Manocha (1965), Kunoh and Akai (1969b), and the zone of apposition (Chou, 1970; Peyton and Bowen, 1963). It is distinct from the collar-like wall apposition termed a sheath by Berlin and Bowen (1964), Bushnell (1972), Calonge (1969), Chou (1970), Hardwick *et al.* (1971), Heath (1971, 1972), Heath and Heath (1971), Peyton and Bowen (1963) and others.

The haustorial sheath, or extrahaustorial matrix (Bushnell, 1972), is literally the environment in which a haustorium exists. It is the medium which coats the haustorium, and to the extent that a haustorium serves as an absorbing organ, it is from or through the haustorial sheath that materials are taken up. Virtually every haustorium is surrounded by a sheath of one sort or another, and often of varying size and extent. Even in examples where there is little or no detectable sheath, thin multimolecular films or matrices may be present beneath the extrahaustorial membrane. Surprisingly, the origin and biochemical nature of haustorial sheaths are still obscure. As will be seen, sheaths have diverse properties and vary according to taxonomic positions of host and parasite, compatibility of host and pathogen, and their development. In spite of the fact that the sheath seems to be a conceptual common denominator among haustoria, the diversity encountered so far makes it nearly impossible to conclude that sheaths are homologous structures among the different groups of hosts and parasites.

Sheaths are usually only a fraction of a micron thick and are thus difficult or impossible to detect by light microscopy. Exceptions are powdery mildews where the sheath either grows or swells (Bracker, 1968; Bushnell, 1971, 1972; Hirata, 1967) to the point that it is easily detected by light microscopy.

Sheath development is most pronounced around the haustorial body and where lobes protrude from the body. The haustorial neck and the distal parts of haustorial lobes usually show the thinnest sheaths. With rust haustoria the sheath matrix gradually tapers off in the transitional region from haustorial body to haustorial neck. The invaginated host plasma membrane is closely appressed to the fungal wall along the proximal portion of the haustorial neck, and no intervening matrix is evident (IT 18, IT 22) (Figs 47, 48, and 52) (Coffey *et al.*, 1972; Ehrlich and Ehrlich, 1971a; Hardwick *et al.*, 1971; Heath, 1972; Littlefield and Bracker, 1972). The wall-membrane junction is especially tight around the neck ring of rust haustoria (Heath, 1972; Heath and Heath, 1971; Littlefield and Bracker, 1972). Heath and Heath (1971) showed partial separation of the membrane from the proximal part of the haustorial neck (IT 24), and Hardwick *et al.* (1971) found partial separation in the same region where wall appositions were being laid down (IT 21). There is evidence that the extrahaustorial membrane is sealed around the haustorial neck, especially in powdery mildews, so that there is no humoral continuity between the sheath and neighbouring regions within or outside the host cell (Bushnell, 1972). The sheath usually does not extend into the collar region around a haustorial neck (Bracker, 1968), but it is found around encased haustoria of rusts (Heath and Heath, 1971; Littlefield and Bracker, 1972) where the wall apposition develops after the haustorium is formed (IT 22, IT 30, IT 31, IT 32). With *Albugo candida* (Berlin and Bowen, 1964) and *Peronospora manshurica* (Peyton and Bowen, 1963) material resembling the extrahaustorial matrix coats the haustorial neck (IT 24) and extends into the collar (IT 27), and through the hole in the host wall to the intercellular space (IT 13). Other examples where the wall of the symbiont contacts the host plasma membrane are with lichens (Roskin, 1970; Webber and Webber, 1970), especially when limited penetration has occurred, and in early stages of mycoparasitism (Armentrout and Wilson, 1969; Manocha and Lee, 1971) where the sheath is greatly diminished or absent. Sheaths did not form around haustoria of *Puccinia carthami* in laticifers that were devoid of cytoplasm (IT 19 or IT 45) (Zimmer, 1970).

The consistency of the sheath matrix is probably flexible in most situations and may vary from a liquid or solution (Bushnell, 1972; Zimmer, 1970) to thickened viscous material, or a gel, and is perhaps even firm where fibrils (Zimmer, 1970) or concentrated layers of material are present.

The sheath is usually distinct in texture and stainability from the haustorial wall or the host wall appositions, although some authors have regarded the sheath as a layer of the haustorial wall (Chou, 1970; Hardwick *et al.*, 1971) or as part of a complex encasement that also involves host wall appositions (Kajiwara, 1971). With all but oomycetous parasites, the sheath is not continuous with wall appositions or the host wall. But in infections by Oomycetes, the distinction between the haustorial sheath and wall appositions has not been clearly established.

The sheath matrix generally has an amorphous homogeneous appearance, suggesting that the major constituents are distributed uniformly throughout the matrix. But there are also clearcut examples showing layering, regions of structural differentiation, and discrete structural entities within the sheath. Frequently, the matrix consists of granular or flocculent material dispersed in an electron-transparent matrix. Reports of fibrils (Kajiwara, 1971; Orcival, 1969; Zimmer, 1970), particulate material (Ehrlich and Ehrlich, 1963a), fragmented material (M. D. Coffey, pers. comm.), remnants of secretory membranes (Peyton and Bowen, 1963), and others, extend the range of structures that occur in the sheath matrix, but we cannot accept any of the interpretations that host or fungal organelles (ER, ribosomes, etc.) are trapped in the sheath.

Sometimes the sheath stains only faintly or not at all with conventional electron stains (Figs 44, 57, 58, 64, and 68) (Coffey *et al.*, 1972; Galun *et al.*, 1970a; Heath, 1972; Heath and Heath, 1971; Jacobs and Ahmadjian, 1971; Littlefield and Bracker, 1972; Manocha and Lee, 1971; Van Dyke and Hooker, 1969). Such images pose the question of whether there is actually any material in the matrix or whether it is just an artefact consisting of an empty space or watery fluid between the fungal wall and the extrahaustorial membrane. It is true that thin watery solutions would not be expected to stain intensely, but the failure of a structure to stain does not necessarily mean organic material is absent, just that it has a low affinity for the stains that were used. For example, many cell walls also fail to stain (Figs 2, 5, and 7) (e.g. Van Dyke and Hooker, 1969). Usually, however, the sheath matrix does stain in a manner demonstrating that there is a layer of material outside the haustorial wall (Figs 60, 61, 72, and 73) (Armentrout and Wilson, 1969; Berlin and Bowen, 1964; Bracker, 1968; Calonge, 1969; Chou, 1970; Coffey *et al.*, 1972; Davison, 1968; Ehrlich and Ehrlich, 1963a, 1971a; Hardwick *et al.*, 1971; Heath and Heath, 1971; Kajiwara, 1969, 1971; Manocha and Lee, 1971; Olah *et al.*, 1971; Peyton and Bowen, 1963; Schnepf *et al.*, 1971a; Zimmer, 1970).

Although structural linkages between the haustorial wall and the invaginated host plasma membrane are rare, Peveling (1968) and Kajiwara (1971) have shown a network of fine fibrils connecting the fungal wall to the host membrane in a lichen and rust respectively. Likewise, we found a coating of fine fibrils that radiated from the hasutorial wall of *Erysiphe graminis*, perpendicular to the wall (Figs 77 and 78). Where the sheath was very thin around the haustorial lobes, the system of fibrils extended from the wall to the extrahaustorial membrane, but where the sheath was substantial the fibrils terminated in the amorphous matrix and did not reach the membrane.

The haustorial sheath often changes with age. Some authors have reported an increase in thickness of the sheath (Armentrout and Wilson, 1969; Bushnell, 1972 and references cited; Manocha and Lee, 1971; Olah *et al.*, 1971; Orcival, 1969; Shaw and Manocha, 1965). An exception is Kajiwara (1971) who found a thick sheath around haustoria that appeared young and vigorous to him, and narrow sheaths occurred around older haustoria. Ehrlich and Ehrlich (1971b) found the sheath to be larger but with less electron-dense material around young haustoria than mature ones. Then, with increasing age, the sheath swelled enormously and finally broke down. In lichens, Galun *et al.* (1970a, c) found the fungal wall and algal plasma membrane to be separated by an electron-transparent region (IT 24) when host cells were intact. They attributed this to a retraction of the algal protoplast from the invading fungus. However, in dead or dying host cells, the algal protoplast was closely pressed to the haustorium and no sheath was present. Contradictory observations about sheath development have not yet been reconciled and similarly, there are contradictory reports that the sheath either did (Shaw and Manocha, 1965; Zimmer, 1970) or did not (Van Dyke and Hooker, 1969) differ depending on host–pathogen compatibility.

From the foregoing it is apparent that the precise role of the sheath in development and in resistance–susceptibility reactions is not uniformly established, but there are enough meaningful observations to show correlations between the nature of the sheath and age or host-parasite compatibility. The changing status of the sheath is at least a result of, if not the cause of, developmental and compatibility phenomena. For example, sheaths around young haustoria of *Puccinia helianthi* and *Melampsora lini* (M. D. Coffey, pers. comm.; Coffey *et al.*, 1972) (Fig. 59) were electron-lucent and lacked stainable contents, but a new layer of electron-dense material was deposited on the haustorial walls when the haustoria aged. Similar material was associated with tubules and the inner surface of the sheath membrane. Orcival (1969) found that the sheath in rust infections was first amorphous and then progressively acquired fibrillar contents. In a resistant reaction to *Puccinia graminis* (Shaw and Manocha, 1965), the haustorial sheath developed more rapidly than in a susceptible reaction. In Zimmer's (1970) study of safflower rust, the sheaths around haustoria in incompatible hosts were more amorphous than in a compatible cultivar. Young haustoria were similar in resistant and susceptible hosts and were surrounded by a homogeneous sheath with granular or finely fibrillar contents considered to be liquid (Zimmer, 1970). As haustoria aged in the compatible host the sheath became stratified into three layers, and glandular appendages with fibrillar contents sometimes formed at the periphery. Sheath debris was also present, suggesting that material had been 'dumped' into the matrix by the host. The fibrillar portions of the sheaths resembled loosely organized cell walls, but it is not clear whether attempted wall formation was a property of the host, the fungus, or both. Collapse of host cytoplasm was accompanied by deterioration of the sheath matrix so that an electron-transparent space was all that remained between the host wall and the extrahaustorial membrane. Sheath deterioration was followed by collapse of haustorial organelles. In immune hosts of *Uromyces phaseoli* (Heath, 1972) the extrahaustorial membrane lost stability and broke down. Then the sheath degenerated and did not remain as a distinct layer around the haustoria. Encased haustoria of *U. phaseoli* in an immune host had a sheath consisting of an electron-dense deposit, in contrast to the electron-lucent sheaths at earlier stages (Heath and Heath, 1971). During early stages of mycoparasitic infections the invaginated host plasma membrane was close to the haustorial wall with little or no intervening sheath, but with time an electron-lucent sheath layer developed and then became filled with electron-dense contents (Armentrout and Wilson, 1969; Manocha and Lee, 1971). Armentrout and Wilson (1969) detected reaction products indicating acid phosphatase activity in the sheath region around haustoria of *Piptocephalis virginiana*. They suggested that lysosomal organelles in the parasite migrate into haustoria and contribute to the sheath matrix by releasing the contents at the surface of the haustorium. Released enzymes may then pass into the host to initiate changes there, or, alternatively, they could act in the sheath matrix to alter materials that could be assimilated by the parasite. Such speculation assumes that Armentrout and Wilson's (1969) localization of the enzyme by light microscopy was correct. Cytochemical studies by electron microscopy should now be done, with adequate safeguards to guarantee no spurious reactions or nonspecific deposition of reaction product, to determine the localization of this enzyme and other biochemical constitutents at the host–pathogen interface.

Although the sheath matrix is generally thought to increase with the age of the haustorium, Hirata (1967, 1971) and Bushnell (1971, 1972) have also shown that in powdery mildews the morphology of the sheath is influenced by the osmotic environment. This becomes important in ultrastructural studies because some fixation procedures also alter the sheath and cause it to swell (Bushnell, 1971) leaving the investigator with a false picture of the host–pathogen interface. Undoubtedly some swelling occurred in a previous study of powdery mildew haustoria (Bracker, 1968), and this may have been further complicated by the age of the haustoria. Recently, however, we have reinvestigated haustoria of *Erysiphe graminis* on a susceptible wheat cultivar, using various aldehyde and osmium tetroxide combinations on specimens 3–5 days after inoculation (Figs 67–82). The sheath matrix is clearly present around every haustorium, and there are no fundamental differences between the conclusions of this study and the previous one. What is clear, however, is that the sheath matrix is not as voluminous as was thought earlier (Bracker, 1968), and the sheath invaginations are not as common. The volume of the sheath matrix did increase with age, and haustoria showing signs of senescence were surrounded by the thickest sheaths. Also, in epidermal cells that were ruptured during dissection of tissue pieces, the sheaths appeared swollen. The evidence of this study demonstrates that the sheaths were not swollen by action of the fixatives. Profiles of haustoria show the extrahaustorial membrane drawn tightly around the haustorial body (Figs 68 and 70) and distal portions of haustorial lobes (Figs 70 and 73), as well as around the perimeter of clusters of haustorial lobes embedded in a common sheath (Figs 71 and 72). The extrahaustorial membrane abuts on the layer of fibrils coating the haustorial wall (Figs 77 and 78). The sheath matrix is granular and with moderate stain intensity (Fig. 72), clearly indicating the presence of organic materials in the matrix. Whether the matrix consists only of a solution (Bushnell, 1972) or also gels, colloids, or other structured forms of matrix is unknown. At least, the layer of fibrils adjacent to the haustorial wall retains its integrity and does not equilibrate with the rest of the matrix.

Within the sheath matrix, haustorial lobes of *E. graminis* are subject to several interface types based on their position. Parts of lobes (Figs 72 and 73) may be close to the invaginated host plasma membrane (IT 18 or IT 24) or may be exposed to portions of other haustorial lobes (IT 42 or IT 43) which subjects them to interactions with cell surfaces of their own kind. Where the haustorial lobes protrude from the bulk of the sheath matrix (Figs 70 and 73), they are always surrounded by the extrahaustorial membrane and a layer of host cytoplasm that may be reduced to as little as 10 nm thick. In these protoplasmically-sparse host cells, organelles proliferate around penetration sites (Figs 70 and 81) and around haustorial lobes (Figs 73 and 77). Still, there is a surprising scarcity of host cytoplasm around haustoria (Figs 68, 71, and 72) when one considers that this is supposedly the site of active interaction around haustoria that are still young enough to be functional.

The extracellular structures around haustoria of oomycetous parasites sometimes differ from those of rusts and powdery mildews and are much more difficult to interpret. There are examples in which a relatively simple sheath matrix bounded by the extrahaustorial membrane is present (IT 24) (Chou, 1970; Peyton and Bowen, 1963), but often the interface is more complicated or has components that are not easily identifiable. The coating around haustoria of *Phytophthora* spp. (Fig. 66) (Ehrlich and Ehrlich, 1966; Hanchey and Wheeler, 1971) has the appearance of a wall apposition (IT 21) and not a sheath. It is continuous with the host wall at the penetration site and resembles a papilla that has not been penetrated. The sheath, when present, seems to be more intimately associated with the haustorial wall than in rusts or powdery mildews and gives the impression of being a layer of the wall (Berlin and Bowen, 1964; Chou, 1970). Sheaths are often stained more intensely than the walls of these pathogens (Berlin and Bowen, 1964; Chou, 1970; Davison, 1968; Kajiwara, 1971; Peyton and Bowen, 1963). Kajiwara (1971) found several structures around downy mildew haustoria, including coatings which appeared to consist of integrated or stratified layers of wall apposition and sheath (IT 27), and an unusual electron-dense coating consisting of columnar particles that formed a palisade layer on the haustorial wall. Haustoria of *Peronospora parasitica* on cabbage (Chou, 1970) were often covered with densely staining porous or vesicular material just beneath the extrahaustorial membrane. We point out these diverse interface components around the haustoria of Oomycetes because they signify different types of interfacial relationships from those usually found with other hyphal and haustorial fungal parasites.

A number of speculations have been made about the origin of the haustorial sheath. As far back as 1900, Smith thought it was debris from the host wall. Others have also thought it was of host origin, but derived from the protoplast (Berlin and Bowen, 1964; Orcival, 1969; Peyton and Bowen, 1963; Shaw and Manocha, 1965) especially when membrane profiles resembling secretory components were seen at the periphery of the sheath. Observations of secretory profiles have been sporadic, however, and this raises two questions: (i) are the secretory components really involved in build up of the sheath, and (ii) if they are involved, are there just certain periods of sheath biogenesis that involve secretion from the host? The parasite has also been implicated in sheath formation. Chou (1970) and Hardwick *et al.* (1971) regarded the sheath as part of the fungal wall. But in view of the frequent extracellular secretions by fungi (see Bracker, 1967) it seems reasonable that secretions by the parasite contribute at least part of the sheath. Such secretions would be distinct from wholesale 'dumping' of material from the pathogen, as we do not have evidence of continuity between haustorial protoplasts and the sheath. Ehrlich and Ehrlich (1971b) queried why the sheath so often resembled haustorial cytoplasm and not host cytoplasm. In fact, it resembles neither host nor parasite cytoplasm, as numerous ultrastructure studies have demonstrated (Berlin and Bowen, 1964; Bracker, 1968; Coffey *et al.*, 1972; Heath, 1972; Heath and Heath, 1971; Littlefield and Bracker, 1972; McKeen *et al.*, 1966; Olah *et al.*, 1971; Orcival, 1969; Peyton and Bowen, 1963; Van Dyke and Hooker, 1969; Zimmer, 1970; and micrographs in this paper). Zimmer's (1970) finding that haustoria in cytoplasm-free laticifers also had no sheath implicates the host protoplast in the formation of the sheath—if not as the sole source of the sheath at least as a contributor. Hence, the final possibility arises that the sheath is a result of the host–parasite interaction (Heath and Heath, 1972; McKeen *et al.*, 1966; Zimmer, 1970), and is maintained by continued interaction. We regard this view as the most plausible and one that is consistent with ultrastructural evidence as well as with the expected mutual secretions by two protoplasts in close association, especially when each partner is known to influence the other

What function does the haustorial sheath perform? Does it facilitate transport of materials from host to pathogen, impede transport, or is it unrelated to transport (Bushnell, 1972)? So far, microscopic autoradiography has not shown accumulation of labelled nutrients in the sheath (Bushnell, 1972). This means that the matrix is probably not a storage pool for those materials tested, but it says nothing about the possibility of transport across the sheath. The suggestion that the haustorium is functional when the extrahaustorial membrane is close to the haustorial wall (Bushnell, 1972) implies a negative correlation between the volume of the sheath and the activity of the haustorium. The sheath could be a 'dumping ground' for materials on their way to a haustorium, as suggested by Ehrlich and Ehrlich (1971b), or vice versa. Hirata's contention that the sheath protected the host cell from the toxic effects of the haustoria (Hirata and Kojima, 1962) deserves considerable attention. This concept can be expanded to regard the sheath as a protective buffer between host and pathogen (Ehrlich and Ehrlich, 1971b), one that could provide for the stability of the extrahaustorial membrane or serve as a binding site for materials from either host or pathogen to keep them from the protoplasts of either partner and hence either accelerate or retard the demise of either partner. It may also be the site of enzymes necessary to convert host constituents into a form compatible with the needs of the pathogen (Kuć, in discussion of Hirata, 1971) or even serve as a source of materials that are unique to either partner and which promote the largely obligate physiological dependence of the parasite upon its host. The evidence that is bound to come with concerted experimental attacks on the nature of the sheath will probably show the sheath matrix to be a multifunctional system. Sheaths in general may have some fundamental characteristics in common that are related to general mechanisms of nutrition of obligate parasites (Zimmer, 1970), but with varied and changing physiological capabilities that can accommodate the progressive development of individual relationships and reflect the taxonomic diversity of parasites and hosts.

EXTRAHAUSTORIAL MEMBRANE

There has been considerable interest in the host membrane surrounding haustoria, and justifiably so. Membranes are known to be biologically active structures, and the extrahaustorial membrane is the invaginated host plasma membrane which makes it the boundary of the living host protoplast. Plasma membranes function in permeability and transport as well as in cell–cell interactions and cell coat formation. The membranes around haustoria have characteristics and specific configurations that suggest functions in the host–pathogen interaction. Recent information on isolated plasma membranes (Hodges *et al.*, 1972; Lembi *et al.*, 1971; VanDerWoude, 1972; see also *Nature, Lond.* **240**, 524) points out biochemical specialization, enzymatic capabilities, and even localization of auxin binding and transport sites and cell wall biosynthetic enzymes on the plasma membrane. Thus, this membrane has considerable functional importance as a component of the host–pathogen interface.

It has been referred to as the **extrahaustorial membrane** by Bushnell (1972) and Ehrlich and Ehrlich (1971a), although in many instances it has been shown to be the **invaginated host plasma membrane**. We use both terms here, and they are considered equivalent. 'Extrahaustorial membrane' is sometimes more convenient, but it has the disadvantage of being restricted to haustoria and thus is not applicable to the membranes around intracellular hyphae, thalli, bacteria, or other parasitic structures. We would prefer a term with broader applicability, especially since the derivation of the membrane in so many diverse systems is the same, but we decline to specify a new term and are uncertain about committing ourselves to other terms such as sheath membrane (Bracker, 1968; Coffey *et al.*, 1972; Dekhuijzen and van der Scheer, 1967, 1969; Smith, 1900; Zimmer, 1970), sac (Hirata and Kojima, 1962), or encapsulation boundary (Ehrlich and Ehrlich, 1966, 1971a) which have also been used as equivalent terms. We would tend to favour sheath membrane which has been in use since the turn of the century and is still widely used, but this term implies that the membrane is a property of the sheath (just as extrahaustorial membrane implies it is a property of the haustorium), when in fact it is a host membrane.

The extrahaustorial membrane surrounds the entire haustorium and separates it from the ground cytoplasm and organelles of the host. Depending on the host–pathogen combination and the stage of development, the extrahaustorial membrane is either close to the haustorial wall (IT 18) or separated from it by one or more layers of additional material (IT 21, IT 24, IT 27). The membrane assumes various profiles from smooth to undulating, or with tubular projections or complex invaginations (Figs 57–66).

Some reports have claimed that the extrahaustorial membrane is absent or disrupted at various sites around haustoria. However, it is necessary to caution that inability to observe a membrane with clarity should not necessarily be interpreted to mean that the membrane is not there. For example, Kajiwara's (1969, 1971) interpretations that the host plasma membrane often disappeared at the apices of haustoria or during host penetration are without foundation. The micrographs show quite clearly that the membrane was intercepted obliquely or tangentially by the sections, and when this happens any membrane will appear as a blurred or diffuse patch and not a clear line. More convincing evidence of disappearance or breakdown of the invaginated host plasma membrane occurs in resistant or immune reactions to rust infections (Heath and Heath, 1971; Van Dyke and Hooker, 1969) and in disorganized host cells (Calonge, 1969; Ehrlich and Ehrlich, 1971b; Heath, 1972).

Origin and continuity of the extrahaustorial membrane. The extrahaustorial membrane is generally acknowledged as the host plasma membrane that is invaginated by the developing haustorium. This was indicated by early light microscopic studies (Rice, 1927; Smith, 1900) and received further support from Thatcher (1939, 1942) and Fraymouth (1956) who plasmolysed host cells and noted that the protoplasts pulled away from haustoria. But proof of the continuity between host plasma membrane and extrahaustorial membrane *in situ* has come from electron microscopy. Clear line continuity is evident for downy mildews (Peyton and Bowen, 1963), lichens (Galun *et al.*, 1970a, c; Jacobs and Ahmadjian, 1971), white rust (*Albugo candida*) (Berlin and Bowen, 1964), infections by *Phytophthora* spp. (Ehrlich and Ehrlich, 1966; Hanchey and Wheeler, 1971), and only recently for several examples of plant rusts (Coffey *et al.*, 1972; Ehrlich and Ehrlich, 1971a; Hardwick *et al.*, 1971; Littlefield and Bracker, 1970, 1972). It is safe to assume that host plasma membrane invagination is a general phenomenon with haustorial parasites, but membranes are often contorted or sectioned obliquely and there is a zone of confusion near the host cell wall that obscures continuity, or else specimen fixation or micrograph quality are insufficient to provide the clear continuity of plasma membrane that is required for definitive proof.

Where a substantial collar surrounds the penetration site it is extremely difficult to evaluate membrane continuity. The problem of tracing plasma membrane continuity under such circumstances has been discussed previously (Bracker, 1968; Littlefield and Bracker, 1970). But if the collar is small or consists only of globular deposits on the host wall, the plasma membrane can be followed along the contour of the wall apposition next to the haustorial neck.

Often the membrane can be seen to double back on itself in the space between the collar and the neck, but still membrane continuity can be confirmed (Fig. 47) (Littlefield and Bracker, 1972). If the plasma membrane fails to adhere to the contour of the collar next to the haustorial neck or passes only part way into the space between collar and neck, the membrane profile may be sufficiently clear that it can be traced with ease (Berlin and Bowen, 1964; Peyton and Bowen, 1963). The serious problems caused by collars are especially evident with powdery mildews (Bracker, 1968) and some examples of rusts (Littlefield and Bracker, 1972; Van Dyke and Hooker, 1969).

With powdery mildews there is little doubt that the extrahaustorial membrane is the invaginated host plasma membrane, but it has not yet been possible to trace the entire continuity in a single micrograph. This is partly because the membrane follows an irregular path as it passes around the collar and up inside the channel between the collar and the haustorial neck (authors' unpublished observations, and Bracker, 1968; Watene, 1968). Furthermore, the material in the channel usually stains very densely (Figs 81 and 82), and the dark-staining components of the membrane are obscured against this dark background. In serial section micrographs, examined at high magnification, it has been possible to trace the membrane up inside the channel toward the host cell wall where it doubles back on itself and then follows the haustorial neck and emerges from the collar region as the extrahaustorial membrane. Clearly, the host plasma membrane and the extrahaustorial membrane converge in the channel and can be traced in parallel where they are not obscured by the dense matrix, and repeated images show a membrane curving over at the top of the channel (see also Bracker, 1968; Watene, 1968).

For powdery mildews, the question of whether the membranes (extrahaustorial membrane and host plasma membrane) retain functional continuity after a haustorium is formed is still open. The dark-staining material in the channel has a necrotic appearance and may seal off the proximal region of the neck and obliterate structural or functional membrane continuity that existed during early stages of haustorium formation. If the haustorial neck became sealed off and the membranes were anchored in place in the channel, it would also explain some of the unusual results of plasmolysis experiments in which the host protoplast does not pull away from the haustorium but appears to be anchored to the haustorium (Bushnell, 1971). Likewise, the fact that isolated haustoria retain the extrahaustorial membrane (Bracker, 1968; Dekhuijzen and van der Scheer, 1967, 1969; Hirata and Kojima, 1962) could be accounted for if the membrane was sealed in place around the haustorial neck. Then, removal of haustoria from host cells would involve severing the neck and tearing most of the haustorial apparatus away from the host plasma membrane, with the tougher reinforced extrahaustorial membrane remaining intact and retaining osmotic capabilities.

Another persistent question is how the host plasma membrane is displaced so that it follows the contour of the channel and doubles back on itself. With rust infections this is relatively easy to understand because the collars develop after the host is penetrated (Coffey *et al.*, 1972; Littlefield and Bracker, 1972), and a plasma membrane that was invaginated along a simple contour without any wall appositions would simply be gradually invaginated again by a developing collar. But the question is more difficult with the powdery mildews because one must assume a mechanism whereby the membrane is displaced upwards inside the channel after the penetration peg has breached the pre-formed papilla. We can speculate about this phenomenon, but what is significant is that it does occur.

Association of host cell components with the extrahaustorial membrane. There is a surprising lack of protoplasmic disorganization by haustorial pathogens in susceptible hosts during early stages of infection (Coffey *et al.*, 1972; Littlefield and Bracker, 1972; Peyton and Bowen, 1963) (Figs 43, 44, 61, 68, 70, and 73). In general, there is a proliferation of host cell organelles after invasion by haustoria so that the host cells return temporarily to a structurally juvenile appearance (Bracker, unpublished; Ehrlich and Ehrlich, 1971a; Shaw and Manocha, 1965; Van Dyke and Hooker, 1969). The further development of organelles and membranes increases the chances of interaction between these host cell components and the haustoria and provides abundant structures which may become part of the interface. The difficulty is in knowing whether or not to include a particular host structure as a part of the interfacial complex. In the absence of data on functional interaction, the question is whether proximity alone (whether a specific interaction or chance association) is sufficient to implicate a structure at the interface.

Nevertheless, numerous host cell components have been implicated as interface components either because of physical closeness to the haustorium or because of suspected continuity between the membranes of these structures and the extrahaustorial membrane. The powdery mildews stand apart as exceptions, however, since no host structures have been consistently observed associated with the haustoria of these fungi.

When a haustorium forms inside a host cell, it displaces whatever is in its way. This invariably leads to a distortion of the profile of the protoplast. Where the host cell contains only a thin peripheral layer of protoplasm (Figs 43, 70, 71, 72, and 78) the haustorium pushes the cytoplasmic layer into the vacuole, and the tonoplast is pressed close to the extrahaustorial membrane. In algae (Bushnell, 1972; Schnepf *et al.*, 1971a), invading haustoria invaginate the chloroplasts as well as the surface of the protoplast. In this way, organelles and membranes may be held in place in a close positional relationship that may also result in a functional relationship.

One of the most intriguing and least understood aspects of host-pathogen interfaces is the role of host cell components in the interaction. It is tempting to propose that there may be interactions between host organelles and haustoria.

The least convincing observations are those in which a haustorium is simply found close to a host mitochondrion, chloroplast, or other organelle. The problem is in determining the specificity of the relationship. Chance associations may not be meaningful, but it is difficult to determine what constitutes a chance association as against a specific and functional association. In view of protoplasmic streaming and organellar motility, it is inevitable that host organelles should come close to large structures such as haustoria, but such associations may represent temporary or accidental relationships. Where haustoria contact and even invaginate organelles such as the algal chloroplasts mentioned above (Schnepf *et al.*, 1971a), it cannot be denied that a close association exists between the fungus and the chloroplast, and perhaps there is a functional relationship. Descriptions of direct continuity between chloroplasts and the extrahaustorial membrane have also been made (Ehrlich and Ehrlich, 1971b), and these interpretations are difficult to accept when the fixation is such that membranes of organelles are ruptured. Nevertheless, there is now a body of ultrastructural and biochemical evidence to implicate structural and functional continuity among seemingly dissimilar membrane systems in eukaryotes (see Bracker and Grove, 1971, and references cited). Therefore, suspected continuities and relationships such as those described by Ehrlich and Ehrlich (1971b), however unlikely they may appear at first, deserve sufficient investigation to confirm or disprove their occurrence.

Commonly, the host nucleus is reported to be closely associated with rust haustoria (Allen, 1928; Coffey *et al.*, 1972; Colley, 1918; Olah *et al.*, 1971; Rice, 1927; Van Dyke and Hooker, 1969). This association does not always exist (e.g. Littlefield and Bracker, 1972), but failure to observe the host nucleus-haustorium association may result from examining sections cut at the wrong angle. When host nuclei are adjacent to haustoria (regardless of the extent or the constancy of this relationship), the host nuclear envelope might well be an important functional component of the interfacial region.

The most obvious and frequent relationship is between host endoplasmic reticulum (ER) and the extrahaustorial membrane. This is especially common in rusts, but rare with powdery mildews. Cisternae of ER are associated with haustoria in a position parallel to the invaginated host plasma membrane (Fig. 57) (Ehrlich and Ehrlich, 1971a, b; Hardwick *et al.*, 1971; Heath, 1972; Heath and Heath, 1971; Littlefield and Bracker, 1972; Manocha and Lee, 1971; Olah *et al.*, 1971; Orcival, 1969; Schnepf *et al.*, 1971a; Shaw and Manocha, 1965; Zimmer, 1970), and in several studies on rusts the ER has been orientated specifically around the neck region of the haustorium (Ehrlich and Ehrlich, 1971a; Hardwick *et al.*, 1971; Heath and Heath, 1971; Littlefield and Bracker, 1970, 1972). The ER-plasma membrane associations usually involve close proximity and sometimes contact between the two membranes. The surface of the ER facing the haustorium usually lacks ribosomes (Hardwick *et al.*, 1971;

Heath, 1972; Heath and Heath, 1971; Littlefield and Bracker, 1972; Orcival, 1969; Schnepf *et al.*, 1971a) much the same as ER that interacts with adjacent Golgi apparatus and mitochondria in eukaryotic cells (Bracker and Grove, 1971; Morré and Mollenhauer, 1973). A smooth section of rough ER is typical at sites where the ER is continuous with or closely associated with other cell components in eukaryotes. Several authors have proposed that host ER could be continuous with the membrane surrounding haustoria (Calonge, 1969; Ehrlich and Ehrlich, 1971a, b; Kajiwara, 1971; Shaw and Manocha, 1965), but the micrographs in support of this hypothesis have not shown clear membrane continuity. We point this out because the possibility of continuity between host ER and the invaginated host plasma membrane poses a potentially significant concept wherein the endoplasmic reticulum could contribute directly to the sheath matrix surrounding the haustorium and thus might be an important cell component as far as transfer of materials to the parasite is concerned. Furthermore, rough ER is known to be active in biosynthesis of materials for export, and smooth ER is often a transition element between rough ER and other endomembrane components (Morré and Mollenhauer, 1973). Thus, it is critical to determine whether or not continuity between ER and the extra-haustorial membrane occurs. We have not observed direct ER–plasma membrane continuity in our specimens. It is highly unlikely that endoplasmic reticulum would normally be continuous with plasma membrane, although recent studies (Heath, 1972; Carothers, 1972) have shown that it is not impossible in unusual circumstances. But it is problematic as a general phenomenon because the structure and chemistry of ER and plasma membrane are known to be different (Grove *et al.*, 1968; Morré and Mollenhauer, 1973), and it is assumed that membrane transformation from ER-like to plasma membrane-like, as in the endomembrane concept (Morré and Mollenhauer, 1973), must occur. Heath's (1972) sensibly cogent statement regarding ER-plasma membrane continuity in diseased cells acknowledged that 'fusion . . . probably reflects a considerable change in the properties of the membranes involved.' Apart from possibilities of direct continuity between ER and plasma membrane, close association and contact between ER and the extrahaustorial membrane may be sufficient to effect intermembrane transfer, perhaps through a 'collision complex' or instant transfer mechanism similar to that proposed for the exchange of materials between ER and mitochondria (see Bracker and Grove, 1971, and references cited). Clearly there is reason to be sceptical about continuities between ER and plasma membrane until they have been documented without question, but there is every reason to be concerned about the frequent close associations observed between ER and haustoria. This phenomenon warrants exploration as a potentially significant functional part of the interface.

The occurrence of cytoplasmic vesicles around haustoria (Ehrlich and Ehrlich, 1963a; Peyton and Bowen, 1963; Orcival, 1969; Shaw and Manocha, 1965) has spawned speculation that the vesicles represent transient stages in transport of material toward or away from the haustoria. Ehrlich and Ehrlich (1971b) correctly pointed out that the presence of vesicles proves only that vesicles exist and not that they are moving in one direction or the other. However, the work of Peyton and Bowen (1963) and Berlin and Bowen (1964) strongly indicates that secretory vesicles and tubules from the host cytoplasm fuse with the invaginated host plasma membrane and deposit their contents into the sheath matrix (Figs 60 and 61). The fact that such 'secretory' structures are formed only in response to the parasite suggests that they play a role in the development of the interface. Transport via ER- or Golgi apparatus-derived vesicles would be a discontinuous mode of transport resulting in functional continuity between the endomembrane system and the extrahaustorial membrane, in contrast to the physically continuous route that would be assumed if cisternae of ER were continuous with the extrahaustorial membrane. Several authors have reported that host Golgi apparatus are stimulated to increased activity in infected cells (Berlin and Bowen, 1964; Ehrlich and Ehrlich, 1971b; Manocha and Shaw, 1967; Shaw and Manocha, 1965; Van Dyke and Hooker, 1969), and this is particularly evident in the cells of wheat and barley leaves infected with *Erysiphe graminis* (Bracker, unpublished). The increase in numbers of Golgi apparatus signifies secretion, by the host. Questions remain about what is secreted, where, and when? As marked as these associations between host structures (including ER) and haustoria are when they are observed, they are not always present, even in a single host–pathogen combination. This observation raises further questions of whether the associated structures are related to particular developmental stages and even whether the associations are essential for the host–parasite interaction.

Specialization of invaginated host plasma membrane. Although the extrahaustorial membrane is continuous with the host plasma membrane, it has some different properties which indicate that it is specialized where it is associated with the haustorium. With conventional stains the extrahaustorial membrane often has the typical appearance of non-invaginated host plasma membrane (e.g. Figs 57 and 64) (Berlin and Bowen, 1964; Coffey *et al.*, 1972; Ehrlich and Ehrlich, 1966; Hardwick *et al.*, 1971; Littlefield and Bracker, 1972; Peyton and Bowen, 1963; Van Dyke and Hooker, 1969) and is distinct from ER, mitochondrial membranes, and other cytomembranes with respect to stainability and dimensions (see Grove *et al.*, 1968 for a comparison of membrane types). However, in some studies the extrahaustorial membrane appears thicker than the plasma membrane (Figs 79 and 80) (Armentrout and Wilson, 1969; Bracker, 1968; Ehrlich and Ehrlich, 1963a; Hirata and Kojima, 1962; Smith, 1900). We will discuss several other lines of evidence indicating that the extrahaustorial membrane is a regional specialization of the host plasma membrane. It is important to note here that membranes are capable of developmental change and differentiation. Ultrastructural evidence shows that membranes have the potential to differentiate in time and space (Grove *et al.*, 1968; Staehelin, 1968), and it is this feature that may be an important determinant in the success or failure of establishing and sustaining a delicate and specific host-parasite relationship.

With powdery mildews the thick extrahaustorial membrane is reinforced. It is tougher and more resistant to stress conditions than any other membrane in either the host or the fungus (Bracker, 1968). This has made it possible to isolate powdery mildew haustoria from host cells with the extrahaustorial membrane intact (Bracker, 1968; Dekhuijzen and van der Scheer, 1967, 1969; Hirata and Kojima, 1962), an important experimental step which some day may permit a characterization of the membrane. Further, Hirata and Kojima (1962) found that applications of calcium made the membrane around haustoria of *E. graminis* more firm and that leaves could be made more susceptible by providing calcium. Lithium, on the other hand, caused the membrane to become unstable. Hirata and Kojima's (1962) experiments suggest a correlation between properties of the extrahaustorial membrane and host susceptibility to powdery mildew and indicate that an unbroken membrane is necessary for the host cell to remain alive. Thus, the contents of the sheath matrix could have adverse effects on the host protoplast if released from the boundary of the sheath. Likewise, a reinforced extrahaustorial membrane, such as occurs around powdery mildew haustoria, permits the sheath environment to be maintained for the haustorium even when other host cell components are severely disrupted. Bushnell (1972) has reviewed experiments on the osmotic and permeability properties of the sheath and extrahaustorial membrane around powdery mildew haustoria.

The extrahaustorial membrane around a mycoparasite, *Piptocephalis virginiana*, was as much as 2–3 times as thick as the non-invaginated host plasma membrane, and it persisted around haustoria after degradation of host cytoplasm (Armentrout and Wilson, 1969). The precise structure of this membrane is difficult to evaluate from published micrographs, but the evidence indicates that it thickened as the relationship developed, since young haustoria (Figs 17 and 18 of Armentrout and Wilson, 1969) were surrounded by thinner membranes that were equivalent to host plasma membrane. The images of later infections suggest that two membranes may be present, similar to the plasmodial envelope of *Plasmodiophora brassicae* (Fig. 16), but the extrahaustorial membrane is separate from the plasma membrane and cell wall of *Piptocephalis*, unlike the close association between protoplasts of *Plasmodiophora* and their host cells.

With rust infections the extrahaustorial membrane is usually the same thickness as the host plasma membrane (Coffey *et al.*, 1972; Littlefield and Bracker, 1970, 1972; Van Dyke and Hooker, 1969), but Heath (1972) showed the extrahaustorial membrane to be thicker and more diffuse around a haustorium of *Uromyces phaseoli* in a non-host plant.

The most clearcut ultrastructural differences between the extrahaustorial membrane and the host plasma membrane in rusts have been shown in flax leaves infected by *Melampsora lini* (Littlefield and Bracker, 1972). Both chemical and structural differences are indicated. When tissues are treated with a special stain that is specific for plant plasma membranes, the non-invaginated portion of the host plasma membrane stains intensely as does the fungal plasma membrane (Fig. 65). But the invaginated part of the host plasma membrane surrounding the haustorium stains faintly or not at all (Fig. 65) in contrast to its comparative ability to be stained with conventional lead citrate stain (Fig. 64). The transition in this property of the membrane occurs in the region of the neck ring on the haustorial wall. This region also corresponds to a change in the nature of the fungal wall (Littlefield and Bracker, 1972). In freeze-etched specimens the invaginated host plasma membrane is characterized by linear cleft-like depressions and a smooth surface (Figs 43 and 62), unlike the non-invaginated plasma membrane which lacks the depressions and is covered with characteristic granules (Fig. 63) that typify plasma membranes of both host and fungus.

Hardwick *et al.* (1971) divided the host plasma membrane into four distinct regions: (i) the area of the original plasma membrane lateral to the limits of the collar which apparently remains unaltered, (ii) the extensive proliferation of new membrane which limits the collar, (iii) the small area around the darkly staining fungal wall (neck band) in the haustorial neck, and (iv) another large area of new membrane around the body of the haustorium. Each region was associated with the presence or absence of particular materials immediately external to it. This led Hardwick *et al.* (1971) to the hypothesis that the membrane is functionally as well as morphologically differentiated, and that in each region the membrane may possess activities (distinct from those which operate in the cytoplasm) essential to the processes of deposition, if not also synthesis, of materials associated with it. The authors went on to state that 'variations in the morphology of different parts of the newly-formed membrane of the invaginated host protoplast may be assumed to be consequences of changes which occur in the interaction of host and parasite during the development of the membrane'.

Other specializations of the invaginated host plasma membrane include distinctive configurations and unique associations with host structures. Heath (1972) and Heath and Heath (1971) found the invaginated host plasma membrane to be highly convoluted and associated with deposits of densely-staining material in cowpea hosts showing an immune reaction to *Uromyces phaseoli* (Fig. 58). As noted earlier, haustoria of *Peronospora manshurica* (Fig. 61) (Peyton and Bowen, 1963) and *Albugo candida* (Fig. 60) (Berlin and Bowen, 1964) had secretory vesicles, secretory bodies, and/or membranous tubules associated with the extrahaustorial membrane and often continuous with it, in contrast to the non-invaginated region of the host plasma membrane. Some haustoria of *Puccinia graminis* (Ehrlich and Ehrlich, 1963a) were surrounded by vesicles next to the extrahaustorial membrane, and tentacles were observed on the invaginated plasma membrane around young haustoria of *Puccinia graminis* (Ehrlich and Ehrlich, 1971b). In a recent investigation of *Puccinia helianthi* and *Melampsora lini* (Coffey *et al.*, 1972; characteristic tubules on the extrahaustorial membrane projected into the host cytoplasm only in older infections before host-cell death. The tubules were continuous with the extrahaustorial membrane, had a membrane type that corresponded to the extrahaustorial membrane, were interspersed with cisternae of rough ER (Fig. 59), and contained material which stained similarly to an outer coating on the haustorial wall.

Around powdery mildew haustoria the extrahaustorial membrane is invaginated into the sheath matrix in simple bulbous or tubular configurations or complex branching clusters of invaginations, especially around the haustorial neck at the distal end of the collar (Bracker, 1968; Dekhuijzen and van der Scheer, 1967, 1969; Ehrlich and Ehrlich, 1963b; Stanbridge *et al.*, 1971; Stavely *et al.*, 1969). The lumina of these sheath invaginations contain host cytoplasm. In a recent study of powdery mildew on wheat (micrographs shown in this paper) in which aldehyde and osmium tetroxide fixations were used on younger infections than in the previous study (Bracker, 1968), the sheath invaginations were much less frequent although still occasionally present.

All of the distinctive features and configurations of the invaginated host plasma membrane signify specialization of the membrane where it is associated with the haustorium. The specific significance of these various specializations is still beyond experimental resolution, but it seems clear that they all have something to do with the interaction between host and parasite. Apart from the various distinctive features of the extrahaustorial membrane, it is important not to forget that the membrane encounters a different external environment than the rest of the host plasma membrane. This alone makes the membrane distinctive because it reflects a region of the host cell surface that differs from the rest of the cell.

Formation of the extrahaustorial membrane. In spite of repeated demonstrations of continuity between the extrahaustorial membrane and the host plasma membrane, questions still remain about how it is formed. These questions are further complicated by the thought that the membrane may be discontinuous or interrupted (at least temporarily) near the penetration site (Ehrlich and Ehrlich, 1971b). But biological membranes virtually always occur *in situ* as continuous structures, and the discontinuities that have been indicated at penetration sites are not supported by studies in which specimen preparation and microscopy have been satisfactory. Therefore, we assume that a continuous extrahaustorial membrane is in place throughout the initiation and development of a haustorium, and the problem is one of increasing the membrane as the haustorium grows.

The notion that the extrahaustorial membrane in powdery mildew infections is at least partly of fungal origin (Dekhuijzen and van der Scheer, 1969; Ehrlich and Ehrlich, 1963b) is not acceptable without some experimental evidence, and the reasons that have been given in support of this hypothesis do not diminish the difficulty in understanding how a haustorium could form an extracellular biological membrane precisely at the boundary of the host protoplast. We do not deny that the formation of the new membrane and acquisition of special properties are induced or stimulated by the pathogen, but there is an important distinction between induction of a host reponse by a pathogen and actual production of a structure by the pathogen.

The extrahaustorial membrane cannot be formed merely by stretching the existing host plasma membrane. New membrane must be synthesized to accommodate the increased surface area of the host protoplast during the growth of a haustorium, and the new plasma membrane that is formed must be of the specialized type that characterizes the host–parasite interface. It may arise by fusion of vesicles, indirectly from ER—via membrane flow and differentiation (Morré and Mollenhauer, 1973), and by whatever other mechanisms are responsible for plasma membrane biogenesis. Two mechanisms are suggested, either alone or in combination, by which the specialization of the extrahaustorial membrane could be achieved: (i) the membrane is first formed as 'normal' plasma membrane and is then transformed specifically around the haustorium, or (ii) during haustorium formation, new host plasma membrane is formed around the haustorium which has a different character from the outset than the non-invaginated plasma membrane (Littlefield and Bracker, 1972).

HOST WALL AND WALL APPOSITIONS

The host wall is a major interface component before and during penetration (IT 8, IT 11, IT 13, IT 16), and sometimes it is altered visibly during the infection process. The most familiar wall modifications are the haloes around penetration sites of powdery mildew fungi. These have been observed by a variety of methods using light microscopy (Akai *et al.*, 1968; Bracker, 1968; Bushnell, 1972; Corner, 1935; Ghemawhat, 1968; Kunoh and Akai, 1969a; Lupton, 1956; McKeen *et al.*, 1969), as well as by electron microscopy (Figs 68–70, 81, and 82) (Akai *et al.*, 1968; Edwards and Allen, 1970; McKeen *et al.*, 1969; Stanbridge *et al.*, 1971). Cytochemical tests show that the haloes contain altered cutin, pectin, polysaccharides, and other carbohydrates in a pattern that radiates from the penetration site. Cellulose is at least altered if not removed in the halo regions. This is accompanied by a modified staining reaction as seen by electron microscopy, but the fibrillar architecture of the wall remains intact even where it shows modified staining. We have observed a broad range of staining patterns around penetration sites of *E. graminis* on a single wheat cultivar. Compare the diffuse uniform haloes in Figs 68 and 69 with the clearly defined patterns of altered wall immediately adjacent to the penetration pegs in Figs 74, 81, and 82. Clearly the haloes represent biochemical alterations in the host wall that are specifically induced by the pathogen, and their existence implies the secretion of enzymes or other biochemical incitants.

Wall elaborations are common responses to trauma in plants, including mechanical injury. Nims *et al.* (1967) showed that a callose wall apposition formed in tobacco callus cells in response to wounding. Within 15 min after cells were penetrated by a needle, callose was deposited as a collar around the base of the needle and then formed a coating around the entire intracellular portion of the needle. Thus, although wall appositions are characteristic of some host-pathogen interactions, it would be a mistake to conclude that induction of wall appositions is solely the result of biochemical interactions between organisms.

We have made repeated reference to host wall appositions induced by haustorial parasites and other pathogens. A number of research reports and reviews have covered details of these structures which will not be included here (Bracker, 1968; Bushnell, 1972; Coffey *et al.*, 1972; Ehrlich and Ehrlich, 1971a; Heath, 1971, 1972; Heath and Heath, 1971). Wall appositions are frequently associated with haustoria (Bushnell, 1972), and they are diverse in their morphology and texture. The appositions vary from small lumpy deposits on the host wall to extensive encasements that completely surround haustoria and wall them off from the host protoplast (Fig. 53). Other forms include collars of various shapes and sizes surrounding the proximal portions of haustoria or haustorial necks and broad plate-like extensions that radiate from the collar and add to the thickness of the host wall (Bracker, 1968).

As noted earlier, papillae are formed in advance of penetration by powdery mildews (Bushnell, 1972; Edwards and Allen, 1970; Smith, 1900) which means that virtually all successful powdery mildew infections require the fungus to breach the host wall and the papilla in order to form a haustorium. The penetrated papilla persists as a collar surrounding the haustorial neck. In contrast, most penetrations by rust fungi do not involve wall appositions until after penetration is accomplished.

The collars surrounding the necks of rust haustoria usually form after the haustoria are established (Figs 50 and 51) (Coffey *et al.*, 1972; Heath, 1971; Littlefield and Bracker, 1972). However, the host wall may thicken somewhat around penetration sites during penetration by rust fungi. The thickenings take the form of lumpy wall appositions (Figs 46 and 47) or more uniform thickenings of the host wall (Fig. 48). Irregular wall appositions do form in cells of immune hosts and non-host plants where the hyphae of rust fungi contact the external surface of the cells (Heath, 1972; Heath and Heath, 1971). Heath (1972) also found wall deposits within the fungal cells where they contacted the plant cell walls, indicating a two-way interaction. When a collar is formed around rust haustoria, the apposition material, apparently secreted by the host protoplast, builds up at the proximal end of the haustorial neck and forms an anchored deposit around the basal one-quarter to one-third of the neck, and usually not past the neck ring. M. D. Coffey (unpublished) found extensive collars developing in older rust infections and noted that the collar material extended deep into the host wall. The haustorial wall fused with the collar near the host wall (IT 21). If deposition of collar material continues, as it sometimes does, the whole haustorium becomes encased and is effectively walled off from the host cell (Fig. 53). When such encasement occurs, the haustorial sheath, extra-haustorial membrane, and host cytoplasm are also trapped by the encasement (Figs 51 and 52), leading to IT 22, IT 30, IT 31, IT 32 or IT 33, depending on the condition of the host and fungal protoplasm. Only a small fraction of rust haustoria in susceptible hosts are encased, however (Heath and Heath, 1971; Littlefield and Bracker, 1972). Often, the protoplast of an encased haustorium becomes necrotic, although Hardwick *et al.* (1971) and Orcival (1969) found occasional encased rust haustoria that were not necrotic. These haustoria had no sheath or membranes trapped between the haustorial wall and the encasement (IT 21) (Fig. 13 of Hardwick *et al.*, 1971), suggesting that they represented rare instances of wall appositions formed in advance of the penetrating rust fungus rather than encasement following penetration.

Viable haustoria of Oomycetes are often surrounded by wall appositions (Ehrlich and Ehrlich, 1966; Hanchey and Wheeler, 1971; Kajiwara, 1971), but occasionally some of the haustoria are necrotic when they are completely encased (Berlin and Bowen, 1964). Haustoria of Oomycetes frequently have a collar-like structure around the base of the neck (Berlin and Bowen, 1964; Peyton and Bowen, 1963), but collar development has not been well documented for these infections, although wall appositions are apparently present around very young haustoria (Chou, 1970; Hanchey and Wheeler, 1971; Kajiwara, 1971).

The texture, morphology, and composition of wall appositions are diverse, as the figures in this paper illustrate (Figs 46, 47, 50, 51, 53, 54, 55, 56, 66, 67, 68, 81, and 82). Some appear amorphous (Berlin and Bowen, 1964; Chou, 1970; Edwards and Allen, 1970; Ehrlich and Ehrlich, 1966; Hanchey and Wheeler, 1971; Peyton and Bowen, 1963), whereas others have definite fibrillar architecture (Coffey *et al.*, 1972; Hardwick *et al.*, 1971; Manocha and Lee, 1971; Orcival, 1969; Watene, 1968). They may have uniform composition, or show distinct layering or zonation (Bracker, 1968; Kajiwara, 1971; Stanbridge *et al.*, 1971; Watene, 1968). With conventional fixatives and stains, wall appositions show stain reactions ranging from faint to intense and dark (Berlin and Bowen, 1964; Bracker, 1968; Edwards and Allen, 1970; Stanbridge *et al.*, 1971; Watene, 1968). In many examples, pockets of densely staining material and membranes are trapped in the appositions (Bracker, 1968; Chou, 1970; Edwards and Allen,

1970; Ehrlich and Ehrlich, 1966; Hardwick *et al.*, 1971; Heath and Heath, 1971; Kajiwara, 1971; Orcival, 1969). Some of the appositions bear striking resemblance to the host wall (Coffey *et al.*, 1972; Watene, 1968) whereas others are distinct and different from wall material.

These differences are not just found among different host-pathogen combinations. We have observed extreme variation in the nature of papillae in a single host-pathogen combination (*Erysiphe graminis* on wheat), and the differences are even apparent among penetration sites within the same host cell. *E. graminis* rarely penetrates guard cells of barley or wheat epidermis, but occasional attempts are made. One of these attempted unsuccessful penetrations is shown in Fig. 56. The papilla stains intensely and is quite different from the papillae and collars found at sites of successful penetrations (Figs 68, 81, and 82). The protoplast of the fungus is withered and retracted in the penetration peg with deposits of densely staining material near the apex of the peg (Fig. 56). We emphasize that the fungus was thwarted as it encountered the papilla and not the host wall. It had successfully penetrated a portion of the epidermal wall that was much thicker than the walls present at normally successful penetration sites. The overall relationship was similar to that found in attempted penetrations of pea root cells by *Verticillium dahliae* (Fig. 55) in which lignitubers form and ward off the pathogen.

It is generally assumed that wall appositions result from localized secretory activity by the host. Several studies have shown cytoplasmic vesicles or dictyosomes to be present near wall appositions (Chou, 1970; Edwards and Allen, 1970; Ehrlich *et al.*, 1968; Littlefield and Bracker, 1972), suggesting that wall appositions are formed at least partly by deposition of material carried in secretory vesicles. However, some of the collars observed around penetration sites appear to be formed as remnants of the host wall pushed aside to form a flange around the haustorial neck (Galun *et al.*, 1970a, c; Peveling, 1968; Roskin, 1970). Other mechanisms of apposition formation are also possible including involvement of the host plasma membrane, and even contributions from the pathogen (Hardwick *et al.*, 1971), but there is not yet enough evidence to clarify the origins of pathogen-induced wall appositions. Research of the sort that is currently under way on mechanisms of cell wall formation and subcellular sites of wall biosynthesis in plants (e.g. VanDerWoude, 1972 and refs cited) will also provide clues for understanding the subcellular origins, mechanisms, and controls of aberrant wall appositions in diseased cells.

The chemical composition of collars and other wall appositions has not been documented extensively, but some constituents are known. Callose has been identified cytochemically in some appositions (Blackwell, 1953; Davison, 1968; Fraymouth, 1956; Hardwick *et al.*, 1971; Heath, 1971; Nims *et al.*, 1967; Stanbridge *et al.*, 1971), and this is not surprising since callose is known to be a wound polysaccharide and could be expected at sites of trauma. But whether callose is the only substance present in such appositions is another question. The diverse stainability of wall appositions would argue against uniform composition. For those that contain fibrils and strongly resemble the host cell wall (e.g. Fig. 49) (Coffey *et al.*, 1972; Manocha and Lee, 1971; Orcival, 1969), there is a good possibility that cellulose or other cell wall polysaccharides are present. Ghemawat's (1968) cytochemical tests indicated that some of the papillae in wheat infected by powdery mildew also contained lignin, and Edwards (1970) reported basic staining material in papillae.

In plants infected by powdery mildews there is a clear demarcation between the host wall and the papilla or collar (Figs 56, 67, 68, 81, and 82) (Bracker, 1968; Edwards and Allen, 1970; Stanbridge *et al.*, 1971; Watene, 1968). An interface, characterized by a thin electron-dense zone, often separates the wall apposition from the wall. By careful examination we have found this electron-dense region to contain trapped membranes (Fig. 74). Membranes between a papilla and the host wall must have been caught there during formation of the papilla and probably represent remnants of secretory vesicles and plasma membrane that were held in place during the rapid formation of the papilla. The membranes trapped in the matrices of the wall appositions of a number of plants infected by fungi indicate similarities between pathogen-induced wall appositions and the lomasomes that are so common in fungal cells and are thought to arise by secretory activity (Heath and Greenwood, 1970). It seems clear that collars such as those found in powdery mildews are formed as deposits on the host wall rather than by swelling or growth of the wall.

However, with many fungal diseases there is little or no demarcation between host walls and wall appositions. For example, the collars and encasements around some haustoria of rusts (Fig. 49), oomycetous parasites, lichen mycobionts, and others (Berlin and Bowen, 1964; Coffey *et al.*, 1972; Hardwick *et al.*, 1971; Littlefield and Bracker, 1972; Roskin, 1970) merge so completely with the wall that no clear distinction can be made.

The functions and significance of wall appositions remain somewhat enigmatic because of the difficulty in obtaining experimental evidence to demonstrate their roles. The suggestion that some encasements limit fungal growth is no doubt valid, especially where haustoria become necrotic or where a young haustorium is arrested and fails to develop. Roles in host-pathogen incompatibility have been proposed (Bushnell, 1972; Heath, 1971, 1972; Heath and Heath, 1971; Littlefield and Aronson, 1969), and formation of encasements around young haustoria in some incompatible hosts could be a form of host protection which retards the hypersensitive response. Encasement may signify greater host tolerance to toxic effects of haustoria than does a necrotic reaction (Heath, 1971). Although wall appositions represent reactions that can be considered 'defensive', we cannot generalize about their role in host resistance. It is true that papillae do bar penetration in some instances, but they are routinely penetrated by powdery mildew fungi, and they remain as compatible components of the haustorium-host interface in some oomycetous infections. Since many types of appositions exist, the nature of the wall apposition is probably critical in regard to the reaction of the pathogen. They are comparable in some ways to the wall ingrowths that coincide with the onset of intensive solute transport in transfer cells of plants (Pate and Gunning, 1972). In the transfer cells, involuted deposits of cell wall increase the surface area of the protoplast (cf. Hardwick *et al.*, 1971) and are thought to facilitate the transmembrane flux of solutes. Therefore, we do not rule out that some wall appositions are actually functional parts of successful interfaces. But if callose has low permeability to small molecules (Heslop-Harrison, 1966), then wall appositions (especially encasements) that consist largely of callose may impede the movement of materials between host and pathogen (Davison, 1968; Hardwick *et al.*, 1971) and serve as effective barriers that alter the nutrition of the parasite. In conclusion, the necrosis so commonly found in encased haustoria signifies a relationship that is detrimental to a balanced and compatible host-parasite interaction, but clearly there are exceptions.

Interface Types

Throughout the text of this paper we have referred to the interface types (IT); these are now presented diagrammatically in this section. Each IT diagram consists of symbolic representations of interface components presented in sequence to form a bar diagram. In keeping with the three-dimensional concept of interfaces discussed on pp. 161-165, the interface types are presented as multi-component systems.

The listing of interface types is essentially an expression of interface taxonomy based on structural components. It should provide a basis for classifying interfaces and analysing similarities and differences among and within various symbiotic relationships. This is a first attempt at such a classification, and as more is learned about host-symbiont interfaces it is hoped the scheme presented will be expanded and modified to reflect new understanding.

Why is it important to identify interface components? Because every component that lies between two interacting protoplasts is potentially functional in the symbiotic interaction. Such components may function as barriers, biochemical pools, sites where materials are altered, lend stability or protection to either host or symbiont, or they may otherwise serve to promote or impede the development of an interaction between a symbiont and its host. At the present stage it would be a mistake to overlook any major component of the interface because each one comprises part of the micro-environment of symbiosis (pathogenesis). Each component deserves sufficient attention to determine its role, if any.

The following explanations will help to clarify the rationale and interpretation of the system of IT diagrams:

(i) The diagrams of interface types are based on a set of symbols which denote the major structural components of the interfacial region. In each of the diagrams the components belonging to the symbiont (pathogen) are at the left, and host components are at the right. Typically, the diagrams extend progressively from symbiont cytoplasm at the extreme left to host cytoplasm at the extreme right, with all intervening structural layers indicated in sequence. The symbol for cytoplasm is a collective symbol designating all cytoplasmic components within the confines of the plasma membrane. Thus, we have not specifically identified intracytoplasmic membranes, inclusions or organelles, even though they are prominent at some host–symbiont interfaces. To facilitate identification of the symbols, the letter S or H is placed beneath most interface components in the diagrams. S indicates structures belonging to the symbiont, and H denotes host structures. The matrix between the parasite and host is not labelled S or H since the origin of matrix materials is not generally known.

(ii) The list of interface types is not comprehensive. We have selected those which occur frequently, are distintive, are particularly well-documented, or are the natural consequence of other interface types. We expect that others will be able to add to the list and modify it as new evidence of other interface types is uncovered. It will be apparent that some interface types are widespread and others are restricted to very few examples. IT 24 is by far the most common interface type among intracellular symbionts. IT 8 and IT 13 are the common ones among intercellular symbionts where the host cells remain alive.

(iii) Many interface types may occur in a single figure at different sites. For example, in Fig. 2, IT 8, IT 13, IT 37, IT 42, and IT 43 are found in different areas of the subcuticular stroma. Likewise, IT 7, IT 13, IT 18, IT 24, and IT 45 are all found in Fig. 44. An example of how these ITs are identified is shown in Fig. 83.

(iv) We include as separate interface types those in which either the symbiont or the host are moribund or dead. These are examples in which the protoplasm or 'cell sap' is disrupted. The decision to include dead cells could be questioned on the ground that such an association is nonfunctional and should be disregarded in a consideration of interfaces. But this objection is not valid because the dead or moribund cell may distinctly affect the living partner. When a cell is disrupted, the interface changes. The structures and barriers of the protoplast are no longer the same, compartmentalization is altered, and the ordered biochemical events of the living cell cease to function. We have used a single symbol to represent the entire disorganized protoplast, without distinguishing between the surface membrane and the cytoplasm. Many of the pathogenic relationships discussed in this paper involve a dead host cell (but with orchid mycorrhizae the symbiont is killed). Consequently, if wood decay and other examples of pathogens in dead or moribund cells are to be included in the system of interface types, provision must be made to include dead or degenerate cells. We realize, however, that it is still extremely difficult to determine by electron microscopy when a cell is dead.

(v) Several interface types are included that do not involve the host. In addition to host components, the symbiont must often contend with cells and products of its own kind as well as with gaseous or liquid surroundings that are not components of the host. These interfaces are concurrent with those that do involve the host. That is, they occur at the same time and on the same thallus as other interface types that include host components. Hence, they comprise part of the total immediate environment that surrounds the symbiotic organism. For example, an intercellular hypha may contact a host cell over part of its surface, but the opposite side of the same hypha may contact the gases in the intercellular space, or it may contact another hypha over part of its surface. The effects of these concurrent interfaces on the host–symbiont interaction are not clear, but they should not be overlooked because they contribute to the micro-environment of the symbiont.

(vi) The explanations of most interface diagrams are followed by descriptions of one or more examples of symbiotic systems and then by citations in which the interface type can be found. There has been no attempt to provide a comprehensive list of examples. Often, the scope and diversity of examples that involve a given interface type are much greater than indicated by the examples cited. For some interface types, no examples are indicated, mainly because we were not aware of a good example at the time this scheme was prepared, although these interface types are ones that logically must occur.

(vii) We distinguish between the host cell wall and wall appositions. In many systems the apposition has properties distinct from the wall and is clearly identifiable. However, the distinction may be artificial for some examples in which the wall apposition appears nearly identical to the wall *per se*.

(viii) Likewise, we distinguish between the host cuticle and the host wall. Although the cuticle is part of the epidermal wall, it has distinctive structure and composition and constitutes a different kind of barrier from the fibrillar portion of the cell wall.

(ix) Where cytoplasm is indicated by the unpatterned symbol in the IT diagrams, this symbol can also be taken to include nucleoplasm if the symbiont is intranuclear. Such a condition would only be expected with prokaryotic symbionts or viruses, however.

(x) The solid black symbol for a membrane pertains mostly to plasma membrane. But where the symbiont is intraprotoplasmic or is attached to a different host membrane (e.g. Figs 23, 27, and 31) the membrane symbol can apply to the nearest host membrane.

(xi) The stippled symbol for matrix applies to a variety of matrices including the sheaths surrounding haustoria (Fig. 57), the extracellular coatings on symbionts in dead host cells (Fig. 5), or other intercellular and extracellular matrices (Figs 8 and 45), regardless of their composition. It is assumed that the matrix material is a secretory product of the host, the symbiont, or both. We realize that matrix regions may consist of multiple constituents and may have differentiated regions, but we do not distinguish among these differences and specializations in the symbolic representations of interfaces. A matrix is considered in the generic sense, apart from walls, wall appositions, and the gaseous or liquid phase that is derived from the external environment and not part of either partner.

Sometimes it is difficult to determine whether a matrix layer is present or not. Substantial and distinct extracellular or intercellular layers are easy to identify, but where the layer is extremely thin (less than 10 nm) or fails to stain distinctively it may escape detection.

(xii) For some interface components there is the question of whether that component terminates precisely at the boundary of the next component in the sequence. For example, the molecular constituents of a matrix layer may also permeate part of an adjacent wall or wall apposition, but ultrastructurally we have no way yet to detect this. In constructing the IT diagrams we have assumed each component to terminate at its boundary with the adjacent component.

(xiii) In several IT diagrams two interface components are integrated into the space of a single symbol. In IT 3, two membranes are integrated as a single 'compound' membrane in accord with the original authors' description. In IT 32 and IT 33 necrotic protoplasm and sheath matrix are integrated between the symbiont wall and the host wall apposition because they become intermixed around encased haustoria.

(xiv) The interface types are intended to represent principally eukaryotic hosts and symbionts. If prokaryotic symbionts are considered, one would have to take into account the special properties and construction of the interface components as they apply to each specific example. For instance, bacterial walls are distinct from plant walls, and the wall symbol should account for the significant differences. Pathogenic macromolecules such as viruses can also be considered in the context of interface types, but a special set of IT designations would have to be erected to accommodate them. For example, if a circle (o) is used to designate a virus, then the following virus–host interfaces could apply to examples illustrated in this paper.

Fig. 30 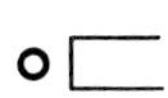

Figs 28 and 29 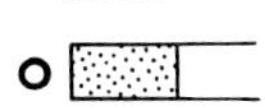

Figs 33 and 34 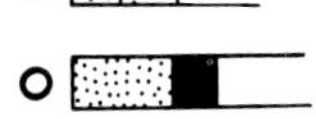

Fig. 31 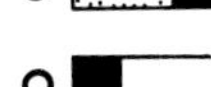

In these instances, the matrix component  would be either vacuolar sap or the clear differentiated matrix surrounding the virus particles; viruses, however, are excluded from the interface diagrams which follow.

KEY TO SYMBOLS USED IN DIAGRAMS OF INTERFACE TYPES

 Symbiont cytoplasm

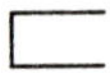 Host cytoplasm

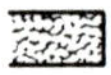 Dead or moribund symbiont protoplasm–degenerate cell sap

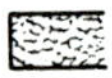 Dead or moribund host protoplasm–degenerate cell sap

 Membrane–usually plasma membrane

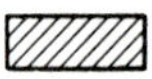 Symbiont cell wall

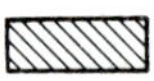 Host cell wall

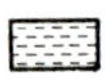 Host cuticle

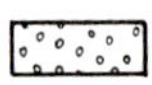 Wall apposition

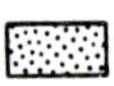 Inter- or extracellular matrix or sheath material–derived from host or symbiont or both

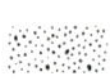 Gas or liquid environment–not a component of host or symbiont

INTERFACE DOES NOT INCLUDE CELL WALLS OF SYMBIONT OR HOST

No intervening matrix between symbiont and host

IT 1

Live, wall-less symbiont and host protoplasm separated only by a membrane–usually the plasma membrane of the symbiont. Example: plasmodium of *Olpidium brassicae* in host cell, see Fig. 20. (Lesemann and Fuchs, 1970b, Figs 3 and 4a; Temmink and Campbell, 1968, Figs 1 and 2)

IT 2 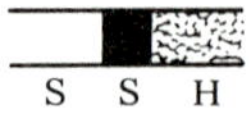

Similar to IT 1, but host protoplast is moribund or dead. Example: young sporangia of *Plasmodiophora brassicae* in host cell. (Williams and McNabola, 1967, Figs 9 and 12)

IT 3 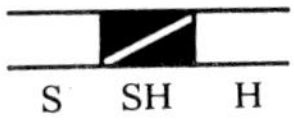

Live, wall-less symbiont and host protoplasm separated by a compound membrane that is formed by an integration of the plasma membranes of host and symbiont. Example: *Aphelidium* thallus in *Scenedesmus* host cell, see Fig. 15. (Schnepf *et al.*, 1971b, Figs 9 and 11)

IT 4 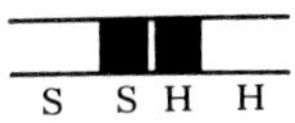

Adjacent protoplasts of live wall-less symbiont and host separated by two closely appressed membranes (probably plasma membranes of host and symbiont). Example: plasmodium of *Plasmodiophora brassicae* in host cell, see Fig. 16. (Aist and Williams, 1971, Fig. 44; Williams and McNabola, 1970, Figs 1 and 2.) (A close variant of this type is shown in Fig. 20, and also in Lesemann and Fuchs, 1970b, Figs 3 and 4 where the host tonoplast is closely appressed to the fungal plasma membrane, although an extremely thin layer of cytoplasm intervenes between the membranes)

Intervening matrix or wall apposition present between symbiont and host

IT 5 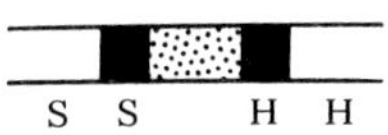

Adjacent protoplasts of live wall-less symbiont and host, similar to IT 4 but separated by a matrix layer. (Possibly Berlin and Bowen, 1964, Figs 2 and 3, if the fungal wall is absent in the neck region)

IT 6 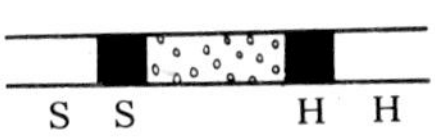

Protoplasts of host and parasite separated by wall apposition layer between the respective plasma membranes. Example: walled-off infection of *Olpidium brassicae.* (Temmink and Campbell, 1969, Fig. 11.)

INTERFACE INCLUDES CELL WALLS OF BOTH SYMBIONT AND HOST

No intervening matrix between the walls of symbiont and host
(i) Wall appositions absent

IT 7 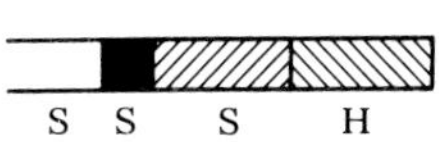

Live, walled symbiont abutting against host wall with no other host cell components beyond the wall. Example: penetration sites where fungi pass through the host wall. This interface is restricted to a plane extending parallel to and within the host wall, see Fig. 83, also Figs 5, 7, 47, 48, 74, 75, and 81.

IT 8 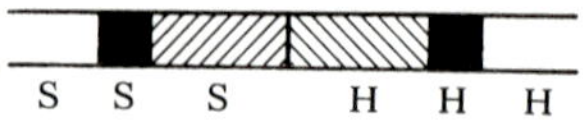

Cell walls of live symbiont and host cell in contact. Example: inter- or extracellular fungal hyphae, and at penetration sites, see Figs 2, 4, 10, and 83.

IT 9 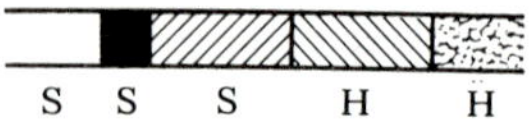

Similar to IT 8 but host cell is moribund or dead. Example: wood-decay fungi and others during host wall penetration. (Chou and Levi, 1971, Figs 1 and 2)

IT 10 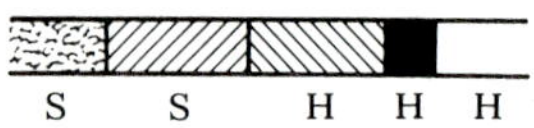

Similar to IT 8, but symbiont is moribund or dead. Example: dead fungal cell on or within a wall of a live host cell.

(ii) Wall appositions present

IT 11 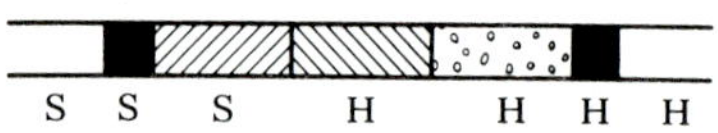

Live walled symbiont in contact with a live host cell that has a wall apposition beneath the point of contact. Example: penetration sites by powdery mildew fungi, see Figs 46, 74, 83, and perhaps also Fig. 54. (Calonge, 1969, Fig. 1; Edwards and Allen, 1970, Figs 8 and 9; Stanbridge *et al.*, 1971, Fig. 3)

IT 12 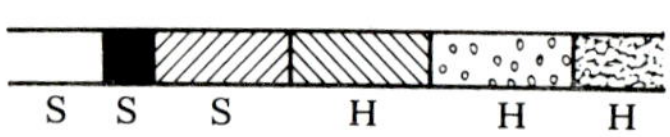

Similar to IT 11 but with host cell dead or moribund. Example: fungal penetration into a host cell that has been killed in advance. (Similar to Hess, 1969, Fig. 22, but at an earlier stage.)

Intervening matrix present between the walls of symbiont and host

(i) Wall appositions absent

IT 13 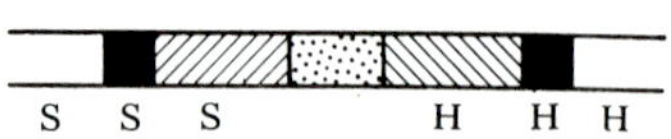

Live symbiont cell and live host cell with a matrix layer intervening between walls of the respective organisms. Example: intercellular symbionts. (Held, 1972, Fig. 3; Olah *et al.*, 1971, Fig. 1; Temmink and Campbell, 1969, Figs 1 and 5)

IT 14

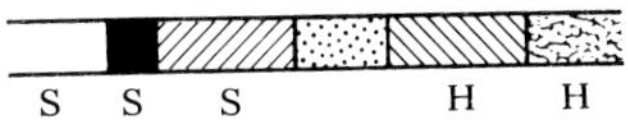

Similar to IT 13, but host cell is moribund or dead. Example: intercellular pathogens that kill in advance; some wood-decay fungi, see Fig. 6. (Chou and Levi, 1971, Fig. 6; Horino and Akai, 1968b, Figs 4 and 7)

IT 15

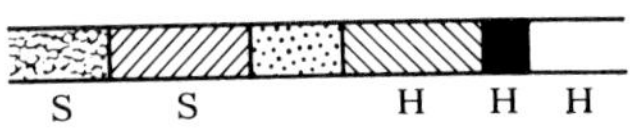

Similar to IT 13 but cell of symbiont is dead or moribund. Example: dead fungal hypha in intercellular space of living host tissue.

(ii) Wall appositions present

IT 16

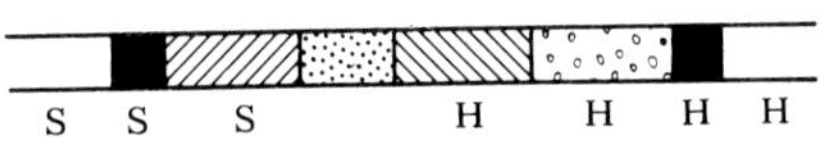

Live, walled symbiont cell adjacent to a living host cell having a wall apposition. A matrix layer intervenes between the walls of the respective organisms. Example: intercellular fungi that have induced wall appositions in the host, and regions lateral to penetration sites, see Figs 47, 54, and 83. (Heath, 1972, Figs 21 and 22; Temmink and Campbell, 1969, Fig. 8)

IT 17

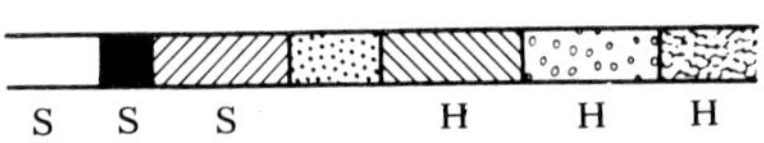

Similar to IT 16, but host cell is moribund or dead.

INTERFACE INCLUDES SYMBIONT CELL WALL BUT NOT HOST CELL WALL

No intervening matrix between symbiont and host

(i) Wall appositions absent

IT 18

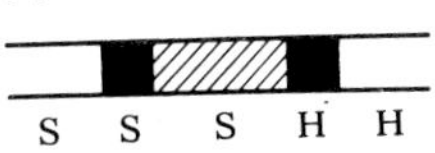

Live, walled symbiont in direct contact with the plasma membrane of a living host cell. Example: the region of the haustorial neck of rust fungi, see Figs 47, 48, and 83. (Heath and Heath, 1971, Fig. 1; Kazama and Fuller, 1970, Fig. 6; Littlefield and Bracker, 1970, Fig. 3; Littlefield and Bracker, 1972, Fig. 10)

IT 19

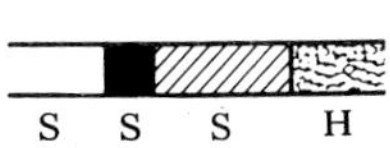

Similar to IT 18, but host cell is moribund or dead. Example: fungal cells in a disrupted host cell. (Hess, 1969, Fig. 3; Horino and Akai, 1968a, Fig. 12; Horino and Akai, 1968b, Fig. 7; Williams and McNabola, 1967, Fig. 13)

IT 20

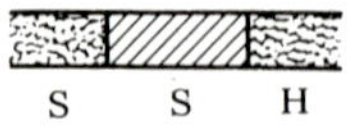

Similar to IT 18, but host and symbiont are both moribund or dead. At such an interface little or no further biological interaction would be expected.

(ii) Wall appositions present

IT 21

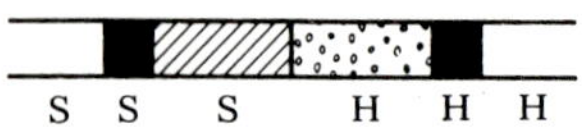

Live, walled symbiont in contact with a wall apposition of a living host cell. Example: some haustoria, encased intracellular hyphae, and sites of host penetration, see Figs 11, 12, 55, 56, 66, and 83. (Edwards and Allen, 1970, Figs 5, 6, and 7; Hardwick *et al.*, 1971, Figs 6 and 13)

IT 22

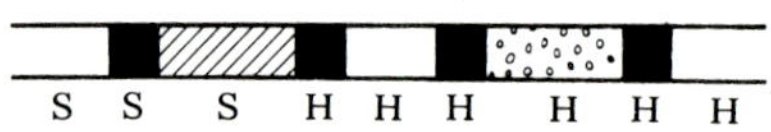

Live, walled symbiont within a living host cell. A layer of host protoplast intervenes between the symbiont wall and a host wall apposition. Example: partially encased haustoria, see Figs 52 and 83. (Fig. 3; Bracker, 1968, Fig. 33)

IT 23

Walled, live symbiont cell in contact with wall apposition of moribund or dead host cell. Example: penetration of fungal hypha into disrupted host cell. (Calonge, 1969, Fig. 13; Hess, 1969, Fig. 22)

Intervening matrix present between symbiont and host

(i) Wall appositions absent

IT 24

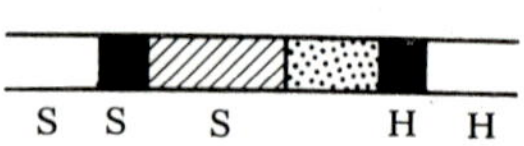

Live, walled symbiont cell separated from plasma membrane of a living host cell by an intervening matrix. This is the most common intracellular interface type. Examples: haustoria, intracellular hyphae including endotrophic mycorrhizae, root nodule bacteria, endobiotic algae, see Figs 13, 14, 21, 22, 44, 57, 58, 59, 60, 61, 64, 65, 72, 73, and 83.

IT 25 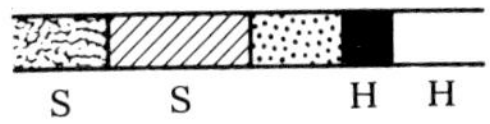

Similar to IT 24, but symbiont is dead or moribund. Matrix intervenes between symbiont wall and plasma membrane of living host cell. Example: necrotic haustoria and degenerate mycorrhizal hyphae, see Fig. 51, i.e. the part of the haustorium not surrounded by an encasement, and Fig. 83. (Dorr and Kollmann, 1969, Figs 2 and 4)

IT 26 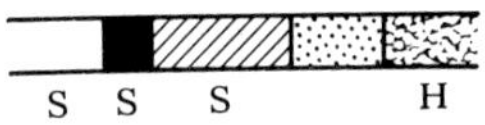

Live, walled symbiont within a moribund or dead host cell. Symbiont coated by a matrix layer. Example: hyphae of intracellular fungal pathogens in disrupted host cells, see Fig. 5. (Hess, 1969, Figs 4 and 5)

(ii) Wall appositions present

IT 27 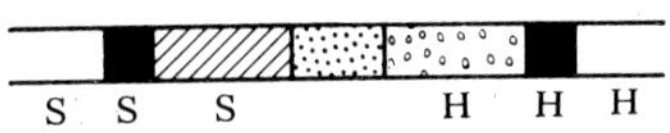

Live, walled symbiont adjacent to wall apposition of a living host cell. Matrix layer intervenes between symbiont wall and the apposition. Example: some downy mildew haustoria. (Berlin and Bowen, 1964, Fig. 5; Chou, 1970, Fig. 4A; Kajiwara, 1971, Figs 10 and 15; Peyton and Bowen, 1963, Fig. 10)

IT 28 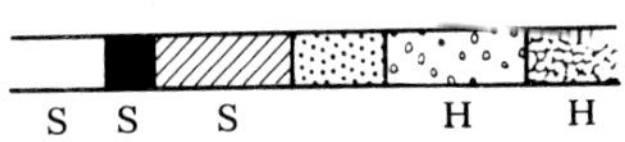

Live, walled symbiont cell separated from wall apposition of a moribund or dead host cell by a matrix layer. Similar to IT 27, but host cell is disrupted. Example: penetration of host cell by hyphae of fungal pathogens that kill in advance. (Hess, 1969, possibly Fig. 23)

IT 29 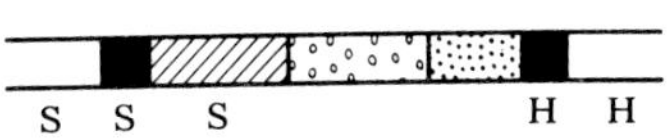

Live, walled symbiont cell in contact with a host wall apposition. Matrix layer separates the apposition from the plasma membrane of a living host cell. Example: intracellular hyphae of smut fungi. (Fullerton, 1970, Fig. 2)

IT 30 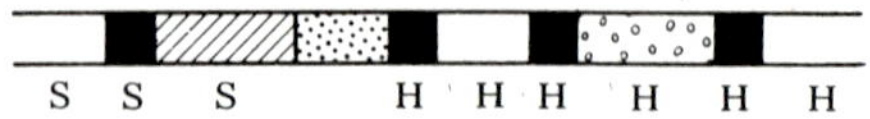

IT 31 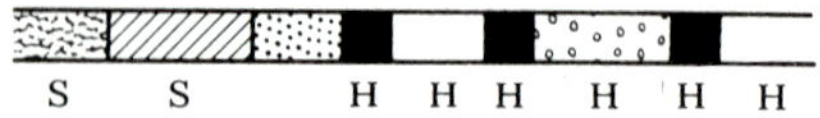

IT 32 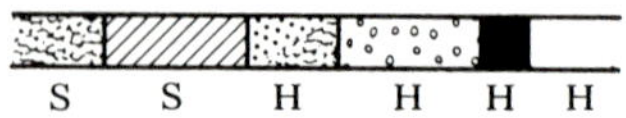

IT 33 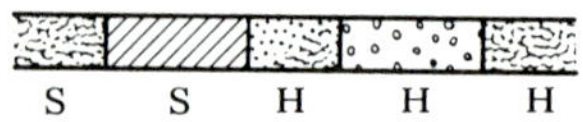

These interface types involve living or dead, walled symbionts separated from living or necrotic host protoplasts by a wall apposition. An additional layer of intact or necrotic host protoplast is trapped between the symbiont and the host wall apposition. Symbiont wall is surrounded by a matrix layer. In IT 32 and IT 33 the matrix layer and necrotic host protoplasm are intermixed. Example: encased haustoria of rust fungi, see Figs 50, 51, 53, and 83. (Heath and Heath, 1971, Figs 15, 17, and 25; Littlefield and Bracker, 1972, Figs 11, 41, and 43)

INTERFACE INCLUDES HOST CELL WALL BUT NOT SYMBIONT CELL WALL

No intervening matrix between symbiont and host

IT 34 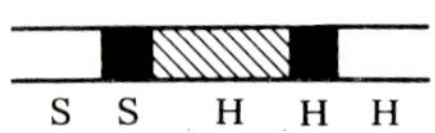

Live, wall-less symbiont in contact with walled, live host cell. Example: fungal zoospores settling on host cells, prior to secretion of fungal wall. (Aist and Williams, 1971, Fig. 8)

Intervening matrix present between symbiont and host

IT 35 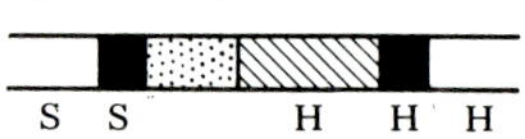

Live, wall-less symbiont cell separated from the wall of a living host cell by a matrix layer. Example: encysting zoospore with adhesive or mucilaginous coating prior to formation of encystment wall.

INTERFACE INCLUDES CUTICLE ON HOST CELL WALL

No intervening matrix between symbiont and host

IT 36 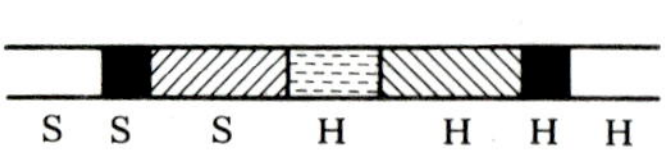

Live, walled symbiont in contact with cuticle of a living host cell. Example: penetration sites of foliar pathogens such as *Venturia inaequalis* at the time of cuticular penetration; also epiphytic hyphae, see Fig. 8, immediately around the penetration site, also Fig. 83. If a wall apposition is present—not illustrated here—Figs 56, 68, 75, and 82 would also apply. (Maeda, 1970, Figs 5A and 6A)

IT 37 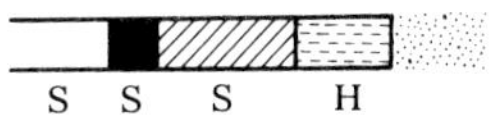

Wall of a living subcuticular symbiont in contact with the inner surface of the host cuticle. Example: *Venturia inaequalis* on apple leaves, see Fig. 2. (Horino and Akai, 1968b, Figs 1 and 2; Maeda, 1970, Fig. 9A)

Intervening matrix present between symbiont and host

IT 38 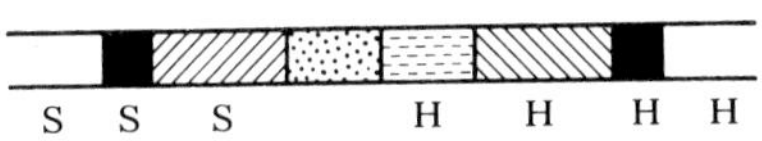

Walled, live symbiont separated from the outer surface of the host cuticle by a matrix layer. Example: epiphytic hyphae; also sites lateral to the infection sac of *Venturia inaequalis* on apple leaves, see Fig. 8, lateral to the penetration site, also Fig. 83.)

IT 39 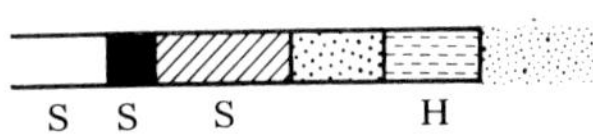

Wall of a living subcuticular symbiont separated from the inner surface of the host cuticle by a matrix layer. Example: subcuticular hyphae of foliar pathogens, see Fig. 9, where dense matrix material is between fungal cell and host cuticle. (Akai *et al.*, 1971, Fig. 2)

CONCURRENT INTERFACES FOR EUKARYOTIC SYMBIONTS BUT NOT INVOLVING HOST CELL COMPONENTS

Symbiont–symbiont interfaces
(i) No cell walls present
(a) No intervening matrix

IT 40 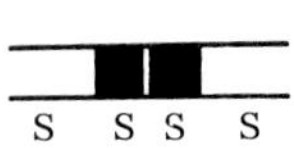

Contact between adjacent, wall-less living cells of a symbiont, not separated by a matrix. Example: sporogenesis of *Plasmodiophora brassicae.* (Williams and McNabola, 1967, Fig. 5)

(b) Intervening matrix present

IT 41 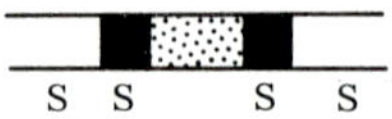

Adjacent wall-less living cells of a symbiont, separated by a matrix layer. Example: sporogenesis of *Plasmodiophora brassicae*. (Williams and McNabola, 1967, Fig. 11)

(ii) Cell walls present

(a) No intervening matrix

IT 42 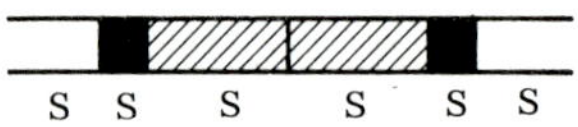

Contact between adjacent, walled, living cells of a symbiont, not separated by a matrix. Example: contact between haustorial lobes of *Erysiphe graminis*; also, adjacent intercellular rust hyphae, see Figs 2 and 72. (Littlefield and Bracker, 1970, Fig. 1)

(b) Intervening matrix present

IT 43 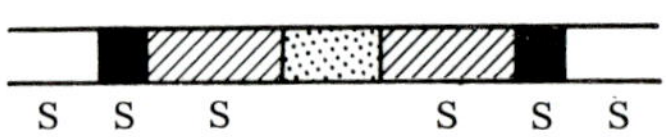

Adjacent, walled, living symbiont cells separated by a matrix layer. Example: adjacent lobes of a haustorium of *Erysiphe graminis* within a common sheath matrix; also adjacent hyphae of intercellular symbionts, see Figs 71 and 72.

Interface between symbiont and gas or liquid environment

(i) Cell wall absent

IT 44 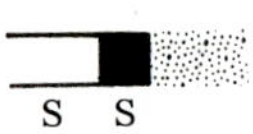

Live, wall-less symbiont interfacing with air or liquid medium. Example: the part of a zoospore surface that is not attached to a plant cell, prior to formation of the encystment wall. (Aist and Williams, 1971, Fig. 8)

(ii) Cell wall present

IT 45 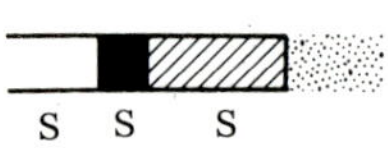

That portion of a live, walled symbiont cell that is exposed to air or liquid medium. No matrix present. Example: encysted cells of *Plasmodiophora* or

Olpidium; also intercellular hyphae of foliar pathogens, see Figs 19, 56, and 83. (Aist and Williams, 1971, Fig. 20; Heath, 1972, Fig. 20)

IT 46

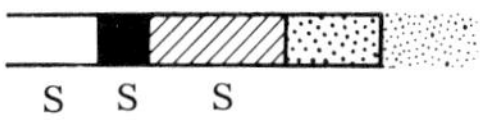

Similar to IT 45, but symbiont wall is coated by a matrix layer which in turn interfaces with air or liquid medium. Example: parts of intercellular hyphae or hyphae on the surface of a plant organ, see Figs 5, 6, 8, and 83. (Hess, 1969, Figs 2 and 3)

To illustrate how these interface types are considered and identified in the course of a developing host–pathogen association, Fig. 83 presents six stages of a hypothetical rust infection from the time of spore germination on a leaf surface until a haustorium has formed and become encased and necrotic. Each IT is marked by a solid black bar that crosses the cell components shown symbolically in the foregoing list of interface types. The changing nature of the interfaces with time is evident through the progression of developmental stages. Also, note that in each diagram, several ITs occur at different sites along the pathogen cell. Hence the time–space consideration noted earlier must be considered in analysing the nature of the host–pathogen interface.

Concluding Comments

SPECIFICATION OF INTERFACES

Held's (1972) work on an intracellular mycoparasite raised an important point regarding the scope and identification of the interfaces that accommodate host penetration. He found limitations on the frequency and time of penetrations as well as on the formation of wall appositions, and on the portion of the host surface that was available for penetration. Although zoospores of *Rozella* encysted all over the hyphae of a susceptible *Allomyces* host, only certain ones penetrated the host cell. Held observed that of two adjacent attached cysts, only one would succeed in penetrating the host. He questioned whether there were fixed sites on the host surface which were intrinsically capable of reacting to the parasite so that the parasite could penetrate, or whether over a given surface area any site could be induced to react in a way that would accommodate penetration by the parasite. Likewise, with other host–parasite systems Maeda (1970) and others have sought explanations for the specific localization of penetration sites. It is outside the scope of this article and of currently available cytological information to answer the questions of determination of penetration sites. But it is a logical extension of the time–space consideration of host–parasite interfaces to include the aspect of interface determination and limitation and to call attention to cell surface specializations, contact phenomena, and microecological features as factors that would influence the establishment of a particular kind or extent of host-parasite interface.

Another question to ask regarding interfaces is whether for a given host-symbiont combination, *any* reaction on the part of the host is required for the parasite to penetrate the host. Evidence involving interactions that result in wall softening by root nodule bacteria suggests that, at times, not only an action by the invader but also a reaction by the host that directly or indirectly involves the interfacial zone is necessary (Dixon, 1969).

Held (1972) noted that wall appositions nearly always accompanied penetration of *Allomyces* by *Rozella* and that the wall appositions formed before penetration. The same is generally true for powdery mildews. Held also found that when wall appositions failed to form, the parasite did not penetrate. Wall appositions have often been assumed to be defence reactions of the host, regardless of when they are formed. But obviously such accretion does not always serve as an insurmountable barrier. He therefore speculated that, although the appositions were commonly associated with successful penetrations of *Allomyces*, some sort of defence reactions might paradoxically be required for penetration. In resistant hosts, he found large wall appositions that actually blocked the penetration by many *Rozella* cysts.

An additional consideration regarding the nature of host-parasite interfaces is the condition of the host protoplast at the time it is confronted by an invader. A possible explanation for the failure of *Rozella* to penetrate cells of *Allomyces* that were already infected is that a 'healthy' host protoplast may be necessary to provide the sort of interaction required to promote penetration by additional parasitic cells. If the interaction, and hence the interface, produced by an infected cell is 'abnormal', then perhaps the new invader would not penetrate. There are of course examples of plant diseases where host cells withstand repeated penetrations by parasitic cells, but this discussion concerns those in which penetration is rare or absent in cells that are already infected. The effect must be mediated through the host-parasite interface.

ENDOMEMBRANE DYSFUNCTION

The discussion of interfaces has repeatedly referred to secretory systems and their involvement in host-symbiont interactions. Cellular secretion accounts for many functional interactions. The transfer of material between protoplasts of two organisms in intimate association must be the result of secretory and uptake processes. Exchange requires that one organism produce and export substances as well as receive substances produced and exported by the 'partner' organism.

However, the fact that secretion of some kind occurs does not specify the secretory mechanism or the materials that are secreted. Among eukaryotes, vesicle-mediated secretion is now known to be widespread. Many major food and fibre commodities of agriculture and commerce are synthesized, stored, and/or released from cells through the cooperative action of membrane systems (Morré and Mollenhauer, 1973). Likewise, normal and abnormal developmental events in eukaryotes are mediated by secretory processes that are membrane-dependent. These include cell growth, division, differentiation, and specification of cell surface (Grove and Bracker, 1970; Morré and Mollenhauer, 1973; Whaley *et al.*, 1972). Already, in work on animal diseases and disorders, attention is being focused on cell membrane components as vital participants in abnormal cell development and cell–cell interaction (Berhsohm and Grossman, 1971; D. J. Morré and T. W. Keenan, unpublished; Richter and Scarpelli, 1971). One of the most promising ideas that underlies such an understanding is the endomembrane concept, an hypothesis which states the essential integrated characteristics of the endomembrane system (Morré and Mollenhauer, 1973).

What is the endomembrane system? In its simplest form it is expressed as a functional and developmental continuum of internal cytoplasmic membranes that characterize eukaryotic cells. The membranes of the nuclear envelope, endoplasmic reticulum (rough and smooth), Golgi apparatus, secretory vesicles, and other transitional membrane elements are the major components of the system, but membrane structures derived from these major components are also included. Derivatives may be vacuoles, lysosomes, plasma membrane, microbodies, and perhaps even parts of the outer membranes of both mitochondria and chloroplasts (but not the inner membrane of these organelles) (Bracker and Grove, 1971; Morré and Mollenhauer, 1972).

The essence of the endomembrane concept is that the membrane components are not regarded as independent or autonomous systems. They each form a part of a highly integrated and interdependent system of cytomembranes, even though each component may have distinctive characteristics which distinguish it from other components of the endomembrane system. There is increasing evidence that the endomembrane system plays a major role in its own biogenesis and multiplication, and is a potential source of new plasma membrane. The endomembrane concept combines the concepts of membrane flow and membrane differentiation (Bennett, 1956; Franke *et al.*, 1971; Grove *et al.*, 1968; Morré *et al.*, 1971; Schnepf, 1969a) to provide a mechanism whereby membranes are synthesized, transferred, and transformed along a chain of cell components in a subcellular developmental pathway. An example of such a pathway would be nuclear envelope → endoplasmic reticulum → Golgi apparatus → secretory vesicles → plasma membrane. Other pathways and interrelationships are also possible. A central feature of the endomembrane concept is the existence of transitional membrane elements which are capable of bridging spatial, temporal, or qualitative gaps between major components of the endomembrane system.

In the sense that the endomembrane system seems to be a major participant in the characteristics of cell surfaces, it is important to our considerations of host-symbiont interfaces. Its participation in the synthesis, modification, transport, and storage of products for export out of the cell is an essential function. Several reviews have dealt extensively with the secretory functions of endomembrane components (Beams and Kessel, 1968; Mollenhauer and Morré, 1966; Morré *et al.*, 1971; Whaley, 1966; Schnepf, 1969b). Such secretory processes may hold vital clues regarding the nature of cell-cell interactions and the ability of two cells to react to and withstand a symbiotic relationship.

Numerous examples already mentioned and in other literature implicate altered functioning of secretory processes and altered endomembrane systems in pathogenic and mutual symbiotic interactions. In plant cells infected by powdery mildews and other fungi, the proliferation of endoplasmic reticulum, Golgi apparatus, or secretory vesicles is clearly a pathological response. Alteration of host plasma membrane in diseased cells shows how strikingly this membrane reacts to invasion or the threat of invasion. Responses include permeability changes, changes in stability, thickness, and ultrastructure. Often a region of altered plasma membrane is accompanied by an altered coating just outside the plasma membrane. Also, the plasma membrane must increase greatly to accommodate the surface area required to surround invading cells. The widespread formation of wall appositions before or during host penetration represents a localized secretory process, and there are indications that vesicles contribute to wall appositions in some plants. Papilla formation would be the end product of an altered secretory (endomembrane) system. Localized secretory activity by symbionts (including adhesive materials, enzymes for penetration, vesicles at penetration sites, infection sacs in appressoria) is another example of altered secretion and changed endomembrane components specifically in relation to the host cell. Secretion may be mutual, and two interacting cells may influence each other by respective secretory processes in such a way that compatible interactions are either made possible or are precluded.

The nature of interface components, their source and mode of formation, and their relation to the integrated processes of symbiosis and disease are significant areas of inquiry that have not been explained. In particular, dysfunction of the endomembrane system may be an important aspect of plant disease which will have conceptual counterparts in those human and animal disorders that alter the qualitative and quantitative functioning of endomembrane pathways and that specify the nature of cell surface characteristics.

Pate and Gunning's (1972) elegant epilogue about the abundance of circumstantial evidence and the dearth of definitive information concerning the functioning of transfer cells applies just as well to the problems of host-symbiont interfaces. It is essential to pursue the nature and role of interface components if we are to understand how hosts and symbionts (pathogens) interact. The studies that will translate descriptive accounts of structural interfaces into an understanding of their function should not be regarded strictly as ultrastructural or biochemical, but rather as micro-ecological investigations approaching their highest degree of resolution.

Acknowledgements

This is Journal Paper No. 4955 of the Purdue University Agricultural Experiment Station, and Journal Paper No. 326 of the North Dakota Agricultural Experimental Station.

Original research reported by the authors was supported in part by National Science Foundation grants GB-3044 and GB-6751 to C.E.B., National Institutes of Health I-F03-GM4348801, and U.S. Department of Agriculture Cooperative Agreement 12-14-100-5560 (34) to L.J.L.

We gratefully acknowledge the contributions of Catalina Montecillo and Anna-Maria Bracker for technical assistance and aid in compiling the manuscript.

We extend special thanks to colleagues who provided unpublished information and ideas, and those who contributed electron micrographs. We would have liked to include many more micrographs from other workers, but this proved impossible in an already extensive descriptive and pictorial documentation of host-pathogen interfaces.

Note added in proof: Since this manuscript was submitted a number of very recent studies have come to our attention. Of these, three deserve special mention. In a paper on evolution of haustoria in tropical rust fungi, R. B. Rajendren illustrates a wide variety of haustorial forms ranging from simple spheroid to highly branched coralloid or digitate, and even some that resemble intracellular hyphae (*Bull. Torrey bot. Club* **99**, 84-88, 1972). A freeze-etching study by J. R. Aist (pers. comm.) of the plasmodial envelope of *Plasmodiophora brassicae* has characterized membrane particles and surface features, and revealed developmental changes at the host–parasite interface based on the fracture properties of the envelope. Aist has considered the possibility that during development an additional membrane is added to the envelope with subsequent partial and selective breakdown of membrane components. R. R. Camp and W. F. Whittingham's ultrastructural study of host–parasite relationships in sooty blotch disease of white clover (*Am. J. Bot.* **59**, 1057-1067, 1972) demonstrated an unusual extracytoplasmic structure, called a **pons**, at the host–parasite interface. The pons is dumbbell-shaped, extends from the host cell to the parasite via an isthmus and 'pores' in the walls of each partner, and is bounded by host plasma membrane on one side and fungal plasma membrane on the other side. Pons are variable—some are digitate, others are simple. They appear structurally similar to wall appositions, but their specific nature is not known. The interface type in the isthmus region of the pons would be similar to IT 6.

Fig. 1. Hypha (H) of *Ceratocystis ulmi* growing from cell to cell through inter-tracheary pit membranes in a two-year-old branch of *Ulmus carpinifolia* five days after inoculation. Note how the hypha conforms to the walls of the pit aperture and is constricted as it penetrates through the inter-tracheary pit membrane (I) from the lumen of one vessel (Ve) to the next. x7000. (From MacDonald and McNabb, 1970.)

Fig. 2. Young subcuticular hyphae (H) of *Venturia inaequalis* growing between the cuticle (Cu) and the epidermal cell wall (W) of a susceptible apple leaf. Lumen of the epidermal cell (Ep). Note the separation of the cuticle from the epidermal cell and its contour over the fungal hyphae. x4000. (From Maeda, 1970.)

Fig. 3. Hyphae (H) of *Ascochyta pisi* growing within the outer epidermal wall (W) of a pea leaf. The host wall has been separated into layers to accommodate the fungus. Lumen of the epidermal cell (Ep). x8000. (From Heath and Wood, 1969.)

Fig. 4. Hypha (H) of *Melampsora lini* growing between and splitting apart the walls (W) of adjacent epidermal cells (Ep) in a leaf of the flax host (*Linum usitatissimum*). Fungal wall (FW). x25 000.

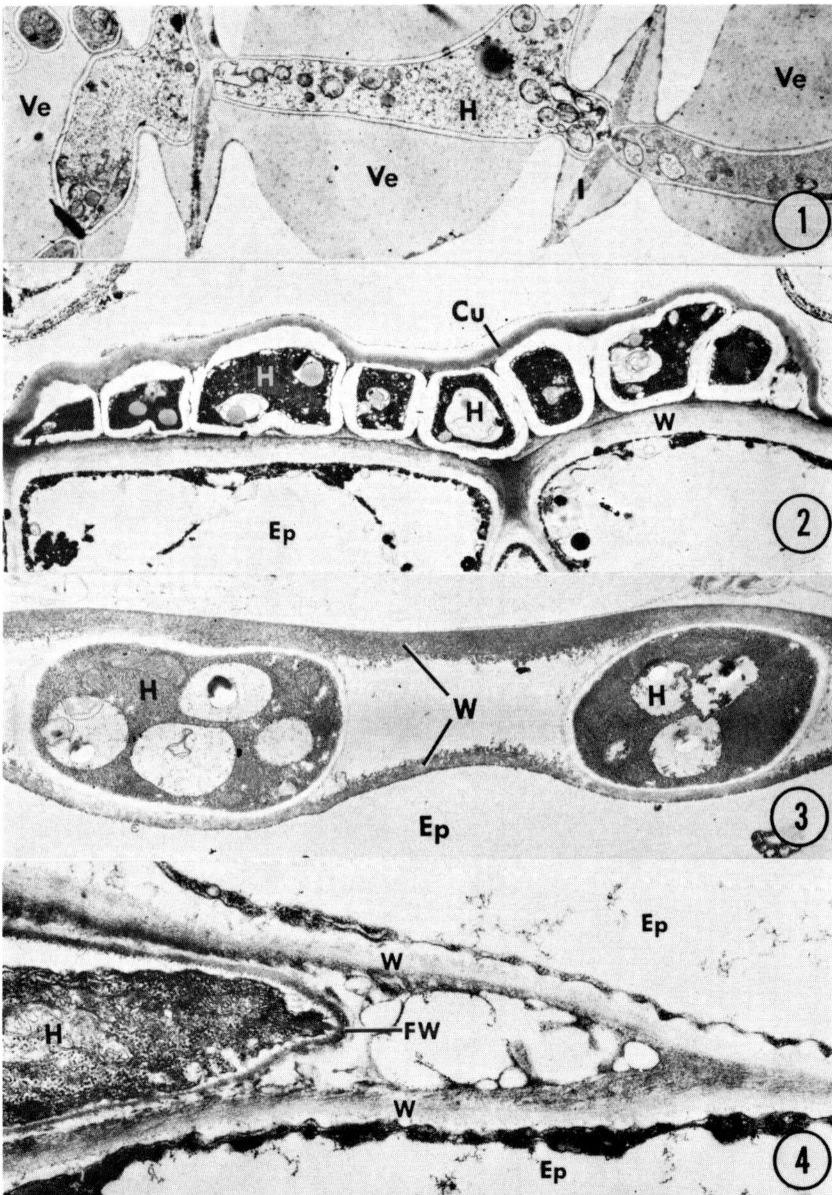
Ve
H
Ve
Ve
I
1
Cu
H
H
W
Ep
2
W
H
H
Ep
3
Ep
W
H
FW
W
Ep
4

Fig. 5. Hypha (H) of *Fusarium solani* f. *phaseoli* which has penetrated into a dead cell (C) of host hypocotyl. The fungus is constricted where it has grown through the host wall (W). Note the granular matrix (Ma) coating the hyphal wall and separating it from the contents of the host cell lumen. The small structures (B) around the intracellular hypha are bacteria. ×10 500. (From Reichle, 1965.)

Fig. 6. Carbon replica of a hypha (H) of *Hypholoma fasciculare* growing on the cell wall (W) of a tracheid of *Picea excelsa*. Note the mucilaginous matrix (Ma) surrounding the hypha. ×8500. (From Schmid, 1966.)

Fig. 7. Penetration of the wall (W) of a bordered pit of *Ulmus carpinifolia* by *Ceratocystis ulmi*. Note expansion of the hypha (H) after penetration, and the zone of greater electron density (arrows) in the host wall on either side of the fungus where the fungus has grown through the wall. Inter-tracheary pit membrane (I), vessel lumen (Ve). ×16 000. (From MacDonald and McNabb, 1970.)

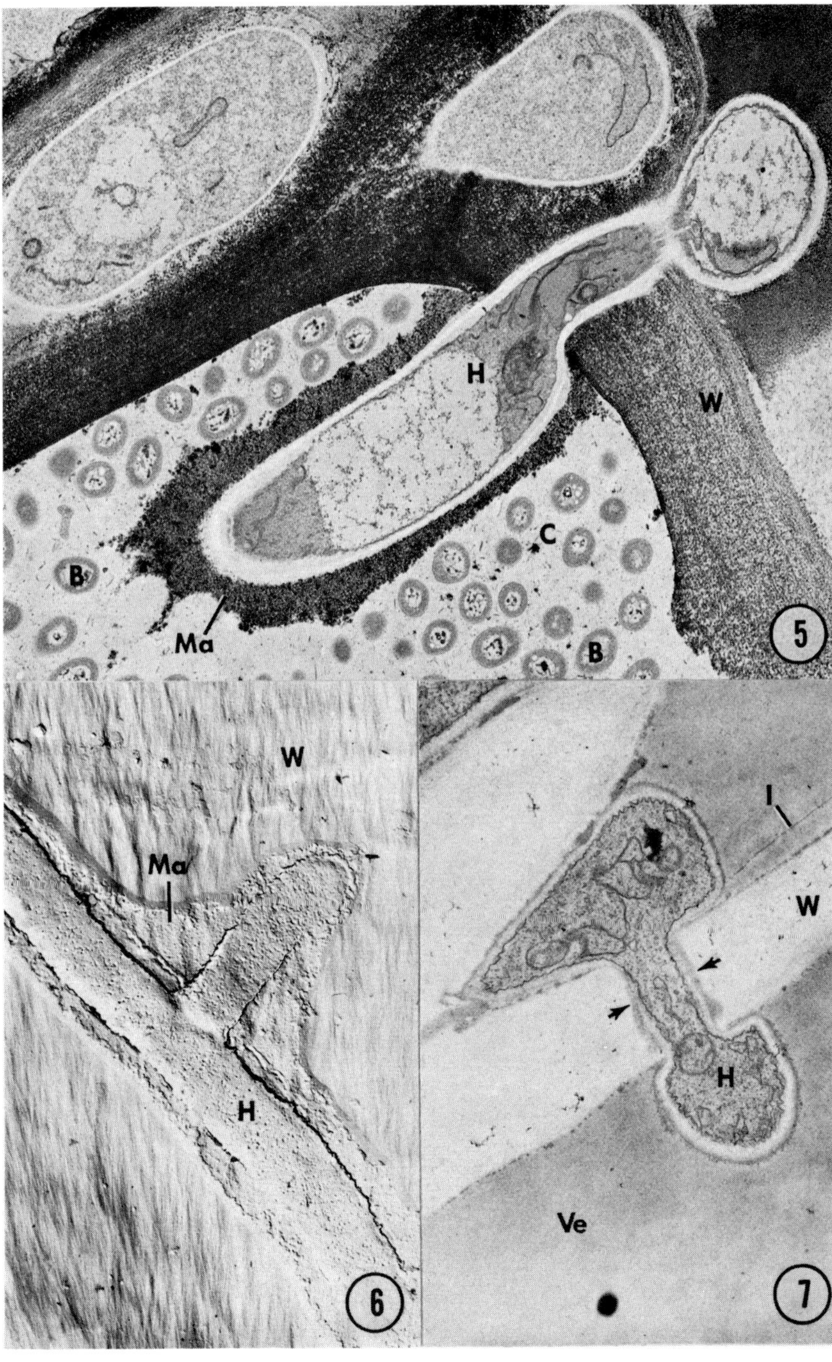
H
W
C
B
Ma
B
5
W
Ma
H
6
I
W
H
Ve
7

Fig. 8. Appressorium (A) of *Venturia inaequalis* on the surface of an apple leaf showing the host–parasite interface immediately prior to penetration of the host cuticle (Cu). Note the extremely thin fungal wall (FW) that separates the host cuticle from the appressorial 'infection sac' (SC) at the site of incipient penetration. The cuticle is already thinned and shows evidence of degradation (arrow) opposite the infection sac. Epidermal cell wall (W), lumen of the epidermal cell (Ep), sheath-like layer (Sh) coating the appressorium. ×15 000. (From Maeda, 1970.)

Fig. 9. Subcuticular cells of *Venturia inaequalis* showing the relationship of the fungal cell walls (FW) to the host cuticle (Cu). Note the dark-staining matrix (Ma) between the fungal cells. The cuticle contains many electron-transparent platelets (Pl) and a web-like network (WN) that extends throughout the cuticle. The cuticle has partially disintegrated near the fungal cells as shown by the separated platelets. ×73 000. (From Maeda, 1970.)

Fig. 10. Part of a subcuticular hypha (transverse section) (H) of *Venturia inaequalis* growing on an etiolated hypocotyl of apple. The irregular profile of the partially disintegrated host wall (W) is evident adjacent to the fungal wall (FW). Loosely arranged fibrillar material (F) occurs in the space between the hyphal wall and the distended cuticle (Cu). Note the etching away of host wall components and the discontinuity of parallel layers of wall fibrils. ×16 000. (From Maeda, 1970.)

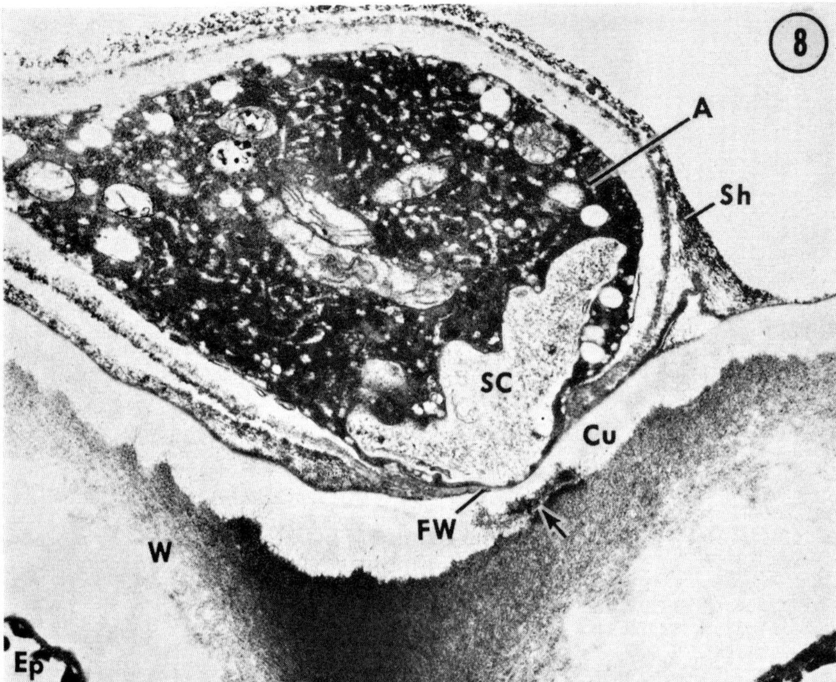
8
A
Sh
SC
Cu
FW
W
Ep

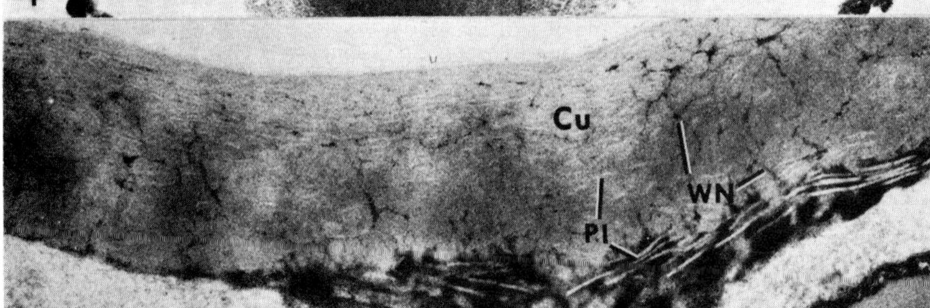
Cu
WN
Pl
FW
Ma
FW
9

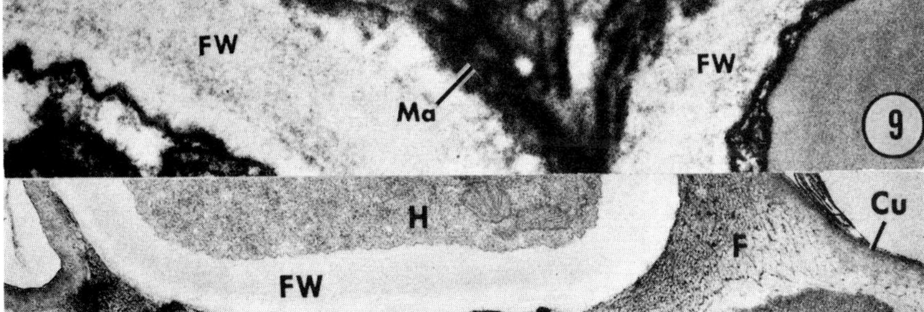
H
Cu
F
FW
W
10

Fig. 11. Intracellular hypha (H) of *Gibberidea heliopsidis* which has grown from one host cell to another in the stem cortex of *Helianthus strumosus*. Note constriction of the fungal cell as it passes through the host cell wall (W). The host plasma membrane (PM) is invaginated and continuous around the invading fungal hypha. A thin appositional layer (Ap) lies between the host plasma membrane and the fungal cell wall (FW). Host cytoplasm (C), host vacuole (Va). ×15 600. (From Mason, 1970.)

Fig. 12. An intracellular hypha (H) of *Gibberidea heliopsidis* encased by a massive wall apposition (Ap) in a host cell (*Helianthus strumosus*). Note the layered and foamy appearance of the apposition. ×6000. (From Mason, 1970.)

Fig. 13. Endosymbiotic cell of the alga *Chlorella* (Chl) within the protozoan *Paramecium bursaria*. Each algal cell is surrounded by a cell wall (W) and is situated within a 'perialgal vacuole' (Ma) which is delimited from the host cytoplasm (C) by a membrane (M). The 'perialgal vacuole' is comparable to a sheath or matrix layer surrounding the invading cells of parasites and symbionts. (Compare Figs 14, 22, 34, 57, 64, 73.) ×19 500. (From Karakashian *et al.*, 1968.)

Fig. 14. Section through an intracellular hypha (H) of an endotrophic mycorrhizal fungus (*Rhizoctonia* sp.) in an orchid (*Dactylorhiza purpurella*) protocorm. The entire fungal cell is surrounded by a membrane (PMI) which is the invaginated host plasma membrane. This membrane nearly contacts the fungal wall (FW) in places, and is separated from it by a space or matrix layer (Ma) in other places. Host cytoplasm (C), host vacuole (Va). ×25 000. (From Hadley *et al.*, 1971.)

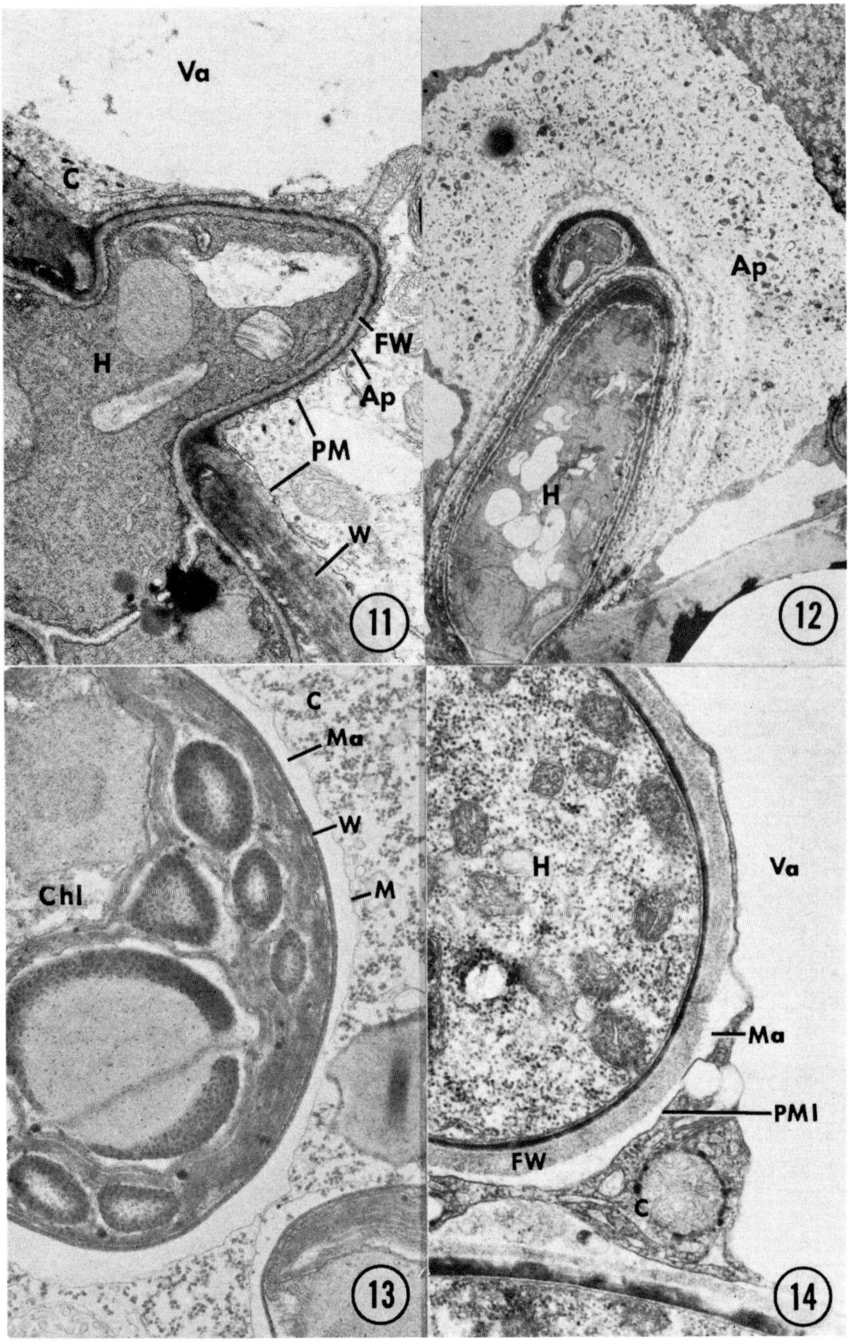
Va
C
H
FW
Ap
PM
W
11
Ap
H
12
C
Ma
W
Chl
M
13
H
Va
Ma
PMI
FW
C
14

Fig. 15. Interfacial zone between the wall-less endoparasitic fungus *Aphelidium* sp. and its algal host *Scenedesmus acutus*. Part of the host plasma membrane is dislocated by the parasite during penetration such that it surrounds the plasmodium of the invading fungal cell. The interface consists of a compound membrane (CM) composed of the associated and integrated plasma membranes of *Aphelidium* and *Scenedesmus*. Cytoplasm of *Aphelidium* (AC), cytoplasm of *Scenedesmus* (SC), plasma membrane of *Scenedesmus* (PM), cell wall of *Scenedesmus* (W). ×240 000. (From Schnepf, 1972.)

Fig. 16. Multilayered plasmodial envelope (PE) separating the cytoplasm of a plasmodium of *Plasmodiophora brassicae* (PC) from the cytoplasm of the cabbage host cell (HC) *Brassica oleracea* var. *capitata*. The multilayered envelope is thought to consist of two closely associated membranes, one derived from the host plasma membrane and the other from the plasma membrane of the parasite. ×150 000. (From Williams and McNabola, 1970.)

Fig. 17. The host-symbiont interface between an intracellular algal endosymbiont, *Nostoc*, within its host, *Geosiphon*. *Nostoc* cytoplasm (NC), *Nostoc* plasma membrane (NPM), *Nostoc* cell wall (NW), *Geosiphon* plasma membrane (GPM), *Geosiphon* cytoplasm (GC), *Geosiphon* tonoplast (GT), *Geosiphon* vacuole (GVa). The arrow labels a connection between the plasma membrane and the thylakoids of the *Nostoc* cell. ×60 000. (From Schnepf and Brown, 1971.)

Fig. 18. A portion of the algal endosymbiont *Symbiodinium* sp. extracted from its jellyfish host, *Casseopeia* sp. A complex 'periplast' surrounds the alga. The periplast comprises several layers, including the plasma membrane (1), a highly convoluted membrane in a space outside the algal cell (2), an amorphous or homogenous layer sandwiched between two membranes (3 and 4), and an outermost membrane (5). Chloroplast (Chl). ×80 000. (From Kevin *et al.*, 1969.)

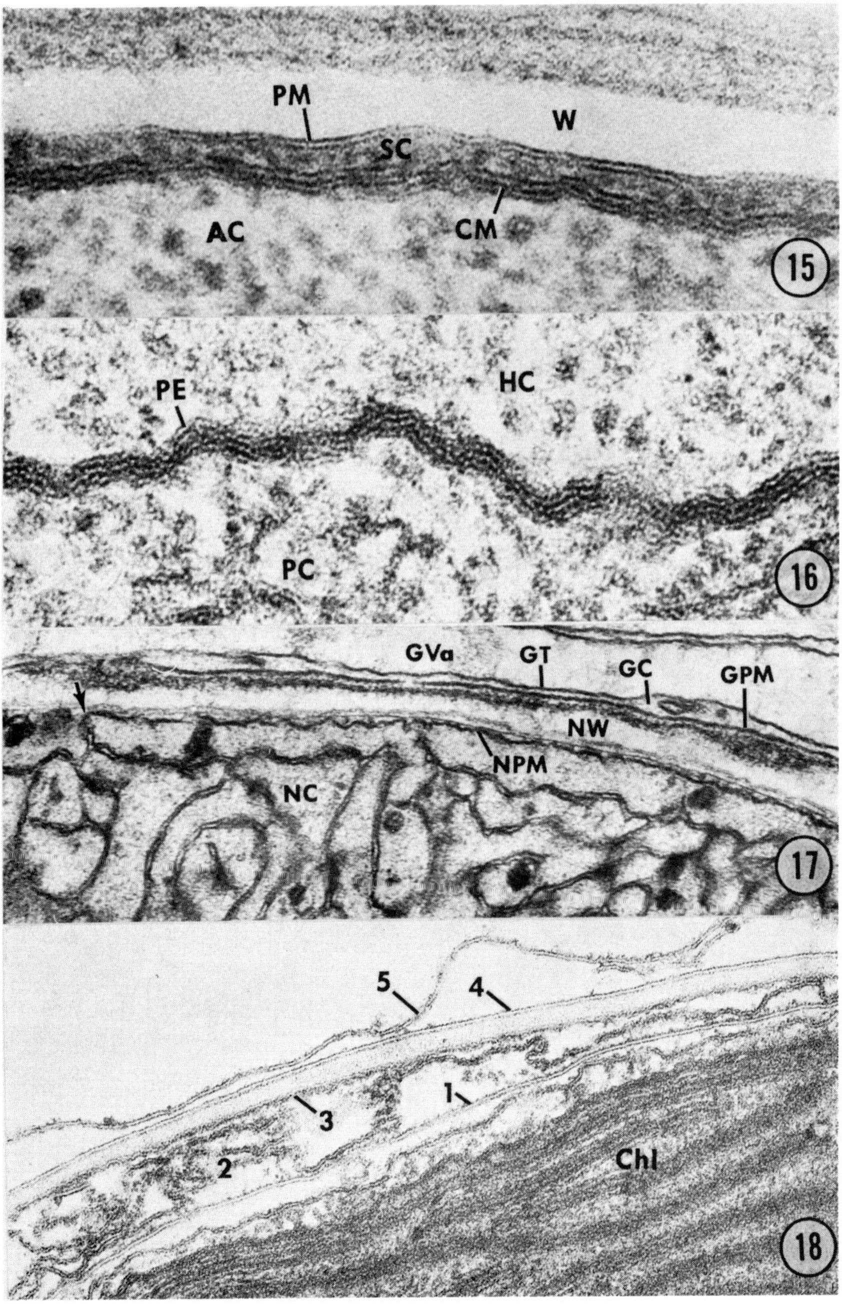
PM
W
SC
AC
CM
15
PE
HC
PC
16
GVa
GT
GC
GPM
NW
NPM
NC
17
5
4
3
1
2
Chl
18

Fig. 19. A cyst of *Olpidium brassicae* on the surface of a root cell of the kohlrabi host, *Brassica oleracea* ssp. *gongyloides*, prior to penetration. Note the accumulation of 'secretory' vesicles (V) and the lomasome-like (Lo) membrane formation within the fungal cell near the point of attachment to the host wall (W). ×36 000. (From Lesemann and Fuchs, 1970a.)

Fig. 20. Young plasmodium of *Olpidium brassicae* within a root cell of the kohlrabi host a few hours after penetration. The fungal plasma membrane (FPM) is in direct contact with host cytoplasm (HC) and constitutes the only distinct structural component of the host-parasite interface. The host tonoplast (T) is distended around the plasmodium, and a thin layer of host cytoplasm lies between the tonoplast and the fungal plasma membrane. Host cell wall (W), host vacuole (HVa), fungal cytoplasm (FC), fungal nucleus (FNu), fungal vacuole (FVa). ×30 000. (From Lesemann and Fuchs, 1970b.)

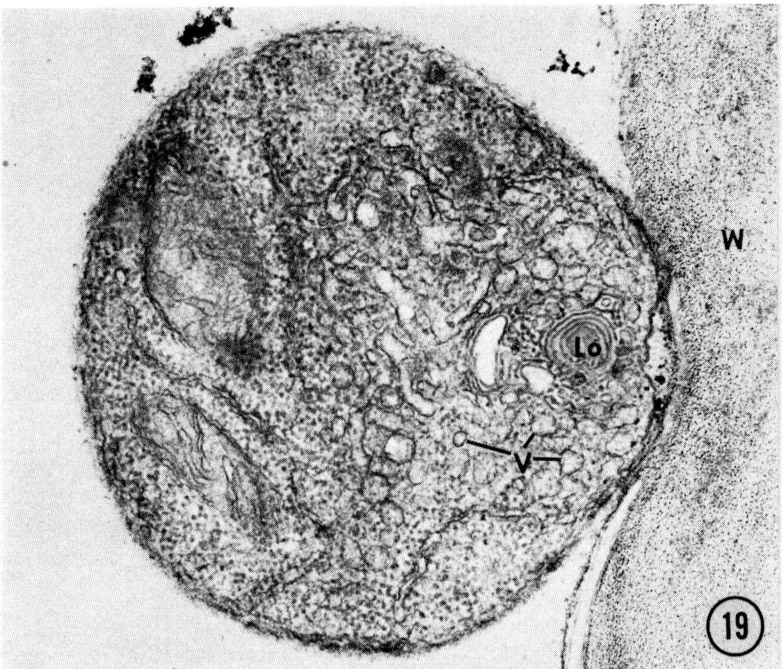
W
Lo
V
19

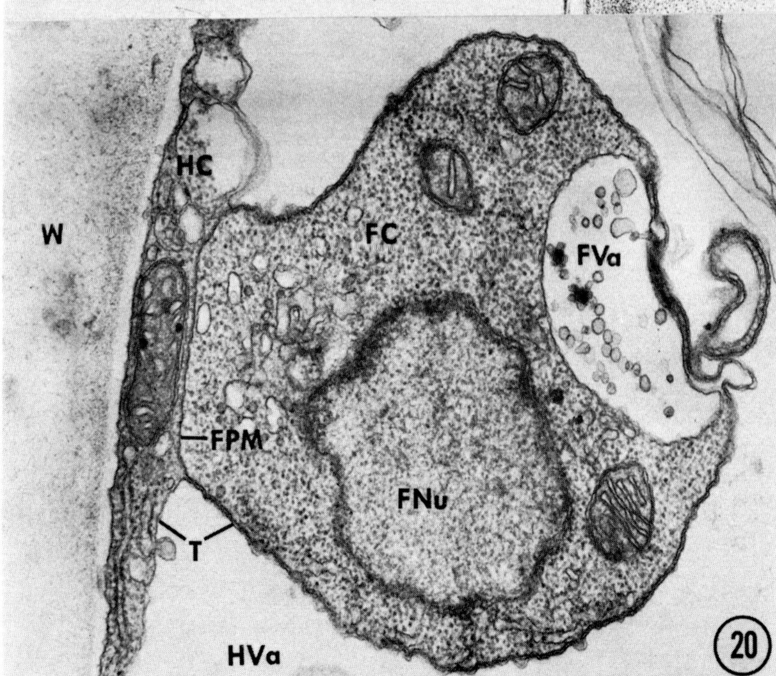
HC
W
FC
FVa
FPM
FNu
T
HVa
20

Fig. 21. *Rhizobium* bacterial cell (B_1) passing from an infection thread into a host cell in a clover root nodule. As the bacterium enters the host cell (C), the infection thread matrix (ITM) is left behind and the bacterium acquires a membrane envelope by invaginating the plasma membrane (PM) of the host cell. Another bacterial cell (B_2), surrounded by a membrane envelope, is outside the infection thread matrix, but the envelope is still attached to the plasma membrane. x32 000. (From Dixon, 1967.)

Fig. 22. *Rhizobium* bacteroid (B) within a host cell (C) of a pea root nodule. The bacteroid is enclosed by a membrane envelope (M). x30 000. (Courtesy of R. O. D. Dixon, University of Edinburgh.)

Fig. 23. Bacterial endosymbionts (B) (epsilon particles) within a cell of *Paramecium multimicronucleatum*. The macronucleus (MaNu) and micronucleus (MiNu) of the host are shown. The bacteria occur within membrane-bounded loculi (L) which are formed by extensions of the nuclear envelopes via channels from the outer membrane of the nuclear envelopes. One loculus (arrow) has multiple connections to the macronuclear and micronuclear envelopes. x33 000. (From Jenkins, 1970.)

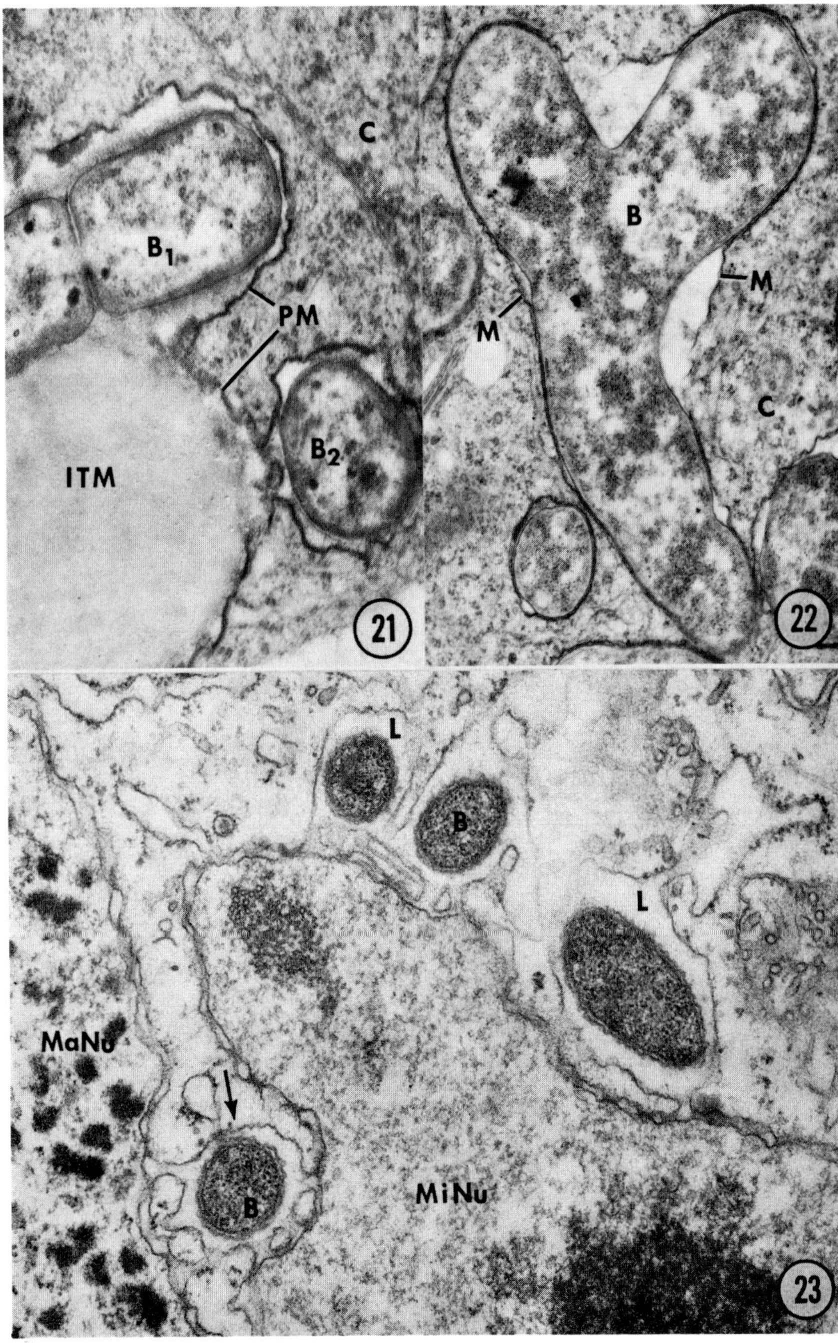
C
B1
PM
B2
ITM
21
B
M
M
C
22
L
B
L
MaNu
B
MiNu
23

Fig. 24. Endonuclear bacteria (B) within a nucleus of the host *Euglena spirogyra*. The bacteria are surrounded by a mucilaginous sheath or matrix layer (S), but this layer is not separated from host plasma (nucleoplasm) (Nu) by any membrane. Host chromosome (Ch). ×40 000. (From Leedale, 1969.)

Fig. 25. Mycoplasma-like bodies (My) associated with the corn stunt disease. The mycoplasma-like bodies are shown within a ganglion of the leaf hopper *Dalbulus elimatus* which acquires them from infected corn plants. The bodies have a distinct limiting membrane and are surrounded by cytoplasm of the leaf hopper cell. ×64 000. (Courtesy of R. Granados, Boyce Thompson Institute for Plant Research, Yonkers, N.Y.)

Fig. 26. Particles of potato yellow dwarf virus (V) located within the lumen of the nuclear envelope of a host cell. The virus particles are found between the two membranes of the nuclear envelope (NE). Host nucleus (Nu), host cytoplasm (C), host vacuole (Va). ×15 000 approx. (Courtesy of R. McLeod, University of Illinois.)

Fig. 27. Similar to Fig. 26, showing an enlarged portion of a nuclear periphery where the virus particles (V) have distended the outer membrane of the nuclear envelope (NE). Host nucleus (Nu), host cytoplasm (C), host vacuole (Va). ×30 000 approx. (Courtesy of R. McLeod, University of Illinois.)

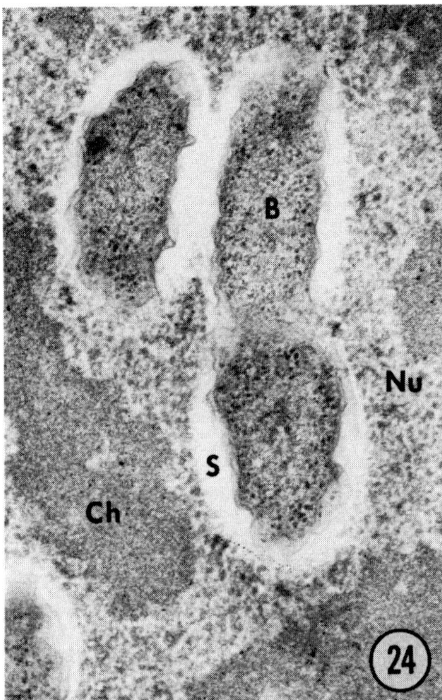
B
Nu
S
Ch
24

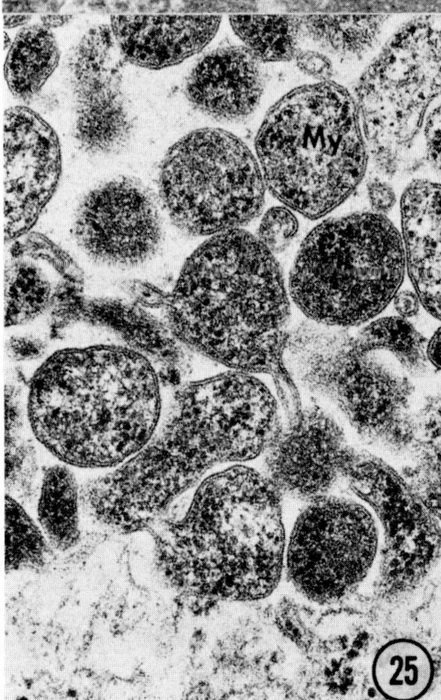
My
25

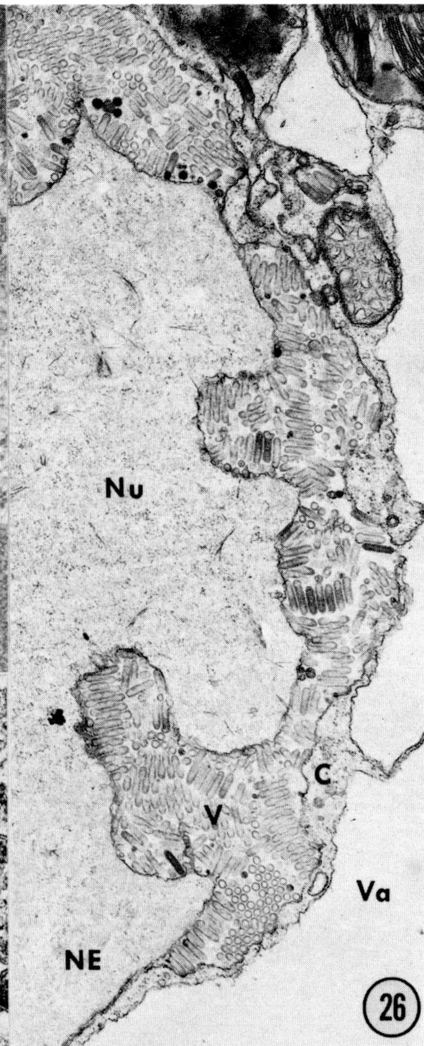
Nu
C
V
Va
NE
26

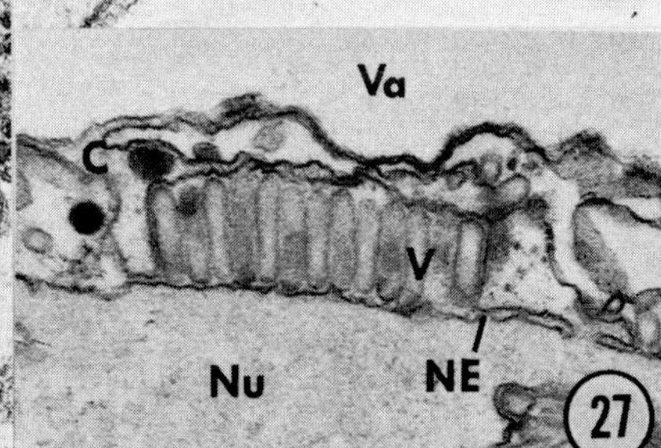
Va
C
V
NE
Nu
27

Fig. 28. Particles of tobacco mosaic virus (V) seen in cross-section (top) and longitudinal section (bottom) within a chloroplast of *Nicotiana tabacum*. The particles are shown in clusters or aggregates within the chloroplast stroma (St). They are surrounded by a light-staining matrix that is distinct from the stroma. Chloroplast grana (G), inner and outer chloroplast membranes (M). ×72 000. (From Esau and Cronshaw, 1967.)

Fig. 29. Tobacco mosaic virus particles (V) occurring in an aggregate in the cytoplasm (C) of a mesophyll cell of *Nicotiana tabacum*. Nucleus (Nu). ×35 000. (From Esau and Gill, 1969.)

Fig. 30. Tobacco mosaic virus particles (V) occurring as scattered particles in the cytoplasm (C) of a mesophyll cell of *Nicotiana tabacum*. Nucleus (Nu), cell wall (W). ×35 000. (From Esau and Gill, 1969.)

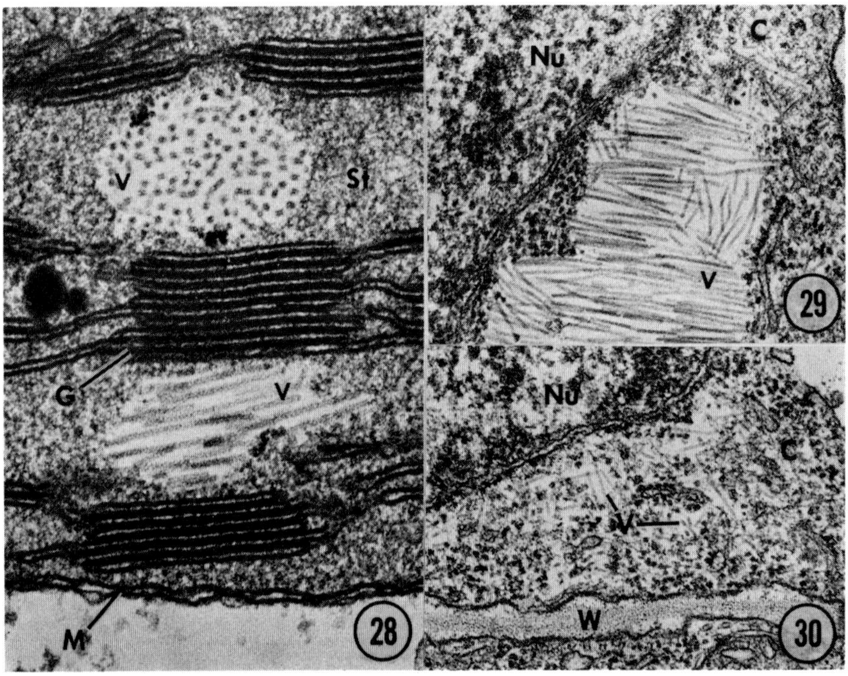
V
St
G
V
M
28
Nu
C
V
29
Nu
C
V
W
30

Fig. 31. Particles of tobacco rattle virus (V) attached by their ends to the outer membrane of host mitochondria (Mi). ×51 000. (From Harrison and Roberts, 1968.)

Fig. 32. Wound tumor virus particles (V) in an infected subesophageal ganglion cell of an insect vector *Agallia constricta.* The particles form linear arrays enclosed by a tubular membranous boundary (M). Some virions are free in the cytoplasm. ×49 000. (From Hirumi *et al.*, 1967.)

Fig. 33. Virus particles (V) in a hypha of the fungus *Penicillium stoloniferum* 2 mm behind the hyphal apex. Virus particles in this portion of the fungal thallus occur in groups that are enclosed by a membrane (M). Fungal cytoplasm (C). ×50 400. (Courtesy of D. Border, Imperial College, London.)

Fig. 34. Similar to Fig. 32 but taken at 4 mm behind the hyphal apex. The virus particles (V) are in crystalline aggregates within a vacuole. Fungal cytoplasm (C). ×32 000. (Courtesy of D. Border, Imperial College, London.)

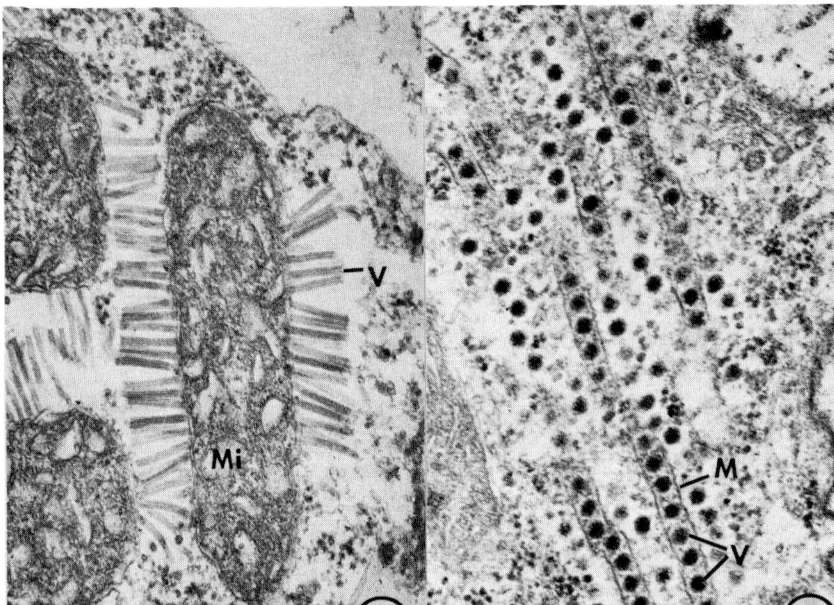
V
Mi
31
M
V
32
C
V
M
33
C
V
34

Figs 35-42. Light micrographs of fixed and stained tissues showing stages in the formation of intracellular haustoria of *Melampsora lini* on flax (*Linum usitatissimum*). Fig. 35. Initial contact of an intercellular haustorial mother cell (MC) with the wall of a host cell (C). The wall of the mother cell appears to thicken slightly in the region of contact (arrow). Fig. 36. The penetration peg (P) is initiated and begins to grow into the host cell, dissolving the host wall at the point of penetration. Fig. 37. The penetration peg (P) continues to elongate and extends farther into the host cell lumen. Fig. 38. The penetration peg (P) reaches a maximum length of about 4 μm before ceasing elongation. Note the dark staining ring (R = neck ring) in the mid-region of the peg. Fig. 39. After the penetration peg stops elongating, the distal end begins to enlarge to initiate formation of the haustorial body (H). Fig. 40. Two immature haustoria (H) in a host cell. What was previously termed the penetration peg has now become the haustorial neck. Note the dark staining ring (R) on the neck of the haustorium on the left. Fig. 41. A slightly later stage of haustorial development than in Fig. 40. The haustorium (H) has lost its spherical shape and has begun to form a lobe on the left-hand side. Fig. 42. A mature haustorium (H) with a single lobe protruding toward the left. Note the prominent neck ring (R). All ×2100. (From Littlefield, 1972.)

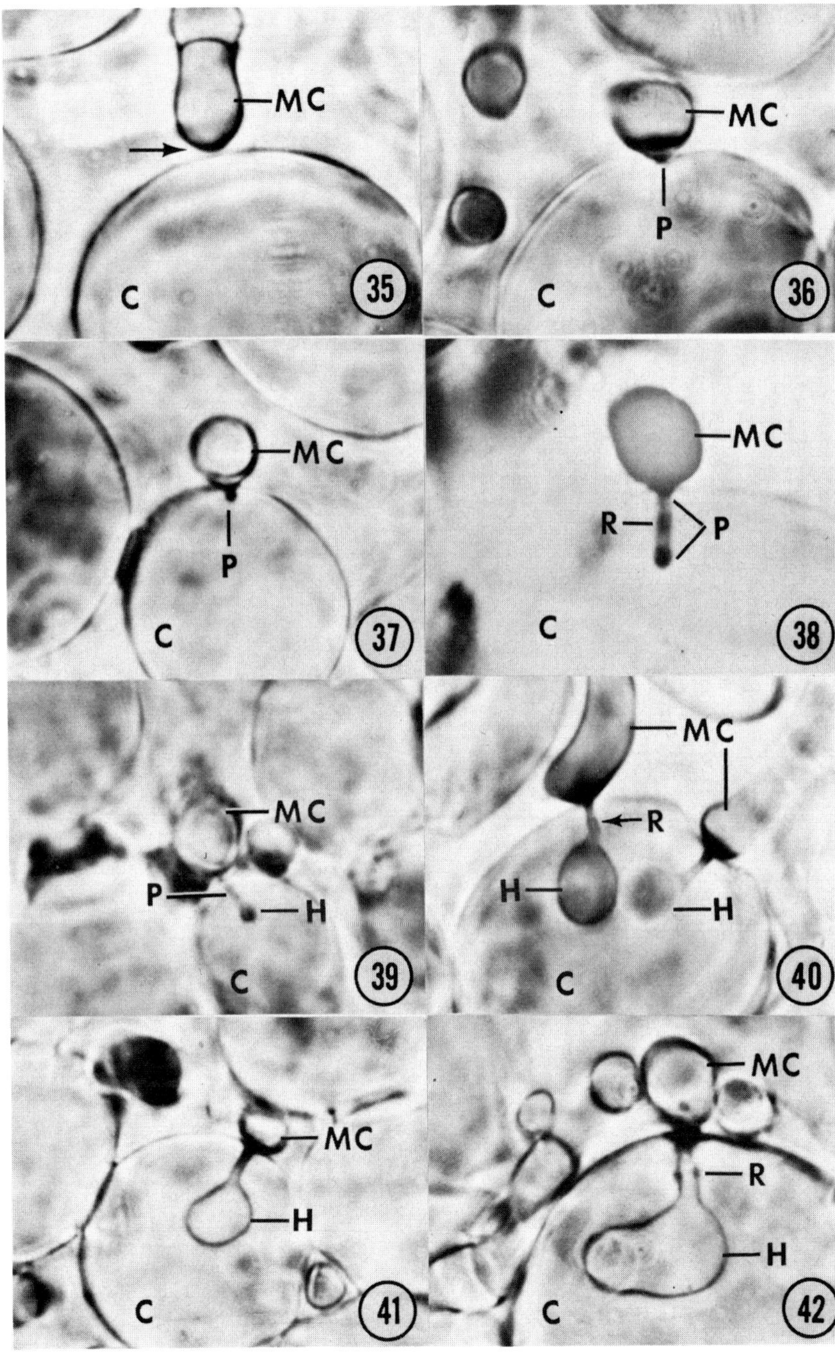
MC
C
35
MC
P
C
36
MC
P
C
37
MC
R
P
C
38
MC
P
H
C
39
MC
R
H
H
C
40
MC
H
C
41
MC
R
H
C
42

Fig. 43. Frozen-etched preparation of a rust-infected flax leaf showing a haustorial mother cell (MC) of *Melampsora lini* and the attached haustorium (H) inside the host cell. The invaginated host plasma membrane (PMI), seen in face view, surrounds and covers the haustorium and is characterized by undulations and cleft-like depressions. A thin layer of host cytoplasm (C) is next to the invaginated host plasma membrane. Host vacuole (Va), host cell wall (W). x15 000. (From Littlefield and Bracker, 1972.)

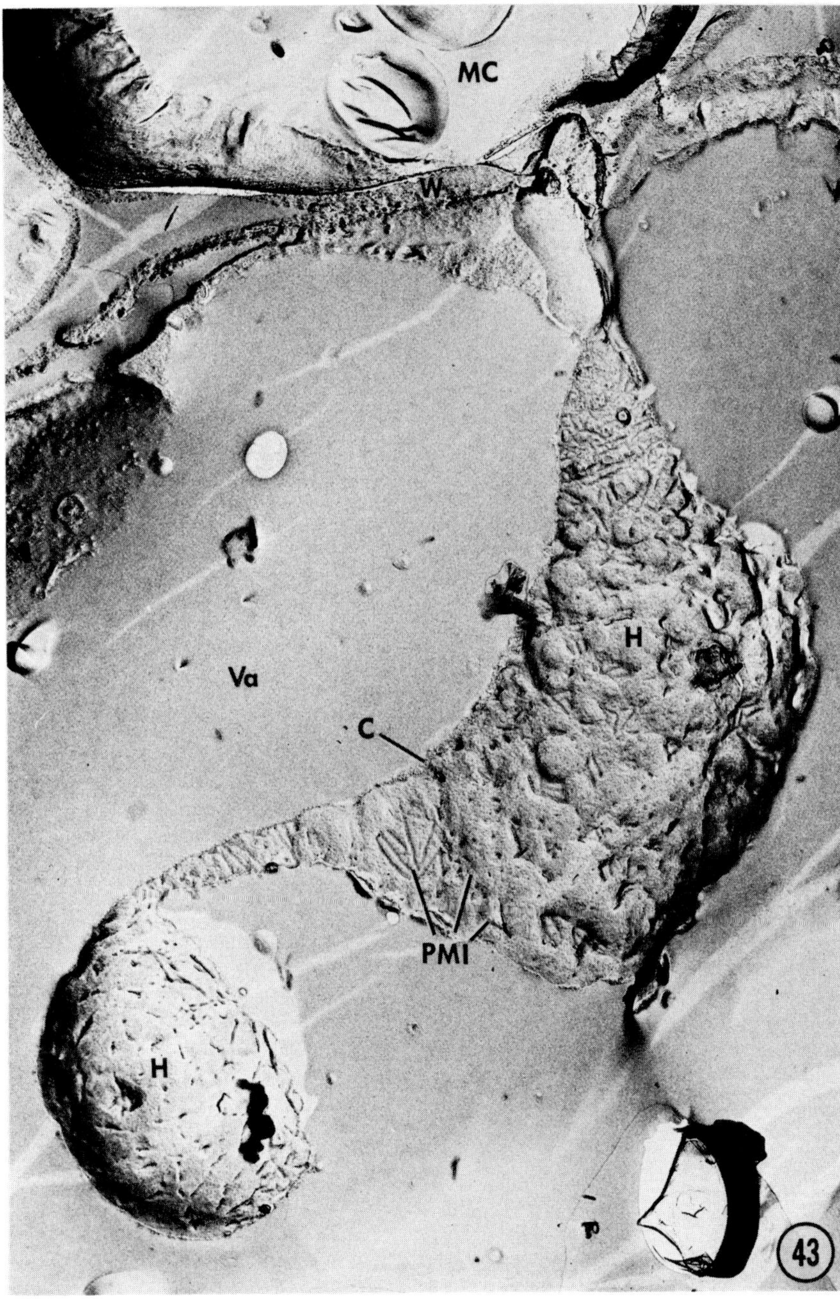
MC
W
H
Va
C
PMI
H
43

Fig. 44. Haustorium (H) of *Melampsora lini* within a mesophyll cell of the host and attached to the haustorial mother cell (MC) via the haustorial neck (N). Note the densely staining neck ring (R) approximately mid-way along the wall of the haustorial neck. A matrix, the sheath (S), separates the haustorial wall (FW) from the invaginated host plasma membrane (PMI) which surrounds the haustorium. Host cytoplasm (C). ×9500. (From Coffey *et al.*, 1972.)

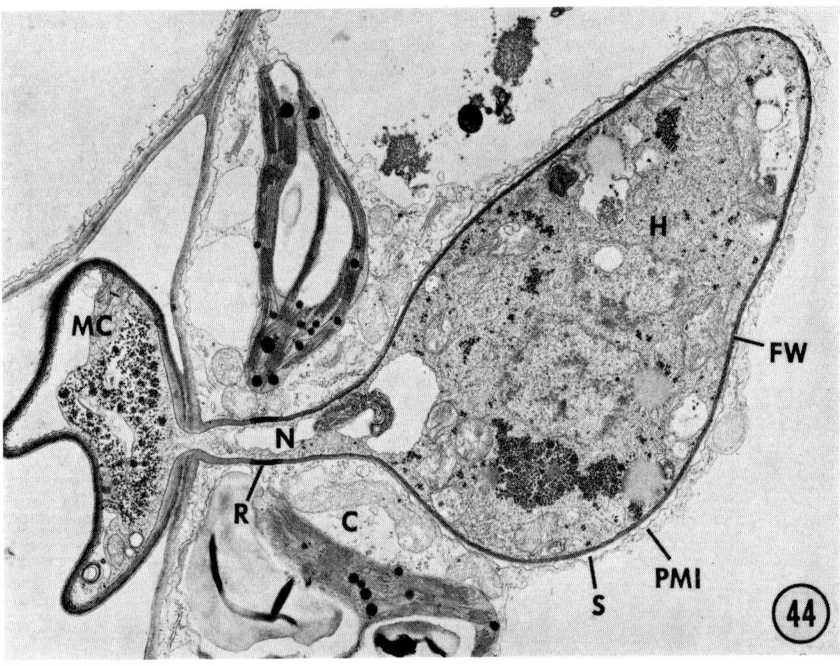
MC
H
FW
N
R
C
S
PMI
44

Fig. 45. A haustorial mother cell (MC) of *Melampsora lini* in contact with a host mesophyll cell (C) during an early stage of host cell penetration. The fungal wall is thickened in the region of contact, and a young penetration peg (P) has begun to form. The arrow indicates amorphous electron-dense material between the walls of host and fungus. ×25 000. (From Littlefield and Bracker, 1972.)

Fig. 46. Enlargement of another section of the incipient penetration peg shown in Fig. 45. The innermost layer (IL) of the fungal wall has grown through the outer portion of the fungal wall and contacts the host wall (W). Wall deposits (Ap = wall appositions) are on the inner surface of the host wall around the penetration site. Host plasma membrane (PM). ×43 000. (From Littlefield and Bracker, 1972.)

Fig. 47. Penetration site where *Melampsora lini* has entered a mesophyll cell of flax. The fungal wall (FW) is continuous between the haustorial mother cell (MC) and the haustorial neck (N). Where the fungus passes through the host wall (W), the fungal wall stains darker (see also Fig. 48) than the host wall, but the boundary between them is indistinct (compare with *Erysiphe graminis*, Figs 75, 81, 82, in which the boundary is distinct). The dark staining amorphous layer (arrow) between the apposed walls of host and fungus extends up to the fungal wall at each side of the penetration site. The host plasma membrane (PM) is invaginated by the penetrating fungus. At the left side of the haustorial neck, the host plasma membrane follows the contours of the wall appositions (Ap), then doubles back on itself and follows the wall of the haustorial neck. At the right side of the haustorial neck where no wall appositions are present, the host plasma membrane is invaginated by the fungus and simply follows the surface of the haustorial neck. Fungal nucleus (FNu). ×67 000. (From Littlefield and Bracker, 1972.)

Fig. 48. Enlargement of part of Fig. 44. Note the absence of sheath matrix around the haustorial neck (N), and the close contact of fungal plasma membrane (FPM), fungal wall (FW), and host plasma membrane (PM) in the region of the neck ring (R). Host wall (W), host cytoplasm (C), haustorial mother cell (MC). ×36 000. (From Coffey *et al.*, 1972.)

Fig. 49. Non-median section through a haustorial neck (N) of *Melampsora lini* near the penetration site. A wall apposition in the form of a fibrillar collar (Co) is continuous with the host wall (W) and surrounds the proximal end of the haustorial neck. Neck ring (R). ×36 000. (From Coffey *et al.*, 1972.)

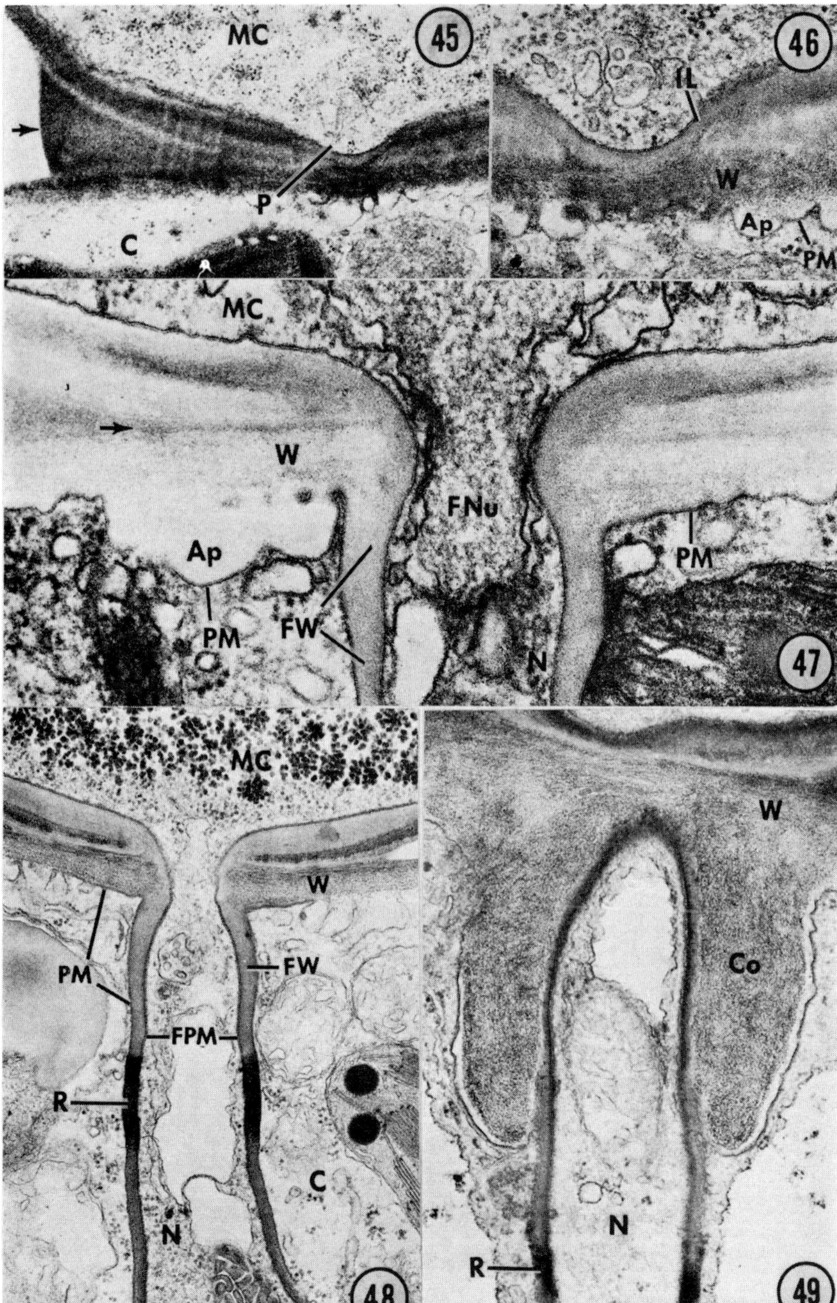
45
MC
P
C
46
IL
W
Ap
PM
MC
W
FNu
PM
Ap
PM
FW
N
47
MC
W
PM
FW
FPM
R
C
N
48
W
Co
N
R
49

Fig. 50. A partially-encased haustorium (H) of *Uromyces phaseoli* var *vignae* in a cowpea leaf. The encasement (En) is a wall-like substance surrounding the haustorial neck and the proximal portion of the haustorial body, and is continuous with the host cell wall (W). It is a type of wall apposition. This structure (a 'collar' by our terminology; a 'sheath' according to Heath and Heath's terminology) is separated from the haustorium by a thin layer of host cytoplasm (arrow). This cytoplasmic layer is seen more clearly at a higher magnification of *M. lini* in Figs 51 and 52. ×4700. (From Heath and Heath, 1971.)

Fig. 51. Higher magnification of a segment of a partially-encased haustorium of *Melampsora lini* similar to that in Fig. 50. The substance of the encasement (En), which is an extension of the collar, is separated from the haustorial wall (FW) by a thin layer of host cytoplasm (HC) sandwiched between two layers of invaginated host plasma membrane (arrows). The haustorium (H) in this figure appears necrotic. A haustorial sheath layer (S) is still present around the haustorial wall. ×29 000. (From Littlefield and Bracker, 1972.)

Fig. 52. Cross-section of a haustorial neck (N) surrounded by a collar (Co) similar to that in Figs 50 and 51. Two layers of host plasma membrane (PM) and an intervening layer of host cytoplasm (HC) separate the collar from the wall (FW) of the haustorial neck. The profiles of host plasma membrane result from the pathway of the invaginated plasma membrane doubling back on itself as it follows the contours of the collar and the haustorial neck (see also Fig. 47). Fungal plasma membrane (FPM). ×60 000. (From Littlefield and Bracker, 1972.)

Fig. 53. Completely encased haustorium (H) of *Uromyces phaseoli* var. *vignae*. The encasement (En) ('sheath', Heath and Heath's terminology) is continuous with the host cell wall and represents a type of wall apposition differing in degree of development from the collar-like apposition in Fig. 50. Haustorial mother cell (MC). ×8400. (From Heath and Heath, 1971.)

Fig. 54. A callosity (Ap) (papilla-like wall apposition) formed on the inner surface of the cell wall (W) of a cowpea plant infected with cowpea rust. This type of deposit stains positively for callose and contains abundant entrapped membranous material. The callosity is found occasionally in a susceptible cultivar of cowpea (Heath and Heath, 1971), but similar callosities are typical responses of non-host plants (e.g. bean) to this same fungus (Heath, 1972). Intercellular hypha (H), host cell protoplast (C). ×9000. (From Heath and Heath, 1971.)

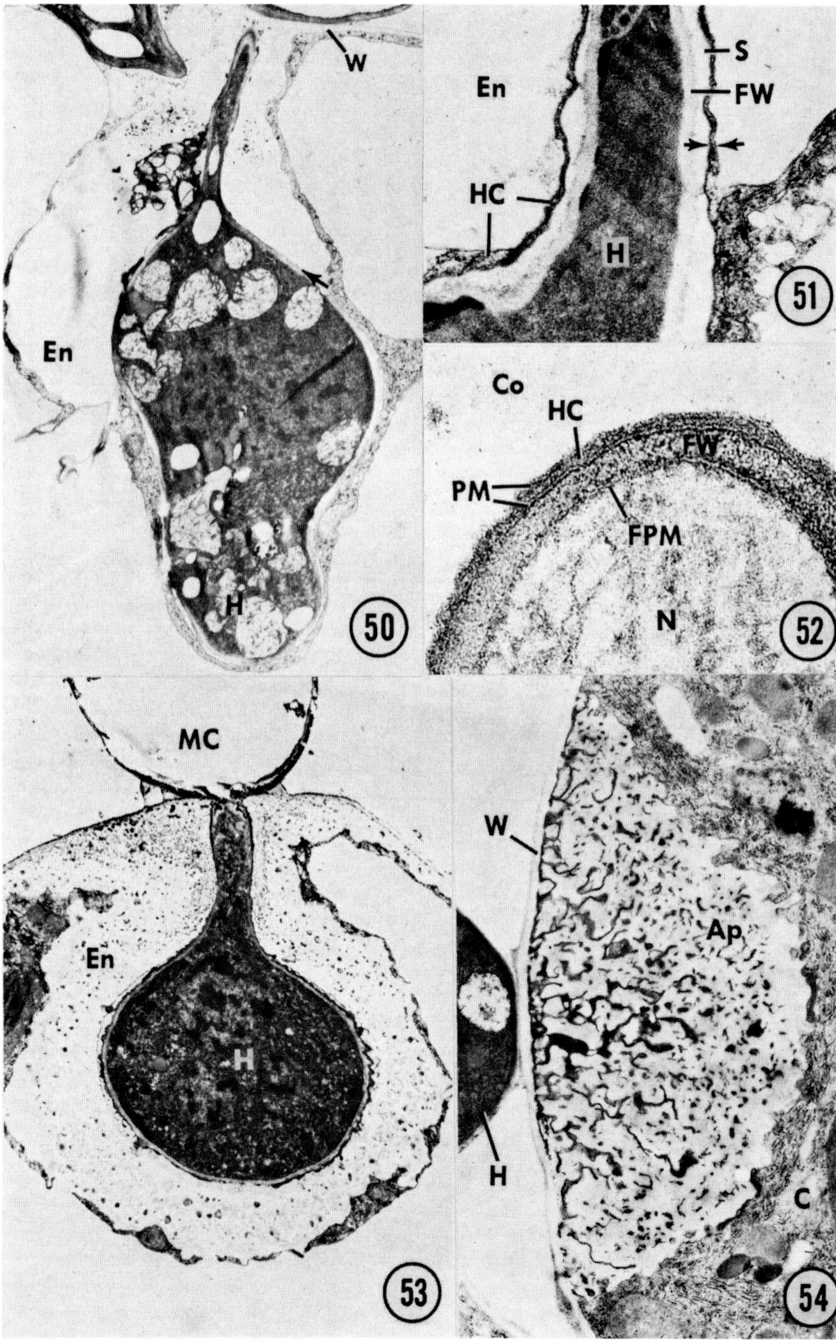
W
En
H
50
En
S
FW
HC
H
51
Co
HC
FW
PM
FPM
N
52
MC
En
H
53
W
Ap
H
C
54

Fig. 55. Lignituber (Ap) (a type of lignin-containing wall apposition) on the inner surface of a pea root cell. The lignituber is formed in response to infection by *Verticillium dahliae* and prevents further colonization of the host by the fungus. Penetration peg (P) of the fungus, fungal wall (FW), host cell wall (W), host cell lumen (C). ×20 000. (From Griffiths, 1971.)

Fig. 56. A papilla (Pa) (=wall apposition) of unknown composition formed on the inner surface of a guard cell wall (W) of a wheat leaf in response to penetration by *Erysiphe graminis tritici*. The fungus rarely penetrates guard cells. This papilla has different staining properties from other papillae or collars at sites of successful penetrations in epidermal cells of wheat. In this example the penetration peg (P) had grown through the host wall and partially into the papilla where it stopped. The cytoplasm in the penetration peg has withered and retreated from the tip, leaving a few electron-dense deposits near the apex of the peg. Appressorium (A), appressorial wall (FW), host cell protoplast (C), host nucleus (Nu). ×12 300.

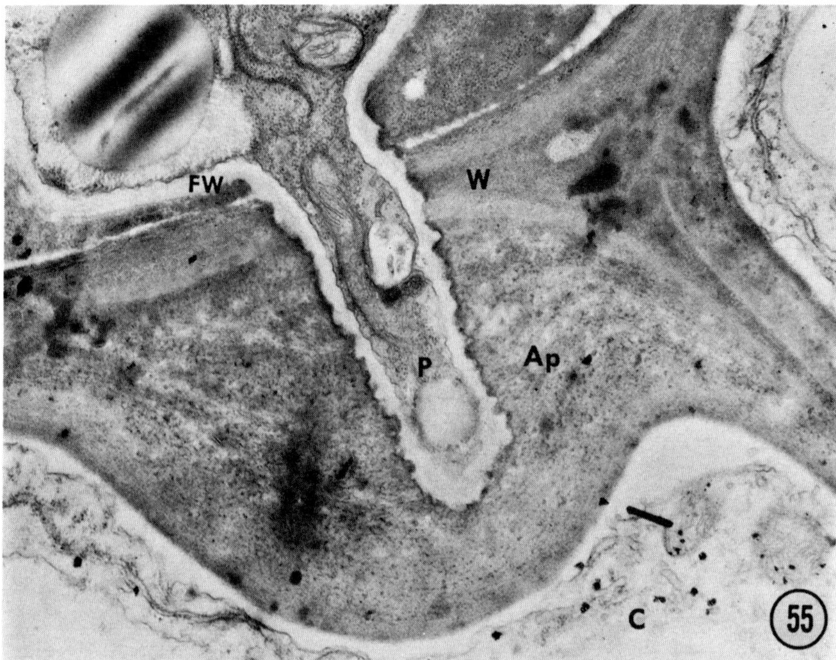
FW
W
P
Ap
C
55

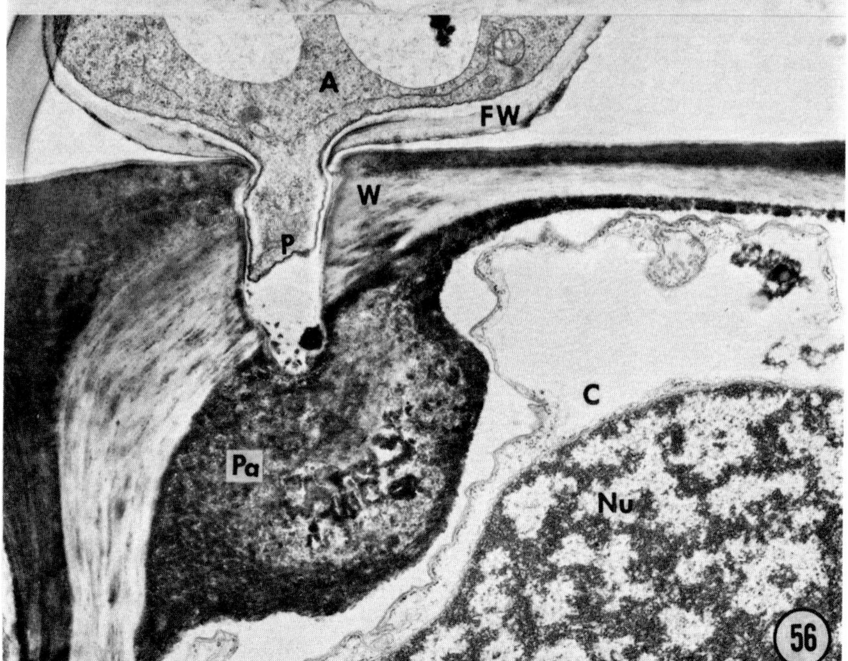
A
FW
W
P
C
Pa
Nu
56

Fig. 57. Cross-section of part of a haustorium (H) of *Melampsora lini* in a flax leaf cell. The haustorial wall (FW) is surrounded by a light-staining matrix, the haustorial sheath (S), and the invaginated plasma membrane (PMI) of the host cell. Host endoplasmic reticulum (ER) is closely associated with the invaginated plasma membrane. The two membranes are in contact at several sites around the haustorial sheath. This close relationship does not constitute continuity, but rather a specialized spatial interaction between host ER and invaginated plasma membrane. Host nucleus (Nu). ×22 500. (From Littlefield and Bracker, 1972.)

Fig. 58. Part of a haustorium (H) of *Uromyces phaseoli* var. *vignae* in an immune cultivar of cowpea. In the immune response the invaginated host plasma membrane (PMI) is commonly convoluted (note that endoplasmic reticulum (ER) and chloroplast (Chl) membranes do not show similar contortions) so that the interface between fungus and host has an undulating, irregular appearance. ×36 000. (From Heath, 1972.)

Fig. 59. Part of a haustorium (H) of *Melampsora lini* showing the interfacial region between haustorium and host protoplast (C). The invaginated host plasma membrane (PMI) surrounding the haustorium has long tentacles (Te) that extend into the host cytoplasm. Continuity between the tentacles and the plasma membrane is clearly established (arrow). The lumen of these tentacles contains material of similar electron density to the inner portion of the haustorial sheath (S_i) as contrasted to the outer portion of the sheath (S_o). Note the difference in membrane thickness and staining characteristics, luminal staining, and ribosome attachments revealed by comparison of the tentacles and host endoplasmic reticulum (ER). Clearly, the tentacles are not host endoplasmic reticulum. Haustorial wall (FW). ×52 000. (Courtesy of M. Coffey, University of Wisconsin.)

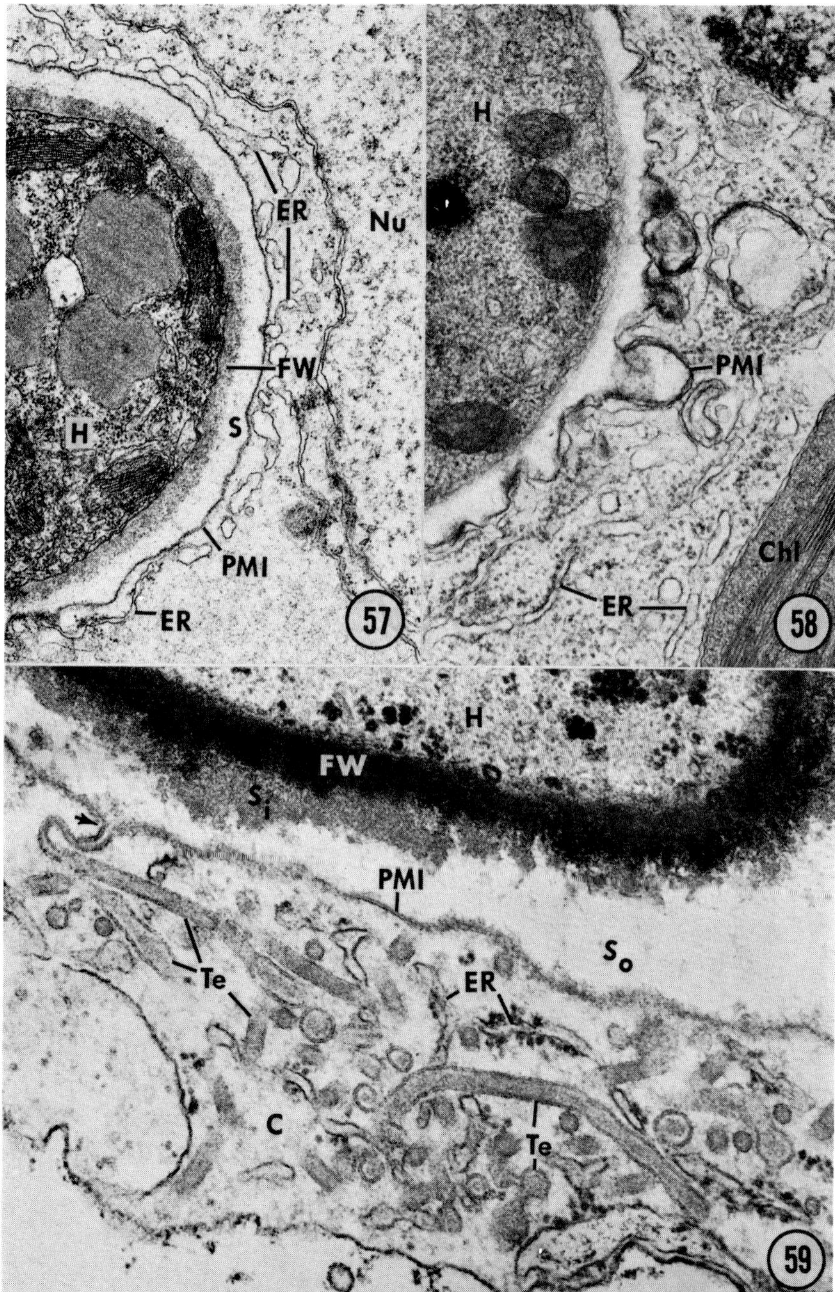
ER
Nu
FW
H
S
PMI
ER
57
H
PMI
Chl
ER
58
H
FW
S_i
PMI
S_o
Te
ER
C
Te
59

Fig. 60. Part of a haustorium (H) of *Albugo candida* in a mesophyll cell (C) of *Raphanus sativus*. A collar-like wall apposition (Co) ('sheath' according to Berlin and Bowen's terminology) is adjacent to the haustorial neck (N). Secretory bodies (Sec) are in the host cytoplasm, and some of these are continuous with the sheath-like layer (S) ('encapsulation', according to Berlin and Bowen's terminology) between the haustorial wall (FW) and the invaginated host plasma membrane (PMI) which surrounds the haustorium. Sometimes these extensions of the haustorial coating resemble the tentacles shown in Fig. 59. x45 000. (From Berlin and Bowen, 1964.)

Fig. 61. Part of a haustorium (H) of *Peronospora manshurica* in a mesophyll cell (C) of *Glycine max*. A sheath-like coating (S) ('zone of apposition' according to Peyton and Bowen's terminology) surrounds the haustorium and the haustorial wall (FW). Host endoplasmic reticulum (ER) is near the haustorium. Structures considered to be secretory bodies (Sec) are shown in various stages of fusion with the host plasma membrane (PMI) around the haustorium. x71 000. (From Peyton and Bowen, 1963.)

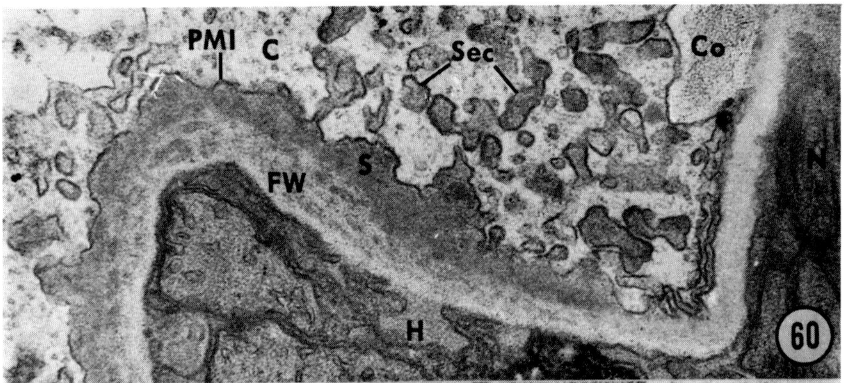
PMI
C
Sec
Co
S
FW
N
H
60

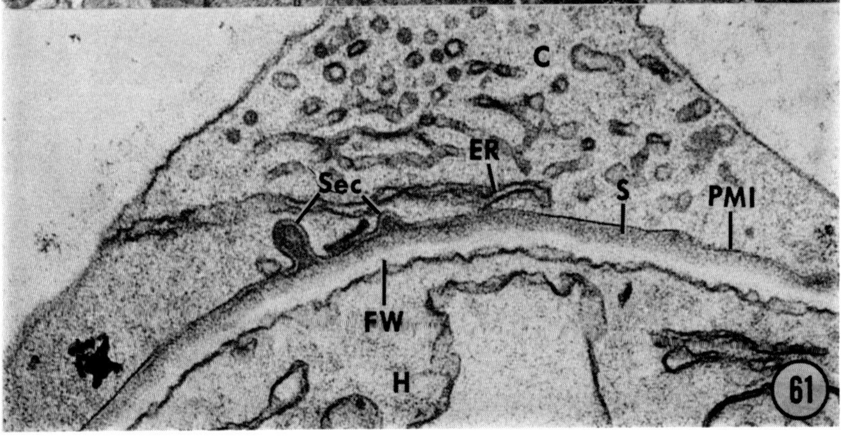
C
ER
Sec
S
PMI
FW
H
61

Figs 62 and 63. Face-view enlargements of frozen-etched preparations of host plasma membrane in rust-infected flax mesophyll. Fig. 62. Part of the invaginated portion of host plasma membrane surrounding a haustorium of *Melampsora lini.* Note the cleft-like depressions of the membrane and the absence of granular structure. Fig. 63. From a non-invaginated portion of the host plasma membrane (i.e. not in association with a haustorium). Note the granular character of the membrane and absence of linear depressions as compared to Fig. 62. Both ×75 000. (From Littlefield and Bracker, 1972.)

Fig. 64. Cross-section near the edge of a haustorium (H) of *Melampsora lini* showing the components of the host–parasite interface in a mesophyll cell of flax. Specimen was stained conventionally with uranyl acetate and lead citrate (see Littlefield and Bracker, 1972). Haustorial plasma membrane (FPM), haustorial wall (FW), matrix of the haustorial sheath (S), invaginated host plasma membrane surrounding the haustorium (PMI), host cytoplasm (C), host tonoplast (T), host vacuole (Va). The fungal and host plasma membranes have equivalent staining characteristics with this staining method. ×105 000. (From Littlefield and Bracker, 1972.)

Fig. 65. Cross-section of part of a haustorium (H) of *Melampsora lini* similar to that in Fig. 64, except sections were post-stained by a procedure which has special affinity for plasma membrane (sections treated with periodic acid, then stained with a mixture containing phosphotungstic acid and chromic acid; see Littlefield and Bracker, 1972, for details). Note the intense staining of the haustorial plasma membrane (FPM) and the non-invaginated portion of the host plasma membrane (PM) that is not associated with the haustorium. By contrast, note that the invaginated portion of the host plasma membrane (PMI), surrounding the haustorium, fails to take the stain. Haustorial wall (FW), matrix of the haustorial sheath (S), host cytoplasm (C), host cell wall (W). ×57 000. (From Littlefield and Bracker, 1972.)

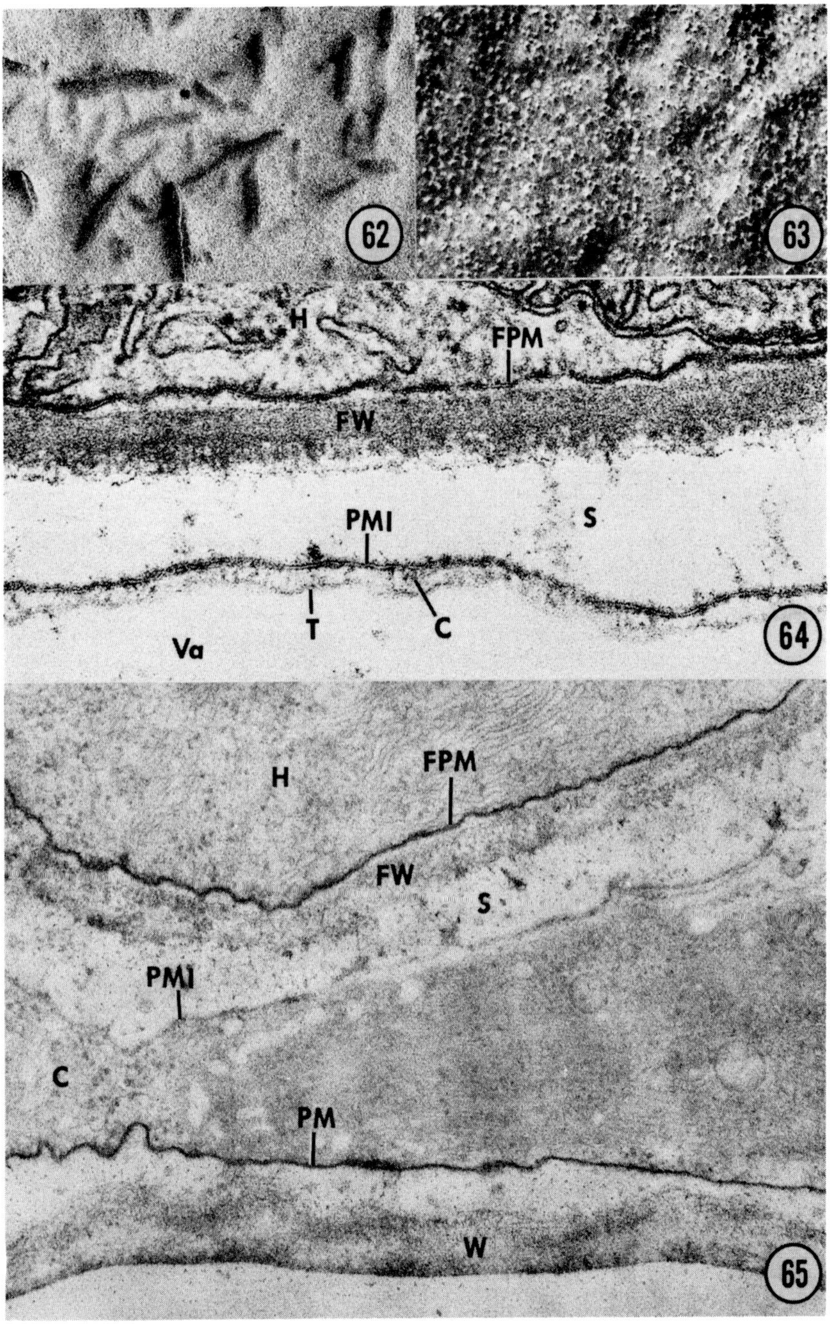
62
63
H
FPM
FW
PMI
S
T
C
Va
64
H
FPM
FW
S
PMI
C
PM
W
65

Fig. 66. Haustorium (H) of *Phytophthora parasitica* var. *nicotianae* in a tobacco root cell. The small, bulbous haustorium of this pathogen is normally surrounded by a wall-like apposition (Ap) that is continuous with the host cell wall (W) and separates the haustorium from the invaginated plasma membrane (PMI) of the host cell. Host cytoplasm (C), vesicles (V) in haustorial cytoplasm. ×30 000. (From Hanchey and Wheeler, 1971.)

Fig. 67. Section through a penetration peg (P) of *Erysiphe graminis* that has penetrated nearly through the outer epidermal wall (W) of a wheat leaf. A wall apposition in the form of a crudely layered papilla (Pa) has been deposited on the inner surface of the host wall in advance of the penetration peg. Note the dark-staining halo (arrow) around the penetration peg which signifies alteration of the host wall and papilla in the immediate vicinity of the penetration peg. Host cytoplasm (C), host vacuole (Va). ×12 500.

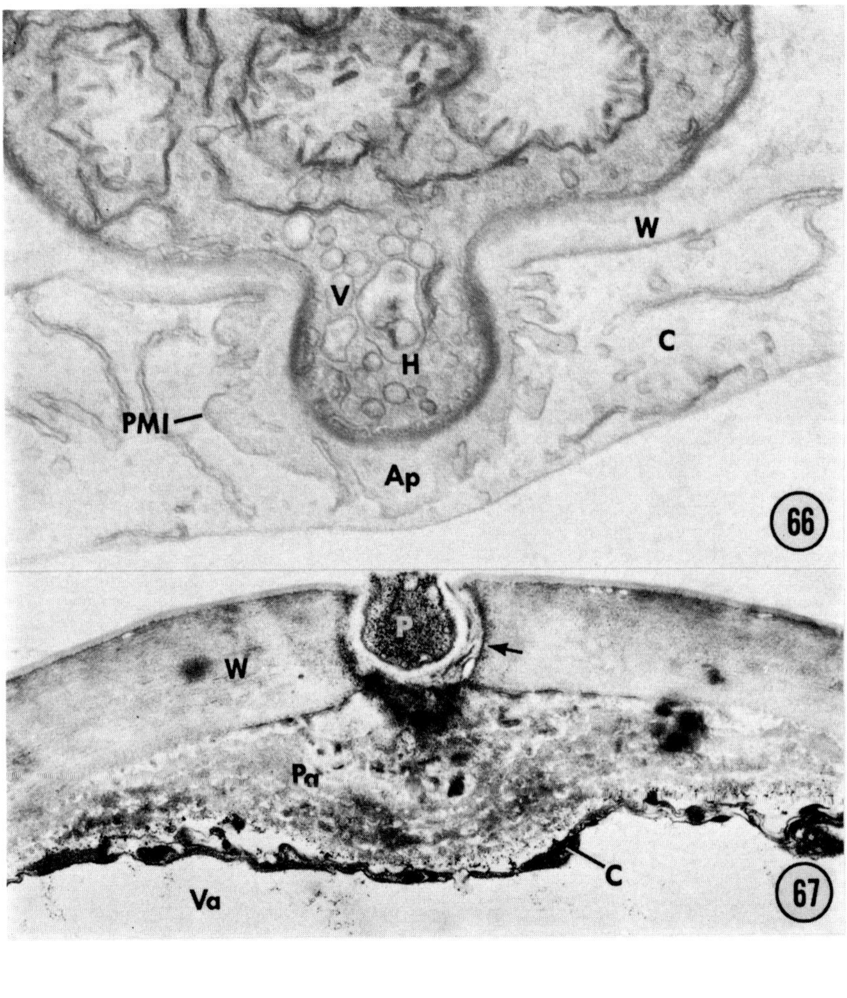
W
V
C
H
PMI
Ap
66
P
W
Pa
C
Va
67

Fig. 68. Cross-section through a wheat leaf epidermal cell showing the site of penetration of *Erysiphe graminis*. Note the densely staining material (Hal) in the host epidermal wall (W) which forms a halo-like region around the penetration site. A collar-like wall apposition (Co) is attached to the host wall and surrounds the proximal region of the haustorial neck (N). Appressorium (A), haustorial body (Bo), host cytoplasm (C), host vacuole (Va). ×11 500.

Fig. 69. Low magnification cross-section through part of an epidermal cell of wheat infected by *Erysiphe graminis*. The section is near a penetration site, but non-median. Part of a collar is evident at Co, and a haustorium (H) is in the lower part of the figure. Note the broad, densely-staining halo (Hal) of altered wall material in the epidermal cell wall (W) surrounding the site of penetration. Fungal hyphae (H) on the leaf surface. ×4000.

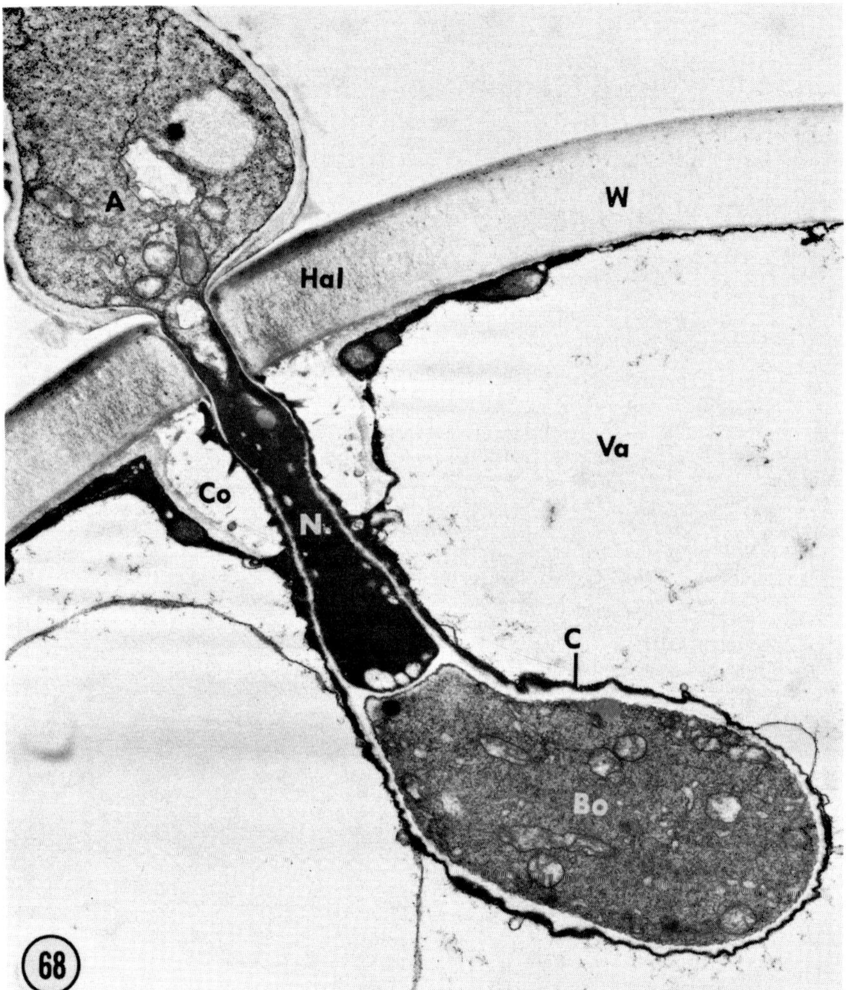
A
W
Hal
Va
Co
N
C
Bo
68

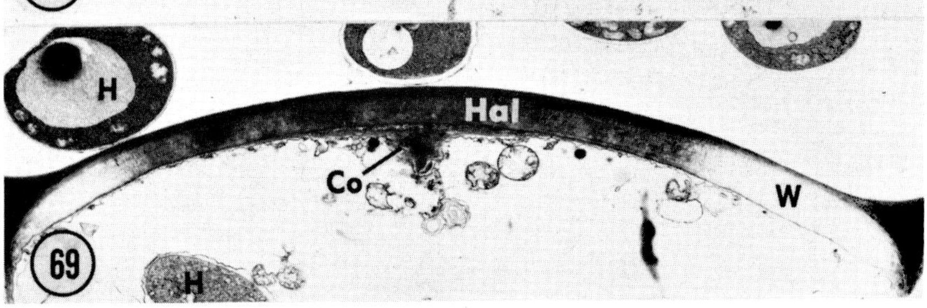
H
Hal
Co
W
69
H

Fig. 70. Haustorium of *Erysiphe graminis* intercepted in longitudinal section in an epidermal cell of a susceptible wheat leaf. Haustorial body (Bo), haustorial nucleus (FNu), finger-like haustorial lobes (Lo), host cytoplasm (C), host vacuole (Va), outer epidermal wall (W), hypha (H) on the leaf surface. This section intercepted the vicinity of three penetration sites, all non-median. They are recognized by the dark-staining haloes (X) in the epidermal cell wall. Two of these penetration sites show parts of the collars (Co) surrounding haustorial necks. x4000.

Fig. 71. Cross-section of an epidermal cell of wheat infected by *Erysiphe graminis*. The haustorial lobes (Lo) are surrounded by the matrix of the haustorial sheath (S) which in turn is bounded by a membrane and the host cytoplasm (C). Host vacuole (Va), host cell wall (W). x4000.

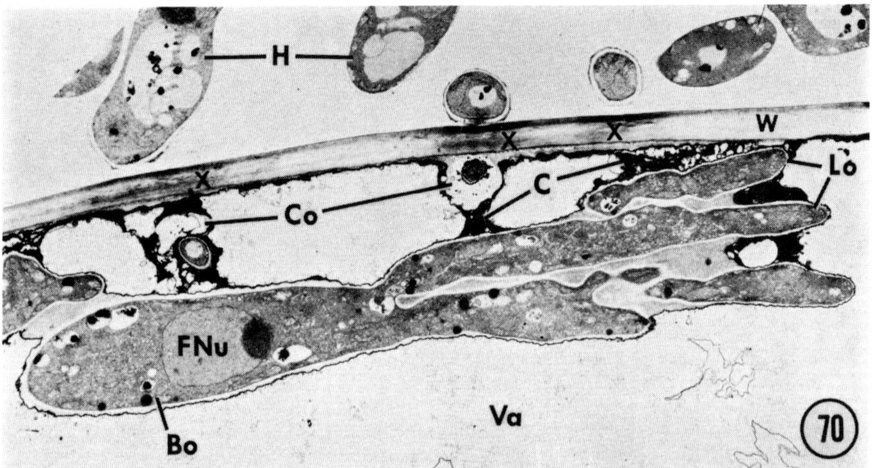
H
W
X
X
X
C
Lo
Co
FNu
Bo
Va
70

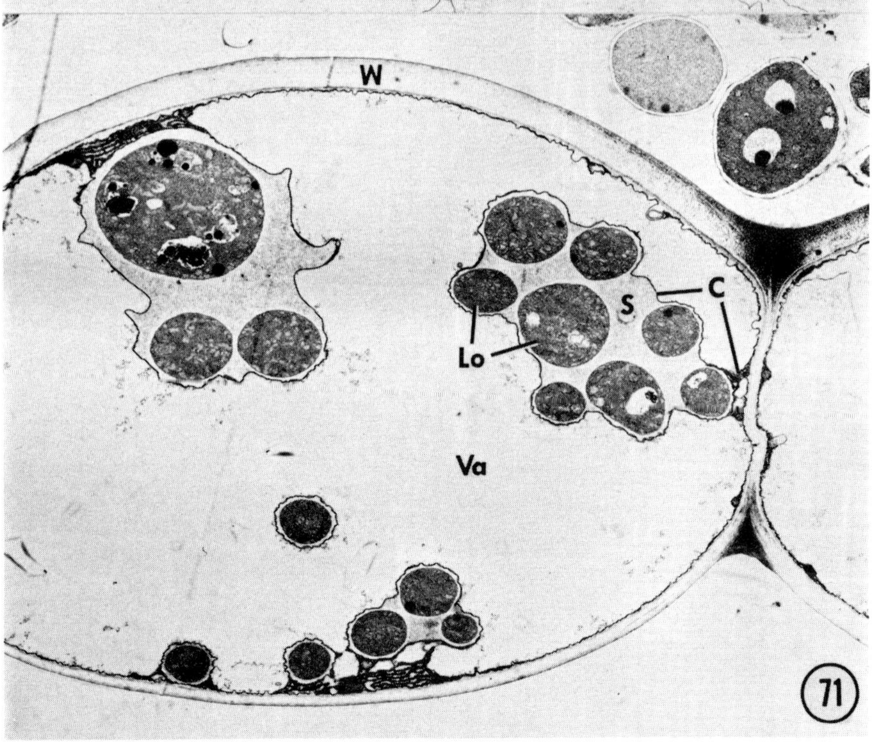
W
S
C
Lo
Va
71

Fig. 72. Cross-section of the lobes (Lo) of one haustorium of *Erysiphe graminis tritici* within a common sheath matrix (S). The haustorial lobes and sheath are bounded by a dark line (arrow) that consists of the invaginated host plasma membrane, a thin layer of host cytoplasm, and the host tonoplast. Host vacuole (Va). Note the several interfaces encountered by portions of haustorial lobes in this figure: 1 = adjacent haustorial walls in contact, 2 = the haustorial wall forms an interface with the sheath matrix, 3 = haustorial wall is closely surrounded by the host protoplast with little or no intervening sheath matrix. The profile of the sheath and surrounding host protoplast (dark line, arrow) indicates close association of the host protoplast with the haustorium and an absence of swelling of the sheath matrix. ×11 500.

Fig. 73. Longitudinal section through two haustorial lobes (Lo) of *Erysiphe graminis* in a susceptible wheat leaf. (Enlargement of a section through the haustorium shown in Fig. 70.) The membrane that bounds the sheath matrix (S) extends around the ends of the lobes even though the sheath is much reduced around the terminal portion of the lobes. Organelle-rich host cytoplasm (C) such as that seen between the lobes is characteristic of infected cells and atypical of non-infected cells. Host vacuole (Va). ×12 500.

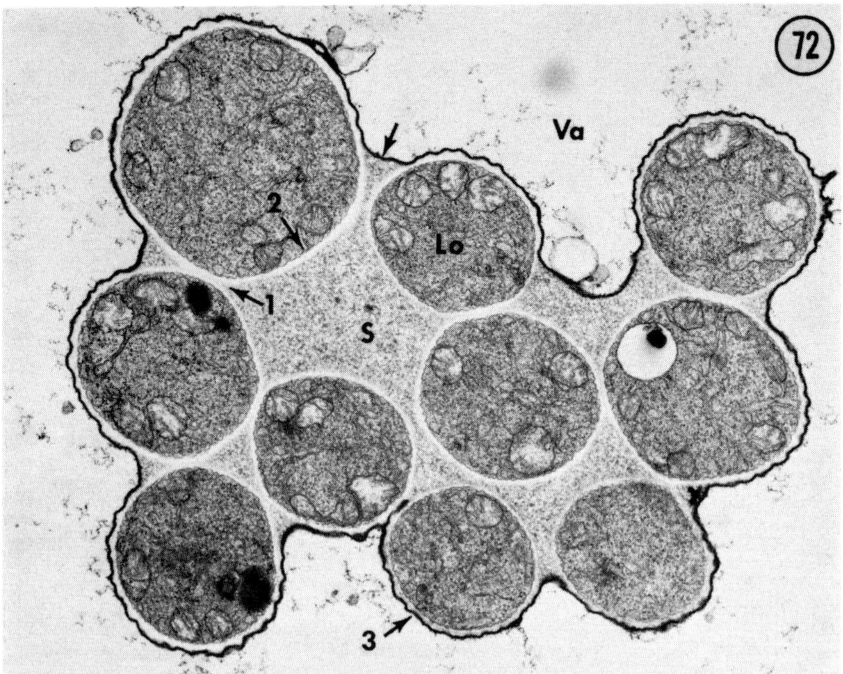
72
Va
2
Lo
1
S
3

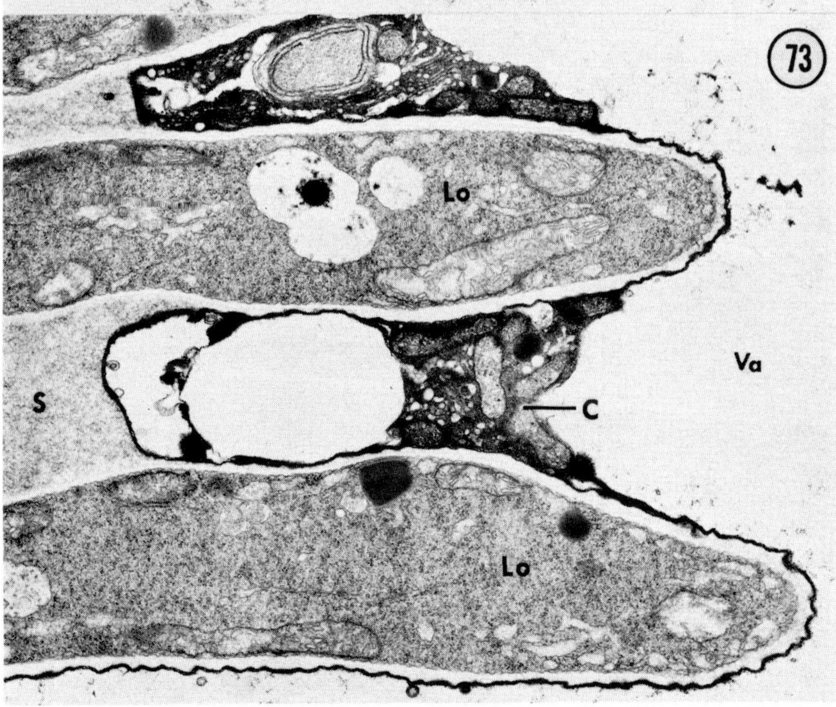
73
Lo
Va
S
C
Lo

Fig. 74. Enlargement of Fig. 67. Note the dark-staining region (unlettered arrow) in the host wall (W) and papilla around the penetration peg (P). Membranes (M) are trapped in the region where the papilla (Pa) joins the epidermal wall. Note the membrane-bounded vesicles (V) in the penetration peg, similar to those found in apices of growing hyphae and germinating spores. Fungal wall (FW), host cuticle (Cu). x69 000.

Fig. 75. *Erysiphe graminis* on wheat. Near-median section through a penetration site (enlargement of Fig. 68). Note the distinct boundary (arrow) between the penetration peg wall (FW) and the host wall (W) as contrasted to the situation with rusts (Figs 47, 48). Around the point of penetration, fibrils (F) of the host wall appear crushed, and that portion of the wall also stains intensely. The host cuticle (Cu) is displaced around the penetration site so that it is pushed partly into the hole around the penetration peg. Such views indicate physical displacement due to mechanical force during host penetration. x86 000.

Fig. 76. Similar to Fig. 75, showing displacement of the host cuticle (Cu) around the penetration site. Note also that the electron-transparent wall fibrils in the outer region of the epidermal wall are discontinuous near the penetration site (arrows), indicating that the fibrils were biochemically degraded in this localized region before or during host penetration. x61 000.

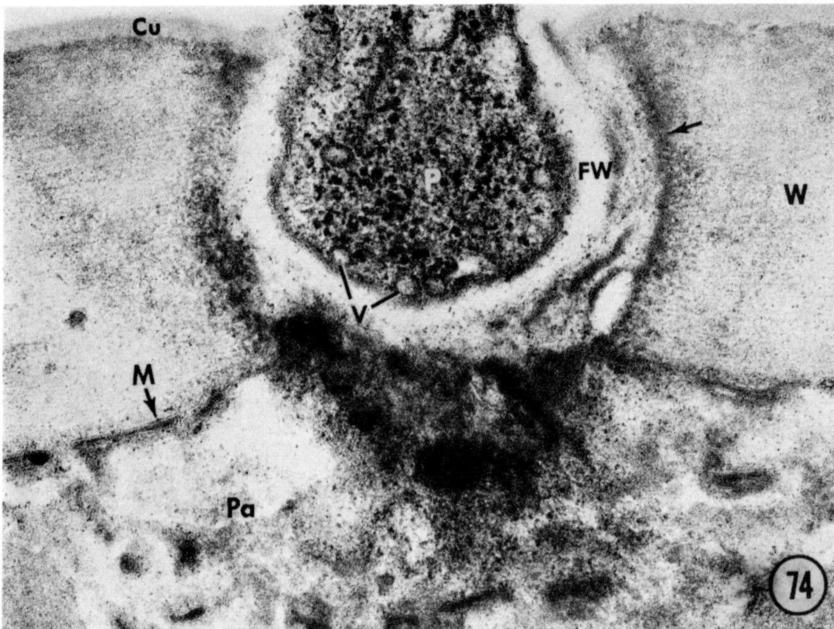
Cu
FW
W
P
V
M
Pa
74

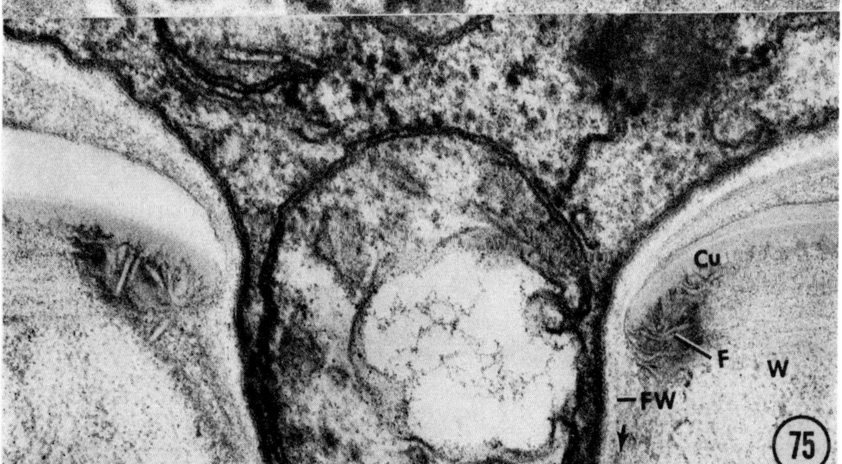
Cu
F
W
FW
75

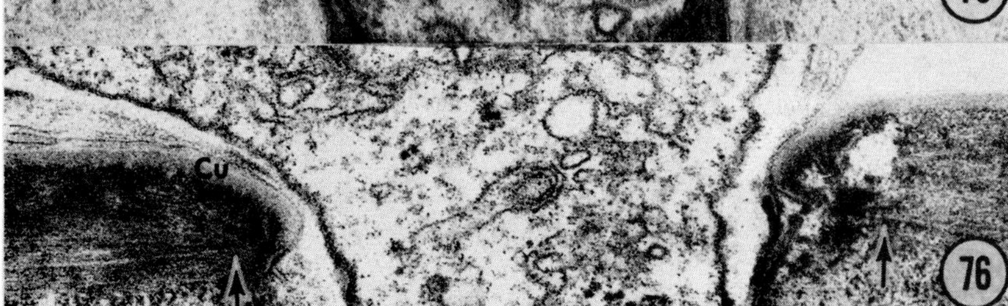
Cu
76

Fig. 77. Median longitudinal section through the apical region of a lobe of a young haustorium of *Erysiphe graminis*. Note the apical vesicles (V) in the tip of the lobe, similar to the organization of growing hyphal tips of fungi. The haustorial wall (FW) and a thin intervening layer (sheath?) separate the plasma membrane of the haustorium from the invaginated plasma membrane (PMI) of the host. Host cytoplasm (C), host vacuole (Va). ×47 000.

Fig. 78. Enlargement of part of a haustorial lobe (Lo) of *Erysiphe graminis* similar to that shown in Fig. 77. Between the haustorial wall (FW) and the invaginated host plasma membrane (PMI) are a number of fine fibrils (arrows) that span the intervening layer and seem to be attached to both the wall and the host membrane. A thin layer of host cytoplasm (C) lies between the host plasma membrane and the tonoplast (T). Host vacuole (Va). ×81 000.

Fig. 79. Plasma membrane (PM) of a barley leaf epidermal cell adjacent to the cell wall (W). Cytoplasm (C). ×200 000. (From Bracker, 1968.)

Fig. 80. A portion of the invaginated host plasma membrane of a barley leaf epidermal cell surrounding a haustorium of *Erysiphe graminis*. The membrane appears thicker than non-invaginated plasma membrane and shows non-homogeneous regions of one of the electron-dense layers (arrows) which indicate addition of material to the membrane. This membrane is far more resistant to adverse conditions and stresses than normal host plasma membrane. Host cytoplasm (C), matrix of the haustorial sheath (S). ×200 000. (From Bracker, 1968.)

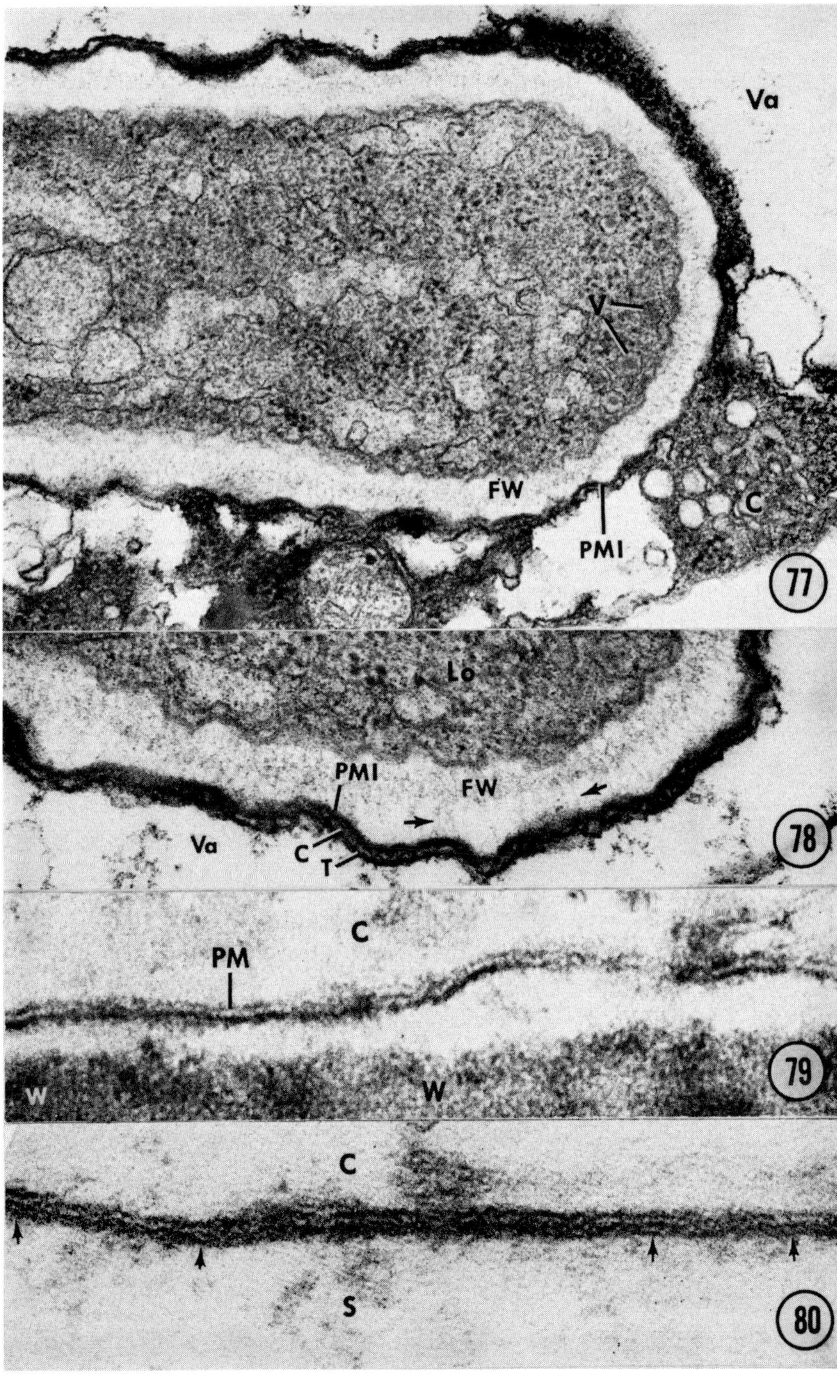
Va
V
FW
PMI
C
77
Lo
PMI
FW
Va
C
T
78
C
PM
W
W
79
C
S
80

Fig. 81. Near-median section through a penetration site of *Erysiphe graminis* on susceptible wheat leaves. Note the pattern of staining in the host wall around the penetration site. Compare with Figs 68 and 82. Haustorial neck (N), host cell wall (W), host cytoplasm (C), collar around the haustorial neck (Co), haustorial lobe (Lo). ×23 000.

Fig. 82. Similar to Fig. 81. Note the staining pattern in the host wall (W) around the penetration site. Diversity in the staining reactions of host walls among penetration sites is common in wheat leaves infected by *Erysiphe graminis*. ×19 000.

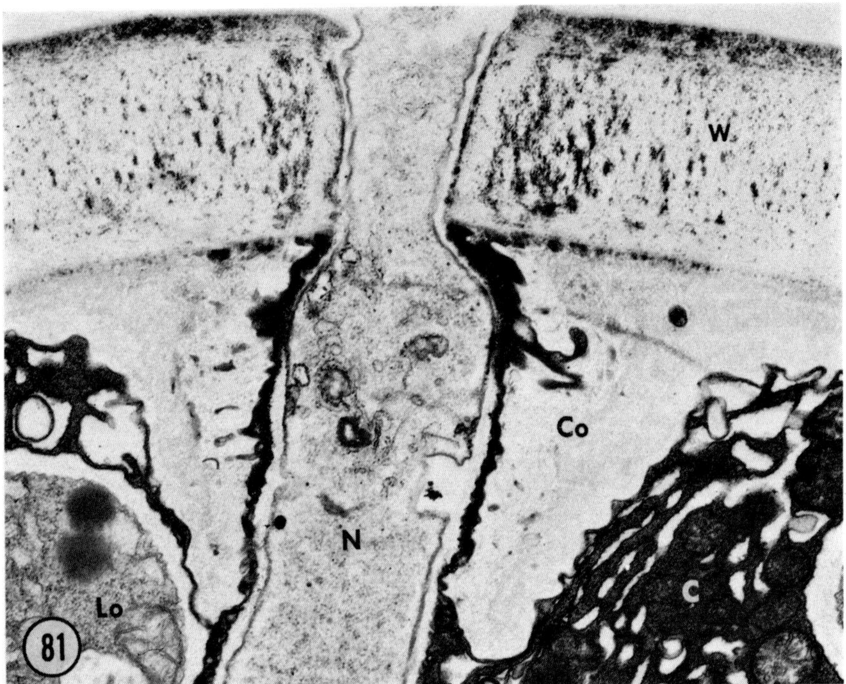
W
Co
N
Lo
C
81

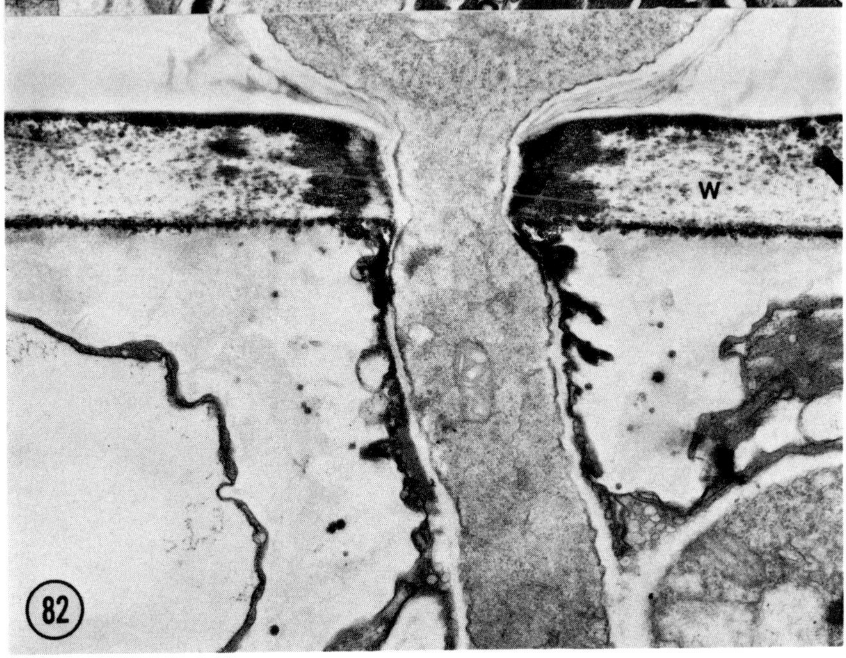
W
82

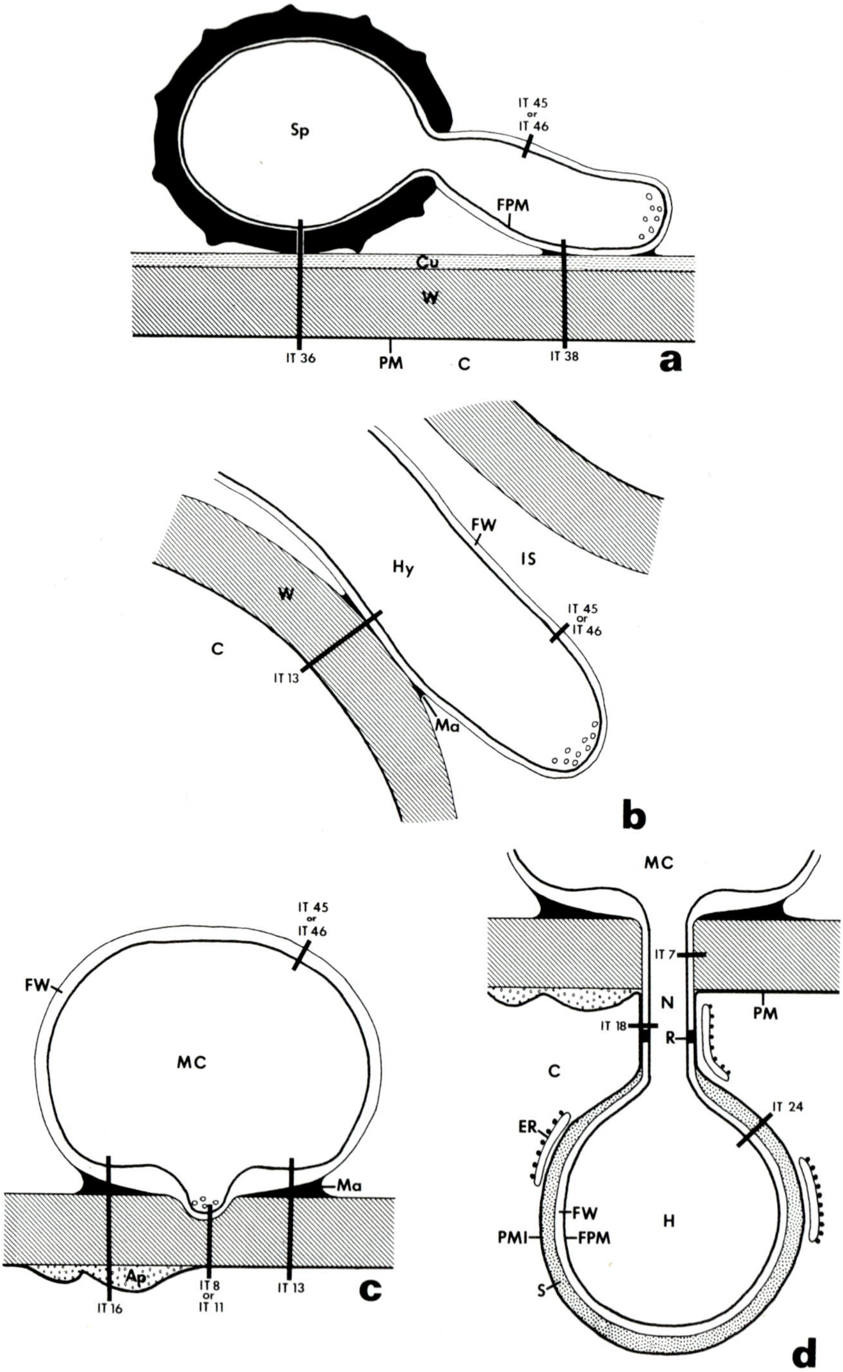
Sp
IT 45 or IT 46
FPM
Cu
W
IT 36
PM
C
IT 38
a
FW
IS
Hy
W
IT 45 or IT 46
C
IT 13
Ma
b
IT 45 or IT 46
FW
MC
Ma
Ap
IT 16
IT 8 or IT 11
IT 13
c
MC
IT 7
N
PM
IT 18
R
C
IT 24
ER
FW
H
PMI
FPM
S
d

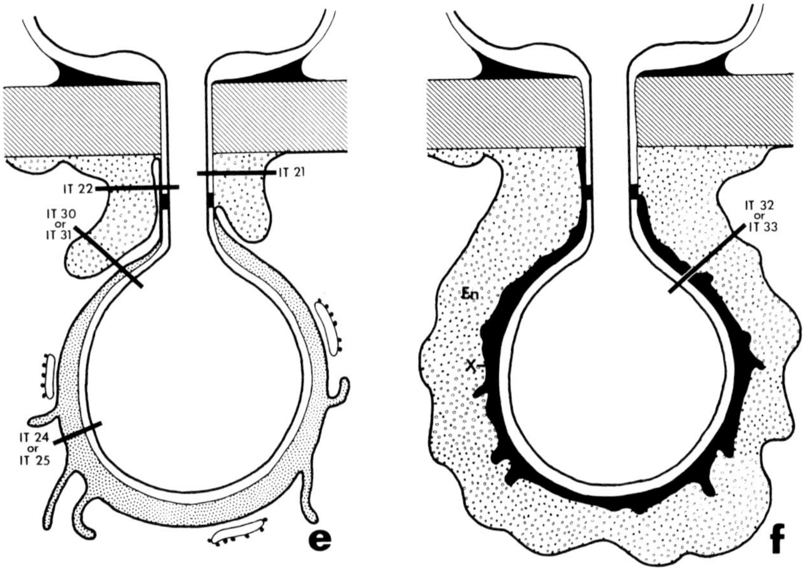

Fig. 83. Six stages in the development of a hypothetical rust infection. In each drawing, the heavy black bar crosses the interface components that are represented in the IT diagrams indicated by the IT number at the end of the bar. See pp. 232-241 for IT diagrams. Multiple interface types occur, and they change with the progression of the relationship. (a) Germinating uredospore (Sp) on an epidermal cell wall of the host. Apical vesicles are in the tip of the germ tube. (b) An intercellular hypha (Hy) in an intercellular space (IS) in a host leaf. The hypha contacts a mesophyll cell wall with an intervening matrix layer (Ma). Apical vesicles are in the hyphal tip. (c) Haustorial mother cell in contact with the host cell wall at the time of penetration. The penetration peg is part way through the host wall. A small wall apposition has formed beneath the haustorial mother cell. (d) A fully expanded, functional haustorium surrounded by a haustorial sheath and the invaginated host plasma membrane. (e) An advanced stage in which the wall apposition has grown to form a collar around the haustorial neck and part of the haustorial body. Membrane-limited tentacles are continuous with the haustorial sheath (M. D. Coffey, pers. comm.). (f) An encased necrotic haustorium that is completely enclosed by the wall apposition. A mixture (X) consisting of degenerate host protoplasm and the degraded haustorial sheath is trapped between the encasement and the haustorial wall. Wall apposition (Ap); lumen of host cell (C); host cuticle (Cu); encasement (En); endoplasmic reticulum (ER); fungal plasma membrane (FPM); fungal wall (FW); haustorium (H); matrix layer (Ma); host plasma membrane (PM); invaginated host plasma membrane (extrahaustorial membrane) (PMI); neck ring (R); haustorial sheath (S); host wall (W).

REFERENCES

Ahmadjian, V. (1967). 'The Lichen Symbiosis'. Blaisdell Publishing Co., Waltham, Mass., Toronto and London.

Ainsworth, G. C. (1971). 'Ainsworth and Bisby's Dictionary of the Fungi', 6th edn. Commonwealth Mycological Institute, Kew, England.

Aist, J. R. and Williams, P. H. (1971). The cytology and kinetics of cabbage root hair penetration by *Plasmodiophora brassicae*. *Can. J. Bot.* **49**, 2023-2034.

Akai, S. (1959). Histology of defense in plants. *In* 'Plant Pathology, An Advanced Treatise' (eds J. G. Horsfall and A. E. Dimond), Vol. I, 392-434. Academic Press, London and New York.

Akai, S., Horino, O., Fukutomi, M., Nakata, A., Kunoh, H. and Shiraishi, M. (1971). Cell wall reaction to infection and resulting change in cell organelles. *In* 'Morphological and Biochemical Events in Plant–Parasite Interaction' (eds S. Akai and S. Ouchi), 329-347. Mochizuki Publishing Co., Japan.

Akai, S., Kunoh, H. and Fukutomi, M. (1968). Histochemical changes of the epidermal cell wall of barley leaves infected by *Erysiphe graminis hordei*. *Mycopath. Mycol. appl.* **35**, 175-180.

Albersheim, P., Jones, T. M. and English, P. D. (1969). Biochemistry of the cell wall in relation to infective processes. *A. Rev. Phytopath.* **7**, 171-194.

Allen, R. F. (1923a). A cytological study of infection of Baart and Kanred wheats by *Puccinia graminis tritici*. *J. agric. Res.* **23**, 131-152.

Allen, R. F. (1923b). Cytological studies of infection of Baart, Kanred, and Mindum wheats by *Puccinia graminis tritici* forms III and XIX. *J. agric. Res.* **26**, 571-604.

Allen, R. F. (1927). A cytological study of orange leaf rust, *Puccinia triticina* physiologic form 11, on Malakoff wheat. *J. agric. Res.* **34**, 697-714.

Allen, R. F. (1928). A cytological study of *Puccinia glumarum* on *Bromus marginatus* and *Triticum vulgare*. *J. agric. Res.* **36**, 487-513.

Armentrout, V. N. and Wilson, C. L. (1969). Haustorium–host interaction during mycoparasitism of *Mycotypha microspora* by *Piptocephalis virginiana*. *Phytopathology* **59**, 897-905.

Beale, G. H., Jurand, A. and Preer, J. R. (1969). The classes of endosymbiont of *Paramecium aurelia*. *J. Cell Sci.* **5**, 65-91.

Beams, H. W. and Kessel, R. G. (1968). The Golgi apparatus: structure and function. *Int. Rev. Cytol.* **23**, 209-276.

Bennett, C. W. (1944). Studies of dodder transmission of plant viruses. *Phytopathology* **34**, 905-932.

Bennett, H. S. (1956). The concepts of membrane flow and membrane vesiculation as mechanisms for active transport and ion pumping. *J. biophys. biochem. Cytol.* **2** (Suppl.), 99-103.

Ben-Shaul, Y., Paran, N. and Galun, M. (1969). The ultrastructure of the association between phycobiont and mycobiont in three ecotypes of the lichen *Caloplaca aurantia* var. *aurantia*. *J. Microscopie* **8**, 415-422.

Bergersen, F. J. (1968). The symbiotic state in legume root nodules: studies with the soybean system. *Proc. 9th int. Congr. Soil Sci.* **2**, 49-63.

Berhsohm, J. and Grossman, H. J. (1971). 'Lipid Storage Diseases: Enzymatic Defects and Clinical Implications'. Academic Press, London and New York.

Berlin, J. D. and Bowen, C. C. (1964). The host–parasite interface of *Albugo candida* on *Raphanus sativus*. *Am. J. Bot.* **51**, 445-452.

Bird, A. F. (1961). The ultrastructure and histochemistry of a nematode-induced giant cell. *J. biophys. biochem. Cytol.* **11**, 701-715.

Blackwell, E. M. (1953). Haustoria of *Phytophthora infestans* and some other species. *Trans. Br. mycol. Soc.* **36**, 138-158.

Border, D. J. (1971). Ultrastructure and intracellular distribution of virus particles in *Penicillium* species. *Proc. 1st int. Mycol. Congr., Exeter* 8 (Abstr.).

Bowyer, J. W. and Atherton, J. G. (1971). *Mycoplasma*-like bodies in French bean, dodder, and the leafhopper vector of the legume little leaf agent. *Aust. J. biol. Sci.* **24**, 717-729.

Bracker, C. E. (1967). Ultrastructure of fungi. *A. Rev. Phytopath.* **5**, 343-374.

Bracker, C. E. (1968). Ultrastructure of the haustorial apparatus of *Erysiphe graminis* and its relationship to the epidermal cell of barley. *Phytopathology* **58**, 12-30.

Bracker, C. E. and Grove, S. N. (1971). Continuity between cytoplasmic endomembranes and outer mitochondrial membranes in fungi. *Protoplasma* **73**, 15-34.

Brown, R. M., Jr. and Wilson, R. (1968). Electron microscopy of the lichen *Physcia aipolia* (Ehrh.) Nyl. *J. Phycol.* **4**, 230-240.

Buchner, P. (1965). 'Endosymbiosis of Animals with Plant Microorganisms'. Interscience Publishers, New York, London and Sydney.

Burnett, J. H. (1968). 'Fundamentals of Mycology'. St. Martin's Press, New York.

Bushnell, W. R. (1971). The haustorium of *Erysiphe graminis*: An experimental study of light microscopy. *In* 'Morphological and Biochemical Events in Plant–Parasite Interaction' (eds S. Akai and S. Ouchi), 229-254. Mochizuki Publishing Co., Japan.

Bushnell, W. R. (1972). Physiology of fungal haustoria. *A. Rev. Phytopath.* **10**, 151-176.

Calonge, F. D. (1969). Ultrastructure of the haustoria or intracellular hyphae in four different fungi. *Arch. Mikrobiol.* **67**, 209-225.

Calonge, F. D., Fielding, A. H., Byrde, R. J. W. and Akinrefon, O. A. (1969). Changes in ultrastructure following fungal invasion and the possible relevance of extracellular enzymes. *J. exp. Bot.* **20**, 350-357.

Carbonell, L. M. (1970). Ultrastructure of human pathogenic fungi and their mycoses. *In* 'Handbuch der Speziellen Pathologischen Anatomie und Histologie' (ed. E. Uehlinger), Vol. III, 38-66. Springer-Verlag, Berlin, Heidelberg and New York.

Carothers, Z. B. (1972). Studies of spermatogenesis in the Hepaticae. III. Continuity between plasma membrane and nuclear envelope in androgonial cells of *Blasia*. *J. Cell Biol.* **52**, 273-282.

Chervin, R. E., Baker, G. E. and Hohl, H. R. (1968). The ultrastructure of phycobiont and mycobiont in two species of *Usnea*. *Can. J. Bot.* **46**, 241-245.

Chilvers, G. A. (1968). Low-power electron microscopy of the root cap region of Eucalypt mycorrhizas. *New Phytol.* **67**, 663-665.

Chou, C. K. (1970). An electron-microscope study of host penetration and early stages of haustorium formation of *Peronospora parasitica* (Fr.) Tul. on cabbage cotyledons. *Ann. Bot.* **34**, 189-204.

Chou, C. K. and Levi, M. P. (1971). An electron microscopical study of the penetration and decomposition of tracheid walls of *Pinus sylvestris* by *Poria vaillantii. Holzforschung* **25**, 107-112

Coffey, M. D., Palevitz, B. A. and Allen, P. J. (1972). The fine structure of two rust fungi, *Puccinia helianthi* and *Melampsora lini. Can. J. Bot.* **50**, 231-240.

Colley, R. H. (1918). Parasitism, morphology, and cytology of *Cronartium ribicola. J. agric. Res.* **15**, 619-660.

Corner, E. J. H. (1935). Observations on resistance to powdery mildews. *New Phytol.* **34**, 180-200.

Cowling, E. B. (1965). Microorganisms and microbial enzyme systems as selective tools in wood anatomy. *In* 'Cellular Ultrastructure of Woody Plants' (ed. W. A. Cote), 341-368. Syracuse University Press, New York.

Dart, P. J. and Mercer, F. V. (1964). Fine structure changes in the development of the nodules of *Trifolium subterraneum* L. and *Medicago tribuloides* Desr. *Arch. Mikrobiol.* **49**, 209-235.

Dart, P. J. and Mercer, F. V. (1966). Fine structure of bacteroids in root nodules of *Vigna sinensis, Acacia longifolia, Viminaria juncea,* and *Lupinus angustifolius. J. Bact.* **91**, 1314-1319.

Davison, E. M. (1968). Cytochemistry and ultrastructure of hyphae and haustoria of *Peronospora parasitica* (Pers. ex Fr.) Fr. *Ann. Bot.* **32**, 613-621.

Dekhuijzen, H. M. and van der Scheer, C. (1967). Electron microscopic observations on haustoria isolated from cucumber leaves infected with powdery mildew. *Neth. J. Pl. Path.* **73**, 121-125.

Dekhuijzen, H. M. and van der Scheer, C. (1969). The ultrastructure of powdery mildew, *Sphaerotheca fuliginea*, isolated from cucumber leaves. *Neth. J. Pl. Path.* **75**, 169-177.

Dilworth, M. J. (1969). The plant as the genetic determinant of leghaemoglobin production in the legume root nodule. *Biochim. biophys. Acta* **184**, 432-441.

Dilworth, M. J. and Kidby, D. K. (1968). Localization of iron and leghaemoglobin in the legume root nodule by electron microscope autoradiography. *Expl Cell Res.* **49**, 148-159.

Dixon, R. O. (1964). The structure of infection threads, bacteria and bacteroids in pea and clover root nodules. *Arch. Mikrobiol.* **48**, 166-178.

Dixon, R. O. (1967). The origin of the membrane envelope surrounding the bacteria and bacteroids and the presence of glycogen in clover root nodules. *Arch. Mikrobiol.* **56**, 156-166.

Dixon, R. O. (1969). Rhizobia (with particular reference to relationships with host plants). *A. Rev. Microbiol.* **23**, 137-158.

Dorr, I. (1969). Feinstruktur intrazellular wachsender *Cuscuta*-Hyphen. *Protoplasma* **67**, 123-137.

Dorr, I. and Kollmann, R. (1969). Fine structure of mycorrhiza in *Neottia nidus-avis* (L). L. C. Rich (Orchidaceae). *Planta* **89**, 372-375.

Drum, R. W. and Pankratz, S. (1965). Fine structure of an unusual cytoplasmic inclusion in the diatom genus, *Rhopalodia. Protoplasma* **60**, 141-149.

Dueck, J., Zeyen, R. J. and Kennedy, B. W. (1972). Ultrastructural observations of soybean leaves affected by bacterial toxemia. *Can. J. Bot.* **50**, 529-531.

Durbin, R. D. (1971). Chlorosis-inducing pseudomonad toxins: their mechanism of action and structure. *In* 'Morphological and Biochemical Events in

Plant–Parasite Interaction' (eds S. Akai and S. Ouchi), 369-385. Mochizuki Publishing Co., Japan.

Durrell, L. W. (1967). An electron microscope study of algal hyphal contact in lichens. *Mycopath. Mycol. appl.* **31**, 273-286.

Echlin, P. (1967). The biology of *Glaucocystis nostochinearum*. I. The Morphology and fine structure. *Br. phycol. Bull.* **3**, 225-239.

Edwards, H. H. (1970). A basic staining material associated with the penetration process in resistant and susceptible powdery mildewed barley. *New Phytol.* **69**, 299-301.

Edwards, H. H. and Allen, P. J. (1970). A fine-structure study of the primary infection process during infection of barley by *Erysiphe graminis* f. sp. *hordei*. *Phytopathology* **60**, 1504-1509.

Ehrlich, H. G. and Ehrlich, M. A. (1963a). Electron microscopy of the host–parasite relationships in stem rust of wheat. *Am. J. Bot.* **50**, 123-130.

Ehrlich, H. G. and Ehrlich, M. A. (1963b). Electron microscopy of the sheath surrounding the haustorium of *Erysiphe graminis*. *Phytopathology* **53**, 1378-1380.

Ehrlich, M. A. and Ehrlich, H. G. (1966). Ultrastructure of the hyphae and haustoria of *Phytophthora infestans* and hyphae of *P. parasitica*. *Can. J. Bot.* **44**, 1495-1503.

Ehrlich, M. A. and Ehrlich, H. G. (1971a). Fine structure of the host–parasite interfaces in mycoparasitism. *A. Rev. Phytopath.* **9**, 155-184.

Ehrlich, M. A. and Ehrlich, H. G. (1971b). Fine structure of *Puccinia graminis* and the transfer of C^{14} from uredospores to *Triticum vulgare*. *In* 'Morphological and Biochemical Events in Plant–Parasite Interaction' (eds S. Akai and S. Ouchi), 279-307. Mochizuki Publishing Co., Japan.

Ehrlich, M. A., Schafer, J. F. and Ehrlich, H. G. (1968). Lomasomes in wheat leaves infected by *Puccinia graminis* and *P. recondita*. *Can. J. Bot.* **46**, 17-20.

Esau, K. (1968). 'Viruses in Plant Hosts. Form, Distribution, and Pathologic Effects'. The University of Wisconsin Press, Madison, Milwaukee and London.

Esau, K. and Cronshaw, J. (1967). Relation of tobacco mosaic virus to the host cells. *J. Cell Biol.* **33**, 665-678.

Esau, K. and Gill, R. H. (1969). Tobacco mosaic virus in dividing mesophyll cells of *Nicotiana*. *Virology* **38**, 464-472.

Esau, K. and Hoefert, L. L. (1971). Cytology of beet yellows virus infection in *Tetragonia*. I. Parenchyma cells in infected leaf. *Protoplasma* **72**, 255-273.

Foster, R. C. and Marks, G. C. (1966). The fine structure of the mycorrhizas of *Pinus radiata* D. Don. *Aust. J. biol. Sci.* **19**, 1027-1038.

Franke, W. W., Morré, D. J., Deumling, B., Cheetham, R. D., Kartenbeck, J., Jarasch, E.-D. and Zentgraf, H.-W. (1971). Synthesis and turnover of membrane proteins in rat liver: an examination of the membrane flow hypothesis. *Z. Naturf. (Sec. B)* **26**, 1031-1039.

Fraymouth, J. (1956). Haustoria of the Peronosporales. *Trans. Br. mycol. Soc.* **39**, 79-107.

Fullerton, R. A. (1970). An electron microscope study of the intracellular hyphae of some smut fungi (Ustilaginales). *Aust. J. Bot.* **18**, 285-292.

Furtado, J. S. and Olive, L. S. (1970). Ultrastructure studies of protostelids: the amoebo-flagellate stage. *Cytobiologie* **2**, 200-219.

Galun, M., Ben-Shaul, Y. and Paran, N. (1971a). The fungus–alga association in the Lecideaceae: an ultrastructural study. *New Phytol.* **70**, 483-485.

Galun, M., Paran, N. and Ben-Shaul, Y. (1970a). The fungus–alga association in the Lecanoraceae: an ultrastructural study. *New Phytol.* **69**, 599-603.

Galun, M., Paran, N. and Ben-Shaul, Y. (1970b). Structural modifications of the phycobiont in the lichen thallus. *Protoplasma* **69**, 85-96.

Galun, M., Paran, N. and Ben-Shaul, Y. (1970c). An ultrastructural study of the fungus–alga association in *Lecanora radiosa* growing under different environmental conditions. *J. Microscopie* **9**, 801-806.

Galun, M., Paran, N. and Ben-Shaul, Y. (1971b). Electron microscopic study of the lichen *Dematocarpon hepaticum* (Ach.) Th. Fr. *Protoplasma* **73**, 457-468.

Gaumann, E. A. and Dodge, C. W. (1928). 'Comparative Morphology of Fungi'. McGraw-Hill Book Co., New York.

Ghemawat, M. S. (1968). Seedling and mature plant resistance of wheat to powdery mildew. Ph.D. thesis, Purdue University, Lafayette, Indiana.

Gipson, I., Kim, K. S. and Riggs, R. D. (1971). An ultrastructural study of syncytium development in soybean roots infected with *Heterodera glycines*. *Phytopathology* **61**, 347-353.

Goodchild, D. J. and Bergersen, F. J. (1966). Electron microscopy of the infection and subsequent development of soybean nodule cells. *J. Bact.* **92**, 204-213.

Goodman, R. N. and Burkowicz, A. (1970). Ultrastructural changes in apple leaves inoculated with virulent or an avirulent strain of *Erwinia amylovora*. *Phytopath. Z.* **68**, 258-268.

Goodman, R. N., Kiraly, Z. and Zaitlin, M. (1967). 'The Biochemistry and Physiology of Infectious Plant Disease'. Van Nostrand Co., Princeton, New Jersey.

Goodman, R. N. and Plurad, S. B. (1971). Ultrastructural changes in tobacco undergoing the hypersensitive reaction caused by plant pathogenic bacteria. *Physiol. Pl. Path.* **1**, 11-15.

Granett, A. L. and Gilmer, R. M. (1971). Mycoplasmas associated with X-disease in various *Prunus* species. *Phytopathology* **61**, 1036-1037.

Gray, W. D. and Alexopoulos, C. J. (1968). 'Biology of the Myxomycetes'. The Ronald Press Co., New York.

Griffiths, D. A. (1971). The development of lignitubers in roots after infection by *Verticillium dahliae* Kleb. *Can. J. Microbiol.* **17**, 441-444.

Grove, S. N. and Bracker, C. E. (1970). Protoplasmic organization of hyphal tips among fungi: vesicles and Spitzenkörper. *J. Bact.* **104**, 989-1009.

Grove, S. N., Bracker, C. E. and Morré, D. J. (1968). Cytomembrane differentiation in the endoplasmic reticulum–Golgi apparatus–vesicle complex. *Science, N.Y.* **161**, 171-173.

Hadley, G., Johnson, R. P. C. and John, D. A. (1971). Fine structure of the host–fungus interface in orchid mycorrhiza. *Planta* **100**, 191-199.

Hall, W. T. and Claus, G. (1963). Ultrastructural studies on the blue-green algal symbiont in *Cyanophora paradoxa* Korschikoff. *J. Cell Biol.* **19**, 551-563.

Hall, W. T. and Claus, G. (1967). Ultrastructural studies on the cyanelles of *Glaucocystis nostochinearum* Itzigsohn. *J. Phycol.* **3**, 37-51.

Hanchey, P. and Wheeler, H. (1969). Pathological changes in ultrastructure: false plasmolysis. *Can. J. Bot.* **47**, 675-678.

Hanchey, P. and Wheeler, H. (1971). Pathological changes in ultrastructure: Tobacco roots infected with *Phytophthora parasitica* var. *nicotianae*. *Phytopathology* **61**, 33-39.

Hanchey, P., Wheeler, H. and Luke, H. H. (1968). Pathological changes in ultrastructure: effects of victorin on oat roots. *Am. J. Bot.* **55**, 53-61.

Hardwick, N. V., Greenwood, A. D. and Wood, R. K. S. (1971). The fine structure of the haustorium of *Uromyces appendiculatus* in *Phaseolus vulgaris*. *Can. J. Bot.* **49**, 383-390.

Harley, J. L. (1968). Mycorrhiza. *In* 'The Fungi. An Advanced Treatise' (eds G. C. Ainsworth and A. S. Sussman), Vol. III, 139-171. Academic Press, London and New York.

Harrison, B. D. and Roberts, I. M. (1968). Association of tobacco rattle virus with mitochondria. *Jnl. gen. Virol.* **3**, 121-124.

Hashioka, Y. and Fukita, T. (1969). Ultrastructural observations on mycoparasitism of *Trichoderma, Gliocladium* and *Acremonium* to phytopathogenic fungi. *Rep. Tottori mycol. Inst. (Japan)* **7**, 8-18.

Hashioka, Y., Ikegami, H., Horino, O. and Kamie, T. (1967). Fine structure of the rice blast. I. Electronmicrographs of *Pyricularia oryzae* and the epidermal cell wall of rice plants. *Res. Bull. Fac. Agric. Gifu Univ. (Japan)* **24**, 66-77.

Heath, M. C. (1971). Haustorial sheath formation in cowpea leaves immune to rust infection. *Phytopathology* **61**, 383-388.

Heath, M. C. (1972). Ultrastructure of host and nonhost reactions to cowpea rust. *Phytopathology* **62**, 27-38.

Heath, I. B. and Greenwood, A. D. (1970). The structure and formation of lomasomes. *J. gen. Microbiol.* **62**, 129-137.

Heath, M. C. and Heath, I. B. (1971). Ultrastructure of an immune and a susceptible reaction of cowpea leaves to rust infection. *Physiol. Pl. Path.* **1**, 277-287.

Heath, M. C. and Wood, R. K. S. (1969). Leaf spots induced by *Ascochyta pisi* and *Mycosphaerella pinodes*. *Ann. Bot.* **33**, 657-670.

Heintz, C. E. and Pramer, D. (1972). Ultrastructure of nematode-trapping fungi. *J. Bact.* **110**, 1163-1170.

Held, A. A. (1972). Host-parasite relations between *Allomyces* and *Rozella*. Parasite penetration depends on growth response of host cell-wall. *Arch. Mikrobiol.* **82**, 128-139.

Henry, S. M. (1966). Foreword, *in* 'Symbiosis, Vol. I. Associations of Microorganisms, Plants, and Marine Organisms' (ed. S. M. Henry), ix-xi. Academic Press, London and New York.

Hertig, M., Taliaferro, W. H. and Schwartz, B. (1937). Supplement to the report of the twelfth annual meeting of the American Society of Parasitologists. *J. Parasitol.* **23**, 325-329.

Heslop-Harrison, J. (1966). Cytoplasmic continuities during spore formation in flowering plants. *Endeavour* **25**, 65-72.

Hess, W. M. (1969). Ultrastructure of onion roots infected with *Pyrenochaeta terrestris*, a fungus parasite. *Am. J. Bot.* **56**, 832-845.

Hess, W. M. and Strobel, G. A. (1970). Ultrastructure of potato stems infected with *Corynebacterium sepedonicum*. *Phytopathology* **60**, 1428-1431.

Hibino, H., Kaloostian, G. H. and Schneider, H. (1971). Mycoplasma-like bodies in the pear psylla vector of pear decline. *Virology* **43**, 34-40.

Hirata, K. (1967). Notes on haustoria, hyphae, and conidia of the powdery mildew fungus of barley, *Erysiphe graminis* f. sp. *hordei. Mem. Fac. Agric. Niigata Univ.* **6**, 207-259.

Hirata, K. (1971). Calcium in relation to the susceptibility of primary barley leaves to powdery mildew. *In* 'Morphological and Biochemical Events in Plant–Parasite Interaction' (eds S. Akai and S. Ouchi), 207-228. Mochizuki Publishing Co., Japan.

Hirata, K. and Kojima, M. (1962). On the structure and the sack of the haustorium of some powdery mildews, with some considerations on the significance of the sack. *Trans. mycol. Soc. Japan* **3**, 43-46.

Hirumi, H., Grandados, R. R. and Maramorosch, K. (1967). Electron microscopy of a plant–pathogenic virus in the nervous system of its insect vector. *Jnl. Virol.* **1**, 430-444.

Hodges, T. K., Leonard, R. T., Bracker, C. E. and Keenan, T. W. (1972). Purification of an ion-stimulated ATPase from plant roots: association with plasma membranes. *Proc. natn. Acad. Sci. U.S.A.* **69**, 3307-3311.

Hofsten, A. von (1969). The ultrastructure of mycorrhiza. I. Ectotrophic and ectendotrophic mycorrhiza of *Pinus silvestris. Svensk bot. Tidskr.* **63**, 455-464.

Hohl, H. R. (1965). Nature and development of membrane systems in food vacuoles of cellular slime molds predatory upon bacteria. *J. Bact.* **90**, 755-765.

Hoitink, H. A. J. and Bradfute, O. E. (1971). Bacterial cell wall triggers plant disease. *Ohio Rep. Res. Dev.* **56**, 78-79.

Holland, A. A. and Fulcher, R. G. (1971). A study of wheat roots infected with *Ophiobolus graminis* (Sacc.) using fluorescence and electron microscopy. *Aust. J. biol. Sci.* **24**, 819-823.

Hollings, M. and Stone, O. M. (1971). Viruses that infect fungi. *A. Rev. Phytopath.* **9**, 93-118.

Honda, Y. and Matsui, C. (1972). Electron microscopy of intracellular radish mosaic virus. *Phytopathology* **62**, 448-452.

Horino, O. and Akai, S. (1968a). Studies on the pathological anatomy of rice plants infected by *Helminthosporium oryzae.* I. Behavior of the causal fungus on the coleoptile of rice seedlings and its ultrafine structure. *Ann. phytopath. Soc. Japan* **34**, 51-55.

Horino, O. and Akai, S. (1968b). Studies on the pathological anatomy of rice plants infected by *Helminthosporium oryzae* Breda de Haan. II. Fine structure of hyphae in tissues of coleoptile of rice plants. *Ann. phytopath. Soc. Japan* **34**, 231-234.

Hosford, R. M., Jr. (1967). Transmission of plant viruses by dodder. *Bot. Rev.* **33**, 387-406.

Huang, C. S. and Maggenti, A. R. (1969). Wall modifications in developing giant cells of *Vicia faba* and *Cucumis sativus* induced by root knot nematode, *Meloidogyne javanica. Phytopathology* **59**, 931-937.

Igwegbe, E. C. K. and Calavan, E. C. (1970). Occurrence of mycoplasmalike bodies in phloem of stubborn-infected citrus seedlings. *Phytopathology* **60**, 1525-1526.

Jacobs, J. B. and Ahmadjian, V. (1969). The ultrastructure of lichens. I. A general survey. *J. Phycol.* **5**, 227-240.

Jacobs, J. B. and Ahmadjian, V. (1971). The ultrastructure of lichens. II. *Cladonia cristatella:* the lichen and its isolated symbionts. *J. Phycol.* **7**, 71-82.

Jenkins, R. A. (1970). The fine structure of a nuclear envelope associated endosymbiont of Paramecium. *J. gen. Microbiol.* **61**, 355-359.

Jordan, D. C. and Grinyer, I. (1965). Electron microscopy of the bacteroids and root nodules of *Lupinus luteus. Can. J. Microbiol.* **11**, 721-725.

Jordan, D. C., Grinyer, I. and Coulter, W. H. (1963). Electron microscopy of infection threads and bacteria in young root nodules of *Medicago sativa. J. Bact.* **86**, 125-137.

Joubert, J. J. and Rijkenberg, F. H. J. (1971). Parasitic green algae. *A. Rev. Phytopath.* **9**, 45-64.

Kajiwara, T. (1969). Ultrastructure of the host–parasite relationships in cucumber downy mildew, caused by *Pseudoperonospora cubensis* (Berk. et Curt.) Rostow. *Bull. natn. Inst. agric. Sci., Tokyo (Ser. C)* **44**, 63-91.

Kajiwara, T. (1971). Structure and physiology of haustoria of various parasites. *In* 'Morphological and Biochemical Events in Plant–Parasite Interaction' (eds S. Akai and S. Ouchi), 255-277. Mochizuki Publishing Co., Japan.

Kaloostian, G. H., Hibino, H. and Schneider, H. (1971). Mycoplasmalike bodies in periwinkle: their cytology and transmission by pear psylla from pear trees affected with pear decline. *Phytopathology* **61**, 1177-1179.

Karakashian, S. J., Karakashian, M. W. and Rudzinska, M. A. (1968). Electron microscopic observations on the symbiosis of *Paramecium bursaria* and its intracellular algae. *J. Protozool.* **15**, 113-128.

Karling, J. S. (1932). Studies in the Chytridiales. VII. The organization of the Chytrid thallus. *Am. J. Bot.* **19**, 41-74.

Kazama, F. and Fuller, M. S. (1970). Ultrastructure of *Porphyra perforata* infected with *Pythium marinum,* a marine fungus. *Can. J. Bot.* **48**, 2103-2107.

Keck, R. W. and Hodges, T. K. (1973). Membrane permeability in plants: changes induced by host specific toxins. *Phytopathology* **63**. In press.

Keskin, B. and Fuchs, W. H. (1969). Der Infektionsvorgang bei *Polymyxa betae. Arch. Mikrobiol.* **68**, 218-226.

Kevin, M. J., Hall, W. T., McLaughlin, J. J. A. and Zahl, P. A. (1969). *Symbiodinium microadriaticum* Freudenthal, a revised taxonomic description, ultrastructure. *J. Phycol.* **5**, 341-350.

Kevin, Sr. P., Zahl, P. A. and McLaughlin, J. J. A. (1966). *In situ* studies of the alga *Symbiodinium microadriaticum* in the sea anemone, *Condylactis* and in the jellyfish, *Casseopeia. J. Protozool.* **13** (Suppl.), Abstr. No. 82.

Kidby, D. K. and Goodchild, D. J. (1966). Host influence on the ultrastructure of root nodules of *Lupinus luteus* and *Ornithopus sativus. J. gen. Microbiol.* **45**, 147-152.

Kim, K. S. and Fulton, J. P. (1971). Tubules with viruslike particles in leaf cells infected with bean pod mottle virus. *Virology* **43**, 329-337.

Kitajima, E. W. and Lauritis, J. A. (1969). Plant virions in plasmodesmata. *Virology* **37**, 681-685.

Kolk, L. A. (1930). Relation of host and pathogen in the oat smut, *Ustilago avenae. Bull. Torrey bot. Club* **57**, 443-507.

Kunoh, H. and Akai, S. (1969a). Histochemical observation of the halo on the epidermal cell wall of barley leaves attacked by *Erysiphe graminis hordei. Mycopath. Mycol. appl.* **37**, 113-118.

Kunoh, H. and Akai, S. (1969b). The electron microscopic observation of haustoria of *Erysiphe graminis hordei. Mycopath. Mycol. appl.* **38**, 337-344.

Leath, K. T. and Rowell, J. B. (1969). Thickening of corn mesophyll cell walls in response to invasion by *Puccinia graminis*. *Phytopathology* **59**, 1654-1656.

Leedale, G. F. (1969). Observations on endonuclear bacteria in euglenoid flagellates. *Öst. bot. Z.* **116**, 279-294.

Lembi, C. A., Morré, D. J., Thomson, K. St. and Hertel, R. (1971). N-l-Naphthylphthalamic-acid-binding activity of a plasma membrane-rich fraction from maize coleoptiles. *Planta* **99**, 37-45.

Leong, P. C., McKeen, W. E. and Smith, R. (1970). Attempted infection of *Erysiphe polygoni* DC. hyphae by its own mycelium. *Can. J. Microbiol.* **16**, 136-137.

Lesemann, D. E. and Fuchs, W. H. (1970a). Elektronenmikroskopische Untersuchung über die Vorbereitung der Infektion in encystierten Zoosporen von *Olpidium brassicae*. *Arch. Mikrobiol.* **71**, 9-19.

Lesemann, D. E. and Fuchs, W. H. (1970b). Die Ultrastruktur des Penetrations -vorganges von *Olpidium brassicae* an Kohlrabi-Wurzeln. *Arch. Mikrobiol.* **71**, 20-30.

Liese, W. (1970). Ultrastructural aspects of woody tissue disintegration. *A. Rev. Phytopath.* **8**, 231-258.

Liese, W. and Schmid, R. (1963). Fibrilläre Strukturen an den Hyphen holzzerstörender Pilze. *Naturwissenschaften* **50**, 102-103.

Liese, W. and Schmid, R. (1964). Über das Wachstum von Blauepilzen durch verholzte Zellwände. *Phytopath. Z.* **51**, 385-393.

Littlefield, L. J. (1972). Development of haustoria of *Melampsora lini*. *Can. J. Bot.* **50**, 1701-1703.

Littlefield, L. J. and Aronson, S. J. (1969). Histological studies of *Melampsora lini* resistance in flax. *Can. J. Bot.* **47**, 1713-1717.

Littlefield, L. J. and Bracker, C. E. (1970). Continuity of host plasma membrane around haustoria of *Melampsora lini*. *Mycologia* **62**, 609-614.

Littlefield, L. J. and Bracker, C. E. (1972). Ultrastructural specialization at the host–pathogen interface in rust-infected flax. *Protoplasma* **74**, 271-305.

Luke, H. H., Warmke, H. E. and Hanchey, P. (1966). Effects of the pathotoxin victorin on ultrastructure of root and leaf tissue of *Avena* species. *Phytopathology* **56**, 1178-1183.

Lupton, F. G. H. (1956). Resistance mechanisms of species of *Triticum* and *Aegilops* and of amphidiploids between them to *Erysiphe graminis* DC. *Trans. Br. mycol. Soc.* **39**, 51-59.

Luria, S. E. and Darnell, J. E., Jr. (1967). 'General Virology', 2nd edn. John Wiley and Sons, New York.

Lutman, B. F. (1910). Some contributions to the life history and cytology of the smuts. *Proc. Wis. Acad. Sci. Arts and Letters* **16**, 1191-1244.

MacDonald, W. L. and McNabb, H. S., Jr. (1970). Fine-structural observations of the growth of *Ceratocystis ulmi* in elm zylem tissue. *Bioscience* **20**, 1060-1061.

MacLeod, R., Black, L. M. and Moyer, F. H. (1966). The fine structure and intracellular localization of potato yellow dwarf virus. *Virology* **29**, 540-552.

Maeda, K. M. (1970). An ultrastructural study of *Venturia inaequalis* (Cke.) Wint. infection of *Malus* hosts. M.S. thesis, Purdue University, Lafayette, Indiana.

Manocha, M. S. and Lee, K. Y. (1971). Host–parasite relations in mycoparasite. I. Fine structure of host, parasite, and their interface. *Can. J. Bot.* **49**, 1677-1681.

Manocha, M. S. and Shaw, M. (1967). Electron microscopy of uredospores of *Melampsora lini* and of rust-infected flax. *Can. J. Bot.* **45**, 1575-1582.

Margulis, L. (1970). 'Origin of Eukaryotic Cells'. Yale University Press, New Haven.

Mason, D. L. (1970). Studies on two phytopathogenic Pyrenomycetes, with observations on host-parasite relations. Ph.D. thesis, University of Wisconsin, Madison.

Matthews, R. E. F. (1970). 'Plant Virology'. Academic Press, London and New York.

McKeen, W. E., Smith, R. and Bhattacharya, P. K. (1969). Alterations of the host wall surrounding the infection peg of powdery mildew fungi. *Can. J. Bot.* **47**, 701-706.

McKeen, W. E., Smith, R. and Mitchell, N. (1966). The haustorium of *Erysiphe cichoracearum* and the host-parasite interface on *Helianthus annuus*. *Can. J. Bot.* **44**, 1299-1306.

Mercer, P. C., Wood, R. K. S. and Greenwood, A. D. (1971). Initial infection of *Phaseolus vulgaris* by *Colletotrichum lindemuthianum*. *In* 'Ecology of Leaf-Surface Micro-organisms' (eds T. F. Preece and C. H. Dickinson), 381-393. Academic Press, London and New York.

Meyer, F. H. (1966). Mycorrhiza and other plant symbioses. *In* 'Symbiosis' (ed. S. M. Henry), Vol. I, 171-255. Academic Press, London and New York.

Mollenhauer, H. H. and Morré, D. J. (1966). Golgi apparatus and plant secretion. *A. Rev. Pl. Physiol.* **17**, 27-46.

Morré, D. J. and Mollenhauer, H. H. (1973). The endomembrane concept: A functional integration of endoplasmic reticulum and Golgi apparatus. *In* 'Dynamics of Plant Ultrastructure' (ed. A. W. Robards). McGraw-Hill Book Co., New York. In press.

Morré, D. J., Mollenhauer, H. H. and Bracker, C. E. (1971). Origin and continuity of Golgi apparatus. *In* 'Results and Problems in Cell Differentiation, Vol. 2. Origin and Continuity of Cell Organelles' (eds J. Reinert and H. Ursprung), 82-126. Springer-verlag, Berlin, Heidelberg and New York.

Nadakavukaren, M. J. (1963). Fine structure of microsclerotia of *Verticillium albo-atrum* Reinke & Berth. *Can. J. Microbiol.* **9**, 411-413.

Nicholson, R. L., Kuć, J. and Williams, E. B. (1972). Histochemical demonstration of transitory esterase activity in *Venturia inaequalis*. *Phytopathology* **62**, 1242-1247.

Nims, R. C., Halliwell, R. S. and Rosberg, D. W. (1967). Wound healing in cultured tobacco cells following microinjection. *Protoplasma* **64**, 305-314.

Olah, G. M., Pinon, J. and Janitor, A. (1971). Modifications ultrastructurales provoquées par *Puccinia graminis* f. sp. *tritici* chez le blé. *Mycopath. Mycol. appl.* **44**, 325-346.

Orcival, J. (1969). Infrastructure des sucoirs et relations hôte-parasite dans des stades écidiens d'Urédinales. *C.r. hebd. Séanc. Acad. Sci. Paris (Ser. D)* **269**, 1973-1975.

Oschman, J. L. (1966). Development of the symbiosis of *Convoluta roscoffensis* Graff and *Platymonas* sp. *J. Phycol.* **2**, 105-111.

Oschman, J. L. and Gray, P. (1965). A study of the fine structure of *Convoluta roscoffensis* and its endosymbiotic algae. *Trans. Am. microsc. Soc.* **84**, 368-375.

Park, H. D., Greenblatt, C. L., Mattern, C. F. T. and Merril, C. R. (1967). Some relationships between *Chlorohydra*, its symbionts and some other chlorophyllous forms. *J. exp. Zool.* **164**, 141-162.

Parke, M. and Manton, I. (1967). The specific identity of the algal symbiont in *Convoluta roscoffensis*. *J. mar. biol. Ass. U.K.* **47**, 445-464.

Pate, J. S. and Gunning, B. E. S. (1972). Transfer cells. *A. Rev. Pl. Physiol.* **23**, 173-196.

Paulson, R. E. and Webster, J. M. (1969). Ultrastructural response of plant cells to gall-forming nematodes. *J. Nematol.* **1**, 22-23 (Abstr.).

Peat, A. (1968). Fine structure of the vegetative thallus of the lichen, *Peltigera polydactyla*. *Arch. Mikrobiol.* **61**, 212-222.

Pedersen, K. J. (1964). The cellular organization of *Convoluta convoluta*, an acoel turbellarian: a cytological, histochemical and fine structural study. *Z. Zellforsch. mikrosk. Anat.* **64**, 655-687.

Peveling, E. (1968). Elektronenoptische Untersuchungen an Flechten. 1. Strukturveränderungen der Algenzellen von *Lecanora muralis* (Schreber) Rabenh. (=*Placodium saxicolum* (Nyl.) *sec.* Klem.) beim Eindringen von Pilzhyphen. *Z. Pflanzenphysiol.* **59**, 172-283.

Peveling, E. (1969a). Elektronenoptische Untersuchungen an Flechten. III. Cytologische Differenzierungen der Pilzzellen. *Z. Pflanzenphysiol.* **61**, 151-164.

Peveling, E. (1969b). Elektronenoptische Untersuchungen an Flechten. IV. Die Feinstruktur einiger Flechten mit Cyanophyceen–Phycobionten. *Protoplasma* **68**, 209-222.

Peyton, G. A. and Bowen, C. C. (1963). The host–parasite interface of *Peronospora manshurica* on *Glycine max*. *Am. J. Bot.* **50**, 787-797.

Preer, J. R., Jr. (1950). Microscopically visible bodies in the cytoplasm of the "killer" strains of *Paramecium aurelia*. *Genetics, Princeton* **35**, 344-362.

Preer, L. B. (1969). Alpha, an infectious macronuclear symbiont of *Paramecium aurelia*. *J. Protozool.* **16**, 570-578.

Reichle, R. E. (1965). An electron microscope study of *Fusarium solani* f. *phaseoli* in bean hypocotyls. Ph.D. thesis, University of California, Berkeley.

Rice, M. A. (1927). The haustoria of certain rusts and the relation between host and pathogene. *Bull. Torrey bot. Club* **54**, 63-153.

Richter, G. W. and Scarpelli, D. G. (eds) (1971). 'Cell Membranes. Biological and Pathological Aspects'. Williams and Wilkins, Baltimore.

Roskin, P. (1970). Ultrastructure of the host–parasite interaction in the basidiolichen *Cora pavonia* (Web.) E. Fries. *Arch. Mikrobiol.* **70**, 176-182.

Russo, M., Martelli, G. P. and Quacquarelli, A. (1968). Studies on the agent of artichoke mottled crinkle. IV. Intracellular localization of the virus. *Virology* **34**, 679-693.

Sachs, I. B., Nair, V. M. G. and Kuntz, J. E. (1970). Penetration and degradation of cell walls in oaks infected with *Ceratocystis fagacearum*. *Phytopathology* **60**, 1399-1404.

Sahlman, K. and Fahraeus, G. (1963). An electron microscope study of root-hair infection by Rhizobium. *J. gen. Microbiol.* **33**, 425-427.

Sarfatti, G. and Bedini, C. (1965). The symbiont alga of the flatworm *Convoluta psammophila* Bekl. observed at the electron microscope. *Caryologia* **18**, 207-223.

Scagel, R. F., Bandoni, R. J., Rouse, G. E., Schofield, W. B., Stein, J. R. and Taylor, T. M. C. (1966). 'An Evolutionary Survey of the Plant Kingdom'. Wadsworth Publishing Co., Belmont, Calif.

Schmid, R. (1966). Studies on extracellular structures of fungal hyphae. *Proc. 6th int. Congr. for Electron Microscopy, Kyoto* **2**, 785-786.

Schmid, R. and Balderman, E. (1967). Elektronenoptischer Nachweis von sauren Mucopolysacchariden bei Pilzhyphen. *Naturwissenschaften* **54**, 521.
Schmid, R. and Liese, W. (1965). Zur Aussenstruktur der Hyphen von Bläupilzen. *Phytopath. Z.* **54**, 275-284.
Schmid, R. and Liese, W. (1968). Structural and histochemical observations on fungal fibre-hyphae. *Proc. 4th Eur. Conf. on Electron Microscopy, Rome* **2**, 415-416.
Schnepf, E. (1964). Zur Feinstruktur von *Geosiphon pyriforme.* Ein Versuch zur Deutung cytoplasmatischer Membranen und Kompartimente. *Arch. Mikrobiol.* **49**, 112-131.
Schnepf, E. (1969a). Membranfluss und Membrantransformation. *Ber. dt. bot. Ges.* **82**, 407-413.
Schnepf, E. (1969b). Sekretion und Exkretion bei Pflanzen. *Protoplasmatologia, Handbuch der Protoplasmaforschung* **8**, 1-181.
Schnepf, E. (1972). Strukturveränderungen am Plasmalemma *Aphelidium* -infizierter *Scenedesmus*-Zellen. *Protoplasma* **75**, 155-165.
Schnepf, E. and Brown, R. M., Jr. (1971). On relationships between endosymbiosis and the origin of plastids and mitochondria. *In* 'Results and Problems in Cell Differentiation, Vol. 2. Origin and Continuity of Cell Organelles' (eds J. Reinert and H. Ursprung), 299-322. Springer-Verlag, Berlin, Heidelberg and New York.
Schnepf, E., Deichgraber, G., Hegewald, E. and Soeder, C. J. (1971a). Elektronenmikroskopische Beobachtungen an Parasiten aus *Scenedesmus*-Massenkulturen. 3. *Chytridium* sp. *Arch. Mikrobiol.* **75**, 230-245.
Schnepf, E., Hegewald, E. and Soeder, C.-J. (1971b). Elektronenmikroskopische Beobachtungen an Parasiten aus *Scenedesmus*-Massenkulturen. 2. Über Entwicklung und Parasit-Wirt-Kontakt von *Aphelidium* und virusartige Partikel im Cytoplasma infizierter *Scenedesmus*-Zellen. *Arch. Mikrobiol.* **75**, 209-229.
Shaw, M. and Manocha, M. S. (1965). The physiology of host-parasite relations. XV. Fine structure in rust-infected wheat leaves. *Can. J. Bot.* **43**, 1285-1292.
Simon, L. D. and Anderson, T. F. (1967). The infection of *Escherichia coli* by T2 and T4 bacteriophages as seen in the electron microscope. I. Attachment and penetration. *Virology* **32**, 279-297.
Sinha, R. C. and Paliwal, Y. C. (1969). Association, development, and growth cycle of *mycoplasma*-like organisms in plants affected with clover phyllody. *Virology* **39**, 759-767.
Sinha, R. C. and Paliwal, Y. C. (1970). Localization of a *mycoplasma*-like organism in tissues of a leafhopper vector carrying clover phyllody agent. *Virology* **40**, 665-672.
Smith, G. (1900). The haustoria of the Erysipheae. *Bot. Gaz.* **29**, 153-184.
Smith, D., Muscatine, L. and Lewis, D. (1969). Carbohydrate movement from autotrophs to heterotrophs in parasitic and mutualistic symbiosis. *Biol. Rev.* **44**, 17-90.
Snell, W. H. and Dick, E. A. (1971). 'A Glossary of Mycology', Revised edn. Harvard University Press, Cambridge.
Sonneborn, T. M. (1938). Mating types, toxic interactions and heredity in *Paramecium aurelia. Science,* **88**, 503 (Abstr.).
Sonneborn, T. M. (1943). Gene and cytoplasm. I. The determination and inheritance of the killer character in variety 4 of *Paramecium aurelia.*

II. The bearing of the determination and inheritance of characters in *Paramecium aurelia* on the problems of cytoplasmic inheritance, pneumococcus transformations, mutations and development. *Proc. natn. Acad. Sci. U.S.A.* **29**, 329-343.

Staehelin, L. A. (1968). Ultrastructural changes of the plasmalemma and the cell wall during the life cycle of *Cyanidium caldarium*. *Proc. R. Soc. (Ser. B)* **171**, 249-259.

Stanbridge, B., Gay, J. L. and Wood, R. K. S. (1971). Gross and fine structural changes in *Erysiphe graminis* and barley before and during infection. *In* 'Ecology of Leaf-Surface Micro-organisms' (eds T. F. Preece and C. H. Dickinson), 367-379. Academic Press, London and New York.

Stavely, J. R., Pillai, A. and Hanson, E. W. (1969). Electron microscopy of the development of *Erysiphe polygoni* in resistant and susceptible *Trifolium pratense*. *Phytopathology* **59**, 1688-1693.

Strobel, G. A. and Hess, W. M. (1968). Biological activity of a phytotoxic glycopeptide produced by *Corynebacterium sepedonicum*. *Pl. Physiol., Lancaster* **43**, 1673-1688.

Strobel, G. A., Hess, W. M. and Steiner, G. W. (1972). Ultrastructure of cells in toxin-treated and *Helminthosporium sacchari*-infected sugarcane leaves. *Phytopathology* **62**, 339-345.

Suzuki, N. (1965). Histochemistry of foliage diseases. *A. Rev. Phytopath.* **3**, 265-286.

Tainter, F. H. (1971). The ultrastructure of *Arceuthobium pusillum*. *Can. J. Bot.* **49**, 1615-1622.

Taylor, D. L. (1968). *In situ* studies on the cytochemistry and ultrastructure of a symbiotic marine dinoflagellate. *J. mar. biol. Ass. U.K.* **48**, 349-366.

Taylor, D. L. (1969). The nutritional relationship of *Anemonia sulcata* (Pennant) and its dinoflagellate symbiont. *J. Cell Sci.* **4**, 751-762.

Temmink, J. H. M. (1971). 'An Ultrastructural Study of *Olpidium brassicae* and its Transmission of Tobacco Necrosis Virus'. H. Veenman and Zonen N. V., Wageningen (Netherlands).

Temmink, J. H. M. and Campbell, R. N. (1968). The ultrastructure of *Olpidium brassicae*. I. Formation of sporangia. *Can. J. Bot.* **46**, 951-956.

Temmink, J. H. M. and Campbell, R. N. (1969). The ultrastructure of *Olpidium brassicae*. III. Infection of host roots. *Can. J. Bot.* **47**, 421-424.

Temmink, J. H. M., Campbell, R. N. and Smith, P. R. (1970). Specificity and site of *in vitro* acquisition of tobacco necrosis virus by zoospores of *Olpidium brassicae*. *Jnl. gen. Virol.* **9**, 201-213.

Thatcher, F. S. (1939). Osmotic and permeability relations in the nutrition of fungus parasites. *Am. J. Bot.* **26**, 449-458.

Thatcher, F. S. (1942). Further studies of osmotic and permeability relations in parasitism. *Can. J. Res. (Ser. C)* **20**, 283-311.

Thoday, M. G. (1911). On the histological relations between *Cuscuta* and its host. *Ann. Bot.* **25**, 655-682.

Tu, J. C. and Hiruki, C. (1971). Electron microscopy of cell wall thickening in local lesions of potato virus-M infected red kidney bean. *Phytopathology* **61**, 862-868.

VanDerWoude, W. (1972). Role of the endomembrane system in cell wall biosynthesis: glucan synthetases of Golgi apparatus and plasma membrane. Ph.D. thesis, Purdue University, Lafayette, Indiana.

Van Dyke, C. G. and Hooker, A. L. (1969). Ultrastructure of host and parasite in interactions of Zea mays with *Puccinia sorghi*. *Phytopathology* **59**, 1934-1946.

Vincent, J. M. (1966). Symbiotic specificity. *Aust. J. Sci.* **29**, 192-197.

Walker, A. T. (1968). Fungus-alga ultrastructure in the lichen, *Cornicularia normoerica*. *Am. J. Bot.* **55**, 641-648.

Watene, A. C. (1968). Ultrastructural investigations of powdery mildew of rose caused by *Sphaerotheca pannosa* (Wallr.) Lev. M.S. thesis, Brigham Young University, Provo, Utah.

Webber, M. M. and Webber, P. J. (1970). Ultrastructure of lichen haustoria: Symbiosis in *Parmelia sulcata*. *Can. J. Bot.* **48**, 1521-1524.

Whaley, W. G. (1966). Proposals concerning replication of the Golgi apparatus. *In* 'Organisation der Zelle. III. Probleme der biologischen Reduplikation. 3. Wissenschaftliche Konferenz der Gesellschaft Deutscher Naturforscher und Arzte' (ed. P. Sitte), 340-371. Springer-Verlag, Berlin, Heidelberg and New York.

Whaley, W. G., Dauwalder, M. and Kephart, J. E. (1972). Golgi apparatus: influence on cell surfaces. *Science, N.Y.* **175**, 596-599.

Williams, P. H., Aist, S. J. and Aist, J. R. (1971). Response of cabbage root hairs to infection by *Plasmodiophora brassicae*. *Can. J. Bot.* **49**, 41-47.

Williams, P. H., Aist, S. J., Aist, J. R. and Bhattacharya, P. K. (1971). Host-parasite relations of *Plasmodiophora brassicae* in root hairs of cabbage seedlings. *In* 'Morphological and Biochemical Events in Plant-Parasite Interaction' (eds S. Akai and S. Ouchi), 309-327. Mochizuki Publishing Co., Japan.

Williams, P. H. and McNabola, S. S. (1967). Fine structure of *Plasmodiophora brassicae* in sporogenesis. *Can. J. Bot.* **45**, 1665-1669.

Williams, P. H. and McNabola, S. S. (1970). Fine structure of the host-parasite interface of *Plasmodiophora brassicae* in cabbage. *Phytopathology* **60**, 1557-1561.

Williams, P. H. and Yukawa, Y. B. (1967). Ultrastructural studies on the host-parasite relations of *Plasmodiophora brassicae*. *Phytopathology* **57**, 682-687.

Wood, R. K. S., Ballio, A. and Graniti, A. (eds) (1972). 'Phytotoxins in Plant Diseases'. Academic Press, London and New York.

Zimmer, D. E. (1970). Fine structure of *Puccinia carthami* and the ultrastructural nature of exclusionary seedling-rust resistance of safflower. *Phytopathology* **60**, 1157-1163.

The preceding contribution was presented at the Symposium as two separate papers, as follows:

"Haustoria and Host–Parasite Interfaces in Powdery Mildews"
(Charles E. Bracker)

"Ultrastructure of *Melampsora lini* Infection in Flax"
(Larry J. Littlefield).

The discussion that followed these papers is given below.

Discussion

Professor N. F. Robertson: I wonder if Dr Bracker sees penetration as taking place by pressure or by the dissolution of the wall?

Dr C. E. Bracker: I do not think it is an either/or situation–it is obvious that the wall is being altered around the site of penetration. It is apparently altered in advance of penetration, and the studies of Stanbridge, Gay and Wood, and also Edwards and Allen on primary penetrations, have also shown that there is a change in the stainability of the wall around penetration sites, as well as a failure to distort the fibrils down in the wall. However, I think that any growth process which involves forward motion of the fungus (whatever it is going to interact with or come in contact with), is probably going to exert some physical force, and so perhaps we should not try to make this an either/or situation where there is obviously some alteration of the wall, but consider that both are involved. The relative importance of these, I really could not assess, but it appears that the cuticles anyway, as Stanbridge also pointed out, are driven down alongside the penetration site, which indicates that it has been moved around a bit.

Dr A. J. Sargent: Would Dr Bracker care to speculate on the origin of the material of the papilla?

Dr Bracker: I would be happy to speculate if you will not hold me to it! Here again, Stanbridge's study and also Edwards's study, have indicated that there are vesicles in the cytoplasm present at or about the time that these form. I have also found around a few haustoria (and I cannot really detect the edge), masses of cytoplasmic vesicles and also Golgi apparatus, which indicate one thing–secretion. There is a dramatic increase in the Golgi apparatus. Just the fact that the Golgi apparatus is there does not mean that it is secreting. It could be secreting now, or we could see the left-overs from what it was doing previously, but my guess, judging from the membranes that are trapped up in the papilla along the host wall and within the papilla, would be that we have some vesicle-mediated secretory process occurring here, which quickly gets that material up against the host wall. This is supported by the indications of vesicles associated with this site, and the bubbling activity that Bushnell has seen in his living preparations in microcultures, just before and during penetration.

Dr Sargent: And you see the whole vesicle going through the plasmalemma?

Dr Bracker: No, I have not seen that particular stage myself, but that would be my speculation, which is consistent with what has been suggested before. I cannot speak for what others have seen.

Dr J. T. Martin: I made a visual calculation of relative thicknesses of some of the surface structures. The cuticle is obviously extremely delicate, and I calculate its thickness as approximately 1/20 of that of the epidermal cell wall. Also the penetration peg as it goes through seems to be of the order of 1/3 of the thickness of the wall. This gives to me, at any rate, a rather different conception, from what I have had in the past, of the relative thickness of the penetration peg and the epidermal wall. The other point I would like to make refers to the cuticle seeming to be first indrawn, and then ruptured, rather than having a neat penetration hole made through it.

Dr Bracker: Stanbridge also arrived at approximately the same conclusion, namely the cuticle itself was probably penetrated mechanically and ruptured. However, you will have noticed from the micrographs that where the cuticle curves in, it also becomes thinner as it is pushed inward alongside the fungal penetration peg. Now this, I imagine, could happen in two ways. The first, if a purely mechanical pressure were applied to the cuticle it would stretch until it ruptured, at the thinnest point, giving the tapering effect. The other explanation would see tapering as arising from some biochemical activity that digests away a portion of the cuticle sufficient for the fungus to grow easily through it. I do not think we can exclude either explanation completely. However, with pathogens such as *Venturia inaequalis* the appressorium comes down to the host cuticle and just beneath the point where the infection sac is formed within the appressorium there is a small area of differentially staining cuticle. The cuticle then gets thinner, and finally the fungus grows underneath it. This penetration seems to be mediated by biochemical breakdown.

Professor Lilian Hawker (to Dr Littlefield): Did you have any evidence of transport of materials across the haustorial-host-cell wall-plasmalemma complex? And secondly, did you try with living material the very simple experiment, which was done in our Department some years ago by Dr Fraymouth, of plasmolysing living material and watching how the cytoplast pulled away from the haustorium, enveloping it again when deplasmolysed?

Dr L. J. Littlefield: The answer to both those questions is no, as far as I am concerned, unless Dr Bracker has done work with the mildews with which I am not familiar. But for rust, we have no evidence to answer the first question, and we have not done the experiments with which to answer the second.

Dr C. E. Bracker: Dr Bushnell has done this with the powdery mildew fungus *Erysiphe graminis* and some of the cells do plasmolyse. The kind of pattern of

plasmolysis that he gets though is unlike that found by Fraymouth and Thatcher. The host cell protoplast plasmolyses, and is anchored around the haustorium and the haustorial neck region, so that it plasmolyses and comes up around the haustorium, rather than pulling away, as occurs with rusts.
rusts.

Professor J. H. Burnett: Referring to that region which you can remove with periodate, presumably at some time that was the actual apical region of the hypha. Have you ever been able to make sections when that part was in fact the apex of the penetrating hypha?

Dr Littlefield: No I have not looked into this yet, but I hope that some day I shall be able to obtain some results by looking at the ring when it is at the apex of an elongating penetration peg.

Professor Burnett: I ask this because in free living fungi when a conidium germinates, the initial apical material seems to be quite different to the apical material of the germ tube as it grows out, and there must be a point when the metabolism changes to the glucan and the chitin, or whatever it is. But the previous material is apparently not any of these, and I wondered if this also applied with your rusts. (Note. The free-living fungus referred to is *Neurospora crassa*.)

Dr Littlefield: We can only speculate because we have done no studies which positively identify any of these regions. Hardwick and coworkers in a recent paper (*Can. J. Bot.* **49**, 383-390, 1971) on bean rust speculated, I think quite correctly, that this ring marks a very major transition in the nature of the wall as it progresses from the intercellular haustorial mother cell down through the penetration zone and then into the initiation of the bulbous haustorial body. That was speculation, but I think it was rather well grounded.

Dr Bracker: I would like to add one thing to that, namely, the neck ring also marks the approximate site of the transition from the stainable host plasma membrane to the non-stainable host plasma membrane where it is invaginated. I think that is a very important transitional area in the system.

Dr Littlefield: Following treatment with the plasma membrane stain procedure it is possible, with really high magnification (which you cannot see very well on a slide) to see that the stained plasma membrane continues down through the length of the etched-out ring. It does not stop above the ring, but it continues on and then fades out at the more distal region of the ring.

Dr E. C. Hislop: I am intrigued with the nature of the material that would be stain- or phase-dense in light microscopy, electron-dense in electron microscopy, and soluble in periodate. Could you please speculate on its nature?

Dr Littlefield: Well, not intelligently. I really cannot speculate on this because we know nothing of its chemical composition. I would like to add that when talking with Dr Tommerup today, she described her own observations that this ring will also stain very nicely with Giemsa stain, which I had not heard of until today. So we really have at present no idea what it is chemically.

Dr Hislop: Were the original pictures phase-contrast?

Dr Littlefield: Yes they were, but the leaves were not living. They were fixed-killed material.

Professor P. H. Williams: Following up Professor Burnett's question, does the timing of the appearance of the haustorial neck-ring coincide with or precede the entrance of a nucleus into this haustorial body?

Dr Littlefield: Judging from the few sections which we have obtained which could give an indication of this, it seems to occur long before, because in the light micrographs we can see the ring present before the body of the haustorium even begins to blow out or form as a body. Then it is not until after this haustorial body is quite large that nuclear migration occurs, so these events are rather distant in time.

Professor Hawker: Could it be a septum that starts to form and is inhibited?

Dr Littlefield: I would rather doubt it, because in the few septa we have seen forming in intercellular hyphae the linear distance of the longitudinal wall which is involved in septum formation is much narrower than the distance of the ring.

Dr Inez Tommerup: In relation to your comment about this septum, I would agree that it was not septa. We have watched the formation of haustoria of *Puccinia versicolor* in living preparations of the fungus in small leaf pieces floated on tissue culture medium with kinetin etc. Using HCl-Giemsa to stain it differentially you can see the appearance of the neck ring. The neck does not appear to develop in the same way as the septum. The septum and ring do not have similar staining properties in Giemsa preparation.

III.3 Structural Concepts of Host–Pathogen Interfaces

CONTENTS

III.4 Means by which Cereal Rusts and Smuts Affect Host Translocation and Growth

J. G. MANNERS AND A. MYERS

Department of Botany, University of Southampton, England

Introduction

When a pathogen directly kills the part of the host plant attacked, i.e. it is necrotrophic, the means by which losses are caused is clear. Many of the most important diseases of cereals, however, are caused by biotrophic pathogens, i.e. ones that exist in contact with living host cells. Such pathogens can cause losses at least as severe as those caused by necrotrophic pathogens, and the means by which such losses are caused is of considerable interest and importance. At present it appears that knowledge of the mechanism by which pathogens cause losses has contributed little or nothing to disease control. However, the recent introduction of sophisticated systemically-acting fungicides may well alter the position. These fungicides have been discovered as a result of mass screening techniques, and little is known of their mode of action. Fungus strains resistant to systemic fungicides have been reported in *Sphaerotheca fuliginea* on cucurbits (Schroeder and Provvidenti, 1969), and plant pathologists would be in a better position to produce fungicides not subject to such resistance if more were known concerning the nature of the interactions between the fungicide, the pathogen and the host.

The mechanisms by which disease losses are caused are also becoming relevant to the plant breeder, since the problems arising with respect to major gene resistance have led breeders to use minor genes involving tolerance, i.e. a situation in which the host, though attacked by the pathogen, is not severely damaged. It is clearly relevant, therefore, to understand the means by which such tolerance is attained.

Plant growth is dependent, *inter alia,* on translocation to the growing organs, and any alteration to the translocation pattern caused by a pathogen will affect the growth of the host as a whole, and of its various organs. Diversion of translocate from such structures as the developing seed will have an important effect on yield of crops such as cereals. In view of these considerations, studies have been made for some years at Southampton on the effect of attack by rusts or smuts on translocation patterns in cereals, in relation to the effects on growth patterns and on other physiological processes. A cereal rust–yellow rust of wheat (*Puccinia striiformis* Westend.)–and a cereal smut–(*Ustilago nuda* (Jens.) Rostr.)–were selected for study as pathogens with contrasting methods of attack on the host.

Yellow Rust of Wheat

Doodson *et al.* (1964) studied the effect, on host growth and development, of infecting various parts of the plant of spring wheat (cv. Jufy 1) with *P. striiformis* race 8b (Table I).

The effect on the host depended on which part of the plant was infected and on the duration of the infection. For example, the number of florets/ear was significantly reduced with complete infection or infection of leaves below the flag leaf, but not when only flag leaf or glumes were infected. Percentage fertility was, however, reduced by infection of the upper parts, so that grain no./ear, as well as single grain weight, was reduced by such infection, which was established by the time that the grain was swelling. A striking feature was the proportional decrease in dry weight of root which was larger than that in the dry weight of any other part of the plant. Final leaf size was reduced and infected leaves senesced prematurely. The maturation of the plant as a whole was retarded by infection. In general, there was a close correlation between the degree of infection and the magnitude of the effects observed.

TABLE I

Effect of rust infection on the growth and yield of wheat (means of 15 plants)

	Infection					
	None	Leaves below flag	Flag only	All leaves	Full	Glumes only
Plant height (cm)	122.7	107.4	120.5	95.2	91.7	121.5
Ear length (cm)	15.1	11.9	14.5	11.2	10.5	14.8
No. spikelets/ear	19.6	19.5	19.7	19.9	19.6	19.5
No. florets/ear	132.4	106.6	131.8	95.8	91.8	133.0
No. grain/ear	74.3	59.6	67.7	50.6	42.6	69.3
% fertility/ear	56.0	55.9	51.4	52.8	46.4	52.1
Wt. of grain/ear (g)	3.9	2.6	3.3	1.8	1.60	3.7
Wt. of single grain (mg)	56.8	44.3	49.0	34.6	37.6	52.7
No. tillers/plant	9.4	4.8	8.4	2.0	2.0	9.4
Dry wt. of roots (g)	1.2	0.40	0.9	0.3	0.3	1.0

In a further series of experiments (Doodson *et al.*, 1965) the effect of infection of the third leaf by *P. striiformis* on the assimilation and translocation pattern was investigated by using $^{14}CO_2$. In an infected leaf the assimilation rate dropped much more sharply than that in a corresponding control leaf, being only 50% of that of the control 14 days after inoculation, i.e. when the infection had fully developed (Figs 1a and b). Translocation from an infected leaf was also

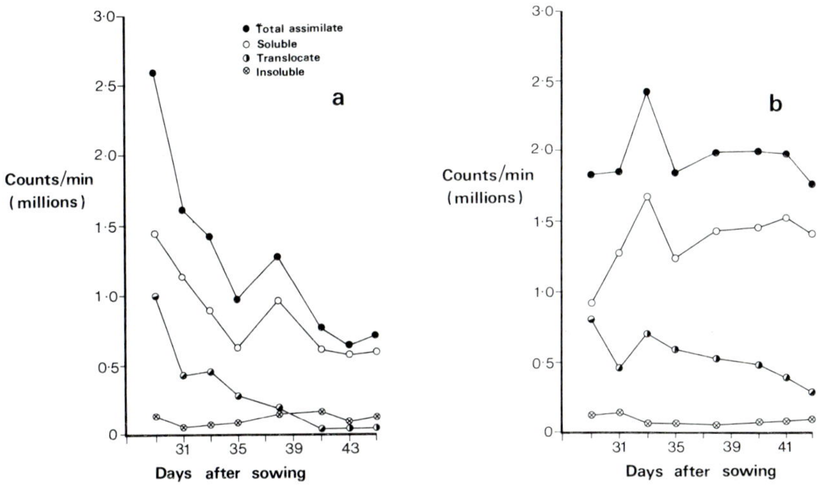

Fig. 1. The amounts of ^{14}C (expressed as counts/min) assimilated by, translocated from and retained in alcohol-soluble or insoluble material (a) in the infected part (lamina) of the third leaf of wheat (L_3) (b) in the lamina of the third leaf of wheat (L_3) of control plants. (Doodson *et al.*, 1965.)

greatly reduced: 14 days after inoculation only negligible amounts (0.4%) of assimilate were leaving the presentation leaf of infected plants, whereas in the control it was 21.0%. However the pattern of distribution of the translocate as between the various plant organs was relatively unaffected, the only important effect of infection being that the proportion going to the roots was much reduced. The combined effect of the reductions in assimilation and translocation caused the amount of assimilate leaving an infected leaf to be, in absolute terms, only 0.87% of that leaving a corresponding control leaf.

The situation in which only one leaf was infected was somewhat artifical, though convenient for experimental purposes. The more usual situation when the whole plant was infected was investigated by Siddiqui and Manners (1971), again using $^{14}CO_2$. Assimilation was affected in the same way as that noted by Doodson *et al.* (1965) but the percentage of assimilate leaving the presentation leaf was much less affected. For example, at 14 days after inoculation, 31% of assimilate was translocated in comparison with 0.4% in Doodson's experiment in which only the presentation leaf was inoculated. Presumably when rust attack reduces the carbohydrate in the plant, some export occurs from a given infected leaf, even though amounts in that leaf may be low, so that little or no export would occur in an otherwise healthy plant. In fully-infected plants the effect on the translocation pattern was greater than when only one leaf was infected: quite consistently the proportion of translocate going to the roots decreased, and that going to the other leaves, stem and tillers increased.

Many of the changes in translocation and growth pattern caused by Yellow Rust attack in wheat can be related to decreases in host assimilation (by what means is not known), increase in host respiration involving the hexose monophosphate shunt (Shaw and Samborski, 1957), and the fungus acting as a sink through its own growth and metabolism. However, the mechanism by which soluble, and, later, insoluble carbohydrates accumulate in infected leaves (Doodson *et al.*, 1965) is difficult to explain. Changes in the translocation pattern are clearly implicated but the factors controlling such changes are not yet fully resolved. The factors controlling normal translocation are not well understood, but there is evidence that growth substances are implicated (Vaadia and Itai, 1969). Furthermore, rust infection in some hosts at least, e.g. certain Leguminosae (Kiraly *et al.*, 1967) is known to affect the concentration of growth substances. Whilst with yellow rusts, growth substances may cause the large reduction of root growth and translocation to the roots, following infection, we cannot postulate whether growth affects translocation or vice versa.

Loose Smut of Wheat

Host–pathogen combinations, such as cereal rusts and mildews, are not ideal for the detailed investigation of the mechanism by which host growth and translocation patterns are altered by the fungus, because the pathogen is normally widespread on the host, and cannot, at least without great difficulty, be grown in culture. Both these obstacles can be overcome by working with a smut fungus, and accordingly Gaunt (1971) studied host–parasite relationships in loose-smut infection of spring wheat (cv. Kloka). *Ustilago nuda,* besides being readily grown on synthetic media, is virtually restricted in the host plants to the nodes and ears (Batts and Jeater, 1958; Dean, 1964). A growth analysis experiment showed (Table II) that smut infection had considerable effects on host growth–in many ways comparable to those produced by rust infection. In particular, root growth at day 40 (at which date the amount of smut mycelium was 0.1% of the total volume of the plant), was reduced by 40%. The phase of delayed growth was followed by a period of rapid development of the infected main stem, and sporulation of the fungus in the ear. This occurred at 50 days, slightly in advance of the development of the main shoot of the healthy plant.

TABLE II

Dry wt. (mg) of healthy wheat plants (H) and plants infected with *U. nuda* (I)

Days after emergence		Total	Roots	Main shoot	Tiller 1	Tiller 2	Tiller 3
10	H	47	8	39			
	I	45	8	38			
20	H	164	26	138			
	I	132*	20	112**			
30	H	302	32	242	29	6	
	I	291	32	232	21	6	
40	H	542	67	439	31	6	
	I	503	40**	445	15		
50	H	1082	71	822	127	62	7
	I	1039**	82*	872**	62**	23*	
60	H	1400	82	1046	151	97	31
	I	1182	85	905**	144	50**	7**

Differences between H and I significant at:
$^*P = 0.1$ $^{**}P = 0.05$ $^{***}P = 0.01$.

Subsequently, at 60 days, the infected main shoot ceased to grow, but the roots developed further. In contrast, the healthy main shoot continued to develop and increase in dry weight after anthesis, and the rate of growth of the roots decreased. Further analysis of the data (Table III) reveals that at 40 days, when ear development had scarcely begun, stem growth was considerably stimulated in infected plants. At 50 days, when the fungus in the infected ear was near sporulation, growth of the rest of the stem in infected plants was still being stimulated. Only at 60 days, when the healthy plant ears were filling, did growth of the healthy stem catch up with that of the infected stem.

Neither the big reduction in root growth at an early stage in the development of the infection, nor the stimulation of host stem growth before and during fungal sporulation can satisfactorily be explained in terms of the fungus acting as a sink.

In a further series of experiments (Table IV) $^{14}CO_2$ was fed to a mature but still active leaf in healthy and infected plants at various stages of growth using a technique similar to that described by Quinlan and Sagar (1962).

The infected plants consistently accumulated a higher proportion of radioactivity in the nodes than the healthy plants. Although this could be caused by the fungus, it was noted that the infected plants also usually accumulated more radioactivity in the internodes and leaves (from which the fungus was

TABLE III

Dry wt. (mg) of the ear and 'rest of stem' in healthy (H) and infected plants (I)

		Days after emergence					
		10	20	30	40	50	60
Ear	H				9	174	355
	I				9	204**	225**
Rest of stem	H	2	8	9	66	180	228
	I	1	4	18**	84**	245**	235

Differences between H and I significant at:
*P = 0.1 **P = 0.05 ***P = 0.01.

TABLE IV

Percentage distribution of recovered radioactivity after feeding $^{14}CO_2$ to wheat, healthy (H) and infected by loose-smut (I)

Days after emergence	40		50		60	
Leaf fed	5		6		7	
	H	I	H	I	H	I
Fed leaf	26.6	28.7	86.3	67.7	52.1	65.1
Other leaves	1.8	6.4	0.9	2.4	0.2	2.4
Nodes	17.7	25.9	2.9	3.7	0.9	3.8
Internodes	28.8	17.7	6.8	17.8	6.6	15.8
Roots	2.0	0.4	2.2	2.8	0.2	4.5
Tillers	20.2	0.7	0.4	1.6	0.4	6.0
Ear	2.9	19.1	0.6	3.9	40.6	2.0

virtually absent) than did the healthy plants. At 40 days, shortly before sporulation, less radioactivity accumulated in the roots of the infected plants. But at 60 days, when sporulation was complete in the infected plants, and the ears were filling in the healthy plants, the roots of the former accumulated more radioactivity. In infected plants a larger proportion of exported radioactivity accumulated in the ear at 40 days (when fungal growth in the ear was most active) than was found in healthy plants. At 60 days the situation was reversed. These results, like those for yellow rust indiciate that the roots are very ineffective sinks, and they only received assimilates, especially from the younger leaves, when all other sinks had little demand for assimilates.

In some instances, assimilates were translocated over long distances, e.g. from the main shoot flag leaf to infected tiller ears. Thus, in a 60-day plant grown under conditions favouring tillering, less than 0.1% of the radioactivity assimilated was found in the ear of tiller 2, but in a comparable infected plant the corresponding figure was 20.5%.

In many associations of fungi with green plants, carbohydrates become available to the heterotroph as a result of the conversion of carbohydrates to a form unavailable to the autotroph. Lewis, Webster and Thorpe (cited by Smith *et al.*, 1969) reported the presence of mannitol and erythritol (substances absent from healthy wheat plants), in infected areas of plants infected by loose smut. We therefore investigated the carbohydrates and polyols of the soluble fraction of the ears of healthy and loose-smut-infected plants, as providing the best opportunity for the isolation of polyols or any special carbohydrates.

In one experiment, ears of 50-day-old plants were analysed (Table V) using the chromatographic methods reviewed by Lewis and Smith (1967b). In the earliest harvest, the majority of the radioactivity was present as sucrose, but after 24 h much of this had been converted in the healthy plants to fructose and glucose, and some to higher molecular weight compounds. In the infected plants however, the conversion was to erythritol, mannitol and trehalose. Growth of the smut in pure culture demonstrated that it could convert sucrose into these three substances, though, surprisingly, they were unable to support the growth of the fungus when supplied as the sole source of carbon. It seems reasonable to assume that in the infected ears these substances were produced by the fungus.

The conversion of sucrose to such substances as erythritol and mannitol, which probably cannot be utilized by the wheat plant (Lewis and Smith, 1967a) means that a sink is being created, in addition to the utilization of sucrose for the growth of the fungus.

Discussion

Throughout this work on yellow rust and loose smut there was, in general, an excellent correlation between the patterns of translocation and growth. As already indicated, it is uncertain to what extent growth patterns determine translocation patterns or vice versa. However, the existence of a sink can be seen to be correlated with the flow of translocate towards that sink in many of our experiments, and in our opinion, the existence of the sink determines the flow of translocate. The extent of yellow-rust infection at relevant times suggests that the existence of the fungal sink is the principal cause of the diversion of translocate. In loose smut infections, however, in the early stages, the amount of smut mycelium present is so small that such a hypothesis is scarcely tenable. The accumulation of carbohydrates around rust pustules, and of polyols in smutted ears will clearly enhance the sink effect (these accumulations themselves pose unsolved problems as far as the mechanism of their accumulation is concerned). The effect of the presence of *U. nuda,* however, in the early stages of infection

TABLE V

Distribution of radioactivity in various carbohydrates and polyols in the ears of healthy and loose-smut-infected wheat plants at several times after feeding leaf-6 with $^{14}CO_2$

	Time after exposure to $^{14}CO_2$ (h)	Origin	Trehalose	Sucrose	Fructose	Glucose	Mannitol	Erythritol
		(% of total soluble activity in the ear)						
Healthy	3			68.1	17.1	14.8		
	24	11.5		16.6	41.2	30.7		
Infected	3			56.7	24.2	17.3	1.0	0.8
	24		2.2	33.3	24.7	13.1	7.6	19.1

is, we feel, much greater than can be accounted for, even with polyol production. A reduction in host photosynthesis caused by a toxic fungal product, and an increase in host respiration may be partly responsible for the observed effects on host growth. However, the possibility that growth factor changes induced by the fungus are involved is particularly interesting, and will be the subject of further investigation at Southampton.

The failure of a simple sink hypothesis to account for the situation in smutted wheat, or even for all the phenomena observed in rusted wheat suggests that such a hypothesis may not be wholly valid for cereal rust infections, because the changes in host development in the two disease are strikingly similar.

It is possible that in biotrophic pathogens all these mechanisms may be operative, although their relative importance may vary both with the host–pathogen combination concerned and the progress of the disease. The further elucidation of such problems will depend on progress not only in studies of the physiology of host–parasite relations, but also in those of the physiology of the healthy plant.

References

Batts, C. C. V. and Jeater, A. (1958). The development of loose smut (*Ustilago tritici*) in susceptible varieties of wheat, and some observations on field infection. *Trans. Br. mycol. Soc.* **41**, 115-125.

Dean, W. M. (1964). 'Some effects of temperature and humidity on loose smut of wheat.' Ph.D. Thesis, University of Nottingham.

Doodson, J. K., Manners, J. G. and Myers, A. (1964). Some effects of Yellow Rust (*Puccinia striiformis*) on the growth and yield of a spring wheat. *Ann. Bot.* **28**, 459-472.

Doodson, J. K., Manners, J. G. and Myers, A. (1965). Some effects of Yellow Rust (*Puccinia striiformis*) on ^{14}carbon assimilation and translocation in wheat. *J. exp. Bot.* **16**, 304-317.

Gaunt, R. E. (1971). 'Host–parasite relations in loose smut of wheat'. Ph.D. Thesis, University of Southampton.

Kiraly, Z., El Hammady, M. and Pozsar, B. I. (1967). Increased cytokinin activity of rust-infected bean and broad bean leaves. *Phytopathology* **57**, 93-94.

Lewis, D. H. and Smith, D. C. (1967a). Sugar alcohols (polyols) in fungi and green plants. I. Distribution, physiology and metabolism. *New Phytol.* **66**, 143-184.

Lewis, D. H. and Smith, D. C. (1967b). Sugar alcohols (polyols) in fungi and green plants. II. Methods of detection and quantitative estimation in plant extracts. *New Phytol.* **66**, 185-204.

Quinlan, J. D. and Sagar, G. R. (1962). An autoradiographic study of the movement of ^{14}C labelled assimilates in the developing wheat plant. *Weed Res.* **2**, 264-273.

Schroeder, W. T. and Provvidenti, R. (1969). Resistance to benomyl in powdery mildew of cucurbits. *Pl. Dis. Reptr.* **53**, 271-275.

Shaw, M. and Samborski, D. J. (1957). The physiology of host–parasite relations: III. The pattern of respiration in rusted and mildewed cereal leaves. *Can. J. Bot.* **35**, 289-407.

Siddiqui, M. Q. and Manners, J. G. (1971). Some effects of general Yellow Rust (*Puccinia striiformis*) infection on ^{14}carbon assimilation, translocation and growth in a spring wheat. *J. exp. Bot.* **22**, 792-799.

Smith, D. C., Muscatine, L. and Lewis, D. H. (1969). Carbohydrate movement from autotrophs to heterotrophs in parasitic and mutualistic symbiosis. *Biol. Rev.* **44**, 17-90.

Vaadia, Y. and Itai, C. (1969). Interrelationships of growth with reference to the distribution of growth substances. *In* 'Root Growth' (ed. W. J. Whittington), Butterworth, London.

DISCUSSION

Dr R. C. Hignett: When you lose photosynthetic activity because of the infection, this may occur during 40 days or so, and really drops right down to zero. Have you tried compensating for this by increasing the light intensity or have you noticed any effect of different light levels on the growth of the fungus?

Dr A. Myers: There is a steady fall in photosynthetic activity immediately after infection, but we have never looked at the effect of light levels. What lies behind your question?

Dr Hignett: I was just wondering, in general terms, if the fungus could be reducing photosynthetic activity for its own purposes, or if this is just some unfortunate byproduct. Obviously it is not a good thing for this to happen, as you pointed out yourself, because it reduces all metabolites. Photosynthetic activity may be cut down for some other reason, for example, the fungus could thereby limit the ability of the plant to produce phytoalexins, or similar compounds. This would then be a protective mechanism and if you increased the light levels, you would boost this protective mechanism Do you think this is a possibility?

Dr Myers: I think it is a possibility. I do not know how correct it is, but it is an interesting idea.

Dr H. M. Dekhuijzen: How do you bring the formation of green islands into this picture of photosynthesis? I think, although I have never worked on photosynthesis, that you used a rather high inoculum which, finally—after 47 days, killed the leaf. But what happens when you use a lower inoculum? I would expect that the photosynthesis would go down for a while, and then go up again.

Dr Myers: There have been reports of a loss of photosynthetic activity and then an increase again, whereby chlorophyll tends to disappear from around the site of infection, and then to re-form this newly formed chlorophyll being effective in photosynthesis. In the sort of experiments that we have been doing we have been looking at the whole leaf, we have not been looking at an area just around a site of infection. Even with a low inoculum containing the right races, etc., green islands will be limited in a sea of yellowing leaf, so that the overall effect is going to be one of decreased activity. If you get a very high inoculum then you will not get a green island effect in any case. So that I think the overall effect is usually, if not always, to lose photosynthetic activity. We have not looked specifically at the green islands.

Dr G. M. Farrell: Could you please comment on the concept of the infection site as a metabolic sink which has developed at least partly because mature rusted leaves of dicotyledons import assimilate from other healthy parts of the plant. Does the fact that this abnormal movement into a rust-infected leaf is not seen with barley yellow rust modify this hypothesis of rust infection as metabolic sinks? Or is it sufficient to consider local redistribution within the infected leaf itself?

Dr Myers: It seems to me that the demands of the pathogen are satisfied by photosynthesis occurring within a given leaf. Certainly at the degree of infection with which we have been dealing this has been true. Perhaps the reduction of photosynthesis is not important to the pathogen on a given leaf, because it has got enough to maintain it. I do not know of any example where infection has turned an exporting leaf into an importer.

Dr Farrell: This is reported to happen with Uromyces infection of bean.

Dr Myers: I am sorry, I was talking about cereals, and it does not happen with them, although it does with other plants. Thank you for pointing this out.

Dr Farrell: In your experiments, rust-infected leaves exported only a very small proportion of the ^{14}C assimilate from $^{14}CO_2$. Have you measured the effect of varying intensities of disease on export out of the infected leaf, or have you just used a single level of disease? Is the export from the infected leaf proportionally reduced as you increase the degree of infection?

Dr Myers: We have generally worked at one level of infection.

Professor P. W. Brian: Have you noticed any effect on water balance? Could this probably be involved to some extent in the effect on photosynthesis?

Dr Myers: It would be well worth investigating this. A big reduction in the growth of roots, for example, will have different effects according to the soil conditions—how much water there is about, the mineral content, and so on. Our work has always been done in pots, and we have kept the plants well supplied with minerals and water, so that presumably a plant can grow well with only a very small root system, provided you are pouring in plenty of water. I should imagine that, on a field scale, a shortage of water could be very serious indeed.

Professor Brian: Could stomatal closure be a possible factor in reducing the rate of photosynthesis?

Dr Myers: Again that is a good idea, but so far, we have not looked at this.

Dr R. Johnson: I was thinking that the amount of fungus in a yellow-rust infection is probably a good deal greater than in a loose-smut infection. Although you said that you did not think that the channels could be blocked, I wondered whether the rather strategic placing of the loose-smut mycelium at the nodes, might block the possible channels for translocation. There seems little possibility of it acting as a sink, in view of the small amount of fungus.

Dr Myers: Yes, it is a very attractive idea that the residue of fungus is left behind at the node acting as a traffic policeman, and shunting the translocate in the direction of the developing smutted ear. However, I do not quite see how it could operate, and there is no evidence that this is what is happening.

Dr Johnson: You did show that there was translocation from the leading tiller leaf right down and up into the secondary tiller leaf, obviously through some infected nodes, and this may not support my suggestion.

Dr Myers: Yes, they would have to be very intelligent infected nodes, knowing that the metabolites must go all the way down and back up again! I do not really see this as feasible.

B. THE PLANT'S RESPONSE

Section IV

Induced and Preformed Resistance Factors

CHAIRMAN'S INTRODUCTION

J. T. MARTIN

Long Ashton Research Station, University of Bristol, England

To define our terms: induced factors are those formed in response to infection, and preformed factors are those normally present, waiting as it were for the attack. Cruickshank, some five years ago, referred to 'natural defence' called into play by the induced factors and to 'natural protection' due to preformed antifungal agents. Differentiation between these defensive mechanisms may be useful but the boundary between them, already narrow, is contracting. The inhibitor in broad bean, for example, occurs preformed but can further accumulate in a phytoalexin-like manner after infection. The papers to be presented at this Session deal overwhelmingly with induced factors; to restore the balance somewhat, may I say something about preformed factors?

The first potential preformed factor met by the invading fungus is the cuticle. The concept that the cuticle acts as a mechanical barrier was set in motion by and has developed since the work by Melander and Craigie in 1927 on the nature of resistance of *Berberis* spp. to *Puccinia graminis.* It is of some interest to refer back to this paper, in which they suggested not one but three morphological factors to account for the inability of the germ tubes to penetrate: in some species, a thick cuticle; in others, thick outer walls of the epidermal cells; and in yet others, thick anticlinal walls of small epidermal cells. They also said that these factors could not account for the resistance of all *Berberis* and that evidently there was also a 'physiological resistance'.

The possibility that chemical inhibitors may occur in cuticles has received less attention. We have found that the antifungal activities of cuticular waxes, and of fractions obtained from them, are small compared with those of cellular extractives. The cuticle has an open, porous structure, and from its chemical composition, of which we are now quite knowledgeable, I see no reason why it should be regarded as unduly tough. A thinner extension of the cuticle lines the stomatal cavity; any penetration must therefore be cuticular. Cuticles differ enormously in heaviness and chemical composition but, in view of the results obtained at Long Ashton, the protection afforded by them either as mechanical or chemical barriers, cannot be great. Sometimes the cuticle, on the flimsiest evidence, has been said to account for resistance to infection when attempts to find other factors have failed.

The cumulative evidence concerning the cellular preformed protectants suggests that they may be of considerable importance. Those so far identified vary considerably in chemical composition; there is no common chemical group to which fungitoxicity may be ascribed. Examples are methoxy-benzoxazolinone from rye and coumaroyl-agmatine from barley. The occurrence of trifolirhizin and two isoflavones, as glycosides, in clover and of other preformed agents will be referred to by Dr Smith. 'Phenolic compounds' have often been said to be implicated in resistance to infection. They are certainly preformed and there is evidence that they are also induced in response to infection. The term 'phenolic compounds', however, embraces many naturally-occurring compounds and so has little meaning. A generalization, based on comparatively few substantiated cases, that phenolic compounds operate in defence seems to me to be unwarranted.

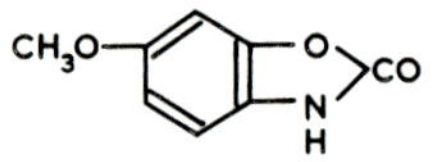

6—methoxy—2(3)—benzoxazolinone

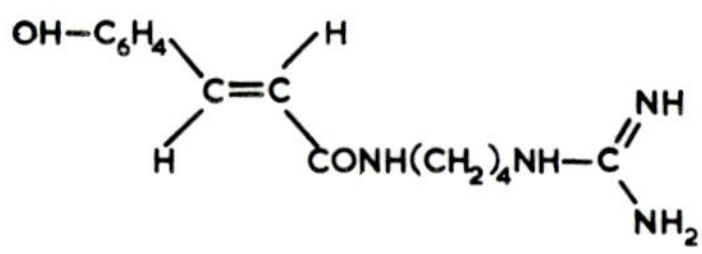

p—coumaroyl—agmatine

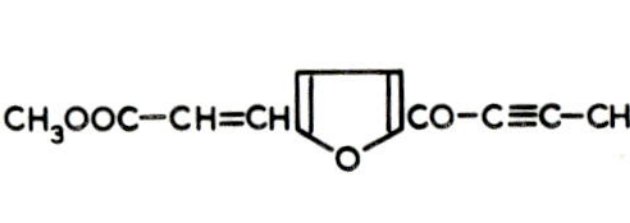

Trifolirhizin R=Glucose

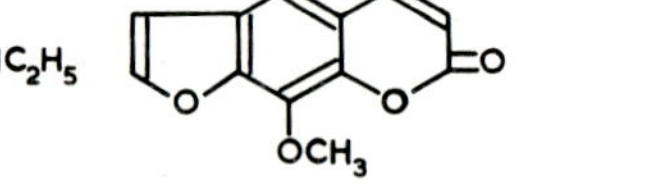

Ipomeamarone

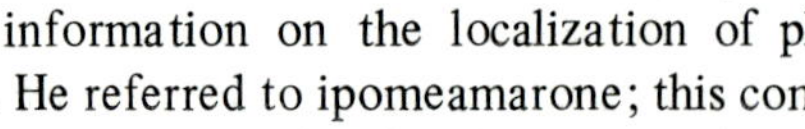

Wyerone

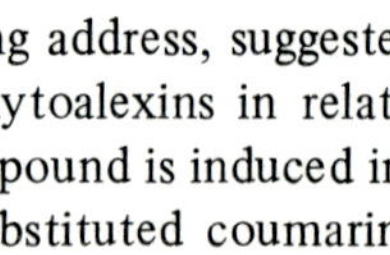

Isopimpinellin

Professor Wood, in his stimulating opening address, suggested that we need more information on the localization of phytoalexins in relation to infected tissue. He referred to ipomeamarone; this compound is induced in infected sweet potato together with related compounds, substituted coumarins and phenolic substances; it seems that the ipomeamarone and related compounds appear chiefly in the infected tissue and the phenolics in the adjacent healthy zone. The inhibitor wyerone in broad bean was originally described as an acetylenic keto-ester. Both ipomeamarone and the keto-ester are derivatives of furan.

Substituted coumarins such as umbelliferone (7-hydroxy-coumarin) have been associated, from time to time, with protective mechanisms without achieving any great status. Combination of the furan and coumarin nuclei gives compounds of considerable biological activity, the furanocoumarins, which have aroused our interest. These occur preformed in many plants, notably Rutaceae and Umbelliferae. The four major furanocoumarins of hogweed–pimpinellin, isopimpinellin, bergapten and sphondin–suppressed growth of the mycelium of *Botrytis cinerea, Sclerotinia fructigena, Stereum purpureum* and *Gloeosporium limetticola* at 500 ppm or less in the culture medium. Isopimpinellin was isolated as pure crystals from the citrus lime leaf; it occurs in the leaf to the extent of at least 100 ppm and shows an ED_{50} of 50 ppm *in vitro* against mycelium of *Gloeosporium limetticola.* I must also refer to unsaturated fatty acids such as linolenic acid, studied by Virtanen and also in Professor Wood's Department, and to hydroxy-fatty acids, e.g. phloionolic acid, which are the building blocks of cutins and suberins. It may yet be found that these acids are significantly involved in resistance complexes.

The furanocoumarins and other preformed factors may contribute significantly to defence. Resistance is obviously a complicated phenomenon not dependent upon any single property. It occurs, in my view, when a delicate balance of a number of interacting factors, which include antifungal agents preformed or induced, is tipped in favour of the host. It will require biochemical research of a high order–on enzymic and other aspects–to unravel it. It remains to be seen whether the preformed defensive agents recede in importance or assume enhanced status as and when new classes of naturally-occurring antifungal agents are found. A vast field of research of great potential importance has hardly been touched.

IV. 1 Phaseollin Accumulation in *Phaseolus vulgaris* Following Infection by Fungi, Bacteria and a Virus

J. A. BAILEY

ARC Plant Growth Substance and Systemic Fungicide Unit
Wye College, Kent, England

INTRODUCTION

The antifungal pterocarpan, phaseollin, was first detected by Müller (1958) and later isolated by Cruickshank and Perrin (1963) from diffusates obtained from seed cavities of pods of bean (*Phaseolus vulgaris*) following inoculation with *Monilinia fructicola*. Since 1963 many other fungi, chemical agents and a few bacteria have also been shown to cause phaseollin formation (Cruickshank and Perrin, 1971). It was on the basis of these results, recently supported by reports that phaseollin was also produced in bean tissue infected with *Rhizoctonia solani* (Pierre and Bateman, 1967) or *Colletotrichum lindemuthianum* (Rahe *et al.*, 1969), that phaseollin has been considered a phytoalexin.

Research into phytoalexins has highlighted two major problems. How does fungal infection incite phytoalexin production and what role do phytoalexins have in controlling disease reactions? Regarding the first question, it has been suggested (Cruickshank and Perrin, 1968; Hadwiger and Schwochau, 1969) that metabolites are released by growing fungi and that these are responsible for altering the metabolism of the host plant in such a way that phytoalexins are produced. On the other hand, Kuć (1968) emphasized that the metabolic changes involved during pathogenesis are very similar to those which occur following cellular injury and he suggested that compounds produced during host–pathogen interactions are the result of an intensification of these changes.

Regarding a role for phytoalexins in disease resistance, Cruickshank (1962) and Cruickshank and Perrin (1971) showed that both pathogens and non-pathogens of peas and beans cause phytoalexin formation in diffusates from pod endocarps. They suggested that pathogens are unaffected by the amounts of phytoalexin produced during the interactions, whereas growth of non-pathogens is completely prevented. Other workers, e.g. Wit-Elshove (1969) and Higgins and Millar (1970) obtained evidence to show that this selective toxicity, and hence pathogenicity, may be explained by the ability of pathogens to convert phytoalexins to non-inhibitory products. They suggested that this ability is absent in non-pathogens.

The production of phytoalexins and their role in the resistance of host plant cultivars to different races of a pathogen have been studied by several workers. Sato and Tomiyama (1969) reported that rishitin was produced only in potato tissue which had been inoculated with an incompatible race of *Phytophthora infestans.* No rishitin accumulated during extensive intracellular growth of a compatible race. Rahe *et al.* (1969), however, working with bean (*P. vulgaris*) infected with *C. lindemuthianum,* obtained evidence which showed that phaseollin and other phenolic compounds were produced during both resistant and susceptible reactions. Similar results were reported for cotton infected with *Verticillium albo-atrum* (Bell, 1969), safflower with *Phytophthora drechsleri* (Allen and Thomas, 1971) and soybean infected with *Phytophthora megasperma* var. *sojae* (Gray *et al.*, 1968; Keen, 1971).

The results discussed in this paper relate to the accumulation of phaseollin in tissue, as distinct from infection droplets, and the importance of phaseollin in resistance to races of *C. lindemuthianum.* Full details of the methods used in the experiments reported here, and summarized below, have been published by Stholasuta *et al.* (1971), Bailey and Deverall (1971) and Bailey and Ingham (1971).

Methods

Spores of *C. lindemuthianum* were suspended in distilled water and inoculated, as 5 μl drops, on to young hypocotyls. The hypocotyls were incubated for required periods under high humidity in an illuminated cabinet at 17 ± 2 °C. The tissue directly affected by the inoculation droplet has been termed the 'inoculated site' which in hypersensitive reactions refers to tissue directly beneath the position of the droplet, and in susceptible reactions, to tissue directly beneath the position of the droplet during the early stages of the reaction, or also to rotted tissue around the position of the droplet during the later stages of the reaction. Uredospores of *Uromyces appendiculatus* were mixed with talc (1 : 25) and dusted on to the surface of unifoliate leaves. After being enclosed in a polythene bag for 48 h the bags were removed and the plants incubated at 22° C. Suspensions of the bacterium *Pseudomonas phaseolicola* were injected under pressure from a spray gun into the intercellular spaces of attached unifoliate leaves through the lower stomatal apertures. The leaves were washed and incubated at 17 ± 2° C in an illuminated cabinet. Partially purified tobacco necrosis virus was suspended in 0.1 M -phosphate buffer and inoculated using a small brush, on to either trifoliate leaves or etiolated hypocotyls. The attached leaves and detached hypocotyls were incubated at 22° C in the light and dark respectively.

Phaseollin was extracted from tissue with 80% ethanol and partitioned into ethyl acetate. The ethyl acetate-soluble material was subjected to t.l.c. on silica and phaseollin was obtained from the appropriate areas of the chromatogram by eluting with ethanol. The amount of phaseollin was measured either from its u.v. absorption spectrum or by g.l.c., the latter technique being particularly useful in measuring small quantities of phaseollin, the limit of detection being between 0.1 and 0.4 μg.

Measurements of the effect of phaseollin on growth of *C. lindemuthianum* were difficult since phaseollin was found to be almost insoluble in aqueous nutrient solutions. However, organic agents were found which at low concentration in nutrient solution dissolved phaseollin and also permitted growth of *C. lindemuthianum*. Ethanol (20% v/v), 2-ethoxy-ethanol (5%) and propane-1,2-diol (2%) were used for assays of spore germination but only 2% propane-1,2-diol was used for assay of germ-tube growth. All solvents produced similar results and none affected *C. lindemuthianum* in the absence of phaseollin.

THE ROLE OF PHASEOLLIN IN RESISTANCE TO *COLLETOTRICHUM LINDEMUTHIANUM*

When assessing the importance of phytoalexins in disease resistance it is necessary not only to demonstrate their existence but also to relate their toxicity *in vitro* to their concentration at the site of fungal growth inhibition. In our work parallel studies were made of biologically observed events and of changes in phaseollin concentration *in vivo*. Attempts were made to calculate the concentration of phaseollin in cells as they underwent interaction with the fungus and to reveal the effects of such concentrations on those stages of fungal development thought to be of most importance in the resistant cell.

The nature of infections of *P. vulgaris* by compatible and incompatible races of *C. lindemuthianum*, were described by Leach (1923) and by Rahe *et al.* (1969) and similar observations were made during the work discussed here (Bailey and Deverall, 1971). Spore germination, appressorial formation and penetration of cells by the germ tubes which were produced were similar on resistant and susceptible hypocotyls. As a result of penetration by an incompatible race, the cell died, cytoplasmic streaming stopped and the cell turned brown. Very little hyphal growth was observed in the epidermal cell and growth into a second cell did not occur. The cellular reactions, which started very soon after penetration, were completed less than 6 days after inoculation. In susceptible cells large hyphae formed without any of the reactions described above taking place. The infected cell remained alive and the hyphae grew into neighbouring cells. Intracellular hyphal growth continued for a further 2 or 3 days, after which time the infected tissue turned brown to form a large lesion. In many interactions, this lesion continued to enlarge beyond the area covered by the inoculation droplet.

The production of phaseollin during interactions of *C. lindemuthianum* and *P. vulgaris* were reported by Cruickshank and Perrin (1963) and by Rahe *et al.* (1969). Results obtained in our work are shown in Tables I and II.

TABLE I

Phaseollin concentration in hypocotyls of *P. vulgaris* cv. Kievit Koekoek at different stages of development of a hypersensitive reaction after inoculation with *C. lindemuthianum*, race δ[1]

Incubation period (h)	Biological observations	No. of 'inoculated sites'	Phaseollin content: Total (μg)	Phaseollin content: Concentration (μg/'inoculated site')
0	None	574	2.9	0.005
44	Appressoria formed; a few cells were responding to infection	475	No phaseollin was detected	
65	Penetrated epidermal cells were dead and turning brown	469	21.2	0.045
93	Penetrated epidermal cells had turned brown	473	158	0.335
117	Penetrated epidermal cells had turned brown	476	212	0.450

[1] From Bailey and Deverall (1971) (refers also to Tables II-VI).

Phaseollin was produced following infection by both compatible and incompatible races but accumulated earlier and to a lesser extent during the hypersensitive reaction. During both interactions phaseollin accumulation was closely correlated with cellular browning. In the hypersensitive reaction, cellular browning and phaseollin accumulation took place soon after penetration, near the time when hyphal growth ceased, but in the susceptible reaction they occurred only after extensive intracellular hyphal growth had taken place.

Further experiments (Table III) showed that phaseollin was localized to the extreme surface of tissue which had reacted hypersensitively. No phaseollin was extracted from the green tissue beneath or between the hypersensitive areas.

A further indication that phaseollin is a product of dying cells was that the highest concentrations were extracted from tissue as they became brown; higher yields were not obtained from tissue after browning was completed. However, phaseollin was not detected, using various histochemical stains, in the brown

TABLE II

Phaseollin concentration in hypocotyls of Kievit Koekoek at different stages of development of a susceptible reaction after inoculation with *C. lindemuthianum*, race δ

Incubation period (h)	Biological observations	No. of 'inoculated sites'	Phaseollin content: Total (μg)	Phaseollin content: Concentration (μg/'inoculated site')
0	None	574	2.9	0.005
43	Appressoria formed; a small number of primary hyphae were observed	434	No phaseollin was detected	
88	A large number of primary hyphae were present in the cells	540	No phaseollin was detected	
118	Extensive hyphal growth in epidermal and cortical cells. Lesions visible at less than 1% of 'inoculated sites'	470	2.7	0.006
142	Lesions visible at 77% of 'inoculated sites'	159	21	0.145
164	Lesions visible at 100% of 'inoculated sites'	161	133	0.83

cells, probably because of the failure of the reagents to penetrate or react with their constituents. Nor was the compound detected in adjacent green cells.

The sensitivity of young germ tubes to phaseollin *in vitro* is probably a relevant indication of activity of phaseollin in cells infected by an incompatible race. Skipp (1971) showed that spores germinated equally well on resistant or susceptible hypocotyls and that hyphal growth was usually limited to a single epidermal cell in resistant hypocotyls. It can be seen from Table IV that after 24 h in nutrient solution spores of *C. lindemuthianum* had produced germ tubes 167 μm in length. The addition of phaseollin at this time, to give a final concentration of 3 μg/ml or greater, not only prevented further germ tube growth but caused the germ tubes to shrink and become distorted and swollen. In the absence of phaseollin, growth continued and extensive mycelium was produced. Germ tubes of *C. lindemuthianum* are thus extremely sensitive to low concentrations of phaseollin.

It has been suggested that selective toxicity of phaseollin towards pathogens and non-pathogens is a determining factor in resistance of *Phaseolus* to disease. In our experiments on the resistance of different cultivars of beans, no evidence was obtained which indicated that the races of *C. lindemuthianum* were not

TABLE III

Distribution of phaseollin in Imuna hypocotyls 6 days after inoculation with *C. lindemuthianum*, race β (a hypersensitive reaction)

Region of hypocotyl extracted	Weight of tissue extracted (g)	Phaseollin content Total (μg)	Concentration (μg/g tissue)
Upper infected half	7.68	88.3	11.5
Lower infected half	6.55	No phaseollin was detected	
Tissue directly beneath 'inoculated site': upper half of hypocotyl only	3.51	92	26.2
Tissue between 'inoculated sites': upper half of hypocotyl only	3.58	No phaseollin was detected	
Extreme surface layers directly beneath 'inoculated sites'	0.775	114	147.0
Tissue remaining after removal of extreme surface layers directly beneath 'inoculated sites'	12.92	No phaseollin was detected	

equally sensitive to phaseollin (Table V). In contrast, the difference between infections by compatible and incompatible races was apparently determined by the initial reaction of the host cell with the invading fungal hypha. During hypersensitive reactions production of phaseollin was associated with an immediate violent reaction of the host cell. This reaction was independent of the host and of the race of *C. lindemuthianum,* occurring whenever any cultivar was infected with an incompatible race. Therefore, from present evidence it seems unlikely that races of *C. lindemuthianum* possess differential sensitivity to phaseollin. Indeed it is not necessary to invoke this concept to postulate a rôle for phaseollin in the resistance to this fungus.

Bearing in mind the toxicity of phaseollin towards *C. lindemuthianum* it can be seen from Table III that when phaseollin was estimated in extracts from the smallest amount of tissue which contained hypersensitive cells, the concentration 5 days after inoculation was greatly in excess of that required to inhibit germ-tube growth. However, the concentration of phaseollin at the site of inhibition of hyphal growth may be even greater since the excised tissue contained a very high proportion of uninfected cells. Less than 20% of the epidermal cells were infected and the tissue also included several layers of uninfected cells. In order to take these facts into consideration an attempt was

TABLE IV

Effect of addition of phaseollin on further growth of pre-existing germ tubes of *C. lindemuthianum*, race δ

Phaseollin concentration (μg/ml)	Length of germ-tubes after 44 h[1] (μm)	Description of hyphae
30	62	Hyphae distorted with large swellings
20	49	Hyphae distorted with large swellings
10	53	Hyphae distorted with large swellings
6	124	Hyphae distorted with small swellings
3	114	Hyphae distorted with small swellings
1	>500	Hyphal mat; small swellings on hyphae
Control with propane-1,2-diol (2% v/v)	>500	Hyphal mat; no swellings observed
Control without propane-1,2-diol	>500	Hyphal mat; no swellings observed

[1] Mean of two replicates, each of 50 germ tubes.
Mean length of germ tubes before addition of phaseollin was 167 μm.

made to measure the volume of infected cells and to calculate the concentration of phaseollin on a cellular basis (Table VI).

This calculation was based on the assumption, as discussed above, that phaseollin only accumulated in infected cells. Hypocotyls were inoculated with *C. lindemuthianum* and five days later the mean volume of an epidermal cell and the mean number of infected cells at each 'inoculated site' was measured. This allowed the total volume of infected cells at an inoculated site to be calculated. The mean amount of phaseollin at each inoculated site was determined and the concentration of phaseollin was expressed as the weight of phaseollin/volume of infected cell. Values of 4250 and 3370 μg/cm^3 infected cell were obtained from the two interactions studied. Thus, even if phaseollin were also present in a few cells adjacent to the infected cell, the amount of phaseollin at the site of hyphal growth five days after inoculation was very much greater than that which would be required to prevent hyphal growth. Whether sufficient phaseollin had accumulated to be effective at the time when hyphal growth was first restricted, requires more precise studies of the events which occur during and immediately after penetration of the host cell by an incompatible fungal germ tube.

No evidence was obtained to indicate that the rate of phaseollin accumulation was different in hypersensitive and susceptible reactions. Results showed that the time of phaseollin production, apparently determined by the time of cellular disorganization, was of great importance. This contrasts with data from soybean

TABLE V

Effect of phaseollin on the germination of *C. lindemuthianum*

Phaseollin[1] concentration (μg/ml)	β Germination[2] (%)	β Germ tube length[3] (μm)	δ Germination[2] (%)	δ Germ tube length[3] (μm)	γ Germination[2] (%)	γ Germ tube length[3] (μm)
50	nil	nil	nil	nil	nil	nil
20	nil	nil	nil	nil	nil	nil
15	nil	nil	nil	nil	nil	nil
10	nil	nil	nil	nil	nil	nil
5	70	102	79	94	81	55
1	81	93	48	87	92	130
0.1	66	109	68	116	85	116
0.0	80	102	94	159	79	102
Nutrient solution only	73	136	54	139	78	106

[1] Solutions of phaseollin were obtained by dissolving in ethanol and adjusting the final concentration of ethanol to 20% with nutrient solution.
[2] Mean of two replicates, each of 100 spores.
[3] Mean of two replicates, each of 30 germ tubes.

TABLE VI

Calculation of phaseollin concentration in hypersensitive cells 5 days after inoculation

	Cultivar-race combination	
	Imuna-β	Kievit-δ
Weight of phaseollin per 'inoculated site' (μg)	0.125	0.057
Mean number of brown cells per 'inoculated site'[1]	1470	445
Mean volume of epidermal cell (μm^3) [2]	2×10^4	3.8×10^4
Phaseollin concentration ($\mu g/cm^3$ brown cell)	4.25×10^3	3.37×10^3

[1] Mean value obtained by counting the number of brown cells in an area of 0.21 mm^2 on 'inoculated sites' whose area was 6.25 mm^2. Fifty areas were chosen from 20 'inoculated sites' obtained from 5 hypocotyls.

[2] The lengths and widths of epidermal cells were measured by light microscopy of epidermal surfaces. The depths of epidermal cells were obtained from electron micrographs of similar hypocotyls.

(Keen, 1971) which indicated that the rate of accumulation of phytoalexin determined whether inhibitory concentrations were produced and hence whether fungal growth was restricted. This difference is probably explained by the fact that both resistance and susceptibility resulted in immediate tissue damage and resistance was expressed as a limitation of lesion size and not as hypersensitivity.

Similar investigations, which have concentrated on the timing of events immediately after inoculation, have been carried out by Tomiyama and his co-workers. They have studied the resistance of different cultivars of potato (*Solanum tuberosum*) to *P. infestans.* After examination of cut surfaces of petioles and tubers, which had been inoculated with an incompatible race of *P. infestans,* they described many details of the infection process and the resulting restriction of hyphal growth (Tomiyama, 1967). With regard to the importance of phytoalexins in this interaction, they isolated the sesquiterpene rishitin from infected tissue and showed it to be markedly antifungal (Katsui *et al.,* 1968). By merging their studies of the biological events with those of rishitin accumulation they demonstrated that death of infected petiole cells did not cause immediate restriction of hyphal growth, but that decreased rate of hyphal growth was only observed when rishitin was first detected several hours after the death of infected cells. Further, they showed that, at the time of lesion limitation, the concentration of rishitin in the surface layers of cells of potato tubers was sufficient to inhibit completely further growth of *P. infestans* (Sato *et al.*, 1971).

Phaseollin Accumulation in Response to other Infections

This discussion of results obtained by use of *C. lindemuthianum* has indicated a very close association between cellular browning and phaseollin production during both hypersensitive and susceptible reactions (Tables I, II and III). Further experiments were thus carried out to show whether this relationship was also true for infections by other agents and to determine whether the results might clarify how phaseollin is produced in infected tissues.

Uromyces appendiculatus. Comparable results were obtained using a strain of *U. appendiculatus*, which in many ways reacted with *P. vulgaris* in a manner similar to *C. lindemuthianum.* Inoculation on to cv. Imuna caused no cellular browning but gave rise to the eruption of uredia two days after appearance of chlorotic flecks. Inoculation on to Line no. 765 also caused localized flecking, but the flecks were brown as a result of disruption of the host cells. From these brown flecks much smaller uredia erupted eight days later. As occurred after infection by *C. lindemuthianum*, phaseollin was only detected in leaves which showed cellular browning. Phaseollin was not detected in uninoculated leaves of either cv. Imuna or Line no. 765, nor in leaves of cv. Imuna which had been inoculated with *U. appendiculatus* (Table VII).

Table VII

Phaseollin content of leaves 6 days after inoculation with *U. appendiculatus*[1]

	Fresh wt. of leaves (g)	Phaseollin content (μg)	Phaseollin content (μg/g leaf)
Imuna, uninoculated	16.0	No phaseollin was detected	
Imuna, inoculated with *U. appendiculatus*[2]	17.5	No phaseollin was detected	
No. 765, uninoculated	24.0	No phaseollin was detected	
No. 765, inoculated with *U. appendiculatus*[3]	25.0	42	1.7

[1] From Bailey and Ingham (1971).
[2] Leaves bore chlorotic flecks.
[3] Leaves bore small superficial brown flecks.

Pseudomonas phaseolicola. Leaves of cv. Red Mexican which had reacted hypersensitively and become brown following inoculation with race 1 of *P. phaseolicola* also contained large amounts of phaseollin. Similar leaves which had been inoculated with race 2 supported bacterial growth and became water-soaked with little browning. These leaves contained considerably less phaseollin (Table VIII).

TABLE VIII

Concentrations of phaseollin in leaves after inoculation with *P. phaseolicola*[1]

Experiment	Days after injection	μg Phaseollin detected/g leaf Race 1 Hypersensitive	Race 2 Susceptible
1	3	220.3	29.7
1	5	217.5	17.6
2	5	183.6	18.4

[1] From Stholasuta *et al.* (1971).

Tobacco necrosis virus. Infection by TNV caused small discrete brown lesions in leaves and similarly coloured lesions which eventually spread throughout the entire tissue in etiolated hypocotyls. Phaseollin accumulated in both infected leaves and hypocotyls. As can be seen in Tables IX and X, phaseollin was again detected only in brown tissue; none was detected in either uninoculated tissue or in virus-infected hypocotyls before browning occurred.

TABLE IX

Phaseollin concentration in tissue 4 days after inoculation with TNV[1]

	Phaseollin concentration μg/g fresh leaf
TNV-infected leaves showing brown necrotic flecking	11.1
Control; leaves treated with 0.1 M phosphate buffer	No phaseollin was detected
TNV-infected hypocotyls showing superficial brown necrosis	3.6
Control; hypocotyl treated with 0.1 M phosphate buffer	No phaseollin was detected

[1] Data from Bailey and Ingham (1971).

TABLE X

Phaseollin concentration in etiolated hypocotyls following inoculation with TNV

Incubation period (h)	Visual symptoms	Phaseollin concentration[1] µg/g hypocotyl
0	None	No phaseollin was detected
32	None	No phaseollin was detected
67	Brown superficial streaks	7.6
74	Brown superficial streaks	9.1
91	Extensive browning of entire hypocotyl	28.2
98	Extensive browning of entire hypocotyl	52.0
115	Extensive browning of entire hypocotyl	49.4

[1] Phaseollin concentration measured by ultraviolet spectrophotometry.

CONCLUSIONS

These experiments with *C. lindemuthianum, U. appendiculatus, P. phaseolicola* and tobacco necrosis virus have produced similar results which indicate a very close relationship between necrosis (cell death), cellular browning and phaseollin accumulation. This relationship was found to be both temporal (i.e. phaseollin accumulated at the time when cells became brown) and also spatial (i.e. phaseollin was present only in brown tissues). Further, they indicate that phaseollin accumulation is not related to the amount of fungal growth; both *C. lindemuthianum* and *U. appendiculatus* grew extensively in susceptible tissue without causing either cellular browning or phaseollin accumulation. If, as has been suggested by Cruickshank and Perrin (1968) and by Hadwiger and Schwochau (1969), metabolites diffusing from the fungus are responsible for inducing phaseollin synthesis, extensive fungal growth would have been expected to result in the formation of large amounts of phaseollin. Moreover, TNV which is unlikely to produce compounds such as monilicolin A (Cruickshank and Perrin, 1968) or other unknown constituents of fungal culture filtrates known to stimulate phaseollin formation (Rathmell and Bendall, 1971) also caused large quantities of phaseollin to accumulate in brown infected tissue. It is thus highly improbable that the production of phaseollin in hypocotyls following infection by *C. lindemuthianum* is directly controlled by diffusible fungal metabolites.

It can also be concluded that the hypersensitive reaction required for rapid hyphal growth limitation, and hence resistance, depended on bean cells undergoing necrosis in response to the presence of incompatible hyphae. It is also suggested that compatible hyphae have the capacity not to cause immediate reactions in the infected cells and as a result not to cause phaseollin accumulation, and that it is this which enables hyphae to colonize tissue extensively. Thus, phaseollin which accumulated in hypersensitive cells and which was probably an important factor in restricting hyphal growth, must be considered as one of many novel metabolites (Rahe *et al.*, 1969; Bailey, unpublished results) arising from general metabolic changes which occur in infected cells as a direct result of necrosis.

References

Allen, E. H. and Thomas, C. A. (1971). Time course of safynol accumulation in resistant and susceptible safflower infected with *Phytophthora drechsleri. Physiol. Pl. Pathol.* **1**, 235-240.

Bailey, J. A. and Deverall, B. J. (1971). Formation and activity of phaseollin in the interaction between bean hypocotyls (*Phaseolus vulgaris*) and physiological races of *Colletotrichum lindemuthianum. Physiol. Pl. Pathol.* **1**, 435-449.

Bailey, J. A. and Ingham, J. L. (1971). Phaseollin accumulation in bean (*Phaseolus vulgaris*) in response to infection by tobacco necrosis virus and the rust *Uromyces appendiculatus. Physiol. Pl. Pathol.* **1**, 451-456.

Bell, A. A. (1969). Phytoalexin production and verticillium wilt resistance in cotton. *Phytopathology* **59**, 1119-1127.

Cruickshank, I. A. M. (1962). Studies on phytoalexins. IV. The antimicrobial spectrum of pisatin. *Aust. J. biol. Sci.* **15**, 147-159.

Cruickshank, I. A. M. and Perrin, D. R. (1963). Phytoalexins of the leguminosae. Phaseollin from *Phaseolus vulgaris* L. *Life Sci.* **2**, 680-682.

Cruickshank, I. A. M. and Perrin, D. R. (1968). The isolation and partial characterization of monilicolin A, a polypeptide with phaseollin-inducing activity from *Monilinia fructicola. Life Sci.* **7**, 449-458.

Cruickshank, I. A. M. and Perrin, D. R. (1971). Studies on phytoalexins. XI The induction, antimicrobial spectrum and chemical assay of phaseollin. *Phytopath. Z.* **70**, 209-229.

Gray, G., Klarman, W. L. and Bridge, M. (1968). Relative quantities of antifungal metabolites produced in resistant and susceptible soybean plants inoculated with *Phytophthora megasperma* var. *sojae* and closely related non-pathogenic fungi. *Can. J. Bot.* **46**, 285-288.

Hadwiger, L. A. and Schwochau, M. E. (1969). Host resistance responses—an induction hypothesis. *Phytopathology* **59**, 223-227.

Higgins, V. J. and Millar, R. L. (1970). Degradation of alfalfa phytoalexin by *Stemphylium loti* and *Colletotrichum phomoides. Phytopathology* **60**, 269-271.

Katsui, K., Murai, A., Takasugi, M., Imaizumi, K. and Masamune, T. (1968). The structure of rishitin, a new antifungal compound from diseased potato tubers. *Chem. Commun.* No. **1**, 43-44.

Keen, N. T. (1971). Hydroxyphaseollin production by soybeans resistant and susceptible to *Phytophthora megasperma* var. *sojae. Physiol. Pl. Pathol.* **1**, 265-275.

Kuć, J. (1968). Biochemical control of disease resistance in plants. *Wld Rev. Pest Contr.* **7**, 42-55.

Leach, J. G. (1923). The parasitism of *Colletotrichum lindemuthianum*. *Bull. Minn. agric. Exp. Stn* **14**.

Müller, K. O. (1958). Studies on phytoalexins. I. The formation and the immunological significance of phytoalexin produced by *Phaseolus vulgaris* in response to infections with *Sclerotinia fructicola* and *Phytophthora infestans*. *Aust. J. biol. Sci.* **11**, 275-300.

Pierre, R. E. and Bateman, D. F. (1967). Induction and distribution of phytoalexins in *Rhizoctonia*-infected bean hypocotyls. *Phytopathology* **57**, 1154-1160.

Rahe, J. E., Kuć, J., Chien-Mei Chuang and Williams, E. B. (1969). Correlation of phenolic metabolism with histological changes in *Phaseolus vulgaris* inoculated with fungi. *Neth. J. Pl. Path.* **75**, 58-71.

Rathmell, W. G. and Bendall, D. S. (1971). Phenolic compounds in relation to phytoalexin biosynthesis in hypocotyls of *Phaseolus vulgaris*. *Physiol. Pl. Pathol.* **1**, 351-362.

Sato, N. and Tomiyama, K. (1969) Localized accumulation of rishitin in the potato tuber tissue infected by an incompatible race of *Phytophthora infestans*. *Ann. phytopath. Soc. Japan* **35**, 202-217.

Sato, N., Kitazawa, K. and Tomiyama, K. (1971). The role of rishitin in localizing the invading hyphae of *Phytophthora infestans* in infection sites at the cut surfaces of potato tubers. *Physiol. Pl. Pathol.* **1**, 289-395.

Skipp, R. A. (1971). 'Factors affecting the resistance and susceptibility of *Phaseolus vulgaris* to races of *Colletotrichum lindemuthianum*'. Ph.D. thesis, University of London.

Stholasuta, P., Bailey, J. A., Severin, V. and Deverall, B. J. (1971). Effect of bacterial inoculation of bean and pea leaves on the accumulation of phaseollin and pisatin. *Physiol. Pl. Pathol.* **1**, 177-183.

Tomiyama, K. (1967). Further observations on the time requirement for hypersensitive cell death of potatoes infected by *Phytophthora infestans* and its relation to metabolic activity. *Phytopath. Z.* **58**, 367-378.

Wit-Elshove, A. de (1969). The role of pisatin in the resistance of pea plants–some further experiments on the breakdown of pisatin. *Neth. J. Pl. Pathol.* **75**, 164-168.

DISCUSSION

Dr E. J. Hewitt: Would it be of interest to use an entirely new approach to obtain cell death, by inducing localized necrotic areas of groups of cells. For example, certain mineral deficiencies produce little groups of necrotic cells which would look very much like a group of the cells infected by a fungus, and which by your elegant methods could be assayed for phytoalexins?

Dr J. A. Bailey: In that situation, probably yes. I could add that we have tried to injure tissue, and we have never obtained any induction of phytoalexins.

Dr Hewitt: Did you try spraying with dilute acid?

Dr Bailey: No. We tried hitting or bruising it. But in these cases I feel death is so quick that none of the necessary reactions take place. But are you suggesting that death resulting from your treatments may in fact be a slow process?

Dr Hewitt: You could get a slow internal necrosis occurring under physiological conditions produced by an entirely different method of injuring the cells.

Dr Bailey: In that situation I think it would be very interesting to look at this.

Dr Hewitt: I should think that with beans, manganese excess or manganese deficiency would both have quite interesting results.

Dr R. B. Drysdale: I am not very happy about the opening statement that in a susceptible plant the fungus grows, and in a resistant one it does not. There are many cases in plant biology of plants which are heavily infected with a virus showing no symptoms, and you can have a plant with a fairly small quantity of a different strain of the virus and this will show very many symptoms. So I do not think that you should accept that because a plant is resistant, the fungus is incapable of growing in it. I do not think that we have a particularly good method of assessing whether or not a fungus can grow in a plant.

Dr Bailey: Yes, I accept that.

Professor P. H. Williams: Do you know whether the continued presence of the fungus is necessary for the production of phytoalexins? Have you attempted to kill a fungus at various stages after putting it on, say with a contact fungicide or a systemic, and seen whether you can continue to induce phaseollin?

Dr Bailey: No, I have not.

Professor Williams: Do you know whether the presence of the fungus is required, or whether a single event is sufficient?

Dr Bailey: In a disease situation of this kind I do not know whether the fungus is necessary once the phaseollin accumulation has started, but there is obviously a lot of evidence that you can cause it to accumulate without the fungus. It would be very interesting to find out.

Dr E. C. Hislop: Do you discount the possibility that the pathogen is inducing a reaction in the host by some diffusible metabolite? Would you consider ethylene to be a possible cause of the hypersensitive reaction, because we would predict that at a very early stage the plants which show a hypersensitive reaction might well produce an excessive amount of ethylene compared with the susceptible ones. This would be very easy to measure.

Dr Bailey: I would certainly expect ethylene to be produced at this time.

Dr Hislop: At a very early stage of infection there would be larger amounts in the resistant tissue than in the susceptible tissue, and this could be the initiator of changed metabolism, before you can see the death of the cell.

Dr Bailey: You would get more ethylene in the resistant plant?

Dr Hislop: This is what I would predict.

Dr Bailey: I am not sure that this would give you a great deal more information, because you have still got to know what triggers off this reaction, and the ethylene may simply be a product of the necrosis as is phaseollin.

Dr Hislop: I would suggest that ethylene may occur long before you get indications of necrosis, and that ethylene may be the stimulator of the phytoalexin production via the phenylalanine–ammonia-lyase pathway.

Dr Bailey: We have not tested this. I could add, however, that we have investigated the effects of endogenous ethylene on both the hypersensitive and susceptible reactions. Ethylene neither broke resistance nor induced susceptibility.

Professor P. W. Brian: I entirely accept that in your particular system the production of the phaseollin appears to be quite closely associated with cell necrosis, but I would like to get this clear; is it not true that you can induce production of phaseollin in *Phaseolus* leaves or stems with fungal diffusates, without cell necrosis?

Dr Bailey: You can induce it, and probably you can do so without necrosis–this is Rathmell and Bendall's work. Also, Cruickshank has isolated monilicolin A from fungal mycelium and shown that it induces phaseollin without causing cell death.

Professor Brian: In the case of other phytoalexins, cell death is not always necessary.

Dr Bailey: Inducing agents may not cause cell death, and I think it may well be that induction by chemicals and induction following fungal infection are separate phenomena. The induction by extraneous chemicals may act directly on the biosynthetic pathway, but during infection, although the same pathway is eventually involved, the control mechanism is different.

Professor Brian: By what means, other than by the effect of some diffusible substance from your fungus, can it induce the formation of the phaseollin? What have you got in mind?

Dr Bailey: It could be a surface phenomenon of the hypha.

Dr D. Price: Do you get the same reactions if you use whole plants rather than excised hypocotyls, and also do you get similar reactions if you alter the concentrations of your inoculum.

Dr Bailey: The answer to the first question is yes; as seen on the slide which was lent by Dr Ian Smith, it was shown that the specificity of the races when sprayed onto a whole plant was identical to the specificity obtained in our system. Whether there has been any detailed investigation of the infection process in his situation, I do not know. As regards the second question, a low concentration of an incompatible race will have very little effect, obviously you get a few infected cells which are very difficult to find. This increases as you increase the inoculum to about 5×10^5.

Dr Price: At these very high concentrations we are moving a long way away from what actually occurs in field infections, aren't we?

Dr Bailey: Yes, this is true, though the cellular responses are probably identical.

Professor R. K. S. Wood: I am rather fascinated by this idea that you can kill cells at different speeds, or that cells can die at different speeds, and that this will mediate an entirely different series of reactions which decide whether or not phytoalexins are produced. You quote in your case *Colletotrichum lindemuthianum,* in which the process of cell death may be rather slow, but I think it is rather different in potato attacked by avirulent hyphae of *Phytophthora infestans,* when I believe the whole sequence of reactions happen very much more rapidly.

Dr Bailey: Yes, I think there must be a time when the cell is alive and then very soon it is dead, but I think it is the processes that occur after the beginning of death and which continue for some time that are important. Is the same true for *Phytophthora*?

Professor Wood: There will be people in the audience who will have seen Tomiyama's work on this. I think it did happen very rapidly, within 30 min or so.

Dr Bailey: Is the complete reaction finished?

Professor Wood: Perhaps not quite complete, but almost. If I may refer to the very provocative question by Professor Brian, that it is very puzzling indeed that you cannot reproduce these reactions with cell-free extracts. Are you suggesting that these are bound substances, for how other than by extra-cellular metabolites do you suggest that the pathogen invokes changes that lead to cell-death?

Dr Bailey: I suggest that cell death may be evoked by phenomena on the surface of the invading hypha interacting with the host cell.

Dr J. P. Blakeman: From your work it would appear that saprophytic fungi are unlikely to induce phaseollin production. If this is so, there would be a marked difference here from the situation in pea where it seems that saprophytic organisms can readily induce pisatin.

Dr Bailey: Cruickshank has shown that if you take a saprophytic organism and put it in an inside cavity of a bean pod you do induce phaseollin formation.

Dr Blakeman: Without the occurrence of the necrosis and cellular browning to which you have referred?

Dr Bailey: Cruickshank does not report whether necrosis occurred.

IV. 2 The Diversity of Phytoalexin-like Responses in Leguminosae*

I. M. SMITH

Department of Botany and Plant Technology, Imperial College, London

Introduction

If the pod cavities of a legume such as French bean are inoculated with a spore suspension of an avirulent fungus, a complex series of changes is initiated (Smith, 1970). The fungal spores germinate and the germ tubes penetrate the endocarp cells, causing discoloration and necrosis. Further growth of the fungus is checked and analysis of the spore suspension liquid (diffusate) shows it to have become inhibitory to spore germination. Many chromatographically distinct compounds accumulate in diffusates by comparison with water controls, and individual compounds account for inhibitory activity (phaseollin and at least one other compound in bean). The fact that these inhibitors are absent from uninfected pods and are induced by fungal infection has led to their classification as phytoalexins, and phytoalexin formation in the pod-diffusate system has been regarded as a primary resistance mechanism (Cruickshank and Perrin, 1961).

However, the observation that the synthesis of phenolic phytoalexins in French bean is closely accompanied by other changes in phenolic metabolism led me to doubt whether a strict resistance mechanism was operating (Smith, 1970). Accordingly, a survey was carried out on a number of leguminous plants to determine their over-all response to pod infection by a non-pathogen (Smith, 1971). The aim was to establish (*i*) whether a phytoalexin system of some sort was of general occurrence in legumes and (*ii*) how phytoalexin production was related to over-all post-infectional changes. An outline of the results of this survey will be given, followed by a discussion of its implications in relation to recent work on resistance mechanisms in legumes.

Results

Details of the methods used in the survey have been given elsewhere (Smith, 1970, 1971). The procedure for all species was essentially the collection and

* The research on which this paper is based was carried out at Makerere University, Kampala, Uganda.

bioassay of diffusates from inoculated and untreated (control) pods. This was followed by paper chromatographic analysis of organic-solvent extracts from diffusates and bioassay of chromatograms to determine which of the accumulating compounds accounted for inhibitory activity. *Colletotrichum lindemuthianum* race δ was used as the infecting fungus.

Table I shows the results of bioassays of diffusates and of successive petroleum ether and diethyl ether extracts taken from them. The species have been grouped according to these results. Group I either gave non-inhibitory diffusates or else the inhibitory factor was not recovered in organic solvent extracts. Group II gave inhibitory diffusates and extracts for the infected but not the control treatment. Group III gave inhibitory diffusates and extracts from both treatments.

Strong necrotic discoloration was observed in infected hyacinth bean, French bean, pigeon pea and cluster bean. Moderate discoloration was observed in green gram, black gram and cowpea, and slight discoloration in the remaining species. Thus necrotic discoloration was not apparently related to inhibitor production (Table I). However, the control/'infected' pattern of Table I was repeated with

TABLE I

Bioassay of diffusates and their fractions

Group	Species	Control Diff.	Control PE	Control DE	Infected Diff.	Infected PE	Infected DE
I	Sunn hemp	–	–	–	–	–	–
	Green gram	+	–	–	+	–	–
	Black gram	–	–	–	–	–	–
II	Jack bean	–	–	–	++	++	++
	Sword bean	+	–	–	++	++	++
	Soybean	–	–	–	+	–	+
	Hyacinth bean	+	–	–	++	++	–
	French bean	–	–	–	++	++	++
	Pea	–	–	–	++	++	–
	Cowpea	–	–	–	++	–	+
III	Groundnut	++	+	+	++	+	+
	Pigeon pea	++	++	–	++	++	–
	Chick pea	++	++	–	++	++	–
	Cluster bean	++	++	++	++	++	++

–, normal germination;
+, reduced germination and germ tubes very short;
++, zero germination;
Diff, whole diffusate;
PE, petroleum ether fraction;
DE, diethyl ether fraction.

respect to necrotic discoloration, so that species in groups I and III gave a similar reaction for both control and infected plants, while group-II species gave a more intense reaction for those infected.

Table II shows the number of compounds detected on paper chromatograms of diffusate extracts. This includes compounds fluorescing under ultraviolet light and compounds reacting with diazotized sulphanilic acid (DSA). This represents only a proportion of the total potential change in phenolic compounds, for compounds not partitioning into ether (e.g. phenolic glycosides) or chromatographically immobile compounds will not have been detected or separated. The figures are arranged to show the number of compounds which increased in concentration after infection. A clear increase was characteristic of all group-II species and even group-III species showed some increase, although with this group the number and intensity of compounds in controls was relatively high. Generally it was the DSA-reacting compounds which showed most change in group II. The pattern of compounds was different for every species.

Finally, Table III shows the number of regions on chromatograms found to be inhibitory to spore germination, and the number of these coinciding with a positive DSA reaction. In group III, these compounds were detected on both control and 'infected' chromatograms, while in group II they were detected as

TABLE II

Number of compounds detected on chromatograms of PE and DE fractions

Group	Species	PE fraction Control[1]	PE fraction Infected	DE fraction Control[1]	DE fraction Infected
I	Sunn hemp	2	2	9	14
	Green gram	1	1	3	7
	Black gram	1	1	4	4
II	Jack bean	0	5	0	10
	Sword bean	2	8	0	10
	Soybean	0	1	3	7
	Hyacinth bean	1	5	0	14
	French bean	1	3	2	12
	Pea	0	2	2	12
	Cowpea	0	0	9	14
III	Groundnut	3	4	6	13
	Pigeon pea	5	6	7	7
	Chick pea	7	7	4	12
	Cluster bean	8	8	4	10

[1] Number of compounds present at the same concentration as on chromatograms of 'infected' fraction.

TABLE III

Number of inhibitory zones detected on chromatograms of PE and DE fractions

Group	Species	PE	DE	DSA[1]
I	Sunn hemp	0	0	0
	Green gram	0	0	0
	Black gram	0	0	0
II	Jack bean	2	1	2
	Sword bean	1	1	1
	Soybean	0	1	1
	Hyacinth bean	1	0	1
	French bean	1	1	2
	Pea	1	0	0
	Cowpea	1	0	0
III	Groundnut	1	0	1
	Pigeon pea	1	0	1
	Chick pea	2	0	1
	Cluster bean	4	1	4

[1] Number of zones coinciding with a positive DSA reaction.

inhibitors only on 'infected' chromatograms, although traces of colour reaction indicated their possible presence in controls in some cases. Several species gave more than one inhibitory zone. A majority of the inhibitors was found in the PE fraction, and most of the inhibitors coincided with a positive DSA reaction.

DISCUSSION

Interpretation of the results of the survey is to some extent limited by the fact that they were obtained by the artificial pod-diffusate system. This system may give misleading results by comparison with the more realistic hypocotyl infection model, particularly when susceptible host-parasite combinations are studied (Bailey and Deverall, 1971). However, the differences are quantitative rather than qualitative, and the pod-diffusate system can be considered to provide a reasonable model of host resistance to a non-pathogen in qualitative terms.

All species, except three in the survey accumulated one or more inhibitors in diffusates after inoculation, at a total concentration sufficient to inhibit further spore germination and germ-tube growth. This result substantiates the general hypothesis that legumes can protect themselves from fungal infection by the formation of antifungal substances. The failure to detect such substances in the three species of group I cannot be explained at present and requires further investigation to determine whether it is real or an experimental artefact.

The group II species evidently formed their inhibitors as a result of infection, so that their reaction was of the phytoalexin type. Group III species gave similar results for control and infected treatments but the high control values for pigeon pea and cluster bean are thought to be due to mechanical damage and possible slight contamination, since necrosis was observed in both control and infected pods. The inhibitors are, therefore, not thought to be pre-formed, and these two species could be considered as giving an easily induced group II reaction. In the other two group III species (chickpea and groundnut), there was little necrosis and fungal spores germinated very poorly in the pod cavities. This clearly suggested the presence of preformed inhibitors and the possibility will be discussed further below.

The common features of the group-II phytoalexin reaction were visible necrosis and the accumulation of many phenolic and other compounds, some of which were inhibitory. This can most simply be interpreted in terms of a general disturbance of phenolic metabolism, presumably involving increases in the activity of enzymes such as phenylalanine ammonia lyase, which controls the early stages of the biosynthesis of all phenolic compounds and is known to increase in activity after infection of pea and bean (Hadwiger *et al.*, 1970). Polyphenol oxidase will also increase in activity and a certain proportion of existing and newly synthesized phenols will be oxidized and polymerized to the accumulating dark pigments.

In most species, only one accumulating compound was inhibitory. The main inhibitory compounds in pea, French bean and soybean were probably the pterocarpans pisatin (Cruickshank and Perrin, 1961), phaseollin (Cruickshank and Perrin, 1971) and hydroxyphaseollin (Keen, 1971) respectively. Some of the inhibitors in other species had similar properties in solvent partition and chromatography and could also be pterocarpans. Superficially at least, there was no indication that altered metabolism was preferentially directed towards phytoalexin biosynthesis, as has been suggested for pisatin in peas (Hadwiger and Schwochau, 1969). However, the method used did integrate events over the whole incubation period and over more or less affected cells. It is possible, therefore, that in at least some species the immediate reaction to infection was rapid synthesis of phytoalexin and that this was obscured by later necrotic changes. Recent biochemical work (Rathmell and Bendall, 1971) has suggested a degree of compartmentation in diseased phenolic metabolism in French bean, isoflavonoid synthesis being stimulated while flavonols were unaffected. Time course experiments with infected French beans (Bailey and Deverall, 1971; Rahe *et al.*, 1969) and soybeans (Frank and Paxton, 1970; Keen, 1971) have strongly suggested, however, that in a situation of true infection phytoalexin accumulation takes place at the same time or later than the accumulation of other compounds and the initiation of necrosis. The results for group II in the survey are explained most simply in these terms.

While a phytoalexin-like response was found in most of the legumes studied, two species (chickpea and groundnut) behaved as though they contained preformed antifungal inhibitors. Such a situation has already been observed in broad bean (Fawcett *et al.*, 1969) and in red clover (Virtanen and Hietala, 1958; Bredenberg, 1961; Bredenberg and Hietala, 1961). The broad bean inhibitor, wyerone, is exceptional in not being phenolic and, though present without infection, wyerone (or the related wyerone acid) can accumulate after infection (Letcher *et al.*, 1970; Fawcett *et al.*, 1971). The antifungal compounds in clover are a pterocarpan glycoside, trifolirhizin, and two isoflavones, biochanin A and formononetin. Both isoflavones are also known to occur in some quantity in chickpea (Barz and Hösel, 1971) and formononetin is present in alfalfa (Olah and Sherwood, 1971). The status of these compounds in disease resistance is uncertain, for they are much less inhibitory than pterocarpan phytoalexins. However, they occur in relatively high concentrations in clover (Wong, 1962), greater than the inhibitory level quoted by Virtanen *et al.* (1957). Schultz (1967) demonstrated that isoflavones are mostly present as glycosides in clover, and Olah and Sherwood (1971) have shown that infection of alfalfa leads to the hydrolysis of isoflavone glycosides. The relative antifungal activity of the glycosides and aglycones is not known, but Perrin and Cruickshank (1969) have shown that maackiain, the aglycone of trifolirhizin, is much more active than its glycoside. Release of antifungal phenolic compounds by hydrolysis has been observed in lima bean (Bell, 1970) and this process may, therefore, contribute to disease resistance in several legumes.

In the present survey, the compound mainly responsible for antifungal activity in chickpea was not one of the major isoflavones, and could be a pterocarpan (present without infection). In alfalfa, the pterocarpan inhibitor medicarpin is formed after infection (Smith *et al.*, 1971). The relative importance of all these isoflavonoid compounds in disease resistance in clover, chickpea and alfalfa is, therefore, still unclear, although it is probable that host-parasite interaction in isoflavonoid-rich species follows a different pattern from that in legumes in which isoflavonoid synthesis is initiated only after infection.

In conclusion, the legumes studied in the survey mostly reacted to infection by a phytoalexin type of response. This response was different in detail for every species, but the general pattern was of many phenolic compounds accumulating, one or several of these being inhibitory to spore germination in bioassays. The response was in most cases not of the classic phytoalexin type, being complex and in some cases induced without infection. Preformed inhibitors may be important in some species, although hydrolysis may be required for their release in active form.

REFERENCES

Bailey, J. A. and Deverall, B. J. (1971). Formation and activity of phaseollin in the interaction between bean hypocotyls (*Phaseolus vulgaris*) and physiological races of *Colletotrichum lindemuthianum*. *Physiol. Pl. Pathol.* **1**, 435-449.

Barz, W. and Hösel, W. (1971). Über den Umsatz von Flavonolen und Isoflavonen in *Cicer arietinum*. *Phytochemistry* **10**, 335-341.

Bell, A. A. (1970). 4-Hydroxybenzaldehyde and vanillin as toxins formed in leaf wound sap of *Phaseolus lunatus*. *Phytopathology* **60**, 161-165.

Bredenberg, J. B. (1961). Identification of an antifungal factor in red clover as biochanin A. *Suomen Kemistilehti B* **34**, 23.

Bredenberg, J. B. and Hietala, P. K. (1961). Investigation of the structure of trifolirhizin, an antifungal compound from *Trifolium pratense* L. *Acta chem. scand.* **15**, 696-699.

Cruickshank, I. A. M. and Perrin, D. R. (1961). Studies on phytoalexins. III. The isolation, assay and general properties of a phytoalexin from *Pisum sativum* L. *Aust. J. biol. Sci.* **14**, 336-348.

Cruickshank, I. A. M. and Perrin, D. R. (1971). Studies on phytoalexins. XI. The induction, antimicrobial spectrum and chemical assay of phaseollin. *Phytopath. Z.* **70**, 209-229.

Fawcett, C. H., Spencer, D. M. and Wain, R. L. (1969). The isolation and properties of a fungicidal compound present in seedlings of *Vicia faba*. *Neth. J. Pl. Path.* **75**, 72-81.

Fawcett, C. H., Firn, D. R. and Spencer, D. M. (1971). Wyerone increase in leaves of broad bean (*Vicia faba* L.) after infection by *Botrytis fabae*. *Physiol. Pl. Pathol.* **1**, 163-166.

Frank, J. A. and Paxton, J. D. (1970). Time sequence for phytoalexin production in Harosoy and Harosoy 63 soybeans. *Phytopathology* **60**, 315-318.

Hadwiger, L. A., Hess, S. L. and von Broembsen, S. (1970). Stimulation of phenylalanine ammonia lyase and phytoalexin production. *Phytopathology* **60**, 332-336.

Hadwiger, L. A. and Schwochau, M. E. (1969). Host resistance responses—an induction hypothesis. *Phytopathology* **59**, 223-227.

Keen, N. T. (1971). Hydroxyphaseollin production by soybeans resistant and susceptible to *Phytophthora megasperma* var. *sojae*. *Physiol. Pl. Pathol.* **1**, 265-275.

Letcher, R. M., Widdowson, D. A., Deverall, B. J. and Mansfield, J. W. (1970). Identification and activity of wyerone acid as a phytoalexin in broad bean (*Vicia faba*) after infection by *Botrytis*. *Phytochemistry* **9**, 249-252.

Olah, A. F. and Sherwood, R. T. (1971). Flavones, isoflavones and coumestans in alfalfa infected by *Ascochyta imperfecta*. *Phytopathology* **61**, 65-69.

Perrin, D. R. and Cruickshank, I. A. M. (1969). The antifungal activity of pterocarpans towards *Monilinia fructicola*. *Phytochemistry* **8**, 971-978.

Rahe, J. E., Kuć, J., Chien-Mei Chuang and Williams, E. B. (1969). Correlation of phenolic metabolism with histological changes in *Phaseolus vulgaris* infected with fungi. *Neth. J. Pl. Path.* **75**, 58-71.

Rathmell, W. G. and Bendall, D. S. (1971). Phenolic compounds in relation to phytoalexin biosynthesis in hypocotyls of *Phaseolus vulgaris*. *Physiol. Pl. Pathol.* **1**, 351-362.

Schultz, G. (1967). Vorkommen und Verbreitung der Isoflavonen als Glycoside bei einigen *Trifolium*-Arten. *Z. Pflanzenphysiol.* **56**, 209-219.

Smith, D. G., McInnes, A. G., Higgins, V. J. and Millar, R. L. (1971). Nature of the phytoalexin produced by alfalfa in response to fungal infection. *Physiol. Pl. Pathol.* **1**, 41-44.

Smith, I. M. (1970). Biochemical changes in French bean pods infected with *Colletotrichum lindemuthianum. Ann. appl. Biol.* **65**, 93-103.

Smith, I. M. (1971). The induction of antifungal inhibitors in pods of tropical legumes. *Physiol. Pl. Pathol.* **1**, 85-94.

Virtanen, A. I., Hietala, P. K. and Wahlroos, O. (1957). Antimicrobial substances in cereals and fodder plants. *Archs Biochem. Biophys.* **69**, 486-500.

Virtanen, A. I. and Hietala, P. K. (1958). Isolation of an anti-*Sclerotinia* factor, 7-hydroxy-4′-methoxyisoflavone, from red clover. *Acta chem. scand.* **12**, 579-580.

Wong, E. (1962). Detection and estimation of oestrogenic constituents in red clover. *J. Sci. Fd Agric.* **13**, 304-308.

DISCUSSION

Dr J. T. Martin: You refer to the diffusates being partitioned into petroleum ether and ether. The phrase 'partitioned into ether', occurs often in the literature and on occasions it is not clear what is meant. Sometimes it clearly means extraction by ether, but I take it that in your work it was partition i.e. you had an aqueous diffusate, which you shook with petroleum ether first, giving you two phases, and you found the compounds in each of them. Did you then do the same thing with ethyl ether?

Dr I. M. Smith: I used the aqueous phase already extracted with petroleum ether, applied the ethyl ether to it, and removed a further batch of material from the same solution.

Dr B. J. Deverall: I would like to ask Dr Smith for his definition of necrosis.

Dr Smith: This is very superficial, because it is necrotic discoloration, visible macroscopically and microscopically. I have not attempted to produce any really quantitative estimate of this, because it is so difficult to do so. I merely talk about a very intense discoloration or a slight discoloration.

Dr D. M. Spencer: Your technique depends on the diffusion of compounds into applied droplets. Was there any question at any time of doing direct extracts of the intact tissue to determine the presence or absence of preformed inhibitors?

Dr Smith: Sometimes I attempted this, especially when considering preformed inhibitors; I was obviously trying to look for these compounds before infection. However, I ran into the difficulty that the methods I used were not applicable readily to extracts from tissue. I was not eager to expand my survey behind its initial limits, and so did not pursue this.

Professor P. H. Williams: During the induction phase of your testing did all the spores or some of the spores germinate and penetrate the pod endocarp cells. What was the condition of the pathogen which was inducing phytoalexin?
Dr Smith: This was checked in a superficial way, certainly not all the spores would have germinated, but a high proportion would.
Professor Williams: Was there general penetration of the tissue or not?
Dr Smith: This was not followed up, but the situation that was observed was more or less the pattern of a single necrotic cell such as Dr Bailey described.
Professor Williams: So that there was a physical contact of the pathogen with the host in each case during the induction.
Dr Smith: I could not say for certain.
Professor Williams: Generally, though?
Dr Smith: I would expect it to be so, but I could not say whether the infection pegs actually got through and made contact with the host cells.
Professor Williams: Did germination occur in each case?
Dr Smith: Germination occurred, yes, except with chick pea and groundnut in which germination was poor, and I think that preformed inhibitors were involved.
Dr D. S. Ingram: Do you have any information on the bacterial population in the infection drops? You mention the possibility of contamination in induction.
Dr Smith: This was not checked specifically. I did do a minor experiment in which I attempted to clean up my procedure to the very utmost, in which everything was autoclaved to try and do it in as near sterile conditions as I could. With pigeon pea under these conditions I was able to cut down the reaction of the control by about 30%, instead of having more or less the same reaction in the control and the infected plants. The normal technique was semi-sterile, and this is why I say that contamination might have contributed to the effect, but I did not check specifically on bacteria.
Dr R. Johnson: I am interested to know why it is that phytoalexin-like substances which diffuse into water droplets, appear not to diffuse out from a lesion into other cells in the leaf, as was suggested by the previous speaker. Has anyone any explanation of this?
Dr Smith: While I was having a discussion with Dr Bailey yesterday I brought up this point. I was thinking that phaseollin should diffuse around, at least over short distances, and this may depend on the tissue. Diffusion may be very much easier in the endocarp than it is in hypocotyl or leaf tissue, and I think that the ease with which this happens may be one of the reasons why the reaction of pod tissues to specific races of *Colletotrichum* say, in bean, is in fact rather abnormal. The phaseollin may diffuse extensively and the reaction is then not the same as one would find in hypocotyls.
Dr Barbara Lund: I was assuming that you pre-treated your tissue to reduce bacterial contamination. Did you do this, and how?

Dr Smith: The pods were surface sterilized with hypochlorite.

K. M. Harrower: Can I ask about the relative age of pods in the different species, because it is known that in the pea–pathogen system, as pods mature the phytoalexin production decreases. Were the pods in the different species at the same relative state of development?

Dr Smith: Yes, I generally attempted to use pods in which the seeds were still enlarging. There was a certain amount of variation in this, which might possibly be an explanation of complete failure to detect any inhibitors in some species. The pods were at the wrong stage of development—they might have been too old.

A. van Dijkman: Is it possible to stimulate the production of these inhibitory substances with things other than *Colletotrichum lindemuthianum,* for example, mercury chloride, copper ions. If this is so, what is the significance of these inhibitory substances in plant pathology?

Dr Smith: I have induced them with mercury ions, and obviously the Australian workers have done so repeatedly. I think I have to fall back on what Dr Bailey said earlier, that there obviously must be different ways of inducing these compounds. Hadwiger would like us to believe that the inducers must interact with DNA, but I do not suppose that mercury ions have any such specific site of action. I think that the mere fact that fungal infection does induce them, and that they do inhibit a fungus that has entered in that situation is a sufficient account of their potential rôle in resistance.

IV. 3 The Resistance of Immature Bramley's Seedling Apples to Rotting by *Nectria galligena* Bres.

T. R. SWINBURNE

Plant Pathology Research Division, Ministry of Agriculture for Northern Ireland and Faculty of Agriculture Queen's University of Belfast, Northern Ireland

INTRODUCTION

Nectria galligena Bres. parasitizes a wide range of hardwood trees and causes wood cankers and fruit rots of many cultivars of apple and pear. Infection of fruit of dessert cultivars of apples occurs at the calyx and an eye-rot develops before or shortly after harvest. This can cause serious losses (Salmon and Wormald, 1915; Dillon-Weston, 1927). Rotting by this organism is the most serious cause of loss in stored Bramley's Seedling in Ireland (Swinburne, 1964; Kavanagh and Glynn, 1966), although it was rarely encountered on this cultivar in earlier surveys (Kidd and Beaumont, 1924). Infection occurs, via lenticels and wounds on any part of the fruit, before harvest (Swinburne, 1971a), but in contrast to dessert cultivars rots only appear after storage (Swinburne, 1970a), and after artificial inoculation, apples are resistant to rotting beyond the normal harvest time (Swinburne, 1964). Conidia, the most probable agents of infection, are discharged from wood cankers throughout the period of fruit development (Swinburne, 1971b), and thus infection of the fruit could occur at any time up to harvest. Rots developed most rapidly in store when unpicked apples were inoculated approximately 100 days after full blossom (i.e. end of August to the beginning of September) than earlier or later. Many inoculations made earlier or later than 100 days from full blossom resulted in necrotic lesions which did not develop into rots, and which the fungus could not be re-isolated (Swinburne, 1964, 1971a).

Storage conditions also influence rot development. Losses in refrigerated gas stored stocks are invariably greater than those in comparable stocks held in barns (Swinburne, 1970a). In a preliminary experiment (Swinburne, 1970b) it was found that the losses were not proportional to the mean carbon dioxide concentrations in stores, as had been anticipated, but were related to the degree of fluctuation of this gas during the storage period.

This paper summarizes investigations made to elucidate the nature of resistance of immature apples and to define the role of the resistance mechanism in the development of the disease.

Reaction of Immature Apples to Infection

Arrested lesions developed approximately 15 days after inoculation with *N.galligena* (by the cork borer method) of apples picked from August to October (Swinburne, 1964; 1971a). Such lesions were 15-19 mm dia. and internally the necrotic cortical tissues remained firm except for a small macerated area around the inoculum. The peel surrounding the lesions became chlorotic. The fungus could be re-isolated from the macerated area within 2 mm of the inoculum disk, but no hyphae were detected beyond this area. Those hyphae furthest from the inoculum appeared distorted. The walls of cells within the necrotic area were suberized, and the cells contained dense clusters of starch granules, whereas healthy cells from apples picked in August and September contained very few starch granules.

No further expansion of these lesions occurred until after 30-50 days incubation at 22° C. When expansion resumed, hyphae were detected at the edge of the rotted tissue. Some lesions failed to develop into rots and the fungus could not be re-isolated. Rots developed unhindered following inoculation of riper apples.

The presence of an antifungal compound within the necrotic tissues from arrested lesions was demonstrated by placing pieces of the tissue on 2% malt agar plates seeded with the spores of *N. galligena* (Swinburne, 1971a). Zones of inhibition developed around the necrotic tissue pieces, but not around comparable tissue from healthy apples (Fig. 1).

Isolation and Identification of the Antifungal Compound

Following the detection of the antifungal compound, an inoculation technique was devised to produce the large quantities of necrotic tissue required to isolate and identify the substance involved (Brown and Swinburne, 1971). Apples, picked in August, were surface sterilized, halved at their equator and the cut surfaces were dipped in a suspension of conidia. After 10 days' incubation large areas of necrosis developed below the inoculated surfaces. The antifungal compound within the necrotic tissue was readily extracted by ethyl acetate. A single antifungal compound was isolated as colourless crystals from the ethyl acetate extracts by liquid–liquid partition between ether and saturated aqueous solutions of sodium bicarbonate (Brown and Swinburne, 1971). This compound was proved, by nuclear magnetic resonance spectroscopy, to be benzoic acid.

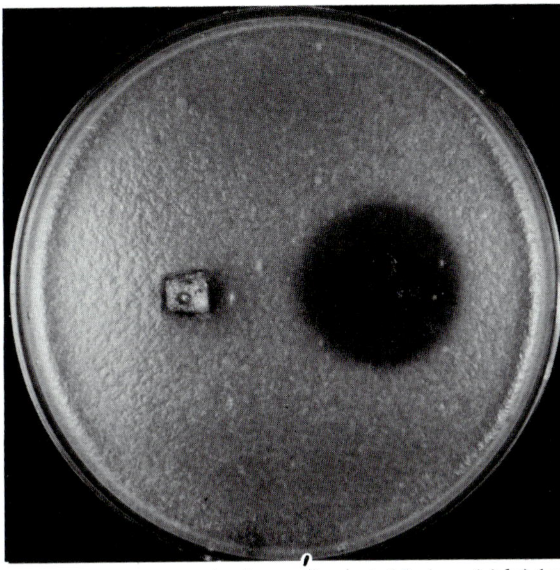

Fig. 1. Antifungal activity in necrotic tissue of arrested lesions (*right*) but not in healthy tissue (*left*). (Swinburne, 1970a.)

For quantitative chemical determination of benzoic acid, aliquots of ethyl acetate extracts of diseased tissue were applied to the origin of t.l.c. plates (Kieselgel G. nach Stahl.). After development with chloroform: ethyl acetate (3 : 1 v/v) the benzoic acid region, located by ultraviolet light, was eluted with methanol and the concentration determined from absorption at λ_{max} (= 273 nm) with reference to a standard curve. In a bioassay procedure 0.1 ml aliquots of a range of concentrations of benzoic acid or solutions of the water soluble solids in the ethyl acetate extracts, were pipetted into wells in 2% malt agar plates seeded with conidia of *N. galligena*. The diameter of the resultant zones of inhibition were directly proportional to the logarithm of the concentration of benzoic acid. In initial experiments there was a considerable discrepancy between the results obtained by these methods; in the bioassay experiments benzoic acid concentrations were usually 10-fold the values obtained by chemical analysis. This difference was shown to be due to acidic compounds in the unpurified extracts which greatly increased the toxicity of benzoic acid. When allowance was made for the effect of these acidic compounds it was shown that benzoic acid accounted for all the antifungal activity present in the tissues.

Benzoic acid could not be detected in extracts of healthy apples at any stage of development, nor in uninoculated sliced apples, and thus if benzoic acid is present in healthy apples the concentrations are less than 1.5 mg/100 g fresh weight, the lower limit of detection by the t.l.c. method.

Effect of Fruit Maturity on Benzoic Acid Production

Further studies (Brown and Swinburne, 1972a) were made of the effect of fruit maturity on the quantity of benzoic acid produced after infection. Apples were picked at approximately weekly intervals between July and November in both 1969 and 1970. Within 24 h of each harvest the apples were halved and inoculated by dipping the cut surface in a suspension of conidia. Inoculated apples were incubated (22° C) for 10 days and were then peeled, and determination was made of benzoic acid in the cortical tissues within 1 cm of the cut surfaces (Fig. 2). Two peaks of benzoic acid production occurred at similar dates in each season; the first approximately 70 days and the second approximately 100 days after full blossom. The greatest quantities were produced in apples picked and inoculated 100 days after full blossom.

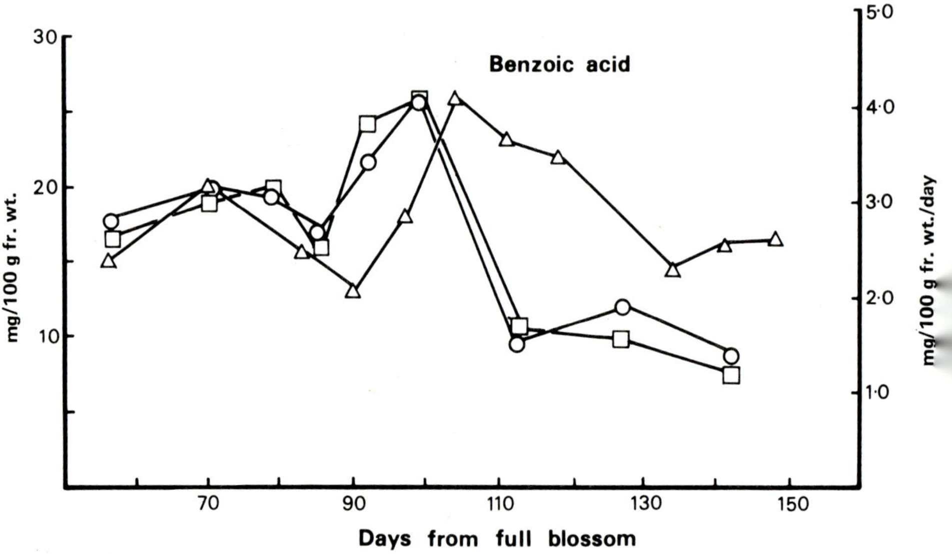

Fig. 2. Quantity of benzoic acid produced, 10 days after inoculation with *N. galligena,* in Bramley's Seedling apples picked at various dates, –△– 1969, –○– 1970; and the rates of benzoic acid production in those apples inoculated in 1970, –□–. (Brown and Swinburne, 1972a.)

In the 1970 experiment sufficiently large numbers of apples were picked and inoculated at each date to enable benzoic acid determinations to be made at daily intervals throughout a 15-day incubation period following inoculation. Benzoic acid was not detected until 2-4 days after inoculation of apples at each date of picking, and the concentrations increased linearly thereafter until reaching a maximum 10-14 days after inoculation. The rates of production of benzoic acid following each inoculation are also shown in Fig. 2. The highest rate of production occurred 90-100 days after full blossom.

EFFECT OF INOCULUM CONCENTRATION ON BENZOIC ACID PRODUCTION

The effect of inoculum concentration was determined by using apples picked 100 days after full blossom (Brown and Swinburne, 1972a). The cut surfaces of half apples were dipped in one of a range of concentrations of conidia in water, and the concentration of benzoic acid in the cortical tissues within 1 cm of the cut surface, determined at intervals after inoculation, is shown in Table I. The maximum concentration of benzoic acid produced appeared to be independent of the concentration of conidia, but the time taken to reach the maximum decreased with increasing spore numbers.

TABLE I

The quantity of benzoic acid in apples at intervals after dipping in suspensions of conidia of various concentration (Brown and Swinburne, 1972a)

No. conidia/ml (thousands)	Benzoic acid (mg/100 g fresh wt.) Days after inoculation 3	6	9	12	18
3000	trace	7.2	8.8	7.1	4.1
1560	nil	6.1	6.1	8.8	4.7
300	nil	2.6	4.7	6.3	5.7
150	nil	trace	3.0	5.5	9.8
25	nil	nil	1.6	3.3	6.4

EFFECT OF CARBON DIOXIDE ON BENZOIC ACID PRODUCTION

The original observation that more rots were found in stores where the carbon dioxide concentration varied over a wide range than in those with stable concentrations (Swinburne, 1970b) has been confirmed in experiments using artificial gas mixtures (unpublished data). The effect of carbon dioxide on benzoic acid production in infected apples was then examined. Apples, picked in mid-September, were halved and inoculated by dipping the cut surfaces in a suspension of conidia. Eight half-apples were placed in each of 18 plastic boxes fitted with gas-tight lids and tubulatures which permitted gas mixtures to be passed through the boxes. Air, or one of two mixtures of air and carbon dioxide (5% and 10% CO_2) were passed (1 litre/min) through six of the boxes, connected in series, and held at 15° C. A switching system enabled three boxes of each set to be connected alternatively, every 12 h, to one of the other gas concentrations, thus six conditions were obtained viz: 0, 5, 10, 0-5, 0-10% and 5-10% CO_2. The CO_2 content of air (0.03-0.04%) was disregarded in this experiment. After 10 days incubation in these conditions the mean benzoic acid content of replicate samples from each treatment were determined (Table II). There was no significant difference in benzoic acid produced between apples incubated in air or 5% CO_2, but only half that concentration was produced by apples held alternately in air and 5% CO_2. Apples held at 10% CO_2 produced significantly less benzoic acid than those held in air, but even lower amounts were produced in apples alternated between air and 10% CO_2.

TABLE II

The production of benzoic acid in inoculated apples incubated in various concentrations of carbon dioxide

Carbon dioxide concn. %	Benzoic acid concn. (mg/100 g fresh wt.)
0	28.6
5	28.4
10	16.5
0-5	14.1
5-10	7.1
0-10	3.8

L.S.D. ($P = 0.01$)5.9

INDUCTION OF BENZOIC ACID IN INFECTED APPLES

Fawcett and Spencer (1967, 1968) demonstrated that the antifungal phenolic acids which accumulate in apples (cv. Edward VII) rotted by *Sclerotinia fructigena* were the products of degradation of host-borne precursors, such as chlorogenic acid, by fungal enzymes. They also found that these antifungal compounds accumulated in cultures of the fungus on autoclaved apple tissue. To determine if benzoic acid arose by a similar mechanism *N. galligena* was cultured on autoclaved apple pulp, apple juice sterilized by heat or filtration and in media, based on Czapek-Dox, containing chlorogenic, quinic or cinnamic acids. After growth of the fungus benzoic acid could not be detected in any of these media.

The production of benzoic acid in tissues remote from those colonized by the fungus suggested that the compound(s) responsible for induction were formed in the macerated area of arrested lesions during the early stages of infection and subsequently diffused into the surrounding healthy tissue. It also seemed probable that these compounds were enzymes which either degraded labile precursors present in healthy cells or caused damage which altered normal metabolism and led to the accumulation of benzoic acid. It was further assumed that such enzymes would be present in the rotted tissue of ripe apples. To test this hypothesis, a concentrate of the water soluble proteins in rot tissue was prepared.

Rotted cortical tissue (1 kg) from ripe apples infected with *N. galligena* was homogenized at 0° C in 1 litre 0.5 M sodium chloride containing 10% w/v polyvinylpyrrolidone (Swinburne and Corden, 1969). The homogenate was pressed through muslin and the filtrate clarified by centrifugation. After dialysis against tap water for 12 h all the protein was precipitated by adding two volumes of acetone at −18° C. The precipitate was removed by centrifugation and dissolved in 100 ml water.

The capacity of this crude protein solution to induce the formation of benzoic acid was tested by pipetting 0.5 ml aliquots into wells (8 mm deep, 8 mm dia.) cut into the equators of immature apples (100-120 days from full blossom); aliquots of the protein solution boiled for 10 min and water served as controls. The wells were sealed with cover slips smeared with petroleum jelly and the apples were incubated at 22° C. After 4-6 days the peel around wells fitted with protein solution had become chlorotic, but not around those filled with the boiled solution or water. After 12 days incubation the apples were dissected and it was found that the cortical tissues up to 6 mm from the wells filled with the protein solution had become necrotic. Microscopic examination of the cells in the necrotic areas showed accumulations of starch. Only slight necrosis, and no accumulations of starch were found in tissues adjoining wells filled with water or boiled protein solution. The tissues surrounding the wells were analysed for benzoic acid; 12-14 mg/100 g fresh wt. were found in those treated with the protein solution, but none in those treated with water or the boiled protein solution.

IDENTIFICATION OF THE INDUCING AGENT

Circumstantial evidence for the identity of the benzoic acid-inducing component in the protein solution came from experiments which tested the ability of other apple rotting organisms to induce benzoic acid. Apples, picked in September, were inoculated, by the cork borer method, with seven species of fungi isolated from natural rots, and after 10 days incubation the tissues around each inoculation were analysed for benzoic acid; the results are shown semi-quantitatively in Table III. The three species, *N. galligena, Pezicula malicorticis* (stat. conid. *Gloeosporium perennans*) and *Diaporthe perniciosa,* which induced benzoic acid were, significantly, those which produce proteolytic enzymes *in vivo* (unpublished data; Porter, 1966; Kuć and Williams, 1962). The

TABLE III

The induction of benzoic acid in immature apples and the production *in vivo* of proteases by various apple pathogens

Organism	Benzoic acid produced	Protease activity
N. galligena	+++	++++
Diaporthe perniciosa	++	+
Pezicula malicorticis	++	++
Aspergillus niger	–	–
Botrytis cinerea	–	–
Penicillium expansum	–	–
Fusarium lateritium	–	–

relative levels of protease activity produced *in vivo* by these organisms is shown in Table III which is based on unpublished data.

The three organisms which induced benzoic acid are also those which initiate latent infections, and produce rots only in ripe apples (Swinburne, 1971a; Ayob and Swinburne, 1970; Edney, 1958). Hulme and Edney (1959) related the resistance of unripe apples to rotting by *G. perennans* to the presence of preformed inhibitors in the peel. The induction of benzoic acid formation by *G. perennans* suggests that compounds formed after infection might also be involved.

In subsequent experiments designed to separate and identify the active component from the protein solution, particular attention was paid to the protease. The various components within the crude protein solution were separated by means of ion-exchange cellulose chromatography, as previously described (Swinburne and Corden, 1969). In a preliminary analysis, 5 ml of the protein solution were applied to a DEAE cellulose column, eluted with 0.01 M tris-HCl buffer (pH 7.0) with a linear gradient of sodium chloride concentration. The collected fractions were assayed for protease and polygalacturonase by a cup–plate method (Dingle *et al.*, 1953) and for protein by measuring the extinction at 280 nm. A typical separation is shown in Fig. 3. The protease was eluted in two peaks; the first, containing approximately 85% of the applied activity, was eluted without adsorption with the void volume of the column, and the second, containing 5-10% of the applied activity was eluted with approximately 0.4 M NaCl, and was only partially resolved from the single peak of polygalacturonase. Most of the protein was eluted as a single peak between 0.1 M and 0.3 M NaCl.

This separation formed the basis of a batchwise treatment of the protein solution with DEAE cellulose. Pre-equilibrated DEAE cellulose was added to

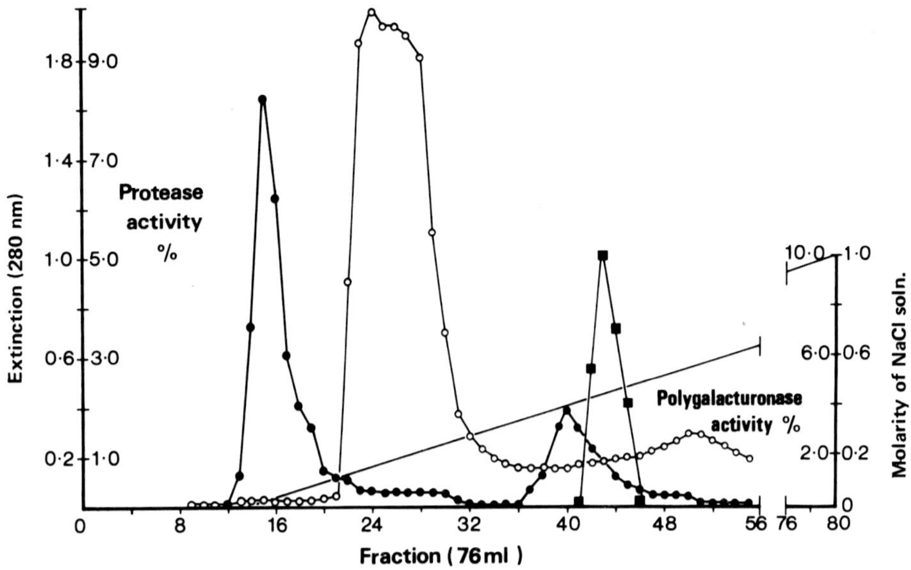

Fig. 3. The separation of components in the crude protein solution extracted from rotted tissue on a column of DEAE-cellulase with tris-HCl buffer (pH 7.0) and a linear gradient of sodium chloride. –●–, protease activity expressed as % of the sample applied to the column; –○–, extinction values at 280 nm; –■–, P.G. activity expressed as % of the sample applied to the column. Approximate salt concentration shown as a solid line.

200 ml of the protein solution, and the supernatant was removed by filtration and retained. The DEAE cellulose was then successively washed with 3 x 500 ml quantities of buffer containing, 0.1, 0.2, 0.3, 0.4 and 1.0 M, NaCl. The supernatants from each stage were concentrated to approximately 200 ml by dialysis against Carbowax 20 M. The protein in each fraction was precipitated with 2 volumes of acetone at −18° C, and each precipitate redissolved in 10 ml water. The protease activity of each fraction was determined, by the method of Anson and Mirsky (1933) (Table IV).

The ability of each fraction to induce benzoic acid in healthy apples was assayed as before. The most active fraction, *a,* was that not absorbed by DEAE cellulose and it contained the highest levels of proteolytic activity (Table IV).

5 ml of fraction *a* were applied to a CM-cellulose column and eluted with sodium acetate buffer (0.01 M, pH 5.0) containing a linear gradient of sodium chloride concentration. Two protein peaks, in addition to the protease were detected in the fractions collected (Fig. 4). Those fractions containing the highest concentrations of each of the protein peaks and the protease were assessed for their ability to induce benzoic acid. Only the protease fraction induced benzoic acid.

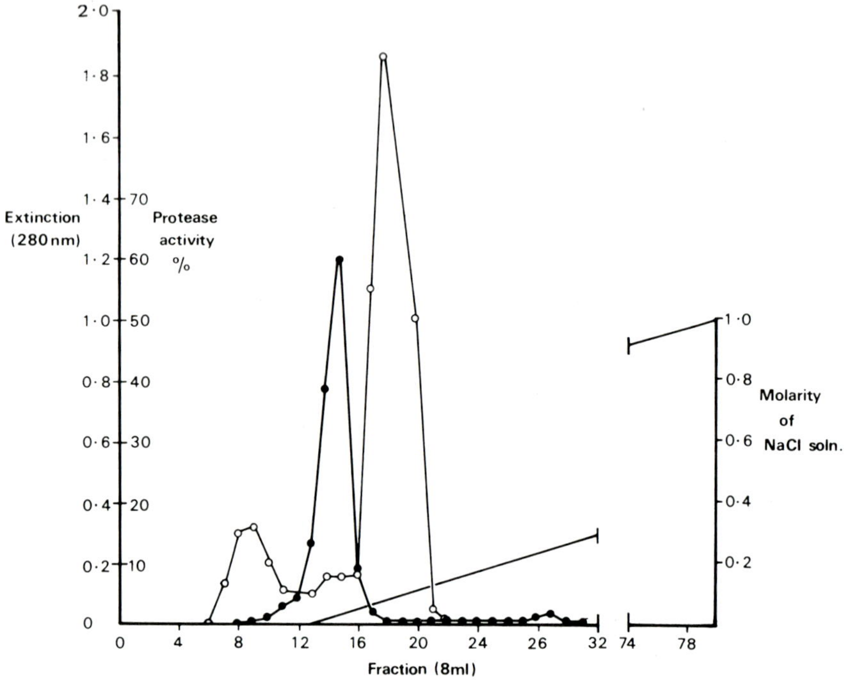

Fig. 4. Purification of the protease, from fraction *a* (see Table IV) on a column of CM cellulose eluted with 0.01 M sodium acetate (pH 5.0) and a linear gradient of sodium chloride. –●–, protease activity expressed as % of the sample applied to the column; –○–, extinction values at 280 nm. Approximate salt concentration shown as a solid line.

TABLE IV

Protease activity and benzoic acid induction of fractions separated by DEAE cellulose adsorption from the proteins extracted from rot tissue

Fraction	Eluant	Protease[1] activity	Benzoic acid induction
a	Buffer alone	21.75	++++
b	Buffer + 0.1 M NaCl	4.93	++
c	Buffer + 0.2 M NaCl	4.14	+
d	Buffer + 0.3 M NaCl	3.66	–
e	Buffer + 0.4 M NaCl	2.00	–
f	Buffer + 1.0 M NaCl	1.52	–

[1] Expressed as m. moles tyrosine liberated from haemoglobin under the standard conditions of Anson and Mirsky (1933).

DEGRADATION OF BENZOIC ACID, *IN VITRO* AND *IN VIVO*

When arrested lesions, formed after inoculation of unripe apples, eventually expanded into progressive rots (30-50 days after inoculation), no antifungal activity could be detected in the diseased tissue (Swinburne, 1971a). Analysis of tissues from lesions at various stages of development (Table V) showed that after reaching a maximum approximately 10 days after inoculation the benzoic acid concentration diminished and none was found in natural rots (Brown and Swinburne, 1972b).

TABLE V

Benzoic acid concentration at various stages of rot development in apples inoculated in October (Brown and Swinburne, 1972b)

Days after inoculation	Stage of development	Benzoic acid (mg/100 g fresh wt.)
10	Arrested lesion	20.6 ± 1.2
25	Lesion expanding	14.7 ± 0.9
56	Progressive rot	8.0 ± 1.1

The ability of healthy apple tissue and *N. galligena* to metabolize benzoic acid was investigated using the labelled compound (Brown and Swinburne, 1972b). Healthy apple tissue was unable to metabolize benzoic acid in any of the conditions tested. The fungus, however, was able to degrade benzoic acid completely with the evolution of carbon dioxide, but the rate of breakdown was dependent on the pH of the medium. Using replacement cultures, containing benzoic acid in buffer solutions at pH 3.4-7.5, it was found that the rate increased with increasing pH, and at pH 3.4, a value comparable to that of apple tissue, the rate was extremely low.

The intermediary products of the degradation of benzoic acid were extracted from the replacement cultures and those identified were *p*-hydroxybenzoic acid, protocatechuic acid and β-oxoadipic acid. The presence of these compounds suggested that *N. galligena* degraded benzoic acid by a similar pathway to that described for the degradation of aromatic acids by other micro-organisms (Cain *et al.*, 1968), as shown in Fig. 5.

These metabolic products were then sought in the tissues of arrested lesions 10 days after inoculation, and in rotted tissue, six weeks after inoculation. There was approximately half the amount of benzoic acid and three times as much *p*-hydroxybenzoic acid in the rotted tissue as found in the arrested lesions, but protocatechuic acid was not detected.

The available evidence suggests that benzoic acid is metabolized *in vivo* by similar mechanisms to those found *in vitro*. Changes in the ripening apple would

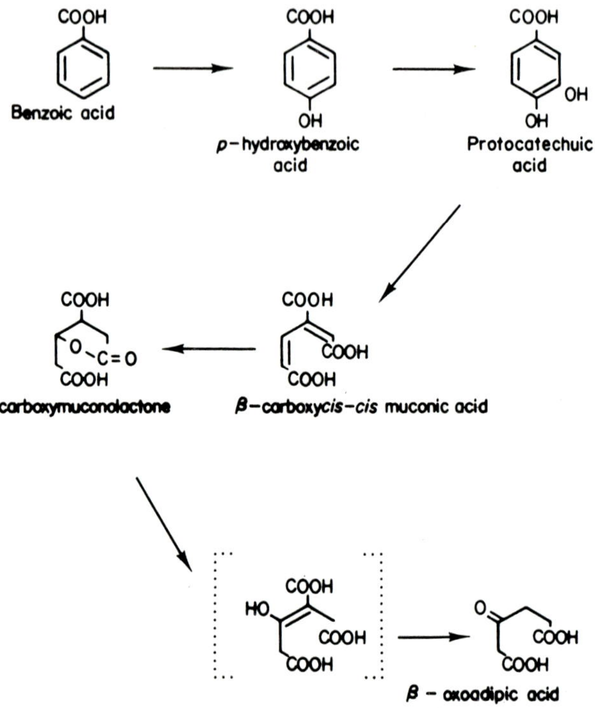

Fig. 5. Metabolic pathway for the degradation of benzoic acid by *N. galligena* (Brown and Swinburne, 1972b).

reduce the effective toxicity of benzoic acid, and conditions would become more conducive to breakdown. The levels of soluble carbohydrate increase with ripening (Hulme, 1958), and Sitterly and Shay (1960) suggested that the cultivars Golden Delicious, Rome Beauty and Grimes Golden became susceptible to rotting by the pathogens *Botryosphaeria ribis* and *Glomerella cingulata* when soluble carbohydrates reached critical levels, sufficient to overcome the presence of inhibitory compounds. The titratable acidity of apples also diminishes with ripening (Hulme, 1958) and although the pH of expressed sap increases only slightly during maturation these changes may be sufficient to increase the rate of breakdown of benzoic acid.

Benzoic Acid as a Phytoalexin

Benzoic acid has so far only been found in apples after infection with certain fungi, and was formed, apparently, only by living cells, probably as a product of necrobiosis, and was only produced in the locality of the infection. These properties conform to the stipulations expressed in the original definition of a phytoalexin proposed by Müller and Börger and restated by Cruickshank (1963).

Other antibiotic compounds formed by various plants in response to infection and referred to as phytoalexins have subsequently been found to be normal constituents of those plants or induced by physical and chemical means (Fawcett and Spencer, 1969). As benzoic acid is a normal constituent of other plants (De Laey and Virtanen, 1957; Clagne and Fellers, 1934) it seems possible that more sensitive techniques would show benzoic acid to be a constituent of healthy apples.

Until the mechanism of synthesis has been elucidated the possibility that benzoic acid is a breakdown product of a host-borne precursor cannot be entirely eliminated. Antifungal compounds with such an origin were termed *false*-phytoalexins by Fawcett and Spencer (1969). The induction of benzoic acid by fungal proteases could be due to the release of a bound form of the compound from a protein complex. The existence of bound forms of aromatic acids in plants has been demonstrated (El-Basyouni and Neish, 1966). However, the induction of phytoalexins by thermolabile substances secreted by pathogens was described by Uehara (1959), and Cruickshank and Perrin (1968) isolated a polypeptide, Monilicolin A, produced by *Monilinia fructicola,* which induced phaseollin production in *Phaseolus vulgaris.*

In the original definition of a phytoalexin (see Cruickshank, 1963) it was proposed that the difference between a susceptible and a resistant reaction was in the speed of formation of the phytoalexin. The rate of production of benzoic acid in apples depended on maturity, and formation was most rapid in apples inoculated approximately 100 days after full blossom. Paradoxically, apples inoculated at this time rotted most quickly in store (Swinburne, 1971a). In the analyses for benzoic acid, no allowance was made for the quantity of unaffected, healthy tissue in the samples, and it was not possible to express the results on the ideal basis of the number of affected cells (Cruickshank *et al.,* 1971). Thus tissues may be more extensively colonized, and more host cells affected following infection at 100 days after full blossom than with earlier or later infections. The quantity of benzoic acid formed by each affected cell may have been relatively small following infection at 100 days from full blossom, but because many more cells were involved, the weight of benzoic acid in a unit volume of the tissue was apparently highest at this time. Further experiments will be required to solve this problem.

REFERENCES

Anson, M. L. and Mirsky, A. E. (1933). Estimation of trypsin with hemoglobin. *J. gen. Physiol.* **17**, 151-157.

Ayob, A. N. and Swinburne, T. R. (1970). Observations on the infection and rotting of apples, var. Bramley's Seedling by *Diaporthe perniciosa. Ann. appl. Biol.* **66**, 245-255.

Brown, A. E. and Swinburne, T. R. (1971). Benzoic acid: an antifungal compound formed in Bramley's Seedling apple fruits following infection by *Nectria galligena* Bres. *Physiol. Pl. Pathol.* **1**.

Brown, A. E. and Swinburne, T. R. (1972a). Factors affecting the production of benzoic acid in Bramley's Seedling apples infected with *N. galligena. Physiol. Pl. Pathol.* In press.

Brown, A. E. and Swinburne, T. R. (1972b). The degradation of benzoic acid by *Nectria galligena* Bres. *in vitro* and *in vivo.* (in preparation)

Cain, R. B., Bilton, R. F. and Darrah, J. A. (1968). The metabolism of aromatic acids by micro organisms. Metabolic pathways in the fungi. *Biochem. J.* **108**, 797-828.

Clagne, J. A. and Fellers, C. R. (1934). Relation of benzoic acid content and other constituents of cranberries to keeping quality. *Pl. Physiol., Lancaster* **9**, 631-636.

Cruickshank, I. A. M. (1963). Phytoalexins. *A. Rev. Phytopath.* **1**, 351-374.

Cruickshank, I. A. M., Biggs, D. R. and Perrin, D. R. (1971). Phytoalexins as determinants of disease reaction in plants. *J. Indian bot. Soc.* **50A**, 1-11.

Cruickshank, I. A. M. and Perrin, D. R. (1968). The isolation and partial characterisation of Monilicolin A, a polypeptide with phaseollin-inducing activity from *Monilinia fructicola. Life Sci.* 7, 449-458.

De Laey, P and Virtanen, A. I. (1957). On antifungal factors in carrots. *Suomen Kemistilehti* **B30**, 218.

Dillon-Weston, W. A. R. (1927). Notes on the canker fungus (*Nectria galligena* Bres.). *Trans. Br. mycol. Soc.* **12**, 5-12.

Dingle, J., Reid, W. W. and Solomons, G. L. (1953). The enzymatic degradation of pectin and other polysaccharides. II. The application of the cup plate assay to the estimation of enzymes. *J. Sci. Fd. Agric.* **4**, 149-155.

Edney, K. L. (1958). Observations on the infection of Cox's Orange Pippin apples by *Gloeosporium perennans* Zeller & Childs. *Ann. appl. Biol.* **46**, 622-629.

El-Basyouni, S. Z. and Neish, A. C. (1966). Occurrence of metabolically-active bound forms of cinnamic acid and its phenolic derivatives in acetone powders of wheat and barley plants. *Phytochemistry* **5**, 683-691.

Fawcett, C. H. and Spencer, D. M. (1967). Antifungal phenolic acids in apple fruits after infection with *Sclerotinia fructigena. Ann. appl. Biol.* **60**, 87-96.

Fawcett, C. H. and Spencer, D. M. (1968). *Sclerotinia fructigena* infection and chlorogenic acid content in relation to antifungal compounds in apple fruits. *Ann. appl. Biol.* **61**, 245-253.

Fawcett, C. H. and Spencer, D. M. (1969). Natural antifungal compounds. *In* 'Fungicides' (ed. D. C. Torgeson). Vol. 2, pp. 637-669. Academic Press, London and New York.

Hulme, A. C. (1958). Some aspects of the biochemistry of apple and pear fruits. *Adv. Fd Res.* **8**, 297-413.

Hulme, A. C. and Edney, K. L. (1959). Phenolic substances in the peel of Cox's Orange Pippin apples with reference to infection by *G. perennans. In* 'Phenolics in plants in health and disease' (ed. J. B. Pridham) pp. 87-94. Pergamon Press: London.

Kavanagh, J. A. and Glynn, A. N. (1966). Brown rot of apples caused by *Nectria galligena* Bres. *Ir. J. agric. Res.* **5**, 143-144.

Kidd, M. N. and Beaumont, B. A. (1924). Apple rot fungi in storage. *Trans. Br. mycol. Soc.* **10**, 98-118.
Kuć, J. and Williams, E. B. (1962). Production of proteolytic enzymes by four pathogens of apple fruit. *Phytopathology* **52**, 739.
Porter, F. (1966). Protease activity in diseased fruits. *Phytopathology* **56**, 1424-1425.
Salmon, E. S. and Wormald, H. (1915). The 'eye-rot' of the apple. *Gdnrs' Chron.* **58**, 289.
Sitterly, W. R. and Shay, J. R. (1960). Physiological factors affecting the onset of susceptibility of apple fruit to rotting by fungus pathogens. *Phytopathology* **50**, 91-93.
Swinburne, T. R. (1964). Rotting of apples of the variety Bramley's Seedling by *Nectria galligena* Bres. *Nature, Lond.* **204**, 493-494.
Swinburne, T. R. (1970a). Fungal rotting of apples. I-A survey of the extent and cause of current fruit losses in Northern Ireland. *Rec. agric. Res. Minist. Agric. Nth. Ir.* **18**, 15-19.
Swinburne, T. R. (1970b). Fungal rotting of apples. II-A preliminary survey of the effect of storage conditions on the development of rots. *Rec. agric. Res. Minist. Agric. Nth. Ir.* **18**, 89-94.
Swinburne, T. R. (1971a). The infection of apples, var. Bramley's Seedling, by *Nectria galligena* Bres. *Ann. appl. Biol.* **68**, 253-262.
Swinburne, T. R. (1971b). The seasonal release of spores of *Nectria galligena* Bres. from apple cankers in Northern Ireland. *Ann. appl. Biol.* **69**, 97-104.
Swinburne, T. R. and Corden, M. E. (1969). A comparison of the polygalacturonases produced *in vivo* and *in vitro* by *Penicillium expansum* Thom. *J. gen. Microbiol.* **55**, 75-87.
Uehara, K. (1959). On the phytoalexin production of the Soy bean pod in reaction to *Fusarium* sp., the causal fungus of pod blight. II. On the effect of conditions of the spore suspension of the causal fungus upon phytoalexin production. *Ann. phytopath. Soc. Japan* **24**, 224-228.

DISCUSSION

Professor J. Friend: Have you looked at the possible biosynthetic mechanisms for benzoic acid formation? This compound is a rather unusual secondary product in plants, since most of the benzoic acid derivatives are hydroxylated. One would assume that cinnamic acid is the precursor. It makes a rather interesting biochemical situation.

Dr T. R. Swinburne: The absence of that hydroxyl group is puzzling. I should add, in answer to what Dr Martin said, that it is interesting that the first product in the metabolism of benzoic acid is in fact *para*hydroxy benzoic acid, which is relatively non-toxic to *Nectria galligena.* I do not know what the precursors of benzoic acid are. We have nothing but negative results on this question. We have been unable to detect benzoic acid as a breakdown product of any precursor which is present in the apple. In other words, no product left in a dead apple, no matter how killed, appears to be a direct precursor. I have looked at the problem of aromatic biosynthesis in apples. In spite of some vigorous searching, and looking at other plants to make sure I have got the technique right, I cannot find phenylalanine ammonia lyase in apples, although we do have some evidence from radioactive studies that phenylalanine might conceivably be used in the formation of benzoic acid, but cinnamic acid is not, as far as we can tell, a very good precursor. It is no better than phenylalanine, and so I am afraid I just do not know how benzoic acid is produced at this stage.

Dr J. A. Kavanagh: Have you looked at the possibility that the benzoic acid production is confined to the outer layers of Bramley's Seedling, or what would happen if you inoculated about 10 mm below the epidermis, would you still get this resistant reaction?

Dr Swinburne: I deliberately chose to avoid going into the complications of the positional effect. The apple is a sphere, and there is a three dimensional variation in the ability of the tissues to produce benzoic acid following infection and, what is worse, that three dimensional variation changes with time. Initially the most productive areas are the core but, with time, the ability to synthesize benzoic acid spreads out towards the outer layers, but there is always a polarization effect, there is a tendency for the rose tissues (around the eye) to be a little more resistant than the stalk. In natural conditions, the fungus is very often introduced by a caterpillar into the rose, grows up through the core, and comes out at the stalk. There is this curious three dimensional relationship, the tissues vary tremendously throughout the apple.

Dr Kavanagh: What would the possibility be of looking at the actual structural changes in these dried out limited lesions?

Dr Swinburne: I think that this will be our next step, particularly now that we have a system whereby we can avoid the use of the fungus. We can in fact induce many of these processes by using the protease. We can now pursue in depth some of these necrotic changes–e.g. swollen nuclei and nucleolus, starch synthesis–which appear to be identical with pure protease as with the fungus itself.

Dr Kavanagh: How do you explain the fact that at harvest time you still get large percentages of mature fruit still showing these stopped lesions, even though your title says that this is confined more or less to immature fruits?

Dr Swinburne: There are paradoxes in all this. I have actually inoculated apples (from gas store) at their equator, and induced a stopped rot, but during incubation a natural rot has developed at the stalk and spread down. So that at one and the same time we have had a natural infection developing, obviously a susceptible reaction, and at the equator a stopped rot. I cannot explain why.

Dr Y. Beyersbergen: This is a useful piece of information for me, because in tulips we have nearly the same problem with *Fusarium* rot during storage. Did you ever determine ethylene concentrations during the storage of the apples?

Dr Swinburne: We have looked at ethylene, but when you have to use the potassium permanganate method for determining ethylene concentrations, the experiments are limited. We have no sophisticated techniques as yet. I would like to think that many of the chlorotic symptoms that we are seeing are good evidence of ethylene, but ethylene is produced by apples infected with all these organisms. It is a little difficult to relate resistance to ethylene production in apples when no matter what you infect them with they are going to produce a lot of ethylene, and we have in fact looked at *Penicillium expansum* infection and ethylene production. The zonate form of rots following artificial inoculation with *P. expansum* seems to be accompanied by pulses of ethylene production with the formation of each new zone. We never get benzoic acid without chlorosis, but we can get chlorosis without benzoic acid. Other fractions within the acetone precipitate of rot tissue induce chlorosis, and therefore perhaps that is an ethylene factor, but we can never get benzoic acid without chlorosis. I do not know whether the presence of benzoic acid is in any way related to ethylene production.

Professor M. A. Stahmann: You showed that the ability to induce benzoic acid was correlated with the protease activity. I wonder if you ever tested the products of protease activity, namely peptides that might be liberated through the action of protease, and their ability to induce benzoic acid.

Dr Swinburne: This is something which we are currently doing. Michael Comer who works with me is back home at the moment doing that very experiment. He is attempting to liberate peptides from healthy apples, by use of a protease, which he will then test as inducers of benzoic acid. The work which I have just described on the induction was completed the day before the paper was sent off, and so it is fairly fresh, and we are very actively engaged in this area at the moment.

Professor Stahmann: It would be interesting to know the breakdown products.

Dr Swinburne: We think it might be a peptide that is liberated. Very often you see in the induction with liquids, necrotic sides to the well, a gap of white (non-necrotic) tissue and then a further band of necrotic tissue, which suggests that there is a two-stage event occurring. A build-up may occur of compounds perhaps liberated by the protease from the first tissues that it encountered, and this may affect the subsequent tissues into which it diffuses. So I believe it is a product of protease degradation of host protein which may be inducing the formation of benzoic acid.

Professor Stahmann: Yes, I would agree.

S. A. Archer: If I understand rightly, you isolated this protease from the crude protein preparation from the apple. Do you get a protease produced in culture by the fungus, and if so, will it induce the benzoic acid production.

Dr Swinburne: Yes, you can get a protease *in vitro.* We have not been able to get it out in anything like the concentration that we obtain from rotted apples, and this has presented us with some difficulties. We have not so far used an enzyme produced *in vitro*. I should refer to the first box of apples that you saw–if you measure the protease activity in that tissue it is as much as 1/10 of the protease activity of duodenal juice. It is extremely active proteolytically.

S. A. Archer: What substrates do you use to assay this enzyme?

Dr Swinburne: Thus far we have used gelatine on a cup-plate basis, and casein and haemoglobin as a standard technique for proteases by Anson's methods. I should add that it will not attack dipeptides, we have not been able to get it to work on anything but large protein molecules as yet.

Dr Kavanagh: To what extent have you any information on the production of phenolic compounds by fungi themselves?

Dr Swinburne: We have not studied this. There are compounds which appear to be of a phenolic nature, and which can be detected chromatographically both from the fungus and of course in a healthy apple, and in greater amounts in a diseased apple. But none of these appear to have very great anti-fungal activity. We do not know the significance of the fungal one, we were only looking at them to eliminate them from the chromatograms at that stage. I am afraid I have no relevant information on phenolics produced by the fungus.

IV. 4 Resistance of Potato to *Phytophthora*

J. FRIEND

Department of Botany, University of Hull, England

INTRODUCTION

It is known from the work of Müller (1953) and Black (1952a and b) that hypersensitive resistance of *Solanum* spp. to *Phytophthora infestans* is controlled by a series of major-genes, called 'R genes', which confer resistance to some but not other races of *P. infestans.* There is now considerable published evidence that R-gene resistance is associated with biochemical changes occurring after infection. The sesquiterpenoid rishitin (Katsui *et al.*, 1968), which inhibits germination of zoospores and growth of germ tubes of *P. infestans* has been isolated from Rishiri potatoes (R_1) after inoculation with an incompatible race (race O) of *P. infestans* (Tomiyama *et al.*, 1968). Rishitin was present only in trace quantities in uninoculated tuber slices, and after inoculation with a compatible race of *P. infestans.* Rishitin thus appears to have some of the features of a phytoalexin (Cruickshank, 1963), especially as it also accumulates in incompatible interactions of four potato cultivars (R_1, R_2, R_3, R_4) inoculated with race O of *P. infestans* (Sato *et al.*, 1968). More recently, Varns *et al.* (1971) have shown that when rishitin accumulates in an incompatible combination, it is accompanied by another terpenoid, phytuberin. There are considerable variations in the amount of rishitin and phytuberin which accumulate and these depend both upon the type of R-gene present and the race of *P. infestans* with which the tuber slice is inoculated. Also it is not yet clear whether terpenoid accumulation is responsible for the hypersensitive response or is a manifestation of it.

For several years now, following work initiated by Professor N. F. Robertson at the University of Hull, we have been investigating various aspects of the biochemistry of the interaction between potatoes and *P. infestans.* We have examined phenolic metabolism in inoculated potato tissue in some detail, and this paper is a presentation of our results from which we have concluded that lignification is an important factor associated with the hypersensitive response. The short section on cell wall hydrolysis is included to put the later studies on lignification into perspective.

Cell Wall Hydrolysis and the Reaction of Potato Tissue Cultures

BIOCHEMISTRY OF CELL WALL PENETRATION BY *P. INFESTANS*

The biochemistry of cell wall hydrolysis was investigated first of all by looking at changes in the cell walls of infected tuber tissue (Friend and Knee, 1969; Knee, 1970); the analyses of the control samples appear to be the first ever published despite the widespread use of tuber slices as test substrates for estimations of so-called 'macerating' activity. The chemical studies were followed by an examination of the properties of extra-cellular enzymes produced by *P. infestans* (Knee and Friend, 1968, 1970; Cole, 1970).

Tuber slices of a susceptible cultivar, King Edward, were inoculated with a spore suspension and incubated in sterile petri dishes; control disks were treated with sterile distilled water. Samples were taken 4, 7 and 14 days after incubation and extracted successively with hot water, 4% NaOH and 16% NaOH to yield the extractives termed respectively pectin and hemi-celluloses A and B; the residual fraction was designated as cellulose. Gravimetric analysis of the individual fractions showed that they all increased with time in control disks, but there was a lower increase in the pectic fraction and a more rapid increase in the extraction residue of the infected disks. The individual fractions were hydrolysed and the monosaccharide composition of the hydrolysates was examined by quantitative paper chromatography. Galactose, which was by far the major component of the pectic fraction, did not increase in the infected disks; at later stages there was also a slight decrease in the pectic galacturonic acid. Glucose increased in the extraction residue and part of this increase was due to an accumulation of hyphal wall material of *P. infestans* which contains mainly an insoluble glucan.

It was possible to demonstrate galactanase activity both in infected tuber tissue and in filtrates from cultures of *P. infestans.* This enzyme degraded potato pectin, white lupin pectin and potato cell walls to yield free galactose. There was a rapid initial release of galactose dependent upon the substrate concentration but after about 24 h a constant proportion of the original substrate had been degraded; then the main products appeared to be galactose dimers, trimers and tetramers.

In view of the high galactose content of the potato pectin measured and the demonstrated galactanase activity it seemed probable that the invasion of tuber cells by *P. infestans* involves enzymatic hydrolysis of the galactan portion of the pectic fraction. Additional confirmatory evidence for this hypothesis was provided when Knee (1970), using a rapid microanalytical method, found that after 48 h some loss of the total pectic fraction was accompanied by a drop of 20% in the galactan component in infected disks, compared with an increase in total pectin and a slight loss in galactan in the uninfected samples.

Although Cole (1970) found that culture filtrates of *P. infestans* and infected tuber extracts contained a polygalacturonase in addition to the galactanase he confirmed that the culture filtrate did not exhibit polygalacturonase activity against potato pectin in incubation periods of up to 24 h. It still seems that galactanase activity is of greater importance in the early stages of infection.

In order to explain fully the mechanism by which the extracellular fungal enzymes assist hyphal penetration, a knowledge of the macromolecular structure of potato pectin will be required. However, on the basis of the limited results we already have we can postulate that a large fraction of the pectin must contain a predominance of 1-4 linked β-D-galactopyranose units. There may be considerable galactan independent of polyuronide because the loss of viscosity of potato pectin corresponds with the release of galactose under circumstances where little, if any, galacturonic acid is released. Galactan could also be attached as side-chains to a polyuronide backbone and removal of the side-chains might be a prerequisite for the hydrolytic cleavage of the polyuronide by the *P. infestans* polygalacturonase; this could explain the decreased galacturonic acid content of the pectin hydrolysates at late stages in infection.

During the measurement of chemical changes in walls of infected tubers, deposition of lignin was found. This result is discussed later in relation to changes in phenolic metabolism.

TISSUE CULTURE EXPERIMENTS

In an attempt to overcome the difficulties of using the whole plant, or fragments of it, which often involve extensive wound surfaces, and the complications of secondary micro-organisms, Ingram and Robertson (1965) and Ingram (1967) investigated the interaction of *P. infestans* with tissue cultures of potato. In particular they used tissue cultures of the two cultivars Majestic (rr) and Orion (R_1) and race 4 of *P. infestans* which is pathogenic to Majestic but which produces a hypersensitive response in Orion.

Tissue aggregates of Majestic but not of Orion stimulated the growth of the fungus on an agar medium which allowed germination but not growth. Killing the cells by boiling had little effect on the stimulatory action of Majestic but the resistance shown by Orion aggregates was inactivated. It was concluded that the resistance manifested in these reactions was a property of living and not of dead tissue.

Ingram (1967) also showed, by a sectioning technique, that there was general and diffuse growth of *P. infestans* race 4 on Majestic, and that there was a network of both inter- and intracellular hyphae permeating the whole aggregate. However, in Orion the fungus was almost totally absent from the tissues except for some isolated cells near the surface of the aggregates. This behaviour resembled that of the fungus on potato plants which had previously been seen by Ferris (1955); similar results have been reported more recently by Kitazawa and Tomiyama (1970). It seemed that the situation observed in the interaction of tissue cultures with the pathogen therefore resembled that of the plant and pathogen.

Suspension cultures of Majestic and Orion were inoculated with *P. infestans* race 4 sporangia and incubated for 7 days. Filtered samples of the liquid culture filtrate were assayed against race 4 zoospores; Majestic filtrate allowed 100% germination of zoospores through the complete experiment but Orion filtrate which had no effect up to 24 h after infection caused a gradually increasing inhibition of zoospore germination from 50% after 2 days to complete inhibition after 7 days. This reaction of the Orion tissue culture suspension resembled the phytoalexin reaction described by Müller (1958) and by Cruickshank (1963) but there were some inconsistencies in that there was no toxicity to spores of *Glomerella cingulata* or *Botrytis allii.*

THE TOXIC MATERIAL FROM INOCULATED SUSPENSION CULTURE OF ORION (SEE ROBERTSON *ET AL.*, 1968)

The toxic fraction could be extracted completely from Orion tissue culture filtrate by shaking with ether; no toxic material could be extracted from Majestic culture filtrates. Toxicity was examined by zoospore tests; it could be extracted from the ether by shaking with either aqueous sodium carbonate or with dilute sodium hydroxide and, after acidification of the alkaline extract, re-extracted back into ether. Only three compounds could be detected on thin-layer chromatograms or by gas-liquid chromatography of a trimethylsilylated extract. The R_F values on t.l.c. and the retention times of the peaks on the g.l.c. corresponded with those for salicylic acid, *para*-hydroxybenzoic acid and vanillic acid and the identity of the compounds was confirmed by mass spectrographic examination of the compounds eluted from the t.l.c. plates.

Quantitative toxicity tests were carried out with the original Orion extract and with an artificial mixture of the three acids in the same proportion as in the Orion extract. The results showed that the natural toxic material had an LD_{50} dose of 12.5 ppm whilst that of the mixture was 25 ppm which indicated the possibility that the extract of Orion tissue culture might have contained small quantities of other materials which increased its toxicity; no sign of any other compound could be detected by either t.l.c. or g.l.c. There was some degree of variability in the test zoospores such that the LD_{50} dose for the artificial mixture measured on nine different occasions varied from 16.5 to 34.5 ppm. However, the possibility still remains that the toxicity of Orion culture filtrate was due to the presence of a compound with such high biological activity that it is present in too low a concentration to be detected by the physico-chemical methods used.

When similar experiments were carried out with slices of potato it was not possible to detect any hydroxybenzoic acids, although traces of them have been found in infected leaf tissue. After hydrolysis of bound phenolic compounds in tubers, only cinnamic acids have been found; some benzoic acids can be found in leaf hydrolysates. The results found for tissue cultures which contain growing potato cells therefore do not necessarily apply to tubers or leaves and the reaction of these tissues has now been re-examined in more detail.

Changes in Phenolic Metabolism in Tubers and Leaves Following Infection

In addition to the accumulation of hydroxybenzoic acids in inoculated Orion tissue cultures and lignin in infected King Edward tuber disks, there was an earlier report (Hughes and Swain, 1960) of increases in both chlorogenic acid and scopolin following infection of Majestic tubers. It was of interest to determine whether infection produced a general increase in phenolic biosynthesis or whether there was a diversion of preformed phenolic compounds to those found to accumulate in the particular disease reaction (hypersensitivity or susceptibility).

Since, according to the scheme in Fig. 1, a key reaction involved in all phenolic biosynthesis is the deamination of phenylalanine to cinnamic acid catalysed by phenylalanine ammonia lyase (PAL) (Koukol and Conn, 1961) we have measured changes in this enzyme and compared them with changes in the phenolic compounds (Friend *et al.*, 1971). The majority of the experiments have been carried out with tuber disks and slices, although some preliminary experiments have also been done with detached leaves. In addition to PAL, we

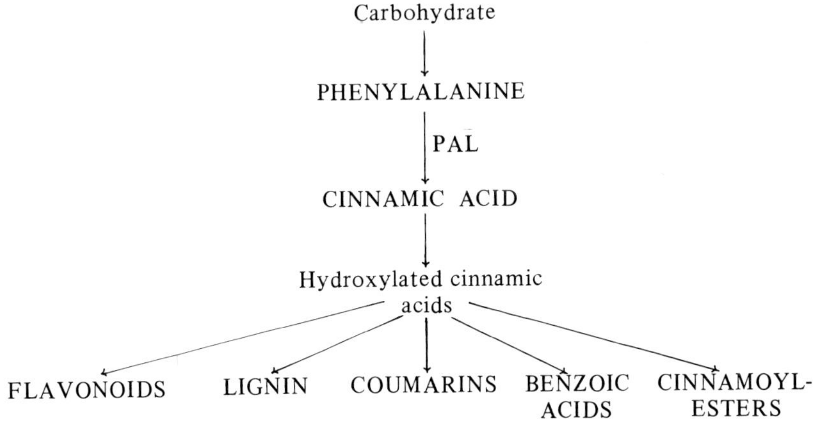

Fig. 1. Biosynthesis of phenolic compounds in higher plants.

have measured the levels of chlorogenic acid, the major phenolic compound of tubers and leaves (Baruah and Swain, 1959) and of lignin.

STUDIES WITH TUBER DISKS

PAL activity was measured using acetone powders of potato disks (Koukol and Conn, 1961), chlorogenic acid extracted with boiling methanol from another sample of disks was measured by the molybdate method of Mapson *et al.* (1963) and lignin, in the methanol residue, by the method of Stafford (1960).

In the first experiment tuber disks were 'cured' by incubating in a dry atmosphere for 24 h, then inoculated with a sporangial suspension of *P. infestans*; controls were treated with sterile distilled water. Samples were taken for analysis during the following 8 days, and the results for PAL, chlorogenic acid and lignin are shown in Tables I, II and III respectively.

TABLE I

Phenylalanine ammonia lyase activity in potato tuber disks (expressed as μg cinnamate produced/g initial fresh wt./h at 40°C), after inoculation with a sporangial suspension of *P. infestans,* compared with the activity in uninoculated disks incubated under identical conditions.

Time (in days)	Majestic Inoc.	Majestic Uninoc.	Orion Inoc.	Orion Uninoc.
0	–	4	–	5
1	40	13	47	29
2	31	20	45.5	42
4	20	15	43	37
6	27	18	35	22
8-9	38	24	67.5	37

TABLE II

Chlorogenic acid in potato tuber disks (expressed as μg chlorogenic acid/g fresh wt.) after inoculation with a sporangial suspension of *P. infestans,* compared with the activity in uninoculated disks incubated under identical conditions

Time (in days)	Majestic Inoc.	Majestic Uninoc.	Orion Inoc.	Orion Uninoc.
0	–	120	–	150
1	170	85	225	365
2	95	25	650	565
4	160	90	535	1080
6	100	180	865	650
8-9	120	180	1505	1285

TABLE III

Lignin content of potato tuber disks inoculated with a sporangial suspension of *P. infestans.* One aliquot of an alkaline extract of a crude cell wall preparation was adjusted to pH 12.0, and another to pH 7.0; the values represent the difference in absorbance ΔA pH 12.0-pH 7.0 at 242 nm and 355 nm/50 mg of crude cell wall fraction. Values for uninoculated disks are *not* included in this table

Time after inoculation (days)	Majestic ΔA at		Orion ΔA at	
	$\lambda 242$	$\lambda 355$	$\lambda 242$	$\lambda 355$
	0.081	0	0.070	0.028
2	0.260	0.088	0.470	0.165
6	0.465	0.185	0.532	0.170
8-9	0.550	0.225	0.522	0.195

There were marked increases in chlorogenic acid in both inoculated and control disks of Orion compared with Majestic. PAL increased more rapidly in Orion than in Majestic; there was a relatively rapid increase in lignin in the early stages in inoculated Orion compared with Majestic, but after 6 days the lignin level in Majestic was higher than that in Orion. These results show that there were considerable complications caused by the measurement of wounding, or rather wound-healing, reactions in addition to those caused by fungal attack and this is one of the disadvantages inherent in the use of tuber disks for this kind of study. It is, however, particularly interesting to note that the very much higher level of chlorogenic acid in Orion compared with Majestic was not found in subsequent experiments carried out on tubers which had been in storage for a longer period but which showed, by visual and microscopic examination, a similar response to fungal inoculation. In all our experiments of this type, the chlorogenic acid level was lower in the early stages in the inoculated than in the uninoculated samples of Orion. It seems unlikely therefore that chlorogenic acid is being produced as an anti-fungal compound. However the lignin values were always higher in the inoculated tissue than in that of the controls and there was always more lignification in Orion than in Majestic. It seemed reasonable, therefore, to postulate that lignification is a direct response to the fungus. An increase in Klason lignin has been found by Sakai *et al.* (1967) for tubers of another R_1 potato cultivar, and it has been suggested that lignification is involved in resistance reactions in other host-parasite combinations (Hijwegen, 1963).

If lignification is involved in the resistance reaction, it would be expected to be concentrated around the small region of infection in Orion and be more diffuse in the large infected portion of Majestic.

LOCALIZATION OF LIGNIFICATION IN TUBER SLICES

In order to determine the localization of lignification in relation to the spread of the fungus, mycelial disks (3 mm dia.) were obtained aseptically from a 7-day culture of *P. infestans* on pea agar and each disk placed centrally on a slice of potato (5 mm thick). In Orion the infection spread to a diameter of 15 mm in 40 h and did not advance any further. The infection in Majestic was still advancing at this time and reached a final diameter of 50 mm after 140 h. Disks (10 mm dia.) from the same relative position in several slices of infected and uninfected tissue were analysed; Table IV shows that there was an increase in lignin close to the centre of the infection site in Orion which reached its maximum after 70 h. However, in Majestic lignification was spread over a wider area, the highest value determined being that of the outer portion of the infected area after 140 h. PAL activity in Orion was highest in the centre during the early stages whereas in Majestic the values were increasing in the later stages both in the centre and at the edges of the infected site (Table V).

We have also started experiments on the incorporation of [U–^{14}C]-phenylalanine into lignin in tuber disks. The preliminary results show that the substituted benzaldehydes obtained by alkaline nitrobenzene oxidation of the

TABLE IV

Increase in lignin across slices of potato which have been inoculated with a mycelial disk of *P. infestans* placed in the centre of the slices

Time after inoculation (h)		Majestic λ242	Majestic λ355	Orion λ242	Orion λ355
40	Centre	0.062	0.020	0.193	0.012
	Surround (U)	– N.M. –		0	0
90	Centre	0.095	0.040	0.160	0.081
	Surround (I)	0.105	0.007	– N.A. –	
	(U)	– N.A. –		0.017	0.029
140	Centre	0.111	0	0.094	0.062
	Surround (I)	0.242	0.024	– N.A. –	

N.M. = not measured N.A. = not applicable.

U and I are uninfected and infected respectively.

In Orion the area surrounding the central infected zone does not become infected whereas in Majestic the infection zone eventually spreads across the surface of the tuber slice.

These values represent the increase in an inoculated slice compared with that in an uninoculated slice and have been calculated by subtracting the values for the centre of an uninoculated slice from those of the area indicated.

The values are expressed in absorbance units/g fresh wt. of tissue.

TABLE V

Increases in phenylalanine ammonia lyase activity across slices of potato which have been inoculated with a mycelial disk of *P. infestans* placed in the centre of the slice.

Time after inoculation (h)		Majestic	Orion
40	Centre	8	67
	Surround (U)	5	42
70	Centre	6	24
	Surround (I)	1	N.A.
	Surround (U)	N.A.	21
90	Centre	46	22
	Surround (I)	18	N.A.
	Surround (U)	N.A.	8

These values represent the increase in an inoculated slice compared with that in an uninoculated slice and have been calculated by subtracting the values for the centre of an uninoculated slice from those in the area indicated.

The values are expressed in μg cinnamate produced/g fresh wt./h at 40°C.

lignin from infected Orion have a higher specific activity than those from Majestic and therefore provide additional confirmatory evidence that lignification linked to PAL activity is greater in Orion than in Majestic.

TABLE VI

Difference in phenylalanine ammonia lyase activity, chlorogenic acid content and lignin content between inoculated detached leaves and uninoculated detached leaves kept under identical conditions.

Time after inoculation		PAL as μg cinnamate/g fresh wt./h at 40°C	CGA μg/g fresh wt.	Lignin ΔA/g initial fresh wt. λ242	λ355
2 days	Majestic	+24.5	N.M.	0.075	0.030
	Orion	+21.5	N.M.	0.165	0.090
5 days	Majestic	+ 3	−63.5	0.175	0.180
	Orion	+ 7	−106.6	0.370	0.180

N.M. = not measured

LEAF EXPERIMENTS

Results which further support the lignification hypothesis have now been obtained in preliminary experiments with detached leaves maintained on benzimidazole solutions. Two days after inoculation there was more lignin in inoculated Orion than in Majestic although the PAL activity was about the same. After 5 days the differences in lignification were more pronounced and although the difference in PAL levels was not large, there was slightly more in the inoculated Orion. Chlorogenic acid, measured only at 5 days, was higher in Majestic than Orion and in both cultivars the inoculated leaves contained much less chlorogenic acid than did the controls (Table VI).

Discussion

THE IMPORTANCE OF LIGNIFICATION IN THE HYPERSENSITIVE REACTION

The results of the experiments with tuber disks and slices and with detached leaves all show that there is more rapid lignification in Orion than in Majestic following inoculation with race 4 of *P. infestans.* Rapid lignification therefore seems to be an important factor in the restriction of fungal growth which occurs in the hypersensitive response. It is known from many histological studies that after penetration of a resistant cell by *P. infestans* the hyphae are confined within that cell and usually die (see Ingram, 1967). Lignin could assist this confinement of the hyphae by acting either as a mechanical or a chemical barrier against fungal penetration. A mechanical-barrier mechanism implies that the lignin is so thick that it impedes physically the progress of the fungal hyphae across the cell wall. This would imply very thick lignification in the penetrated and adjacent cells. If lignification is forming a chemical barrier either by cross-linking the galactan or modifying it in some other way so that it can no longer act as a substrate for the fungal galactanase, then the lignin might not need to be deposited so thickly. We have histological evidence for thickening of the walls of Orion cells around the infected site but so far we have not demonstrated conclusively lignin deposition; potato lignin does not stain well with phloroglucinol. Autoradiography may reveal the site of lignification and we are now starting such experiments.

THE ROUTE OF LIGNIN BIOSYNTHESIS

In the tuber-slice experiments lignification was correlated with a rise in PAL activity similar to the one demonstrated in lignifying sycamore cell tissue cultures by Rubery and Northcote (1968). However the correlation was not as good in the disk or leaf experiments and there are two possible explanations. The first postulates at least two forms of PAL, one necessary for lignin and the other for soluble phenolic biosynthesis (Swain and Williams, 1970; Ahmed and Swain, 1970). If so, measurements of total PAL would include both forms, and it would be necessary to use other methods of assay which could distinguish between the two. The second would see lignin as synthesized from pre-existing soluble phenolics, such as chlorogenic acid. Taylor and Zucker (1966) have shown that chlorogenic acid can be converted to lignin-like insoluble polymers in both *Xanthium* leaves and potato tuber disks. This pathway could be operating in the early stages of tuber infection and in later stages of leaf infection in Orion, where an increase in lignin appears to be correlated with a decreased amount of chlorogenic acid.

If the latter explanation is correct, lignification need not be controlled by PAL levels but these would reflect the activity of other enzymes catalysing reactions closer to the actual polymerization reaction. Since little is known of the enzymatic reactions involved in the later stages of lignification it is not yet possible to suggest at which stage the regulation might occur.

TERPENOID METABOLISM

In addition to the rôle of rishitin in the hypersensitive reaction, which has already been mentioned briefly, the possible rôle of sterols in the host-parasite interaction should also be considered.

There is now abundant evidence that sterols are required for sexual reproduction of several *Phytophthora* spp. and that they increase the growth rate and are required for production of viable zoospores. Elliott and Knights (1969) have pointed out that resistance of several cultivars of potatoes to infection by *P. infestans* appear to be correlated with a high ratio of cyclo-artenol to β-sitosterol in uninfected tissue.

We have been examining changes in sterols after inoculation, and we have found that the cyclo-artenol: β-sitosterol ratio is much higher in Orion than in Majestic. Inoculation of detached leaves gives a 20% increase in total sterol of Orion compared with a slight decrease in Majestic, whereas in the uninoculated controls there is a decrease in Orion and an increase in Majestic. This might indicate that the actively-growing fungus is utilizing the sterols in Majestic. Preliminary experiments with labelled mevalonate show that, in addition to sterols, it is incorporated into a fraction with the same R_F value as rishitin but that there is little difference in the amount of radioactivity in this fraction between Majestic and Orion. In other experiments, we have found small amounts of chemically detectable rishitin in infected Orion tubers; the amounts are much less than those reported by Tomiyama *et al.* (1968) for 'Rishiri' tubers.

Conclusion

There are considerable changes in phenolic metabolism in potatoes after inoculation with *P. infestans.* It appears that the production of a lignin-like polymer is an important biochemical manifestation of the hypersensitive response of the R_1-gene expressed in Orion when challenged by race 4 of *P. infestans.*

However further work is needed to determine whether this biochemical situation holds for other combinations of R-genes and fungal races and in addition whether the altered patterns of terpenoid metabolism are significant in terms of disease resistance and whether they are correlated with the changes in phenol metabolism.

Acknowledgements

The work described in this paper was initiated by Professor N. F. Robertson and was carried out in collaboration with Dr D. Ingram, Dr M. Knee, Dr A. L. J. Cole, Mrs M. A. Aveyard, Mr S. B. Reynolds, Mr M. H. Asquith, Mrs M. Huffee and Mrs A. Stones. Financial support was provided by the Agricultural Research Council and the Science Research Council.

References

Ahmed, S. I. and Swain, T. (1970). The effect of light on the activity of enzymes of the aromatic pathway in peas and mung beans. *Phytochemistry* **9**, 2287-2290.

Baruah, P. and Swain, T. (1959). The action of potato phenolase on flavonoid compounds. *J. Sci. Fd Agric.* **10**, 125-129.

Black, W. (1952a). Inheritance of resistance to blight (*Phytophthora infestans*) in potatoes: inter-relationships of genes and strains. *Proc. R. Soc. Edinb.* **B64**, 312-352.

Black, W. (1952b). A genetical basis for the classification of strains of *Phytophthora infestans. Proc. R. Soc. Edinb.* **B65**, 36-51.

Cole, A. L. J. (1970). Pectic enzyme activity from *Phytophthora infestans. Phytochemistry* **9**, 337-340.

Cruickshank, I. A. M. (1963). Phytoalexins. *A. Rev. Phytopathol.* **1**, 351-374.

Elliott, C. G. and Knights, B. A. (1969). Interactions between steroids in the growth of *Phytophthora. J. Sci. Fd Agric.* **20**, 406-408.

Ferris, V. R. (1955). Histological study of pathogen-suscept relationships between *Phytophthora infestans* and derivatives of *Solanum demissum. Phytopathology* **45**, 546-552.

Friend, J. and Knee, M. (1969). Cell wall changes in potato tuber tissue infected with *Phytophthora infestans. J. exp. Bot.* **20**, 763-765.

Friend, J., Reynolds, S. B. and Aveyard, M. A. (1971). Phenolic metabolism in potato tuber tissue after infection with *Phytophthora infestans. Biochem. J.* **124**, 29P.

Hijwegen, T. (1963). Lignification, a possible mechanism of active resistance against pathogens. *Tijdsch. PlZiekt.* **69**, 314-317.

Hughes, J. C. and Swain, T. (1960). Scopolin production in potato tubers infected with *Phytophthora infestans. Phytopathology* **50**, 398-402.

Ingram, D. S. (1967). The expression of R-gene resistance to *Phytophthora infestans* in tissue cultures of *Solanum tuberosum. J. gen. Microbiol.* **49**, 99-108.

Ingram, D. S. and Robertson, N. F. (1965). Interaction between *Phytophthora infestans* and tissue cultures of *Solanum tuberosum. J. gen. Microbiol.* **40**, 431-437.

Katsui, N., Murai, A., Takasugi, M., Imaizumi, K. and Masamune, T. (1968). The structure of rishitin, a new antifungal compound from diseased potato tubers. *Chem. Comm.* **No. 1**, 43-44.

Kitazawa, K. and Tomiyama, K. (1970). Microscopic observations of infection of potato cells by compatible and incompatible races of *Phytophthora infestans. Phytopath. Z.* **66**, 317-324.

Knee, M. (1970). The use of a new, rapid micro-method for analysing changes in the carbohydrate fractions of potato tuber tissue after invasion by *Phytophthora infestans. Phytochemistry* **9**, 2075-2083.

Knee, M. and Friend, J. (1968). Extracellular "galactanase" activity from *Phytophthora infestans* (Mont.) de Bary. *Phytochemistry* **7**, 1289-1291.

Knee, M. and Friend, J. (1970). Some properties of the galactanase secreted by *Phytophthora infestans* (Mont.) de Bary. *J. gen. Microbiol.* **60**, 23-30.

Koukol, J. and Conn, E. E. (1961). Metabolism of aromatic compounds in higher plants. IV. Purification and properties of phenylalanine deaminase of *Hordeum vulgare. J. biol. Chem.* **236**, 2692-2698.

Mapson, L. W., Swain, T. and Tomalin, A. W. (1963). Influence of variety, cultural conditions and temperature of storage on enzymic browning of potato tubers. *J. Sci. Fd Agric.* **14**, 673-684.

Müller, K. O. (1953). The nature of the resistance of the potato plant to blight, *Phytophthora infestans. J. nat. Inst. Agric. Bot.* **6**, 346-360.

Müller, K. O. (1958). Studies on phytoalexins. I. The formation and immunological significance of phytoalexin produced by *Phaseolus vulgaris* in response to infection with *Sclerotinia fructicola* and *Phytophthora infestans. Aust. J. biol. Sci.* **11**, 275-300.

Robertson, N. F., Friend, J., Aveyard, M. A., Brown, J., Huffee, M. and Homans, A. L. (1968). The accumulation of phenolic acids in tissue culture combinations of *Solanum tuberosum* and *Phytophthora infestans. J. gen. Microbiol.* **54**, 261-268.

Rubery, P. H. and Northcote, D. H. (1968). Site of phenylalanine ammonia-lyase activity and synthesis of lignin during xylem differentiation. *Nature, Lond.* **219**, 1230-1234.

Sakai, R., Tomiyama, K., Ishizaka, N. and Sato, N. (1967). Phenol metabolism in disease resistance of potato tubers. 3. Phenol metabolism in tissue neighbouring the necrogenous infection. *Ann. phytopath. Soc. Japan* **33**, 216-222.

Sato, N., Tomiyama, K., Katsui, N. and Masamune, T. (1968). Isolation of rishitin from tubers of interspecific potato varieties containing late-blight resistance genes. *Ann. phytopath. Soc. Japan* **34**, 140-142.

Stafford, H. A. (1960). Difference between lignin-like polymers formed by peroxidation of eugenol and ferulic acid in leaf sections of Phleum. *Pl. Physiol., Lancaster* **35**, 108-118.

Swain, T. and Williams, C. A. (1970). The role of phenylalanine in flavonoid biosynthesis. *Phytochemistry* **9**, 2115-2122.

Taylor, A. O. and Zucker, M. (1966). Turnover and metabolism of chlorogenic acid in *Xanthium* leaves and potato tubers. *Pl. Physiol., Lancaster* **41**, 1350-1359.

Tomiyama, K., Sakuma, T., Ishizaka, N., Sato, N., Katsui, N., Takasugi, M. and Masamune, T. (1968). A new antifungal substance isolated from resistant potato tuber tissue infected by pathogens. *Phytopathology* **58**, 115-116.

Varns, J. L., Kuć, J. and Williams, E. G. (1971). Terpenoid accumulation as a biochemical response of the potato tuber to *Phytophthora infestans*. *Phytopathology* **61**, 174-177.

DISCUSSION

Dr D. S. Ingram: Do you think that your lignification hypothesis is an explanation for resistance in Orion only, or an explanation for resistance in all R-gene potato reactions? Have you also examined other R-gene reactions?

Professor Friend: As we have not looked at any other R-gene potatotes we have to say that this hypothesis is for Orion only. We would like to look at a range of other R-gene potatoes, but of course the large amounts of rishitin in some of these others may be more important. Neither have we looked at what happens when Orion is invaded by a race which will infect it, and we are hoping to do this quite soon.

A. van Dijkman: Do you have another race of *Phytophthora* to which Majestic is resistant, but Orion is susceptible? That would sustain your theory about resistance if you have this cross relation.

Professor Friend: Majestic does not have any R-gene at all, it is completely susceptible, and so we have to find a race which will grow on Orion, or some other tubers as well.

Professor J. H. Burnett: Is anything known about the galactanase activity of different races of *Phytophthora,* because such differences are a necessary corollary to your ideas?

Professor Friend: No, there is nothing known about them. Dr Cole has done some work on the extracellular enzymes. However one could invoke lignin as creating a mechanical barrier rather than causing an alteration to the substrate and under these circumstances galactanase activity would not be too important. So one can build on the lignification hypothesis without much effort and really embellish it if one wants to.

Professor R. K. S. Wood: I think my question is probably related to the last but one, and this is a general problem of methodology in the study of all resistance problems. I refer particularly to the possible explanation of the resistance of Orion in terms of the ratios of those two sterols you mentioned. The difficulty is that it is almost certainly going to be possible to get a race of *Phytophthora infestans* to which Orion is susceptible. How then do you explain the significance of this balance of sterols in Orion? You have then got to implicate the new race of *Phytophthora infestans.*

Professor Friend: I realize that we will probably have to change our ideas completely when we do our experiments with a different race of *Phytophthora.* Maybe this is just an answer for one particular race, and one particular cultivar.

Dr H. M. Dekhuijzen: In relation to Dr Ingram's paper given yesterday, I would like to ask you if it is really possible to use tissue culture for the extraction experiments. Can you really transfer the results obtained with tissue culture to what is going on in normal tissue?

Professor Friend: Obviously the difficulty we have found with tissue culture is common to most other tissue cultures, i.e. they do not produce the same secondary products that the whole plant does. Here the tissue cultures are producing benzoic acids and the plant produces cinnamic acids in the form of esters, that is mainly chlorogenic acid. I think there might be an explanation for this benzoic acid production, it might be a spill-over after the lignification, and this may explain the excess of benzoic acids but it does mean that the tissue culture has got some β-oxidation method of converting cinnamic acids into benzoic acids, which the plant itself does not have.

Dr Dekhuijzen: And is the tissue culture polyploid, is it normal or abnormal?

Professor Friend: I am sure it is highly abnormal. The Orion was forming a nice white sector which was growing much faster, and so we started picking up the faster growing one, and then it lost its resistance.

Dr Dekhuijzen: It lost its resistance?

Professor Friend: Yes, it will produce sectors, and if you choose one of the sectors which you think is growing faster, and so will be better to use for more experiments, then it loses its resistance, and so you have picked the wrong one. I do not think you would ask me to pick a winner in a horse race!

Professor M. A. Stahmann: I was very much interested in your pointing out the increases in phenylalanine ammonia lyase associated with increased lignification and production of these aromatic acids. It is possible that another race of *Phytophthora* may not incite this increase, so that your explanation for specificity might hold with other races. We find marked changes in many enzymes as a result of infection, and just how these enzymes are integrated might determine whether or not the host is resistant or susceptible.

Professor Friend: I should perhaps point out that PAL is induced in potatoes by illumination. Zucker showed this six years ago, and we have looked at the effect of light on Majestic and Orion. The rate of induction of PAL activity is much faster in Orion than it is in Majestic, and so this is inbuilt for the potato–it is not just a response to infection. There is a great deal of difficulty here in distinguishing between a wounding reaction and the infection situation, and this is why we want to start looking at the possibility of isoenzymes, or different locations for them. But as you say, there are fantastic biochemical changes in potatoes when they are cut, so it is really a matter of trying to work out which ones are significant in terms of resistant reaction.

Professor Burnett: One item in your data which I do not quite understand is in the table for lignin production. In the Orion data, although it is perfectly true the lignin went up initially, it then dropped far below anything in the Majestic.

Professor Friend: This value was the difference in lignification between the inoculated and the uninoculated, so it does not refer to the total amount of lignin that is formed. The total amount goes up to a peak and more or less stays there. I have taken the results and doctored them, as it were, by subtracting the values for the uninoculated. Majestic at the later stage is producing lignin—quite a lot of lignin. The point we would suggest is that it is producing the lignin in an area where fungus is no longer growing, it is producing it in the centre of the infected zone, and the fungus is growing around the edge of the slice at this stage.

Professor Burnett: But am I not right that in the Orion data you have two occasions where you took samples, and in the second one, for Orion, the lignin content had dropped right down. This is the point which puzzles me, it should have stayed constant, surely?

Professor Friend: I agree that the value given in Table IV for Orion does drop in the second case. However the total amount of lignin in Orion does not drop. The values given at 90 and 140 h in Orion reflect that whereas lignification has more or less ceased in the centre of the inoculated slice, it is still increasing in the uninoculated slice, so that the values expressed in Table IV as inoculated minus uninoculated are decreasing. The increases in the total amount of lignin in the uninoculated control are part of the wounding response. The situation in Majestic is different because at 90 h there is far less lignin in both inoculated and uninoculated slices compared with Orion. In addition the difference between inoculated and uninoculated is less than in Orion. At 140 h the total amount of lignin in the infcted surround of Majestic is as high as that found in Orion at earlier stage; however because the amount of lignin in the uninoculated slice is still low, the value (shown in Table IV) for inoculated minus uninoculated Majestic surround at 140 h is higher than any of the values shown for Orion.

I have expressed the results as values for inoculated tissue minus those for uninoculated tissue in order to try and distinguish reactions caused by infection from wounding reactions.

A. van Dijkman: I should like to ask you if this lignification, this high activity of PAL is a so-called primary determinant, or is it a secondary effect. Is it possible that you can have the same effect when you treat the tissue with another substance which can damage the membrane, e.g. nystatin, or a little bit of chloroform? The second question is have you looked for any peroxidase activity in this system?

Professor Friend: No we have not looked at peroxidase, and I am pretty sure that one can get induction of PAL by a variety of things. Certainly one can do it by putting tuber slices in the light and making measurements at different times, and one detects an increase and then a decrease. Zucker has done this, and we have found it to be faster in Orion than in Majestic. Whether this is a primary response to the fungus or not, I do not know. I suppose I ought to say something about ethylene. We have not done any experiments with ethylene, but Dr Rhodes at the Food Research Institute who has been looking at the effect of ethylene on PAL induction in several different types of plant tissue, has tried it with potato tuber tissue, and he finds that ethylene does not induce PAL formation in potato tuber tissue, whereas it will do so in a lot of other plants. The antibiotics which we have looked at are the ones which inhibit protein synthesis, and these suppress the induction of PAL when you put the potato tuber tissue in actidione.

A. van Dijkman: No, I meant the polyenic ones.

Professor Friend: No, we have not looked at nystatin, and we have not tried the effects of chloroform. But if you do just cause a general wounding reaction, e.g. by slicing the potato, you get very little induction of PAL, and you have either to put it in the light to get induction, or you have to infect it with a fungus.

General Discussion on Section IV

S. B. Reynolds: We have heard Dr Bailey and Dr Smith discussing phaseollin, and several other speakers considering whether the induction is the actual necrosis or the hypersensitive death of the cell, or whether in fact phenolics have nothing to do with hypersensitive cell death in resistance, as they merely result from the death of the cell and are therefore involved in the reaction between the host and the pathogen.

Professor M. A. Stahmann: May I make two general comments, first in regard to phytoalexins. I have often thought the production of phytoalexins might involve two steps, first the stimulation of aromatic biosynthesis, and then a stimulation of enzyme systems which form free-radicals. The free-radicals produced by the enzymes could be captured by aromatic residues to induce their condensation to give compounds with phytoalexin activity. This presumably might happen only in plant species in which the proper precursor phenols are produced, and when these two events occur you might have phytoalexin formation. I think we should give more consideration to the biosynthesis of these compounds. In the first Session we talked about the involvement of fungal proteins and discussed the possible action of pectolytic enzymes, but very little consideration has been given to the effects of the products of these enzymes. I wonder if the polyuronides which are produced as pectins or other polysaccharides are degraded, might have some physiological effects. These polyuronides are polyanions and there may be receptor sites on host enzymes that bind them. In other words, I would suggest that further studies be made on the possible biological activity of the intermediate products of hydrolytic enzymes. So I would like to suggest that these gaps be considered before the next Session which deals with altered metabolism.

Dr I. M. Smith: I want to comment on this question of the alteration of phenolic biosynthesis, and one of the observations which I did not emphasize this morning was the interesting uniqueness of the pattern of compounds which was found in every species I looked at. It appears that there ought to be common substrates in different species, that the same sorts of enzymes would be induced, and you ought to get common products to some extent, and superimposed on this one might get a few specific products, including specific phytoalexins, but in my experience this was not so. I tended to get a distinctly unique pattern in every species. Also if necrosis and discoloration damage the cell organelles—this damage being seen at quite an early stage corresponding to phytoalexin production—this must self-evidently correspond to massive biochemical changes. We cannot pick out a little portion of it leading to one phytoalexin, as being of any particular significance in the overall pattern.

Dr B. J. Deverall: When we are discussing phytoalexin-like substances, we should not just talk about phenolic substances. Some of them are non-phenolic, and some are non-aromatic.

Professor P. H. Williams: When considering concepts surrounding preformed versus induced forms of resistance, we should take into account the type of cell that is reacting. In the tissue as a whole this may be one thing, but there may be different types of cells which have either the capability of forming new compounds, or which already have preformed compounds in glucosidic form, or non-reactive form, let us say, and I wonder how much these types of cells play a part in resistance. Around the vascular strands of many plant tissues there are cells which have the capability of reacting dramatically to the presence of a pathogen by providing or releasing anti-fungal or anti-bacterial materials. Other tissues or cells very close to these responsive cells may not react to the pathogen. As to Dr Bailey's photographs of specific cells in the leaf reaction, I wonder whether this was a function of genetically-selected cells, or whether any cell in a leaf would have reacted this way. We were talking last night about the colonization of cells by obligate parasites, and it was commented that we rarely see such colonization around vascular systems. I wonder how much has been done at the cellular level, or how much work needs to be done.

Professor R. K. S. Wood: In systems such as the *Phytophthora infestans*/R-gene and the *Colletotrichum*/γ,δ races, we must beware of concentrating most of our studies on post-infection events, whether these be the actual patterns of biosynthesis of the phytoalexin, or else lignin or suberin formation. I am not saying these are not important. These are the ways in which resistance is ultimately expressed. But they tell us little about the really important critical events which happen very much earlier. The vogue word 'recognition' may not be the best term, but it describes a very important aspect of resistance. What is it, in fact, that stimulates all these responses? Because I think the evidence is quite clear that in the *Phytophthora infestans*/R-gene or *Colletotrichum* systems, the subsequent reactions are very similar. What differs is the triggering response, or the way in which it is triggered.

Professor J. H. Burnett: I would like to make a comment on what Professor Wood has just said. I think it is a fact that all the cases which have been described this morning involve penetration before you get any reaction. I do not know if this is a generalization. Now the hyphal tip (or whatever you may call it) which penetrates–if it is like the apex of the hyphae of free-living fungi–is, chemically, going to be different from the walls of the rest of the fungus. Almost certainly it is going to be protein in its outermost layer, so that the first contact on penetration is going to be between wall protein of fungus and cytoplasmic protein of host; and protein-protein interactions in other spheres can give rise to many various kinds of reactions. Of that protein (i.e. fungal wall protein), if our data on free-living fungi are anything to go by, about 50% will be enzymatic. The other 50% seems to be structural protein, whatever that means. At any rate, it is not enzymatic. Of that protein, quite a lot is fairly easily separated off in ionic solvents and so on, and I think therefore, if you are going to go back to the very first starting point, you should perhaps try to find out really what is the nature of the fungal, bacterial, or any other surface, which penetrates the cell. What is its composition and its properties? As I understand it, this is the start of everything.

Professor J. Friend: I would certainly agree with Professor Burnett's comments, and I think the point is that these studies present so many technical problems that we are all looking at the much easier side of the later stages of post-infection events. I should think it is fairly obvious that one is getting a great deal of enzymatic change, either the actual induction of enzymes, or control of allosteric sites to alter these metabolic pathways, and these really are the events we should be looking at.

Dr J. A. Kavanagh: There is just one thing which I think is related to a lot of studies on the physiology of parasitism. I think sometimes we pay great attention to seeking out a system that is workable under laboratory conditions, but that sometimes does not altogether resemble the situation under natural conditions. I think that in some of the systems which have been used we should just try and relate what is going on in the field to what actually goes on in the systems in the laboratory.

Dr J. T. Martin: With regret I must draw the meeting to a close. When I looked at the title of the Session 'Preformed and induced resistance factors', I wondered, resistance to what? Resistance to infection or resistance to disease? Sometimes I think we may be a bit confused. Infection is the act of penetration of a pathogenic micro-organism; disease is the result of such penetration. Sometimes the difference is not entirely clear. Resistance to infection obviously is a complicated phenomenon and, as I view it, the result of a delicate balance of interacting factors which is tipped in favour of the host. We have progressed very much from the stage when people were looking for a single factor to account for resistance; obviously many interacting factors are involved.

Section V
Altered Metabolism

V. 1 Changes in Enzymes of Host and Pathogen with Special Reference to Peroxidase Interaction

M. A. STAHMANN AND D. M. DEMOREST

Department of Biochemistry
College of Agricultural and Life Sciences
University of Wisconsin, Madison, 53706 U.S.A.

INTRODUCTION

I (M. A. S.) began studies on the biochemistry of plant diseases and resistance in the late thirties just after Link *et al.* (1933) had isolated protocatechuic acid and catechol from the outer scales of onion bulbs resistant to onion smudge. They suggested that disease resistance in plants was a passive character conferred by the presence in resistant cultivars of phenols or other toxic substances that blocked the growth of the pathogen. As a graduate student, I was asked to study the mustard oils of crucifers which were claimed to be the basis for resistance to clubroot. I isolated a mustard oil from both resistant and susceptible turnips and although the oil was very toxic I could not show that it was related to resistance (Stahmann *et al.*, 1943). After much unsuccessful searching for other preformed toxic substances that might confer resistance, I was forced to conclude that the factors that control resistance or susceptibility might not be expressed until after the pathogen had contacted the host, or that resistance was an active rather than a passive character.

Plant breeders had shown that the resistant character was often under the control of genes of the host and since genes control protein synthesis, I concluded that the problem in resolving the nature of the genetic resistance of plants would be to identify the proteins whose synthesis was controlled by the resistant genes. However, since each cell may contain thousands of proteins, this is very difficult.

During the 1950s, we looked at some plant proteins by free electrophoresis, but the resolving power was too low. Gel electrophoresis gave greater resolution and when, in the 1960s, this was combined with biological detection tests for specific proteins we clearly saw changes in proteins following infection. The biological test first used was that of antigen-antibody interaction; this utilized antisera prepared against protein extracts from healthy or inoculated, resistant and susceptible plants. New antigens were seen after inoculation of cabbage with *Fusarium oxysporum* f. *conglutinans* (Heitefuss *et al.*, 1960) and sweet potato roots with *Ceratocystis fimbriata* (Uritani and Stahmann, 1961). These new antigens were detected in sweet potato tissue adjacent to the area invaded by the fungus. They were produced in response to the infection and were more concentrated in the tissues of resistant sweet potatoes. One of these new antigens was identified as a peroxidase.

When white potato tuber tissue was inoculated with *Phytophthora infestans* there was also an increase in both peroxidase and polyphenol oxidase in the cells a few millimetres below the inoculated surface (Tomiyama and Stahmann, 1964). This increase was greater and extended deeper into the inner tissue when the incompatible race was used. Two new isoenzymes of peroxidase were formed after inoculation with the incompatible race to which the tissue was resistant but not with the compatible race to which it was susceptible.

In a study of enzymes in susceptible bean leaves after infection by the bean rust fungus, Staples and Stahmann (1964) observed an increased number of isoenzymes of acid and alkaline phosphatase, succinate dehydrogenase and malate dehydrogenase. Peroxidase activity increased 150%.

A study of isoenzymes of bean leaves after infection with *Pseudomonas phaseolicola* showed increased activities of peroxidase, polyphenol oxidase and dehydrogenases of glucose-6-phosphate, isocitrate, malate and glutamate (Rudolph and Stahmann, 1966) and changes in isoenzyme patterns. Virulent bacteria showed strong catalase activity which was thought to depress the activity of peroxidases involved in the defence reactions of the host.

Thus, by the middle 1960s, changes in several enzymes of the host plant had been shown to follow inoculation with fungal and bacterial pathogens. Such changes have now been studied in greater detail.

Enzyme Changes Following a Virus Infection

Dr G. L. Farkas and I wondered if the increase in enzyme activity following inoculation was due to enzyme activation or synthesis. We decided to study enzyme changes following a virus infection. A marked change in peroxidase isoenzymes of bean leaves resulted from inoculation with southern bean mosaic virus (Farkas and Stahmann, 1966). Young healthy bean leaves contained two peroxidase isoenzymes. Associated with lesion development, two additional isoenzymes appeared which were most pronounced at the site of lesion development. Purification of these four components by gel filtration and column chromatography showed them to be different proteins. The formation of the new peroxidases in the virus-infected tissues was blocked by inhibitors of protein synthesis. We concluded that some of the increase in peroxidase following virus infection is due to protein synthesis.

Enzyme Changes in Bacterial Diseases

PEROXIDASE IN THE RESISTANCE OF TOBACCO TO *PSEUDOMONAS TABACI*

Injection of heat-killed cells of *Pseudomonas tabaci* into tobacco leaves induced a protection against the wildfire disease (Lovrekovich *et al.*, 1968a). The right half of a leaf was injected with a suspension containing 10^9 killed cells/ml; the opposite half was injected with water. The next day, both halves were injected with a suspension containing 10^7 living cells. Four days later the right side which had been injected with heat-killed cells showed no disease symptoms; in contrast, the left side which had been injected with water showed severe symptoms.

In the half-leaves injected with heat-killed bacteria, peroxidase was more than doubled within four days. The injection of heat-killed bacteria also resulted in the production of two additional isoenzymes of peroxidase that were produced by the host in response to the infection or to the injection of dead bacteria.

Injection of peroxidase also produced a marked protection against the wildfire disease. Half-leaves were injected with 50 μg/ml of a commercial, purified peroxidase; the opposite halves with water. Inoculation of both halves was made the next day. The injected peroxidase protected against the development of disease symptoms. Boiled peroxidase gave no protection. There was no protection when peroxidase and bacteria were injected at the same time, and peroxidase did not suppress *P. tabaci* growth in culture. We believe that the disease was suppressed by products formed by or induced by the injected peroxidase.

These results, which resemble vaccination and the passive transfer of immunity, suggest that an increase in peroxidase of the host may be responsible for increased resistance. Since there was no protection when peroxidase was injected at the same time as the living bacteria and no inhibition of bacterial growth by peroxidase, we suggest that increased resistance may be the result of peroxidase action or the induction by peroxidase of other enzymes involved in resistance.

TOBACCO MOSAIC VIRUS-INDUCED RESISTANCE TO *PSEUDOMONAS TABACI*

Virus infected plants often develop resistance to another virus or sometimes to fungal pathogens (Lovrekovich *et al.*, 1968b). Resistance to *Pseudomonas tabaci* was induced by local-lesion tobacco mosaic virus infection. Tobacco leaves were rubbed with buffer, or with tobacco mosaic virus. Three days later they were inoculated with *P. tabaci.* Severe symptoms of wildfire developed in the leaves rubbed with buffer. There was no bacterial symptoms in the leaves inoculated with virus. Plate counts showed that the multiplication of *P. tabaci* was suppressed by the virus inoculation.

There was an increase in peroxidase in tobacco leaves infected with tobacco mosaic virus compared with a control consisting of leaves on separate plants rubbed with buffer. The increase was greatest in tissue close to virus lesions but an increase also occurred in tissue between lesions.

From these results it was concluded that tobacco mosaic virus increases resistance to *P. tabaci* and that this resistance was associated with a virus-induced increase in host peroxidase. Simons and Ross (1970) have confirmed the enhanced peroxidase activity following inoculation with tobacco mosaic virus, and shown that it is associated also with the virus-induced resistance to tobacco mosaic virus in hypersensitive tobacco.

Enzyme Changes in Fungal Diseases

INDUCTION OF ENZYME CHANGES AND ACQUIRED IMMUNITY IN SWEET POTATOES

Sweet potato roots were cut into pieces and inoculated on two surfaces with a nonpathogenic or a pathogenic isolate of *Ceratocystis fimbriata.* The pathogens formed abundant mycelium on the surface but penetrated into roots of only very susceptible cultivars. In contrast there was only little surface growth by the nonpathogens. After two or three days, sections were cut parallel to the infected surface. The upper section containing the fungus was discarded and enzymes were extracted from the underlying sections.

Gel electrophoresis patterns of peroxidase from resistant and susceptible sweet potatoes were altered by inoculation with both the pathogenic and nonpathogenic isolates. Inoculation produced an increase in the number and intensity of the isoenzyme bands of peroxidase. Some nonpathogens produced changes similar to the pathogen. Growth of the fungus on the surface induced changes in the enzymes at a distance up to 3 mm below the infection.

On the basis that induced enzyme changes represent an immune response, we carried out experiments (Weber and Stahmann, 1966) to determine whether or not a nonpathogenic isolate from almonds which induced similar enzymatic changes would induce resistance. Tissue pieces from a resistant and a susceptible cultivar were inoculated with the nonpathogen. Two days later the pieces were challenged by inoculation with the pathogenic isolate. Only the susceptible tissue that was not inoculated with a nonpathogen developed severe symptoms of black rot; in contrast, the susceptible pieces which were first inoculated with the nonpathogen before challenge showed the resistant reaction and remained free of internal symptoms. Fungal growth was confined to the surface.

We concluded that inoculation of the surface of susceptible sweet potatoes with some nonpathogenic isolates of *C. fimbriata* induced resistance or immunity to subsequent infection by the pathogenic isolate. This immunity was limited to a few cell layers below the surface and could be induced on one side of the section. If the upper cells were scraped away, the pathogen was able to reach the underlying susceptible tissue and rot the entire piece.

In many ways this induced immunity or resistance resembles vaccination. It differs in two respects. First there is no demonstration of antibody formation in the sense that specific precipitating or neutralizing agents are formed. Secondly, this immunity is confined to a few cell layers around the infection site.

We examined enzymatic changes associated with induced and natural resistance (Weber *et al.*, 1967). There was only slight increase in enzyme activity when healthy tissue was sliced or when it was inoculated with an isolate that did not induce resistance. However, there was an increase in peroxidase, polyphenol oxidase, and alkaline phosphatase with the pathogen or nonpathogenic isolates which induced resistance. Malic dehydrogenase, glucose-6-phosphate dehydrogenase, and alkaline phosphatase decreased. Both the pathogen and nonpathogen that induced resistance caused similar changes in seven out of eight of the enzymes.

It seems that the ability of the nonpathogens to induce changes in the enzymes of the tissues is associated with their ability to induce immunity or resistance. We suggest that whenever these enzymatic changes occur sufficiently far in advance of penetration, the pathogen is unable to invade the tissue. We conclude that these enzymatic changes represent a defence reaction of the plant.

THE INDUCER THAT INCREASES RESISTANCE AND ENZYME ACTIVITY

It was unexpectedly observed that uninoculated pieces of sweet potato incubated in closed chambers with infected pieces showed an increase in peroxidase activity. This suggested that some volatile material from the infected tissue was involved. We considered ethylene because it is a common product of infected tissue and can produce an increase in respiratory activity. We first tested this possibility by incubating sweet potato tissue in the presence of an apple, a known source of ethylene. The volatile material given off by the apple increased the peroxidase content and the disease resistance.

We then looked for an increase in peroxidase and polyphenol oxidase in sweet potato tissue treated with ethylene (Stahmann *et al.*, 1966). There was an 11-fold increase in peroxidase following exposure to 8 ppm of ethylene. Polyphenol oxidase was very low before ethylene treatment and increased after exposure to ethylene.

Resistance in a susceptible sweet potato was increased by ethylene. Pieces of susceptible sweet potato root tissue were exposed to 0, 8, or 150 ppm of ethylene for two days prior to inoculation with *C. fimbriata.* Severe symptoms of black rot developed in the pieces that had been incubated in an atmosphere containing no ethylene. In contrast, the pieces incubated in ethylene (8 or 150 ppm) showed a resistant reaction similar to that of resistant cultivars in which fungal growth was confined to the surface.

Ethylene production was measured from pieces of uninoculated sweet potato root tissue, and from tissue inoculated with fungal spores of *C. minor*, a non-inducer that does not cause resistance, and with the pathogenic isolate. The tissue pieces were incubated for three days in closed chambers and ethylene determined by gas chromatography. A volatile compound with the same retention time as ethylene was demonstrated above the infected sweet potato tissue. Uninoculated tissues formed very little ethylene. Ethylene production was larger with the nonpathogenic strain which induced resistance than with non-inducers; it was largest with the pathogen. More ethylene was formed by the resistant Sunnyside than by the susceptible Julian. Ethylene was not detected above cultures of *C. fimbriata* on potato dextrose agar. This suggests that the infected host tissue produced ethylene and that ethylene is one of the factors that regulates induction of resistance to black rot which is associated with an increase in enzyme activity.

THE EFFECT OF PEROXIDASE ON GERMINATION AND GROWTH OF WHEAT RUST

We measured the peroxidase level in a resistant (Kapli) and a susceptible wheat (Little Club) before and after inoculation with *Puccinia graminis* f. sp. *tritici* (Macko *et al.*, 1968). Peroxidase activity in healthy leaves of both showed almost no change and no difference during the experimental period. After inoculation, there was a small increase in peroxidase in the susceptible wheat, but this was more marked in the resistant wheat.

When rust spores were germinated on nutrient media supplemented with peroxidase and hydrogen peroxide, the elongation of germ tubes was very slow. Growth of mycelium was altered and small discrete colonies composed of short branched mycelia formed. In many ways colonies grown in the presence of peroxidase resembled the fleck reaction in resistant plants. The large increase in peroxidase in the resistant host after inoculation and the alteration of mycelial growth on nutrient agar by peroxidase may indicate that host peroxidase is an important factor in the regulation of resistance, or the incompatible reaction of wheat rust.

ISOENZYME CHANGES IN PEAS INFECTED WITH FUSARIUM WILT

Isoenzyme patterns of 16 different enzymes were examined during development of wilt disease in peas caused by *Fusarium oxysporum* f. sp. *pisi* race 1, and were compared with patterns obtained from non-infected plants and from the culture grown fungus (Reddy and Stahmann, unpublished results). The isoenzyme bands from extracts of stem tissue 12-15 days after inoculation were generally more intense than those from the non-infected plants. The intensity of the single band of catalase, alkaline phosphatase and NAD-dependent glutamate dehydrogenase was increased. With peroxidase, acetylesterase, acid phosphatase, glucokinase and aldolase, the intensity of some isoenzyme bands increased and others decreased following infection. The number and intensity of peroxidase bands varied with the type of the substrate used. Soluble isoenzymes for fumarase, succinate dehydrogenase and NADP-dependent isocitrate dehydrogenase were detected in the infected plants but not in the non-infected plants; these bands of the infected plants did not correspond to fungal bands. New isoenzymes which could not be found in extracts from healthy plants or the fungus were detected with peroxidase, aldolase, glucokinase, glucose-6-phosphate dehydrogenase, NADP-dependent glutamate dehydrogenase, NAD-dependent malate dehydrogenase and NADP-dependent malate dehydrogenase (decarboxylating) following infection. Table I summarizes the isoenzyme changes in *Fusarium*-infected pea stem tissue.

The change of malate dehydrogenase has been studied in more detail. *Fusarium* infection causes a 280% increase in activity 12 days after inoculation. A new fast-moving isoenzyme band appeared in the soluble fraction within six days. This band contained 21% of the total malate dehydrogenase activity. On heating at 55° C, all fungal malate dehydrogenase bands were destroyed within 5 min, those from healthy tissues within 22 min while 40 min was required for total loss of activity of the new band from infected tissue. The binding affinity of the malate dehydrogenase from stem tissue was increased on infection; the K_m value for extracts from infected tissue was about half that for extracts from healthy tissue. Such increases in binding affinity of enzymes after infection may be the biochemical basis for the metabolic sink often observed about infection sites and which make it possible for nutrients to accumulate in or around infected areas.

CHANGES IN PEROXIDASE IN BARLEY LEAVES INFECTED WITH MILDEW

With Dr E. C. Hislop we studied peroxidase and ethylene production by barley leaves infected with *Erysiphe graminis* f. sp. *hordei,* (Hislop and Stahmann, 1971). We were interested in factors related to resistance or susceptibility which is determined within about 24 h after inoculation.

Inoculation of primary leaves of barley of differing compatibilities to race 3 of *Erysiphe graminis* f. sp. *hordei* resulted in a 3–5-fold increase in peroxidase activity. This increase was usually evident within 24 h of inoculation and was accompanied by the appearance of one new major isoenzyme band. This new band was not seen in extracts of conidia of the pathogen, which contained little peroxidase. It was concluded that the increase in peroxidase was a host response to infection.

TABLE I

Summary of the number of isoenzymes from healthy pea stem tissue, *Fusarium*-infected stems and from mycelium of the pathogen *Fusarium oxysporum* f. sp. *pisi* race 1 and the change in the number or intensity of isoenzymes 15 days after inoculation.

Enzyme	No. bands from:– Healthy	Infected	Fungus	No. bands changed after inoculation[1] Intensity (+)	(–)	New isoenzyme bands
I. ENZYMES SHOWING AN INCREASE IN INTENSITY WITH NO CHANGE IN THE NUMBER OF ISOENZYMES						
Catalase	1	1	4	1	0	0
Alkaline phosphatase	1	1	1	1	0	0
NAD-glutamate dehydrogenase	1	1	1	1	0	0
II. ENZYMES SHOWING AN INCREASE IN THE NUMBER OF ISOENZYMES AND AN INCREASE OR DECREASE IN INTENSITY						
Peroxidase (*p*-ansidine)	6	10	4	6	0	2
Peroxidase (benzidine)	7	10	4	4	2	2
Peroxidase (chlorogenic acid)	6	9	4	6	0	1
Peroxidase (pyrogallol)	6	8	6	4	1	1
Acetylesterase	6	7	3	2	2	0
Acid phosphatase	7	8	3	4	2	0
Glucokinase	1	4	1	0	1	3
Aldolase	1	3	3	0	1	2
III. ENZYMES SHOWING BANDS ONLY AFTER INFECTION						
Fumarase	0	6	3	0	0	6
Succinate dehydrogenase	0	4	2	0	0	2
Isocitrate dehydrogenase	0	2	0	0	0	2
IV. ENZYMES SHOWING AN INCREASE IN THE NUMBER AND INTENSITY OF ISOENZYME BANDS						
NADP-glutamate dehydrogenase	1	3	1	1	0	2
NAD-malate dehydrogenase	1	4	4	1	0	1
NADP-malate dehydrogenase (decarboxylating)	0	1	1	0	0	0
NADP-malate dehydrogenase (decarboxylating)[2]	1	3	1	1	0	2
Glucose-6-phosphate dehydrogenase	1	4	1	1	0	2
Glucose-6-phosphate dehydrogenase[2]	1	3	1	1	0	2
Phosphogluconate dehydrogenase	1	2	1	0	0	1

[1] The intensity of isoenzymes in the infected plants was visually graded as increase (+), or decrease (–) when compared to those from the healthy stem tissue. Isoenzymes were considered new when their position did not correspond to those from either non-infected stems or the fungus.

[2] The substrate concentration in the staining solution was increased 2-4 fold.

There was a rapid initial increase in peroxidase activity in both susceptible (S) and resistant (R) lines to 50 h after inoculation. The Atlas (S) plants developed greater activity than the Atlas 46(R) from 50 h to 160 h. This condition was reversed for the Ml-g(R) and ml-g(S) material, where the immune line developed greater activity than the susceptible line in the later stages of infection. Fresh leaf extracts of this latter material made 96 h after inoculation confirmed that for these lines peroxidase activity in immune leaves was considerably higher than in susceptible leaves. Since both the Atlas 46 and the Ml-g line contain the Goldfoil gene for resistance it appeared that changes in peroxidase activity were associated with factors independent of these genes. Table II indicates that the four pairs of near-isogenic lines all showed a considerable increase in peroxidase activity within 24 h of inoculation. The results also show that in all cases there was a slightly more rapid increase in peroxidase activity in resistant leaves compared with susceptible leaves.

The peroxidase isoenzyme patterns of all of the susceptible and resistant lines 24 h after inoculation were very similar and contained one major isoenzyme band not seen in extracts of any of the uninoculated plants. The isoenzyme patterns of the uninoculated plants were similar. The new isoenzyme band was not seen in extracts of conidia of the pathogen which contained very little peroxidase. Further, when the bulk of the superficial mycelium was wiped from seven-day-old infections, the peroxidase levels and isoenzyme patterns in wiped and unwiped leaves were similar, indicating that the increased production of peroxidase was a host response.

TABLE II

Peroxidase activity in healthy and infected near-isogenic lines of barley with different genes for resistance, 24 h after inoculation.

Plant selection	Infection type[1]	Peroxidase activity[2]		
		Healthy (−)	Infected (+)	(+)−(−)
ml-a	4	0.05	0.20	0.15
Ml-a	0	0.04	0.22	0.18
ml-g	4	0.05	0.17	0.12
Ml-g	0-1	0.04	0.20	0.16
ml-p	4	0.05	0.19	0.14
Ml-p	2(1-3)	0.04	0.22	0.18
ml-k	4	0.07	0.20	0.13
Ml-k	2H	0.07	0.23	0.16

[1] 0–immune, 2–semi-resistant, 2H–delayed hypersensitive, 4–susceptible.

[2] ΔE_{240}/min/0.2 mg acetone powder.

Conidia of *E. graminis* f. sp. *hordei* germinate to produce haustoria equally well on susceptible and resistant leaves. Under the growing conditions used in the present work penetration of susceptible and resistant cells occurred about 11-16 h after inoculation. Abundant haustoria were seen developing in the susceptible within 24 h of inoculation but very few were seen on the highly resistant or immune lines (e.g. Atlas, Ml-a, Ml-g). Masri and Ellingboe (1966) examined the development of race 3 of *E. graminis* f. sp. *hordei* on the same near-isogenic lines and gave the percentage of infections which develop haustoria in the resistant Ml-a, Ml-g, Ml-p and Ml-k lines as 4, 14, 36, and 34 respectively, while 90% of penetrations on susceptible lines developed haustoria. These data indicate that at least for immune lines major factors determining a compatible or incompatible interaction are operative within 24 h of inoculation. It was therefore of interest to find that peroxidase was altered both quantitatively and qualitatively and that ethylene production was stimulated in immune lines within the same period. Further, there was some indication in several experiments that peroxidase activity increased more rapidly in resistant plants than in susceptible ones. The fact that peroxidase was altered in susceptible and resistant lines does not preclude its involvement either directly or indirectly in resistance, since the production of phytoalexins in response to infection also occurs in susceptible and resistant plants.

Multiple molecular forms of fourteen enzymes (isoenzymes) from near-isogenic barley lines inoculated with powdery mildew were studied by polyacrylamide disk electrophoresis (Sako and Stahmann, unpublished). Seven days after inoculation of the susceptible line (ml-g), the number of isoenzyme bands of acetylesterase, acid phosphatase, malate dehydrogenase (NADP), succinate dehydrogenase and peroxidase were increased (Table III). These new bands were not detected in extracts of healthy tissue or mycelium and conidia from infected leaves; their intensity was not reduced by removing mycelium and conidia before preparing extracts. Only peroxidase showed a new band within one day after inoculation. Eleven enzymes from inoculated susceptible lines showed an increase in intensity of one or more bands within seven days; four enzymes showed a decrease. A hypersensitive line (Ml-k) showed changes after inoculation that were similar to those of the susceptible line. With a resistant line (Ml-g), there was an intensity increase in one or more bands of seven enzymes within seven days after inoculation. Such changes in the multiple molecular forms and activity of enzymes are biochemical symptoms of disease, may be a basis for the increased metabolism associated with infection and these changes suggest profound interactions between parasite and host.

Alteration of Proteins and Histones by Peroxidase

As we saw an increase in the activity or number of peroxidase isoenzymes following inoculation with every fungal, bacterial or viral disease that we

TABLE III

Isoenzymes from healthy and mildew infected leaves of susceptible (ml-g) and resistant (Ml-g) lines of barley[1].

Enzyme	Isoenzyme bands from susceptible leaves				Isoenzyme bands from resistant leaves			
	Healthy	Inoculated	Intensity changes[2]	New bands[3]	Healthy	Inoculated	Intensity changes[2]	New bands[3]
Acid phosphatase	4	5	+3	1	4	4	0	0
Acetylesterase	9	11	+2	2	9	9	+2	0
Peroxidase	5	6	+2	1	5	6	+2	1
Succinate dehydrogenase	4	5	−3	1	4	4	0	0
Malate dehydrogenase	5	5	−1	1	5	5	0	0
Malate dehydrogenase (NADP)	7	8	+3	1	7	7	+3	0
Glucose-6-phosphate dehydrogenase	7	7	+1,−5	0	7	7	+1	0
Phosphogluconate dehydrogenase	2	2	+1,−1	0	2	2	+2	0
Glutamate dehydrogenase	1	1	+1	0	1	1	+1	0
Glutamate dehydrogenase (NADP)	1	1	+1	0	1	1	+1	0
Leucine aminopeptidase	3	3	+1	0	3	3	+1	0
Alcohol dehydrogenase	3	3	0	0	3	3	0	0
Glucokinase	6	6	+1	0	6	6	0	0
Glucosephosphate isomerase	4	3	+2,−1	0	4	4	0	0

[1] Inoculated leaves were sampled 7 days after inoculation; ml-g and Ml-g give infection type 4 and 0-1, respectively.

[2] Number of bands showing an increase (+), decrease (−) or no change (0) in intensity of isoenzymes from inoculated tissues as compared to those from healthy tissues.

[3] Number of new bands seen in gels from infected plants which were not visible in those from healthy plants.

studied, I wondered if peroxidase might play an important role in disease resistance and if it could have an effect upon nucleic acids or proteins. Because peroxidase forms free radicals and quinones which can react with proteins, I thought that peroxidase might be able to alter their properties and thereby exert some degree of regulation of protein synthesis or enzyme activity. I suggested that experiments be carried out to determine if peroxidase could have an effect upon proteins, particularly the regulatory proteins or histones that bind to nucleic acids. I suspected that a reaction might occur with amino or sulphydryl groups which could change the mobility of the proteins.

Preliminary experiments involving gel electrophoresis of polylysine and several proteins before and after exposure to a peroxidase system revealed changes in mobility and formation of a substance, probably an aldehyde, which was oxidized to α-amino adipic acid. This was evidence for reaction with the amino group of lysine. We then studied the reaction of peroxidase systems with histones.

Experiments were conducted to test the hypothesis that peroxidase systems can alter the chemical and physical properties of histone, and that the altered histone is a less effective repressor of DNA-dependent RNA synthesis (Demorest and Stahmann, unpublished results). If such an alteration occurred in the cell, peroxidase might cause an increase in growth and metabolism by stimulating RNA synthesis leading to an enhanced protein synthesis. We have found that two different horseradish peroxidase systems can alter the chemical and physical properties of calf-thymus histone. First, we have shown that the peroxidase oxidation product(s) of indole-3-acetic acid (IAA) bind to calf-thymus histone. In particular, the data suggest that one product, 3-methyleneoxindole, binds to the sulphydryl groups of arginine-rich histone. Secondly, we have shown that a system of peroxidase, catechol, and hydrogen peroxide (H_2O_2) can oxidize lysine residues in a lysine-rich histone to the δ-semialdehyde and can alter the electrophoretic mobility of a number of histone types, such as the arginine-rich histone.

Evidence for the binding of the peroxidase oxidation product(s) of IAA to commercial calf-thymus histone is shown in Tables IV and V. Table IV shows that when crude histone is added to the peroxidase + IAA incubation mixture, there is a decrease in the optical density at 250 nm. This decrease is known to occur when sulphydryl groups (such as in glutathione) conjugate with 3-methyleneoxindole, a peroxidase oxidation product of IAA (Still *et al.*, 1965). Arginine-rich histone also reacts with 3-methyleneoxindole in the presence of urea. Table V shows that there is a 10-fold increase in binding of IAA-2-^{14}C to crude histone after oxidation by peroxidase. This binding is probably due to the conjugation of the 3-methyleneoxindole with the sulphydryl groups in the histone since the binding was decreased significantly by alkaline pH, decreased by glutathione, and increased by heating the peroxidase and IAA mixture. It is

TABLE IV

The reaction of calf-thymus histone with the peroxidase oxidation product(s) of indole-3-acetic acid.

Addition	Change in optical density with urea	without urea
Buffer	0.00	0.00
Crude histone	−0.05	−0.03
Arginine-rich histone	−0.03	0.00
Glutathione (reduced)	–	−0.45

Peroxidase (10 μg/ml) and indole-3-acetic acid (2.0×10^{-4} M) were incubated together at pH 5.0 for 60 min. The mixture was then heated at 100°C for 10 min and cooled to room temperature. An equal volume of histone (calf-thymus, 2.0 mg/ml, containing 4.0 M urea or no urea) or reduced glutathione (2.0×10^{-4} M) was then added and after 30 min the optical density at 250 nm was determined.

TABLE V

The binding of the peroxidase oxidation product(s) of indole-3-acetic acid-2-^{14}C (IAA) to crude calf-thymus histone separated on Sephadex G-25.

Incubation mixture	Counts/min incorporated into high mol. wt. fraction[1]	%
Peroxidase + IAA + histone (pH 5)	133 000[2]	100
Peroxidase + IAA + buffer (pH 5)	3 500	3
IAA + histone (pH 5)	12 400	9
Peroxidase + IAA + histone (pH 8)[3]	84 600	64
IAA + histone (pH 8)[3]	6 090	5
Peroxidase + IAA + histone (pH 5)[4] + glutathione	90 300	68
Peroxidase + IAA + histone (pH 5)[5] (heated)	337 000	254

[1] The high mol. wt. (>5000) fraction was eluted at 13-23 ml and the IAA was eluted at 33-43 ml at pH 8.0 and 37-46 ml at pH 5.0

[2] The 133 000 counts/min incorporated is equal to about 6.0×10^{-9} mole of IAA

[3] The histone was incubated at pH 8.0 and chromatographed at pH 8.0

[4] Reduced glutathione (2.0×10^{-4} M) was included with the histone

[5] The peroxidase + IAA mixture was heated after incubation at 100°C for 10 min and cooled to room temperature before adding histone.

Peroxidase (10 μg/ml) and IAA-2-^{14}C (2.0×10^{-4} M, 4.1×10^{6} counts/min/ml) were incubated at room temperature for 60 min at pH 5.0 before adding an equal volume of crude calf-thymus histone (8.0 mg/ml) to make 1 ml total volume. After 30 min at room temperature, the mixtures were flushed with nitrogen, stored at −20°C and chromatographed on a 30 ml Sephadex G-25 column.

known that the sulphydryl conjugation product is unstable at alkaline pH, that it is formed with glutathione (Still *et al.*, 1965) and that the formation of 3-methyleneoxindole is increased non-enzymatically by heating (Hinman and Lang, 1965). Binding may occur with arginine-rich histone since the arginine-rich histone contains sulphydryl groups (Fambrough and Bonner, 1968).

Evidence for the alteration of calf-thymus histone by the peroxidase + catechol + H_2O_2 system is shown in Table VI and Fig. 1. Table VI shows that when histone very rich in lysine is incubated with the complete peroxidase system three times as much α-amino adipic acid is formed and twice as much catechol is found in the high-molecular weight protein as when peroxidase is omitted. The peroxidase system may oxidize ε-amino groups of lysine residues to an aldehyde, which is then further oxidized to α-amino adipic acid by performic acid. Figure 1 shows that when crude histone is incubated with the complete peroxidase system and subjected to electrophoresis, fast-moving types of histones are converted to a heterogeneous group of slower moving proteins.

The above data suggest that peroxidase systems can alter significantly the physical and chemical properties of histone. Future experiments will attempt to show that this altered histone is less effective in repressing DNA-dependent RNA synthesis. Some experiments have shown that the template activity of isolated pea internode chromatin is increased by treatment with peroxidase and IAA.

TABLE VI

Content of α-amino adipic acid and catechol oxidation products in peroxidase treated calf-thymus histone, very rich in lysine.

Incubation mixture	μmole α-amino adipic acid/μmole histone[1]	% catechol[2]
Histone	nil	nil
Histone + peroxidase + H_2O_2	nil	nil
Histone + peroxidase + catechol	nil	19
Histone + H_2O_2 + catechol	0.3	28
Histone + peroxidase + H_2O_2 + catechol	1.0	67
Peroxidase + H_2O_2 + catechol	nil	nil

[1] The μmole of histone was determined from the alanine and glycine content and the known molecular weight of histone very rich in lysine.

[2] The % catechol or catechol oxidation products bound to histone in the high mol. wt. fraction (>5000) was calculated as the % of material absorbing at 280 nm not due to histone, peroxidase, or unbound catechol oxidation products, which was recovered from the original mixture.

The mixtures (histone, 1.0 mg/ml; peroxidase, 0.1 mg/ml; H_2O_2, 2.5 mM; catechol, 0.25 mM) were incubated for 2 h at room temperature and then passed through a Sephadex G-25 column. The high mol. wt. fraction was well separated from the catechol and H_2O_2, and then dialysed at 0°C for 48 h. The α-amino adipic acid content in the dialysed preparation was determined by standard amino acid analysis after performic acid oxidation.

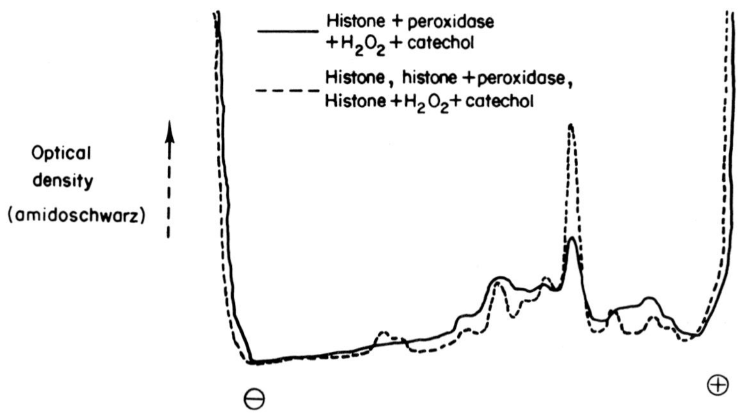

Fig. 1. The figure shows the densiometer tracing of amidoschwarz stained crude calf-thymus histone which was treated with a peroxidase + H_2O_2 + catechol system. The mixture (histone, 0.4 mg/ml; peroxidase, 0.04 mg/ml; H_2O_2, 0.2 mM; catechol, 0.2 mM) was incubated for 3-5 min at room temperature at pH 8.0, and then about 38 μg of histone was subjected to electrophoresis on acrylamide gels containing 6.0 M urea according to the method of Panyim and Chalkley (1969). The three controls gave the same tracing shown by the dashed line.

The results give support to the idea that some of the hormonal effects of IAA are due to the binding of its peroxidase oxidation product(s) to histones and that peroxidase systems may play a pivotal role in the de-repression of the genome during injury and disease. We have suggested that de-repression by ribosomal peroxidase may stimulate ribosome synthesis (Stahmann and Demorest, 1972).

References

Fambrough, D. M. and Bonner, J. (1968). Sequence homology and role of cysteine in plant and animal arginine-rich histones. *J. biol. Chem.* **243**, 4434-4439.

Farkas, G. L. and Stahmann, M. A. (1966). On the nature of changes in peroxidase isoenzymes in bean leaves infected by southern bean mosaic virus. *Phytopathology* **56**, 669-677.

Heitefuss, R., Buchanan-Davidson, D. J., Stahmann, M. A. and Walker, J. C. (1960). Electrophoretic and immunochemical studies of proteins in cabbage infected with *Fusarium oxysporum* f. *conglutinans. Phytopathology* **50**, 198-205.

Hinman, R. L. and Lang, J. (1965). Peroxidase-catalyzed oxidation of indole-3-acetic acid. *Biochemistry* **4**, 144-158.

Hislop, E. C. and Stahmann, M. A. (1971). Peroxidase and ethylene production by barley leaves infected with *Erysiphe graminis* f. sp. *hordei. Physiol. Pl. Path.* **1**, 297-312.

Link, K. P., Angell, H. R. and Walker, J. C. (1933). The isolation of catechol from pigmented onion scales and its significance in relation to disease resistance in onions. *J. biol. Chem.* **100**, 379-383.

Lovrekovich, L., Lovrekovich, H. and Stahmann, M. A. (1968a). The importance of peroxidase in the wildfire disease. *Phytopathology* **58**, 193-198.

Lovrekovich, L., Lovrekovich, H. and Stahmann, M. A. (1968b). Tobacco mosaic virus-induced resistance to *Pseudomonas tabaci* in tobacco. *Phytopathology* **58**, 1034-1035.

Macko, V., Woodbury, W. and Stahmann, M. A. (1968). The effect of peroxidase on the germination and growth of mycelium of *Puccinia graminis* f. sp. *tritici.* (1968). *Phytopathology* **58**, 1250-1254.

Masri, S. S. and Ellingboe, A. H. (1966). Primary infection of wheat and barley by *Erysiphe graminis. Phytopathology* **56**, 389-395.

Panyim, S. and Chalkley, R. (1969). High resolution acrylamide gel electrophoresis of histones. *Archs Biochem. Biophys.* **130**, 337-346.

Rudolph, K. and Stahmann, M. A. (1966). Multiple hydrolases in bean leaves (*Phaseolus vulgaris* L.) and the effect of halo blight diseases caused by *Pseudomonas phaseolicola* (Burkh) Dowson. *Pl. Physiol., Lancaster* **41**, 389-394.

Simons, T. J. and Ross, A. F. (1970). Enhanced peroxidase activity associated with induction of resistance to tobacco mosaic virus in hypersensitive tobacco. *Phytopathology* **60**, 383-384.

Stahmann, M. A., Clare, B. G. and Woodbury, W. (1966). Increased disease resistance and enzyme activity induced by ethylene and ethylene production by black rot infected sweet potato tissue. *Pl. Physiol., Lancaster* **41**, 1505-1512.

Stahmann, M. A. and Demorest, D. M. (1972). Changes in isoenzymes of host and pathogen following some fungal infections. *Proceedings of Conference on Nucleic Acids and Proteins in Higher Plants,* Tihany, Hungary, *Symp. Biol. Hung.* **13**, 355-356.

Stahmann, M. A., Link, K. P. and Walker, J. C. (1943). Mustard oils in crucifers and their relation to resistance to clubroot. *J. agr. Res.* **67**, 49-63.

Staples, R. C. and Stahmann, M. A. (1964). Changes in proteins and several enzymes in susceptible bean leaves after infection by the bean rust fungus. *Phytopathology* **54**, 760-764.

Still, C. C., Fukuyama, T. T. and Moyed, H. S. (1965). Inhibitory oxidation products of indole-3-acetic acid. Mechanism of action and route of detoxification. *J. biol. Chem.* **240**, 2612-2618.

Tomiyama, K. and Stahmann, M. A. (1964). Alteration of oxidative enzymes in potato tuber tissue by infection with *Phytophthora infestans. Pl. Physiol., Lancaster* **39**, 483-490.

Uritani, I. and Stahmann, M. A. (1961). Changes in nitrogen metabolism in sweet potato with black rot. *Pl. Physiol., Lancaster* **36**, 770-782.

Weber, D. J., Clare, B. and Stahmann, M. A. (1967). Enzymic changes associated with induced and natural resistance of sweet potato to *Ceratocystis fimbriata. Phytopathology* **57**, 421-424.

Weber, D. J. and Stahmann, M. A. (1966). Induced immunity to Ceratocystis infection in sweet potato root tissue. *Phytopathology* **56**, 1066-1070.

DISCUSSION

Dr A. Kaars Sijpesteijn: Where there was increased peroxidase formation did you ever find increased lignification, and could that be a reason for resistance?

Professor M. A. Stahmann: We have not looked for that, but I would suspect that since peroxidase is an important enzyme in the formation of lignin, it may well act in this way.
Dr Kaars Sijpesteijn: We have done experiments with cucumbers to which we fed phenyl thiourea and this caused increased peroxidase activity. At the same time we found lignification and resistance to *Cladosporium fulvum,* so this might fit into your pattern.
Professor P. H. Williams: Do you have any evidence that DNA de-repression might lead to increases in protein and oxidative enzymes. Is this a cyclic system?
Professor Stahmann: I suggest that the reaction with the ϵ-amino group of repressor proteins or histones would reduce the ionic binding to DNA and that this may have an activating effect. We have no evidence that the new bands we see are histones. I doubt that very much, because we tested for enzymic activity, and certainly the histones would not have these specific enzyme activities.
Professor Williams: Would this apply to the new protein bands that you see? Are you suggesting that all these new enzymes that show up are the product of DNA de-repression of histones?
Professor Stahmann: We have considered two or three possibilities as to how these new bands may arise. We proposed, at a symposium in Japan, that it might be possible to have an exchange of information between the pathogen and parasite, at different levels. One would be at the nucleic acid level—through exchange of genomes. Secondly, there may be exchange at the enzyme sub-unit level.

In the intimate contact between haustoria and cell it may be possible that enzymes dissociate, and sub-units are exchanged between host and parasite to produce hybrid enzymes which would account for new bands. Thirdly, it may be the result of an exchange of allosteric regulators. At the moment I cannot say which occurs. I am sure that there is a great deal of interaction between host and parasite which is manifest at the enzyme level. These are really biochemical symptoms that later give rise to the gross morphological symptoms that the plant pathologists have described for many years.
Dr G. A. Kamerbeek: There are dwarf plants (*Phaseolus, Zea mays*) which have an extremely high natural content of peroxidase. Did you ever test these plants to see whether they are resistant or not compared with the normal plants?
Professor Stahmann: No. Horseradish for example is loaded with peroxidase, but we have never worked with it.
Dr Kamerbeek: The *Phaseolus* dwarf plant has an extremely high peroxidase content, and you could compare the dwarf plant with the normal plant, to see if one is resistant and the other not.
Professor Stahmann: We have not done this; it would be interesting. Perhaps I should also point out that peroxidase is an enzyme which exists with many isoenzyme forms. Dr H. Stegemann in Germany has studied this and has shown

that in potato as many as 20 or 25 isoenzymes of peroxidase may be detected by a combination of isoelectric focusing and gel-electrophoresis. Many of them are different proteins, and show different enzyme specificities.

Dr J. C. M. Beyersbergen: You found that in uninfected tissue the peroxidase activity increased if this tissue was enclosed with infected tissue. Do you have an explanation for the fact that after infection of the tissue by a parasite the infection does not stop? Do you think that ethylene does not function in the neighbourhood of infected cells?

Professor Stahmann: In resistant cultivars of sweet potato the infection was confined to the surface layers–it did stop. Only in very susceptible cultivars was it able to penetrate and turn the whole tissue black. When we treated eight different susceptible cultivars with ethylene we did stop the infection. This was with sweet potatoes, it did not seem to work with some plants, e.g. with wheat and rust infection.

Dr Beyersbergen: So you found that in the infected tissue the parasite produced ethylene?

Professor Stahmann: Yes, both the parasite and host tissue.

Dr Beyersbergen: Then I cannot imagine that when the infection progresses, those neighbouring healthy cells are infected by the parasite, because they should also become resistant as ethylene is present there, having been formed by the infected cells. The infection should stop.

Professor Stahmann: This may depend upon the rate at which the subsequent changes occur. Just as a man may get a disease and die from it, even though he produced the antibodies in defence of this, the antibodies may come too late to save him. I think a similar situation occurs in the plant. There is a time element in all these events which I think is extremely important.

Dr Beyersbergen: Thank you.

Dr H. M. Dekhuijzen: If some of the hormonal effects of IAA are due to the binding of the oxidation product to histones, I would expect that this compound itself also has some hormonal effects. Is it a stable compound?

Professor Stahmann: Do you mean is the IAA active?

Dr Dekhuijzen: The methylene oxindole.

Professor Stahmann: Oh yes, it has been claimed that the methylene oxindole is more active than IAA.

Dr R. C. Hignett: I wondered about the induced immunity in tobacco when you inject heat-killed cells and various other agents. It seems to be non-specific. I wonder if this is a mechanical effect–if you inject say, a suspension of silica, would you get similar changes occurring?

Professor Stahmann: I do not know, we have never injected silica. When we inject buffer we do not get it.

Dr Hignett: If you kill the cells in any other way than by heat do you get any difference? Streptomycin will kill cells, for example.

Professor Stahmann: We have not studied this.

V.2 Response of Tomato to Infection by *Fusarium oxysporum* f. *lycopersici*

R. B. DRYSDALE AND P. LANGCAKE*

Department of Microbiology, University of Birmingham, England

INTRODUCTION

During the development of any organism, complex series of biochemical reactions proceed in an orderly, highly integrated manner. In disease, the normal developmental sequence is replaced by another sequence of biochemical and physiological changes which have a detrimental effect on the host.

While resistance mechanisms can exist in a host plant before it comes into contact with a pathogen most resistance mechanisms are induced in the host after the contact and thus involve changes, either qualitative or quantitative, in the host's metabolism. These changes may result from the interaction of fungal products with compounds already present in the host or with the host's genome. Unfortunately, most of the information on host–pathogen relationships is superficial and does not deal in precise terms with the biochemical interactions between pathogen and host. The reasons for this situation are historical, technical and conceptual. Many of the technical problems have been resolved and application of newer concepts should lead to the deeper knowledge of the molecular bases of interactions between host and pathogen which will be necessary for effective crop protection in the future.

To obtain information about the basis of pathogenesis and the mechanism of resistance in fusarial wilt of tomato, we have been investigating, during the past 3-4 years, various aspects of the biochemistry of the interaction between race 1 of the imperfect fungus *Fusarium oxysporum* f. *lycopersici* Snyd. and Hans. and the tomato cultivars Homestead (HS; resistant) and Bonny Best (BB; susceptible). We will consider two aspects, firstly the production of pectic enzymes in infected susceptible plants and secondly the production, after infection, of tomatine, an inhibitor of the fungus. Pectic enzymes and tomatine are normal metabolic products of healthy tomato plants.

* Present address: Woodstock Agricultural Research Centre, Sittingbourne, Kent

Pectic Enzymes

The importance of pectic enzymes in wilt pathogenesis in tomato has been recognized widely (e.g. Gothoskar *et al.*, 1955; Paquin and Coulombe, 1962; Matta and Dimond, 1963) but not universally (Husain and Dimond, 1960; McDonnell, 1962; Mann, 1962) and the literature on these enzymes in relation to the disease is noteworthy for its inconsistencies.

POLYGALACTURONASES (PG)

Waggoner and Dimond (1955) found that the PG produced *in vitro* by the fungus liberated monogalacturonic acid from polypectate (i.e. it is an exo-PG) but other workers (e.g. Gothoskar *et al.*, 1955; Heitefuss *et al.*, 1960) reported that the enzyme produced *in vitro* is a depolymerase, i.e. an endo-PG, which does not produce monogalacturonic acid.

Polygalacturonase does not appear to be present in healthy stems and leaves of tomato (Blackhurst and Wood, 1963; Matta and Dimond, 1963; Patil and Dimond, 1968) although it is a normal constituent of tomato fruit (Lee and Macmillan, 1968). Some workers (Waggoner and Dimond, 1955; Matta and Dimond, 1963) failed to find PG in infected plants but Patil and Dimond (1968) reported that infected plants contained an exo-PG which released monogalacturonic acid from both pectin and polypectate. Deese and Stahmann (1962) had previously identified a pectate deploymerase, i.e. an endo-PG, which did not release monogalacturonic acid, in Bonny Best plants infected with *F. oxysporum.* These workers also noted depolymerase activity in juice from healthy stems. We have not found PG activity in either healthy or infected tissue but have detected an exo-PG produced *in vitro* by *F. oxysporum* f. *lycopersici.*

The variation in the nature of the PGs produced *in vitro* may be due to the use of different strains of the fungus. The nature of the enzyme produced *in vivo* could be important in pathogenesis if, as suggested by Deese and Stahmann (1962), endo-PG releases pectic fragments within infected plants. These fragments could, with divalent cations, form the pectic gel plugs observed in wilting plants (Pierson *et al.*, 1955).

The apparently normal progression of the disease despite, firstly, the presence or absence of PG in infected and healthy tomato plants and, secondly, the variation in the nature of the PG produced by the fungus *in vivo* and *in vitro,* makes it unlikely that PG is of major importance in pathogenesis.

PECTINMETHYLESTERASES (PME)

Superficially at least the picture regarding the production of PME is much more uniform. The enzyme is produced *in vitro* by the fungus (e.g. Waggoner and Dimond, 1955; Winstead and Walker, 1954), it is present in healthy plants (e.g. Deese and Stahmann, 1962), and its activity increases in infected plants (Waggoner and Dimond, 1955; Deese and Stahmann, 1962; Mussell and Green, 1970). Attempts to identify the origin of pectinmethylesterase in infected plants have relied on a difference in the pH optimum of host and fungal enzyme and on the differential effect of detergent on enzyme from the two sources. We have used chromatography on DEAE-cellulose to separate host and fungal pectinmethylesterase from infected tomato plants and find that there is a substantial increase in enzyme activity of the host. Our results on the effect of detergent and pH on the activity of unfractionated enzyme from infected plants support this conclusion (Langcake and Drysdale, 1973a).

Effect of pH on pectinmethylesterase activity. Pectinmethylesterases of plant and fungal origin often differ in their pH optima (Wood, 1960) affording a possible means of distinguishing between them. The activity of pectinmethylesterase from *F. oxysporum* f. *lycopersici* and in expressed juice of stems of healthy and infected plants was measured at pH 5.5 and pH 7.0, the pH optimum of fungal and plant enzymes respectively (McColloch and Kertesz, 1947). Table I shows the activity of pectinmethylesterase at pH 5.5 expressing the activity at pH 7.0 as 1.00. Enzyme from fungal culture filtrates has about the same activity at both pH values whilst that from healthy plants is about 50% as active at pH 5.5 as at pH 7.0. Pectinmethylesterase from infected plants appears to have the same pH characteristics as that from healthy plants.

TABLE I

Effect of pH on activity of pectinmethylesterase (PME).

PME from	pH	Relative activity[1]
Fungal culture filtrate	7.0	1.00
	5.5	1.05
Healthy tomato	7.0	1.00
	5.5	0.50
Infected tomato	7.0	1.00
	5.5	0.43

[1] Activity/activity at pH 7.0

Effect of detergent on pectinmethyleserase activity. Preliminary experiments with various concentrations of sodium lauryl sulphate showed that addition of 1 ml of 1.5% sodium lauryl sulphate to the assay system gave virtually complete inhibition of the enzyme from healthy plants but only about 40% inhibition of enzyme from fungal culture medium. Table II shows the results of experiments

TABLE II

Effect of sodium lauryl sulphate (NaLS) on activity of PME.

PME from	PME activity Without NaLS	With NaLS[3]	% Inhibition
Fungal culture filtrate	36.5 ± 1.9[1]	22.1 ± 1.9[1]	39.5
Healthy tomato	58.2 ± 2.7[2]	0.6 ± 2.7[2]	99.0
Infected tomato	109.6 ± 4.3[2]	2.8 ± 4.3[2]	97.4

[1] units/ml filtrate.
[2] units/g fresh wt.
[3] 1 ml of 1.5% NaLS added to assay mixture.

to measure the effect of this concentration of detergent on pectinmethylesterase from fungus grown *in vitro* and from stem juice of healthy and infected Bonny Best plants. The increase in activity, over controls, in infected plants was 51.4 units/g. If this increased activity were due to fungal enzyme then the activity expected in the presence of detergent should have been about 31 units/g. However, in the presence of sodium lauryl sulphate only 2.8 units/g were detected, making it unlikely that the additional enzyme in infected plants is fungal in origin.

Fractionation of pectinmethylesterases on DEAE-cellulose. Preliminary experiments with pectinmethylesterase from fungal culture medium and from healthy plants established conditions for the adsorption and selective elution of enzyme from the two sources.

Table III shows the results of experiments on the adsorption on to and elution from DEAE-cellulose of pectinmethylesterase from fungal culture medium and from healthy and infected tomato plants.

TABLE III

DEAE-cellulose fractionation of PME from fungus grown *in vitro* and from healthy and infected Bonny Best stems.

PME from	PME units in fractions from DEAE-cellulose				Input	% Recovery
	4	5	6	7		
Fungal culture medium	15	0	0	0	18.7	80
Healthy stem	0	0	44	23	75	89
Infected stem	45	0	383	67	697[1]	84

[1] Includes 90 units not absorbed, and recovered in fractions 1 and 2.

Enzyme from all three sources adsorbed to DEAE-cellulose equilibrated in 0.01 M, pH 8.2, tris-HCl (cf. Lee and Macmillan, 1968). While fungal enzyme was eluted with 0.025 M NaCl, plant enzyme remained adsorbed but was eluted by 0.5 M NaCl. The minimum concentration of sodium chloride to elute plant enzyme was not determined.

Further treatment of tissue residue with 5% saline extracted only small amounts of host enzyme and no evidence was found for binding of fungal enzyme to plant tissue.

Tables I, II and III indicate that most of the increase in pectinmethylesterase activity is due to host enzyme. As yet there is no evidence to indicate whether this increase is due to the synthesis of new enzyme or to the release or activation of preformed enzyme. Preliminary experiments indicate that addition of fungal culture filtrate to plant extracts stimulates the PME activity of these extracts (Langcake and Drysdale, 1973b). The significance of this observation to the situation *in vivo* remains to be established.

Fungal enzyme activity accounts for a maximum of 5-10% of the total activity in infected plants (Tables II, III). Because of the relatively small amount of fungal pectinmethylesterase present in infected plants it appears unlikely that the fungal enzyme has an important role in wilt pathogenesis. Further information on the specificity of fungal enzyme and on its location in the host plant is necessary to substantiate this suggestion.

Tomatine

Gottlieb (1943) found that *F. oxysporum* was inhibited by expressed juice from healthy tomato stems. α-Tomatine was later shown to be responsible for this inhibition (Fontaine *et al.*, 1948) and is present in healthy susceptible, and in both mono- and multi-genic resistant cultivars (Beckman, 1964; Uhle and Moore, 1954). Kern (1952), however, found that most of the tomatine was present in leaves and the concentration in roots and stems was insufficient to inhibit the fungus appreciably.

While phytoalexin-like responses occur in tomato plants inoculated with *formae* of *F. oxysporum* other than *lycopersici* (Davis, 1968; Langton, 1969) fungal inhibitors produced following infection, i.e. phytoalexins (Cruickshank, 1963) have not yet been isolated from the tomato/*F. oxysporum* f. *lycopersici* system. However, evidence for a phytoalexin, with a role in resistance, has been obtained in cotton plants infected with the wilt fungus *Verticillium albo-atrum* (Bell, 1969).

We have investigated the production of inhibitors following the infection of both susceptible and monogenic resistant tomato plants with *F. oxysporum* f. *lycopersici* (Langcake *et al.*, 1972).

Examination of crude extracts. Extracts made in 50% methanol of roots, lower stems (the first 10 cm), upper stems and leaves of healthy and infected tomato plants were examined using a hyphal extension bioassay (Strange and Smith, 1971). None of the extracts from roots or stems gave a hyphal extension value less than that in the water controls, though leaf extracts gave somewhat lower values. Nevertheless, the presence of compounds inhibitory to the growth of *F. oxysporum* f. *lycopersici* was suggested by the asymmetry of fungal growth around the wells. Growth toward the centre well, containing the test solution, was considerably less than that away from the centre well. The ratio of growth in one direction to that in the other direction gave a measure of this asymmetry (Table IV). The asymmetry suggested that the extracts contained a mixture of substances–some stimulating, the other(s) inhibiting growth of *F. oxysporum* f. *lycopersici.*

TABLE IV

Asymmetry[1] of fungal growth in the bioassay (by hyphal extension of *F. oxysporum*) of methanol extracts of Homestead (resistant) and Bonny Best (susceptible) tissue.

Origin of sample		Days after infection	Volume of sample	
Cultivar	Tissue		20 μl	30 μl
Homestead	Lower stem	9	–	0.62
Bonny Best	Lower stem	6	–	0.68
Bonny Best	Leaf	uninfected	0.64	–
	Control (water)		0.86	0.92

[1] Fungal growth towards central well/fungal growth away from central well.

No inhibition of spore germination or hyphal extension was detected using tracheal fluids from healthy or infected plants in the bioassay.

Chromatography and electrophoresis of extracts. Confirmation that extracts contained both inhibitor(s) and stimulants of hyphal extension was obtained by chromatography (butan-1-ol-acetic acid-water) of samples of the extract followed by bioassay of the chromatograms (Fig. 1).

These results indicate clearly that while the roots and stems of uninfected plants do not contain inhibitors, such compounds develop after infection and are present two days later in lower stems and 3-4 days later in roots.

Electrophoresis (pH 5.3) and chromatography of extracts from stems of infected plants in several systems gave single peaks of inhibitory activity. In other solvents and on electrophoresis (pH 4.0) all inhibitory activity was lost.

Identification of inhibitor. The loss of inhibitory activity in alkaline conditions and the presence of an inhibitor in the leaves of healthy plants suggested that inhibition of hyphal extension might be due to tomatine. Various tests were carried out to compare the inhibitor with tomatine.

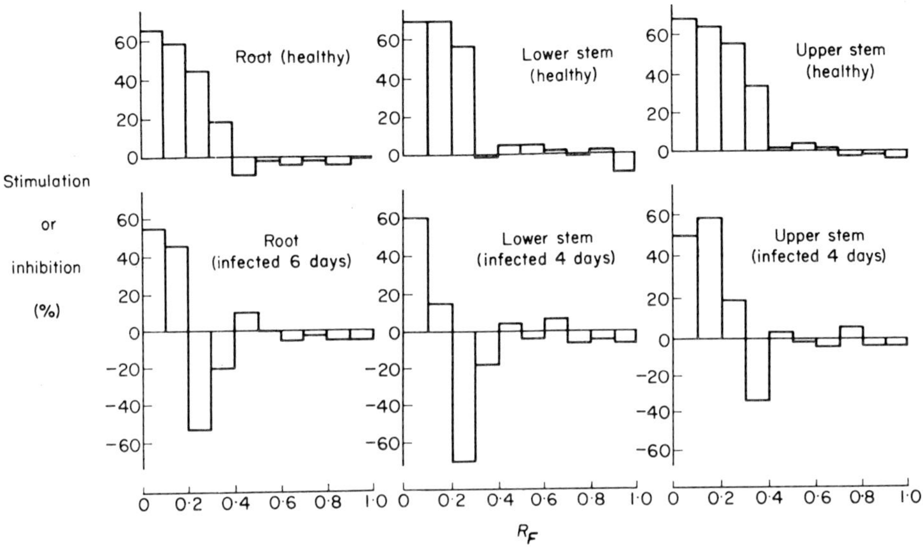

Fig. 1. Paper chromatography (butan-1-ol-acetic acid-water, 6/1/2, by vol.) and bioassay by hyphal extension of methanol extracts of healthy and infected Homestead tissue. Results for Bonny Best were similar. Stimulation (+) and inhibition (–) of hyphal extension were measured relative to a water control (i.e. water control = 0%).

i. Tomatine behaved in the same way as the inhibitor during chromatography, co-chromatography and electrophoresis. In addition, following paper chromatography both tomatine and the inhibitor gave a positive colour reaction with iodine and bromocresol green, reagents which have been used for locating alkaloids (Smith, 1968).

ii. When tomato tissue (roots and stems at various times after inoculation) was subjected to the purification procedure for tomatine, inhibitory activity was recovered. In these preparations the tomatine was measured by an anthrone method for total carbohydrate (Morris, 1948). Each preparation gave only one anthrone-positive spot following thin layer chromatography (silica gel G). This had the same R_F value as tomatine, and the amount of inhibitor present in these preparations was that expected if all of the anthrone positive material was tomatine.

iii. A sample of the inhibitor, prepared from stems of infected tomato plants using the method for tomatine, and authentic tomatine were compared using an MS9 high resolution mass spectrometer. The spectra obtained were very similar. There was no peak corresponding to the molecular ion (m/e = 1033) but both spectra had peaks at m/e = 415, probably the aglycone, and strikingly similar patterns of peaks between m/e = 250 and m/e = 460.

Tomatine levels in plants. The concentration of inhibitor in roots and stems of tomato plants was measured at various times after inoculation of the plants with *F. oxysporum* f. *lycopersici* (Fig. 2). There was a substantial increase in the amount of a glycosidal alkaloid, inhibitory to the fungus, following inoculation or root injury (control plants). The amount of inhibitor present appeared to increase for at least three days after inoculation. The properties of the inhibitor suggest that it is either α-tomatine (Fig. 3) or a similar compound (cf. solanine

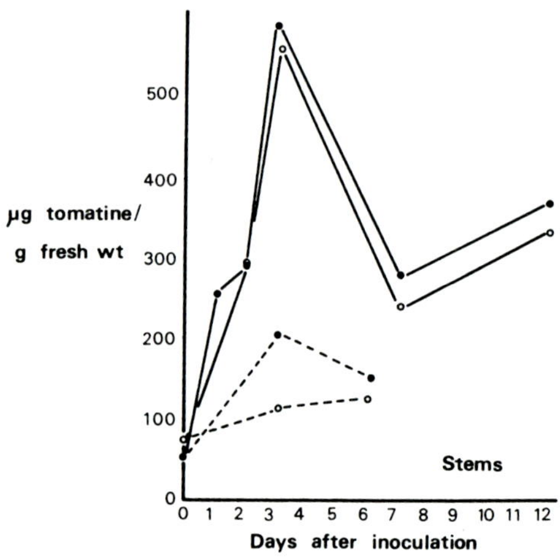

Fig. 2. Variation in tomatine concentration in tomato tissues.
Homestead–control . . . o . . . Bonny Best–control . . . ● . . .
Homestead–infected ——o—— Bonny Best–infected ——●——

and chaconine from potato (Allen, 1970) and demissine from *Solanum demissum* (Kern, 1952)).

The variation of about +0.05 units observed in the R_F value of the inhibitory peak in paper chromatograms (see Fig. 1) was probably due to overloading of the papers. Although authentic tomatine has an R_F value of about 0.5 in butan-1-ol-acetic acid-water when mixed with plant extract prior to chromatography its R_F value decreased to about 0.3, i.e. the approximate R_F value of the inhibitor present in plant extracts (Fig. 1). Only a single peak having inhibitory activity was obtained on paper chromatography (Fig. 1) and this inhibitory material was not separated completely from stimulatory substances.

Kern's observations on the distribution of tomatine in healthy plants have been confirmed. Tomatine was present mainly in the leaves (0.5-1% of the dry wt.) while the concentration in roots or stems was $<1/10$ of this value.

Kern (1952) suggested two reasons to explain why tomatine is not involved in resistance of tomato to *F. oxysporum* f. *lycopersici* (*i*) the compound is not very

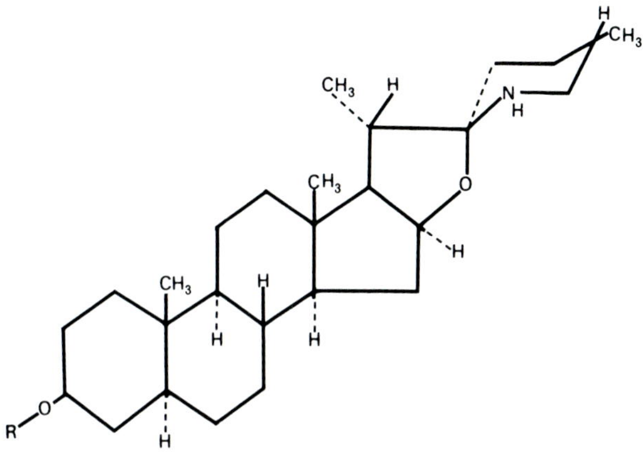

Fig. 3. Structure of α-tomatine. R = xylosyl-(glucosyl)-glucosyl-galactosyl-.

inhibitory to the fungus and (*ii*) the concentration in roots and stems is insufficient to inhibit the fungus. Our results show that, on the medium used, authentic tomatine is quite inhibitory to hyphal extension with an ED_{50} of 1.4×10^{-5} M (assuming that the compound diffuses into only 2 ml of the bioassay medium). Since both the solubility and toxicity of tomatine are markedly influenced by pH (solubility decreases and toxicity increases as the pH rises (Arneson and Durbin, 1968a)) it is possible that *F. oxysporum* f. *lycopersici* is less sensitive to tomatine when growing in Richard's solution as used by Kern (1952). The ED_{50} value quoted was calculated from experiments *in vitro* and may not be applicable to the situation *in vivo* where factors such as pH, the precise cellular location of tomatine and the presence of stimulatory substances will determine whether fungal growth is inhibited by a given concentration of tomatine.

Following Kern's conclusion, little interest was shown in tomatine until the more recent demonstration that it may be involved in resistance to tomato leaf spot caused by *Septoria lycopersici* (Arneson and Durbin, 1967; 1968b) and bacterial wilt of tomato caused by *Pseudomonas solanacearum* (Mohanakumaran *et al.*, 1969).

Our results show that, immediately following infection, there is an increase in the tomatine concentration in stem and roots of infected plants. Cruickshank (1963) suggests that a broad interpretation of the phytoalexin theory 'does not exclude post-infectional increases in toxic compounds which are normal plant metabolites'. However, in our case, the response occurs in both resistant and susceptible plants and thus, unless further work reveals a difference in the distribution of tomatine in the stems of infected plants of the two cultivars, it appears unlikely that tomatine is involved in monogenic resistance of tomato to *F. oxysporum* f. *lycopersici*.

References

Allen, E. H. (1970). The nature of antifungal substances in the peel of Irish potato tubers. *Phytopath. Z.* **69**, 151-159.

Arneson, P. A. and Durbin, R. D. (1967). Hydrolysis of tomatine by *Septoria lycopersici*: a detoxification mechanism. *Phytopathology* **57**, 1358-1360.

Arneson, P. A. and Durbin, R. D. (1968a). Studies on the mode of action of tomatine as a fungitoxic agent. *Pl. Physiol. Lancaster* **43**, 683-686.

Arneson, P. A. and Durbin, R. D. (1968b). The sensitivity of fungi to α-tomatine. *Phytopathology* **58**, 536-537.

Beckman, C. H. (1964). Host response to vascular infection. *A. Rev. Phytopath.* **2**, 231-252.

Bell, A. A. (1969). Phytoalexin production and *Verticillium* wilt resistance in cotton. *Phytopathology* **59**, 1119-1127.

Blackhurst, E. M. and Wood, R. K. S. (1963). *Verticillium* wilt of tomatoes–further experiments on the role of pectic and cellulolytic enzymes. *Ann. appl. Biol.* **52**, 89-96.

Cruickshank, I. A. M. (1963). Phytoalexins. *A Rev. Phytopath.* **1**, 351-374.

Davis, D. (1968). Partial control of Fusarium wilt in tomato by formae of *Fusarium oxysporum. Phytopathology* **58**, 121-122.

Deese, D. C. and Stahmann, M. A. (1962). Pectic enzymes in *Fusarium*-infected susceptible and resistant tomato plants. *Phytopathology* **52**, 255-260.

Fontaine, T. D., Irving, G. W., Ma, R. M., Poole, J. B. and Doolittle, S. P. (1948). Isolation and partial characterisation of crystalline tomatine, an antibiotic agent from the tomato plant. *Archs Biochem. Biophys.* **18**, 467-475.

Gothoskar, S. S., Scheffer, R. P., Stahmann, M. A. and Walker, J. C. (1955). The role of enzymes in the development of *Fusarium* wilt of tomato. *Phytopathology* **45**, 381-387.

Gottlieb, D. (1943). Expressed sap of tomato plants in relation to wilt resistance. *Phytopathology* **33**, 1111.

Heitefuss, R., Stahmann, M. A. and Walker, J. C. (1960). Production of pectolytic enzymes and fusaric acid by *Fusarium oxysporum* f. *conglutinans* in relation to cabbage yellows. *Phytopathology* **50**, 367-370.

Husain, A. and Dimond, A. E. (1960). Role of cellulolytic enzymes in pathogenesis by *Fusarium oxysporum* f. *lycopersici. Phytopathology* **50**, 329-331.

Kern, H. (1952). Uber die Beziehungen zwischen dem Alkaloidgehalt verschiedener Tomatensorten und ihrer Resistenz gegen *Fusarium lycopersici. Phytopath. Z.* **19**, 351-382.

Langcake, P. and Drysdale, R. B. (with Bratt, P. M.) (1973a). Pectinmethylesterase in *Fusarium*-infected susceptible tomato plants. *Physiol. Pl. Path.* **3**, 101-107.

Langcake, P. and Drysdale, R. B. (1973b). The role of pectic enzyme production in the resistance of tomato to *Fusarium oxysporum* f. *lycopersici. Physiol. Pl. Path.* (in press).

Langcake, P., Drysdale, R. B. and Smith, H. (1972). Post-infectional production of an inhibitor of *Fusarium oxysporum* f. *lycopersici. Physiol. Pl. Path.* **2**, 17-25.

Langton, F. A. (1969). Interactions of the tomato with two formae speciales of *Fusarium oxysporum. Ann. appl. Biol.* **62**, 413-427.

Lee, M. and Macmillan, J. D. (1968). Mode of action of pectic enzymes. I. Purification and certain properties of tomato pectinesterase. *Biochemistry N.Y.* 7, 4005-4010.

McColloch, R. J. and Kertesz, Z. I. (1947). Pectic enzymes VIII. A comparison of fungal pectinmethylesterase with that of higher plants especially tomatoes. *Archs Biochem. Biophys.* **13**, 217-229.

McDonnell, K. (1962). Relationship of pectic enzymes and pathogenicity in the Fusarium wilt of tomatoes. *Trans. Br. mycol. Soc.* **45**, 55-62.

Mann, B. (1962). Role of pectic enzymes in the Fusarium wilt syndrome of tomato. *Trans. Br. mycol. Soc.* **45**, 169-178.

Matta, A. and Dimond, A. E. (1963). Symptoms of Fusarium wilt in relation to quantity of fungus and enzyme activity in tomato stems. *Phytopathology* **53**, 574-578.

Mohanakumaran, N., Gilbert, J. C. and Buddenhagen, I. W. (1969). Relationship between tomatine and bacterial wilt resistance in tomato. *Phytopathology* **59**, 14.

Morris, D. L. (1948). Quantitative determination of carbohydrates with Dreywood's anthrone reagent. *Science, N.Y.* **107**, 254-255.

Mussell, H. W. and Green, R. J. (1970). Host colonisation and polygalacturonase production by two tracheomycotic fungi. *Phytopathology* **60**, 192-195.

Paquin, R. and Coulombe, L. J. (1962). Pectic enzyme synthesis in relation to virulence in *Fusarium oxysporum* f. *lycopersici* (Sacc.) Snyder and Hansen. *Can. J. Bot.* **40**, 533-541.

Patil, S. S. and Dimond, A. E. (1968). Repression of polygalacturonase synthesis in *Fusarium oxysporum* f. sp. *lycopersici* by sugars and its effect on symptom reduction in infected tomato plants. *Phytopathology* **58**, 676-682.

Pierson, C. F., Gothoskar, S. S., Walker, J. C. and Stahmann, M. A. (1955). Histological studies on the role of pectic enzymes in the development of *Fusarium* wilt symptoms in tomato. *Phytopathology* **45**, 524-527.

Smith, I. (ed.) (1968). 'Chromatographic and Electrophoretic Techniques', 3rd edn. Vol. 1, p. 519. Heinemann, London.

Strange, R. N. and Smith, H. (1971). A rapid assay of fungal growth stimulants. *Trans. Br. mycol. Soc.* **56**, 485-488.

Uhle, F. C. and Moore, J. A. (1954). The partial synthesis of tomatidine *J. Am. chem. Soc.* **76**, 6412-6413.

Waggoner, P. E. and Dimond, A. E. (1955). Production and role of extracellular pectic enzymes of *Fusarium oxysporum* f. *lycopersici. Phytopathology* **45**, 79-87.

Winstead, N. N. and Walker, J. C. (1954). Toxic metabolites of the pathogen in relation to Fusarium resistance. *Phytopathology* **44**, 159-166.

Wood, R. K. S. (1960). Pectic and celluloytic enzymes in plant disease. *A. Rev. Pl. Physiol.* **11**, 299-322.

DISCUSSION

A. van Dijkman: How did you measure the content of tomatine in tomato tissue?

Dr R. B. Drysdale: I think that the method in the literature is the gravimetric one. We did not like this, and so we attempted to purify tomatine by a method which is basically Kern's, and we then measured anthrone-positive material having previously checked that we had only a single anthrone-positive spot by thin-layer chromatography.

A. van Dijkman: How do you extract your tomatine from the healthy and infected stems?—because I think that if the tissue in the infected stems is weak and the cells are damaged you will get the tomatine out of the vacuoles of the plant cells. Would it not be better to use a lipophilic organic solvent?

Dr P. Langcake: Tomatine was extracted with 1% acetic acid which is a fairly drastic procedure, so I think the release of tomatine from vacuoles would not explain the increase, because we should have extracted this from healthy tissue.

A. van Dijkman: So you think you have damaged cells in both healthy and infected stems?

Dr Langcake: Yes.

A. van Dijkman: There is one thing which it is very difficult for me to understand because I used tomatine in the *Fusarium* tests in our routine roll-culture test. I used potato dextrose agar, and I found no inhibition at all even above 1000 ppm. That is quite a difference from your 14 ppm, if I have calculated this correctly on a mol. wt. of 1031 for tomatine.

Dr Drysdale: What was the pH of your medium?

A. van Dijkman: 6.5.

Dr Langcake: I think this must remain unexplained, because we have used commercial preparations of tomatine, and we have found that this was just as toxic as our purified preparations, based on their anthrone reaction. I do not understand why people get different sensitivities of fungi to this.

A. van Dijkman: I used different strains of *Fusarium oxysporum* from tomato, peas and bulb flowers.

Dr Drysdale: We have not looked at anything other than race 1 of *F. oxysporum lycopersici.*

Professor P. H. Williams: You have just answered my question, I was wondering if you ever used race 2 or 3, with respect to the sensitivity to the tomatine.

Dr Drysdale: We are rather reluctant to get involved with using race 2, in case we get contamination, because there is no real way of separating the races except by doing host range tests.

Professor Williams: It would be interesting to know whether race 2 could detoxify tomatine.

Dr Langcake: We are not actually suggesting that tomatine is involved in resistance to race 1, because as you have seen, we have not really got any evidence to support this, therefore one would expect, I think, a similar sensitivity of race 2 to the compound as you would with race 1.

Dr Drysdale: There certainly are fungi which will chop off the sugars, or at least some of the sugars and the compound is then not inhibitory to the growth of the fungi.

S. A. Archer: Do I understand you said you found no polygalacturonase etc., in infected tomato tissue? Do you find it in cultures of the fungus?

Dr Drysdale: If the fungus is grown on pectin *in vitro,* polygalacturonase is produced. I cannot tell you whether it is an exo- or an endo- PG.

S. A. Archer: Have you looked for inhibitors of this enzyme in tomato tissue?

Dr Drysdale: Yes, unsuccessfully.

Dr Langcake: We have tried mixing extracts of tissue with culture-produced PG, and there is a very slight effect, and I would suggest that this effect was due to precipitation of the polypectate substrate by some component of the extract.

S. A. Archer: Do you think the pH in the lumen of the xylem vessels is wrong for induction of the enzyme?

Dr Langcake: I really cannot comment on this, but I think it unlikely that conditions within the xylem are unsuitable for the induction of pectic enzymes.

Professor R. K. S. Wood: Inevitably one must ask this question, as one always does about vascular parasites–they have a very unusual distribution in plants. Perhaps you will confirm first that *Fusarium oxysporum lycopersici* is substantially confined to the xylem vessels.

Dr Drysdale: Yes it is.

Professor Wood: But in a whole stem, the only cells *Fusarium* is in contact with are xylem itself plus the xylem parenchyma. Inevitably one must ask what is the significance of a whole plant extract for a fungus which is confined to the xylem parenchyma. Secondly, and yet possibly more important, the fungus is growing in the xylem parenchyma, therefore something must be operating against the hyphae in this tissue. Is there any tomatine in xylem exudates?

Dr Drysdale: We would like to study two things basically, as far as tomatine is concerned. Firstly, we would like to see if it is exported from the leaves, or is in fact newly synthesized in the stem. Secondly, we would like to do some histochemistry, if possible, to try and locate precisely the part of the stem in which the tomatine resides. While we find the same gross concentration in resistant and susceptible plants, we do not know the location of it, or indeed if the location is is the same in the two cultivars.

Dr Langcake: Could I add, that we have tested xylem sap which we collected by normal methods, and this does not seem to contain things which we can detect that are inhibitory to the fungus.

Professor M. A. Stahmann: You mentioned the variation in results reported in the literature concerning PG activity, and you suggested that this might be due to differences in the source of the enzyme. Another possibility might be a difference in substrates used, which could differ in the degree of methylation. What substrate did you use for PG?

Dr Drysdale: We have used two substrates, citrus pectin, and apple pectin.

Professor Stahmann: These may vary in the degree of methylation, and this may affect the activity of the PG. In our studies we methylated in order to get a uniform methoxyl content.

Dr Langcake: We used sodium polypectate for the PG assays, but pectin from two sources. I think the apple pectin had a very low methoxyl content, and this was not very suitable for use in PME assays. The other pectin was Koch-Light citrus pectin.

Professor Stahmann: Such substrates may be variable, and hence might give different results. I would also like to suggest that if you really want to produce pectic enzymes you grow the organism on pectin. You suggest that the pectin-degrading enzymes of the fungus might not be important. However, the fungus releases pectin in the vascular system to induce pectinase synthesis by the host plant.

Dr Drysdale: Would not this depend on the nature of the pectic enzyme which was actually produced? One of the other conflicts in the literature is whether or not it is an exo- or an endo-PG which is produced. Now if it is an exo-PG it is going to produce basically only monogalacturonic acid residues.

Professor Stahmann: Fungi often form mixtures of pectic enzymes.

Dr Drysdale: I do not think that in the literature there is anyone who claims that there is a mixture. The claims are either for an exo- or an endo-PG. Now I would accept that the assay methods used may not be critical enough to distinguish between the two, but I do not think that there is any suggestion from any of the papers that I have read that there is in fact a mixture produced *in vivo.*

Professor Stahmann: Did it make any difference in the amount of enzyme produced in the host plant–whether it was resistant or susceptible. I recall from some work we did on resistant and susceptible banana tissue, there was quite a difference in the amount of enzyme produced when the fungus was grown on each.

Dr Drysdale: I think the susceptible one usually produced more.

Dr Langcake: Yes, we can only talk about PME *in vivo* because it is the only one which we have detected, but definitely in the susceptible plant there was a two-fold increase of this PME compared with the monogenic resistant tissue.

Dr Drysdale: What is perhaps even more interesting, there is considerably less fungus in the resistant ones, so that the increase in PME/unit weight of fungus is much greater in the resistant than in the susceptible plant.

V.3 The Host–Parasite Interactions in Resistance of Tomatoes to *Cladosporium fulvum*

A. KAARS SIJPESTEIJN AND A. VAN DIJKMAN

Institute for Organic Chemistry, TNO, Utrecht, The Netherlands

INTRODUCTION

Leaf mould caused by *Cladosporium fulvum* Cooke is an economically important disease in tomatoes. By breeding and by introduction of resistance factors from wild *Lycopersicon* species, resistant cultivars have been obtained (Persiel, 1967; Williams, 1964). When inoculated with an incompatible race of *C. fulvum* they show hypersensitivity under favourable conditions. During this breeding work it was shown that resistance of *Lycopersicon esculentum* to *C. fulvum* is determined by four independent genes which have been called Cf 1, Cf 2, Cf 3 and Cf 4 (Bailey and Kerr, 1964; Kooistra, 1964). The dominant allele of each of them determines resistance to certain races of the pathogen but is quite ineffective towards other races. To illustrate this fact some data, largely derived from Hubbeling (1966, 1971) have been summarized in Table I.

The cultivars are indicated by the dominant resistance alleles present; the tomatoes presented here are homozygous for these genes. As the authors cited

TABLE I

Relation between some tomato cultivars and races of *Cladosporium fulvum*.

Tomato	Dominant resistance genes	*Cladosporium fulvum*, physiological race 0	1	2	1.2	1.2.3	1.2.4	4
Moneymaker	none	S	S	S	S	S	S	S
LMR	Cf1	R	S	R	S	S	S	R
Vetomold	Cf2	R	R	S	S	S	S	R
V473	Cf1 Cf2	R	R	R	S	S	S	R
V121	Cf3	R	R	R	R	S	R	R
Purdue 135	Cf4	R	R	R	R	R	S	S
Vagabond	Cf2 Cf4	R	R	R	R	R	S	R

R–resistant S–susceptible

could not then designate the physiological races of the pathogen by distinctive genotypes, the races were given the indices of those resistance alleles of the tomato which are ineffective towards them. The symbol 0 has been given to the race which can only attack tomatoes that are recessive to all resistance genes, e.g. the cultivar Moneymaker.

The complicated relation between host cultivars and races of the pathogen in tomato has been recognized as a 'gene-for-gene' relation by Day (1954) by analogy with similar relations earlier described for other diseases, e.g. flax rust (Flor, 1942) and potato late blight (Black *et al.*, 1953; Toxopeus, 1956). Such relations were later also described for apple scab (Boone and Keitt, 1957) and rusts and smuts (cf. Fincham and Day, 1963).

The pattern of resistance and susceptibility of tomato to *C. fulvum* at first sight looks very complicated. We have tried to unravel the biochemical mechanism of resistance to this disease because a former guest worker of our Institute—Dr J. Raa—has studied the biochemical mechanism of resistance to one of the diseases just mentioned, namely apple scab (Raa, 1968a, 1968b). For a certain strain of *Venturia inaequalis* he obtained strong indications that it was able to excrete a compound into the medium which is toxic selectively to resistant apples in such a way as to cause cell damage and a hypersensitive reaction. To apples which were susceptible to the same strain of *Venturia,* preparations containing this compound were not toxic. It was proposed that the different avirulence genes of Venturia (cf. Fincham and Day, 1963) are responsible for the production of various compounds each of which reacts selectively with specific membrane constituents of the host cells, thus leading to the hypersensitive reaction (Raa and Kaars Sijpesteijn, 1968; Kaars Sijpesteijn, 1969). The different resistance genes in apple are supposed to control the presence of such specific membrane constituents.

We now reasoned that the same principle might underlie the resistance reaction in tomato to *C. fulvum* (Van Dijkman and Kaars Sijpesteijn, 1971). What does this mean?

Let us first look at Table II which considers only the first four tomato cultivars mentioned in Table I and the physiologic races 0, 1, 2 and 1.2.

According to our hypothesis, race 1 should be able to produce a compound which is toxic selectively to a tomato cultivar which it cannot attack, like Vetomold or V473 with the gene Cf2; but it should not be toxic to a susceptible cultivar such as Moneymaker or LMR which lack the gene Cf1. The pattern of resistance towards race 2 is the reverse. Therefore we suppose that this race produces a different compound which is toxic selectively to tomato LMR or V473 with gene Cf1 giving a hypersensitive reaction; but it should not be toxic to the susceptible cultivars Moneymaker or Vetomold which lack Cf1.

In Table II we have indicated with A_1 this presumed ability to form a compound toxic to tomato Cf1, and with A_2 the ability to form a compound

TABLE II

Presumed toxin production by *Cladosporium fulvum.*

Tomato	Dominant resistance genes	*Cladosporium fulvum,* physiological race 0	1	2	1.2
		presumed genotype for toxin production A_1A_2	a_1A_2	A_1a_2	a_1a_2
Moneymaker	none	S	S	S	S
LMR	Cf1	R	S	R	S
Vetomold	Cf2	R	R	S	S
V473	Cf1 Cf2	R	R	R	S

gene A_1 –ability to form a toxin for tomato Cf1
gene A_2 –ability to form a toxin for tomato Cf2
S–susceptible R–resistant

toxic to tomato Cf2; these abilities have tentatively been written as a genotype. Race 0 cannot attack tomatoes which possess either gene Cf1 or Cf2; therefore it might produce both toxins and should be indicated as $A_1 A_2$.

Table II is a simplified scheme which considers only the genes Cf1 and Cf2. The same reasoning can, however, be extended to the genes Cf3 and Cf4 as well as to the ability of certain physiologic races to produce compounds toxic to tomatoes which possess the dominant allele of gene Cf3 or that of gene Cf4. A_3 and A_4 would then indicate the ability to form a compound toxic to a tomato with Cf3 and to a tomato with Cf4 respectively.

METHODS AND RESULTS

To obtain evidence for our hypothesis of the production of various selective toxins by the fungus, a study was made of the toxicity of certain constituents of culture filtrates from various races of *C. fulvum* towards different tomato cultivars was studied (van Dijkman and Kaars Sijpesteijn, 1971). The physiological races of the fungus and seeds of the tomato cultivars used, were kindly made available to us by Ir. N. Hubbeling from the Institute of Phytopathological Research and by Ir. E. Kooistra from the Institute of Horticultural Plant Breeding at Wageningen.

In the first experiment, properties of the interaction of races 1 and 2 with the tomatoes LMR (Cf1) and Vetomold (Cf2) were compared in the following way. The compounds excreted by the fungus were obtained by growing shake cultures of the two races for about three weeks. Thereafter the culture filtrate was freed from low-mol. wt. material by filtration over Sephadex G25. The high-mol. wt. fraction was freeze-dried and stored until use.

Meanwhile plants of LMR and Vetomold were grown. Mature leaves were cut off and placed, for several hours, with their petioles dipped into a solution of $^{32}PO_4$ to label the leaf cells. Then disks were prepared from these leaves. They were transferred to a buffered solution of the fungal material. To ensure proper contact between the labelled plant cells and the fungal material the liquid was infiltrated into the disks by evacuation of the flask. After infiltration air was slowly admitted again.

Our hypothesis suggested that the infiltrated fungal material would contain a compound that would be toxic selectively to the cells of a resistant host plant, but not to those of a susceptible host plant. Hence we expected that in the case of *resistance* the host cells would be damaged and that consequently the labelled compounds would leak out of the cells and out of the disks into the surrounding liquid. But in the case of *susceptibility* we expected no leakage by fungal products. And this is indeed what we found. The amount of leakage was determined by measuring radioactivity of the liquid at different intervals after infiltration. The percentage of leakage of the total ^{32}P present could be calculated.

Figure 1 gives the results obtained with tomato LMR (Cf1) and with Vetomold (Cf2). The extent of leakage of labelled compounds from the disks is given in relation to the time elapsed after infiltration of the excretion products of the fungi. LMR (Cf1) is susceptible to the race $a_1 A_2 A_3 A_4$ and infiltration with products of this race does not cause a leakage which exceeds that caused by infiltration of the buffer solution alone. The same fungal products, however, caused strong leakage in excess of the buffer control after infiltration into Vetomold (Cf2), which is resistant to this race $a_1 A_2 A_3 A_4$. Quite the opposite situation was found for the race $A_1 a_2 A_3 A_4$ which is able to attack Vetomold

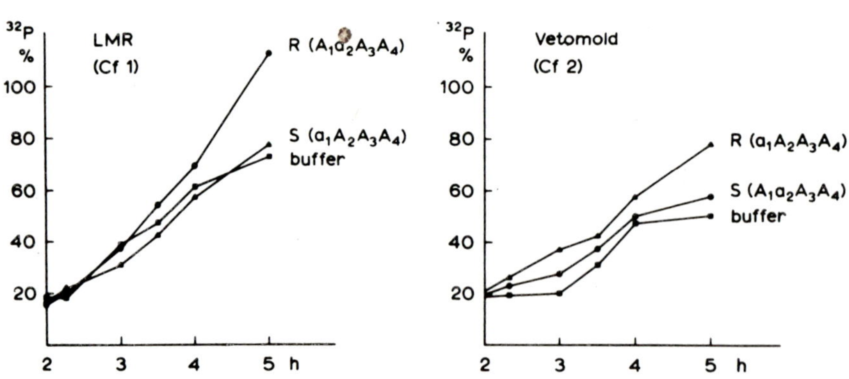

Fig. 1. Leakage of ^{32}P from tomato leaf disks infiltrated with the void volume fraction of culture filtrate of two races of *C. fulvum*. *Left:* Tomato 'Leaf Mould Register No. 1' (Cf1). *Right:* Tomato 'Vetomold' (Cf2) R: incompatible combination; S: compatible combination; Buffer: buffer control.

(Cf2) but not LMR (Cf1): we found strong leakage of LMR but not of Vetomold. These results are strongly in favour of our hypothesis of selectively-toxic products being excreted by the parasite.

A similar correlation between resistance *in vivo* and leakage in the model experiment was found for the tomato V473 which carries the resistance genes Cf1 and Cf2 (Fig. 2-*left*). Again infiltration with material from two fungal races

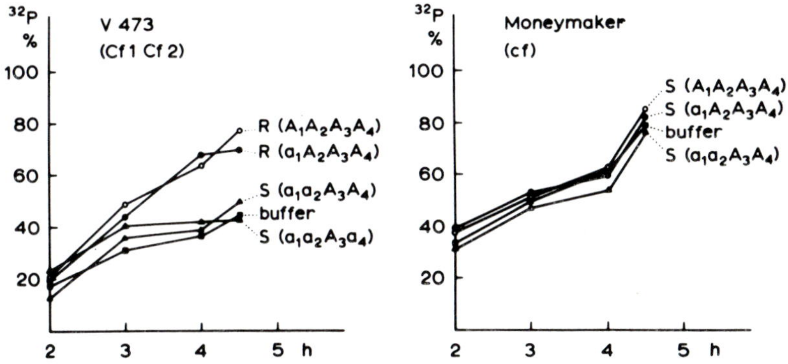

Fig. 2. Leakage of ^{32}P from leaf disks of tomato cultivars infiltrated with void volume fraction of culture filtrate of *C. fulvum* races R: incompatible combination; S:compatible combination; Buffer: buffer control.
Left: 'V 473' (Cf1 Cf2).
Right: 'Moneymaker' (cf).

to which this plant is resistant–in this case $A_1A_2A_3A_4$ and $a_1A_2A_3A_4$ –causes strong leakage in excess of the control. In contrast the high molecular material excreted by the two physiologic races $a_1a_2A_3A_4$ and $a_1a_2A_3a_4$ which are both able to attack this tomato cultivar does not cause any extra leakage.

From three of these races the products were also infiltrated into the tomato Moneymaker which is susceptible to all races of the pathogen; it is recessive to all resistance genes. According to expectation no leakage in excess of the control was observed (Fig. 2-*right*).

So far we have been dealing with the resistance genes Cf1 and Cf2. The cultivar Purdue 135 carries the dominant allele Cf4. Results of infiltration of leaf disks with the high-mol. wt. fraction of culture filtrates of various physiologic races entirely supported our hypothesis (Fig. 3). The races $A_1A_2a_3a_4$ and $a_1a_2A_3a_4$ attacked this tomato and accordingly their culture filtrates were unable to cause any extra leakage of the cells after infiltration. In contrast preparations of the physiologic races $A_1A_2A_3A_4$ and $A_1a_2A_3A_4$ which cannot attack this tomato caused a leakage of the host cells which greatly exceeded that effected by the buffer alone.

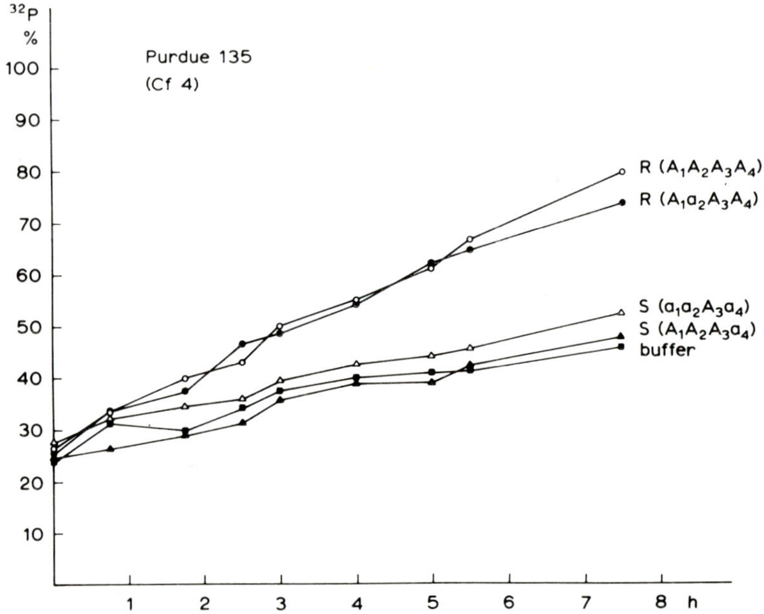

Fig. 3. Leakage of ^{32}P from leaf disks of Purdue 135 (Cf4), infiltrated with the void volume fraction of culture filtrate of *C. fulvum* races.
R: incompatible combination; S: compatible combination; Buffer: buffer control.

An experiment carried out with Vetomold and Purdue 135, and the races $a_1 a_2 a_3 A_4$ and $A_1 A_2 A_3 a_4$ also was in full agreement with the hypothesis (Fig. 4).

So far, no experiments have been undertaken with tomatoes carrying the dominant allele of gene Cf3.

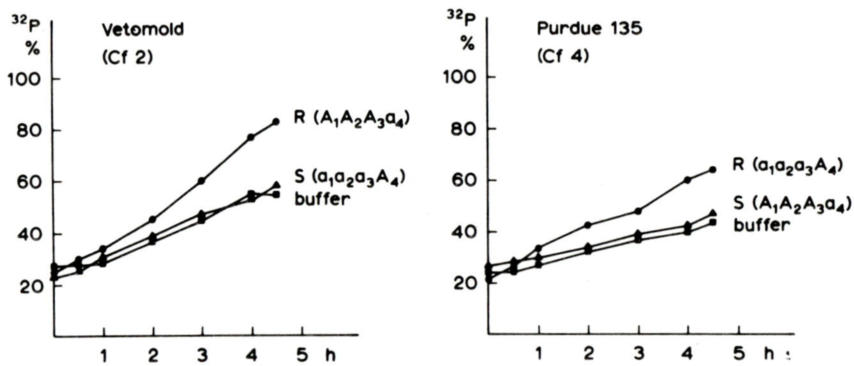

Fig. 4. Leakage of ^{32}P from leaf disks of Vetomold (Cf2) and Purdue 135 (Cf4) with the void volume fraction of culture filtrate of *C. fulvum* races.
R: incompatible combination; S; compatible combination; Buffer: buffer control.

TABLE III

Observed correlation between resistance *in vivo* and leakage by selective toxins.

Tomato	Dominant resistance genes	*Cladosporium fulvum*, physiological race 0	1	2	1.2	1.2.3	1.2.4	4
		Proposed genotype for avirulence						
		$A_1A_2A_3A_4$	$a_1A_2A_3A_4$	$A_1a_2A_3A_4$	$a_1a_2A_3A_4$	$a_1a_2a_3A_4$	$a_1a_2A_3a_4$	$A_1A_2A_3a_4$
Moneymaker	none	S/N	S/N		S/N		S/N	S/N
LMR	Cf1		S/N	R/L				
Vetomold	Cf2	R/L	R/L	S/N		S/N		R/L
V473	Cf1 Cf2	R/L	R/L		S/N		S/N	
Purdue 135	Cf4	R/L		R/L		R/L	S/N	S/N
Vagabond	Cf2 Cf4	R/L				R/L	S/N	R/L

R–resistant
S–susceptible
L–leakage in excess of control
N–no leakage in excess of control

Discussion and Conclusions

Results of these leakage experiments and others carried out so far have been summarized in Table III. These show a striking correlation between the occurrence of a hypersensitive resistance reaction *in vivo* (R) and leakage in the model experiments (L) as well as between susceptibility (S) and the absence of leakage (N). This correlation shows that the various physiologic races of Cladosporium are distinguished by their ability to produce one or more compounds, each of which is toxic selectively only to those tomato cultivars which carry the appropriate resistance gene.

We believe that the various resistance genes in the tomato control the presence of different receptor sites in the cell membranes each of which is sensitive to one of the fungal toxins only. The presumed genes in the fungus which control toxin production may then be called *avirulence genes.* Each of these corresponds to one resistance gene in the tomato host in such a way that the toxin causes leakage of the cell membranes of the appropriate host resulting in a hypersensitive reaction.

Yet the question remains–why does the occurrence of a hypersensitive reaction in the tomato plant stop further development of *C. fulvum,* a facultative parasite, which grows well on a homogenate of the host plant? It is true that by destruction of the tomato cells the compound tomatine, which is toxic to some fungi, is liberated and partly converted into its aglycone tomatidine. However, neither tomatine nor tomatidine proved to be fungitoxic to *C. fulvum.* Further investigations are required to elucidate this point. Possibly the tissue dries out after the hypersensitive reaction.

There is much reason to believe that in other host–parasite combinations which display a gene-for-gene relation, as for example potato blight and flax rust, this relation is accomplished in a way similar to that of leaf mould of tomato, namely by resistance genes in the host plant which control the presence of receptor sites, these in their turn being selectively sensitive to the various fungal toxins elaborated by avirulence genes.

References

Bailey, D. L. and Kerr, E. A. (1964). *Cladosporium fulvum* race 10 and resistance to it in tomato. *Can. J. Bot.* **42**, 1555-1558.

Black, W. B., Mastenbroek, C., Mills, W. R. and Peterson, L. C. (1953). A proposal for an international nomenclature of races of *Phytophthora infestans* and of genes controlling immunity in *Solanum demissum* derivatives. *Euphytica* **2**, 173-178.

Boone, D. M. and Keitt, G. W. (1957). *Venturia inaequalis* (Cke) Wint. XII. Genes controlling pathogenicity of wild-type lines. *Phytopathology* **47**, 403-409.

Day, P. R. (1954). Physiologic specialization of *Cladosporium fulvum* in England and Wales. *Pl. Path.* **3**, 35-39.

Fincham, J. R. S. and Day, P. R. (1963). 'Fungal genetics.' Blackwell Scientific Publications, Oxford.

Flor, H. H. (1942). Inheritance of pathogenicity in *Melampsora lini. Phytopathology* **32**, 653-669.

Hubbeling, N. (1966). Identificatie van nieuwe fysio's van *Cladosporium fulvum* en selectie op resistentie daartegen bij de tomaat. *Meded. LandbHogesch. OpzoekStns Gent* **21**, 925-930.

Hubbeling, N. (1971). Determination trouble with new races of *Cladosporium fulvum* Cooke. *Meded. Rijksfac. Landbouwwet. Gent* **36**, 300-305.

Kaars Sijpesteijn, A. (1969). Aspects of natural disease resistance. *Meded. Rijksfac. Landbouwwet. Gent* **34**, 379-391.

Kooistra, E. (1964). Recent experiences of breeding leaf mould resistant tomatoes. *Euphytica* **13**, 103-109.

Persiel, F. (1967). Resistenz und Resistenzzüchtung gegen die Braunflecken-krankheit, *Cladosporium fulvum* Cooke, bei Tomaten. *Z. PflZücht.* **57**, 325-360.

Raa, J. (1968a). Polyphenols and natural resistance of apple leaves against *Venturia inaequalis. Neth. J. Pl. Pathol.* **74**, 37-45.

Raa, J. (1968b). Natural resistance of apple plant to *Venturia inaequalis*–a biochemical study of its mechanism. Dissertation. State University Utrecht, The Netherlands.

Raa, J. and Kaars Sijpesteijn, A. (1968). A biochemical mechanism of natural resistance of apple to *Venturia inaequalis. Neth.J. Pl. Pathol.* **74**, 229-331.

Toxopeus, H. J. (1956). Reflections on the origin of new physiologic races in *Phytophthora infestans* and the breeding for resistance in potatoes. *Euphytica* **5**, 221-237.

Van Dijkman, A. and Kaars Sijpesteijn, A. (1971). A biochemical mechanism for the gene-for-gene resistance of tomato to *Cladosporium fulvum* Cooke. *Neth.J.Pl. Pathol.* **77**, 14-24.

Williams, W. (1964). 'Genetical principles and plant breeding'. Chap. XI. Blackwell Scientific Publications Oxford.

DISCUSSION

P. W. Wilkins: Do you intend to find out the nature of the substances that cause this leakage reaction in the resistant plants?

Dr A. Kaars Sijpesteijn: We think they might be proteins, as by their nature they have a rather large molecule. But that is all we know about them, we would like to know more, but of course the concentration is very low.

P. W. Wilkins: Mutations which result in a failure of synthesis of a compound, e.g. an enzyme, are far more common than positive mutations, e.g. for an enzyme which can degrade a host product. This might explain the peculiarity of this type of resistance, which seems to break down very quickly.

Dr Kaars Sijpesteijn: If I have understood you, there is a rapid breakdown of resistance of tomato plants and this can be explained by the hypothesis that the fungal races might turn from dominance to recessiveness–then it would lose the capacity to form the toxin, and the tomato will become susceptible to this race.

Dr P. Langcake: A similar effect has been shown with *Fusarium* wilt of tomato and monogenic resistance. This is Keyworth's work, and I think it is true to say metabolites responsible for this were low molecular weight compounds. Have you looked at low molecular weight fractions from the culture filtrates, or did you have any particular reason at the outset to look at the high molecular weight compounds?

Dr Kaars Sijpesteijn: We found no selective effect with the low molecular weight fractions.

Dr B. J. Deverall: Have you seen any visible effects of these products on your resistant plants?

Dr Kaars Sijpesteijn: Do you mean if we applied the fungal material immediately on to the plants? We think the large molecules have difficulty in penetrating, and they are probably proteinaceous in nature, so if they stay for several days on the plant, they are probably decomposed by bacteria.

Dr Deverall: Have you attempted the experiment to see what happens?

Dr Kaars Sijpesteijn: We have attempted it, but it becomes confused.

A. van Dijkman: We have applied these materials to gauze on the leaf of a resistant plant, and then you see hypersensitivity reactions. But, if you inoculate a tomato with compatible races you do not see any symptoms before 10-14 days. So it will take a long time, and naturally it is very difficult to infiltrate the substance into the intercellular system of the intact leaf.

Dr R. C. Hignett: If you could get your toxin in, would you expect to be able to induce resistance in a susceptible cultivar by applying the appropriate toxins?

Dr Sijpesteijn: We have not tried this.

Dr Hignett: Suppose, for example, you put on a mixed inoculum containing a pathogenic strain and a non-pathogenic strain, would the effect prevent the pathogenic strain from infecting?

Dr Sijpesteijn: This might be something to try. I thought you were thinking of model experiments, but you are thinking of experiments *in vivo.*

Dr I. M. Smith: You said, I think, that you used culture filtrates, taken from three-week-old cultures. Have you looked for the same toxins in germination fluids, i.e. in a situation a little closer to the *Cladosporium* directly infecting the leaf?

Dr Sijpesteijn: Even in the resistant combinations, *Cladosporium* spreads in the intercellular cavities, so it is infecting hyphae that come into contact with the cells.

Dr Smith: Yes, so that the culture filtrate is a reasonable model for the situation.

Dr Sijpesteijn: But one needs quite a quantity of the compound to do these experiments, and if one starts with spore germination fluids, then you need a very high concentration.

Dr Deverall: Skipp attempted to do similar experiments with *Colletotrichum lindemuthianum,* and he failed to get any form of specificity. He was able to damage both resistant and susceptible cells in apparently the same way, but he did not separate the fungal products as much as you have done.

Dr Sijpesteijn: One has to fractionate rather carefully to remove unspecific toxic material.

A. van Dijkman: We were rather careful with our products. They were never above 0° C, and we freeze-dried them, and kept them in the deep freeze all the time. In diluting the protein or the fraction, if you keep it too long and stir it too much until it is foaming, you get a low effect. So that is probably one of the reasons that some of my results were negative.

Dr R. J. W. Byrde: I wonder if there is any possibility that the receptor site is in the cell wall. I believe that if Peter Albersheim were here he would say that. In view of the paper by Dr Hall and Professor Wood, and the general finding that wall-degrading enzymes seem to be the ones implicated in cell leakage, is this not a possibility to be considered? I agree, of course, that we will know much more when we know the nature of the material.

Dr Sijpesteijn: You imagine that the receptor would be in the cell wall, instead of in the cell membranes?

Dr Byrde: I think this could be so, because so many of the leakage phenomena seem to have been associated with wall-degrading enzymes.

Dr Sijpesteijn: Yes, but would you get a loss of turgidity if the receptor were in the cell wall instead of in the cell membrane? The hypersensitive reaction suggests a loss of turgidity.

Dr Byrde: I was suggesting that activation of the receptor in the cell wall would be followed by membrane changes. I agree that if the membrane is altered, this would finally lead to hypersensitivity.

Dr R. Johnson: I have done one cross-inoculation experiment with yellow rust on wheat, using two cultivars, one of which gives a very small fleck to a virulent race, and another which gives a rather large chlorotic lesion. Although I have not done the microscopic studies, it seems you can get infection with a virulent race after using the avirulent race, anywhere except where the actual mycelium has penetrated. Therefore where you have the tiny chlorotic fleck, you can easily get infection with the virulent race over the remainder of the leaf. It is only as the mycelium expands in producing the large chlorotic lesion that the tissue becomes immune. Your system may be the same as this, since a large molecule is presumably involved. There is no transmissibility of this type of resistance, and therefore one could not use it to immunize a plant.

Dr Sijpesteijn: If you mix up your compatible with the incompatible race you would only get the resistant reaction.

Dr Johnson: Yes, but if you leave it and inoculate on a subsequent day, you cannot see the chlorotic area at this time because it is too early for it to be shown—but nevertheless changes have taken place which prevent further infection over an increasing area as the days go by. Where there is a small chlorotic fleck, a mixture would appear as a completely virulent race, because the fleck is too small to influence the infection.

Dr Sijpesteijn: I think we should try this.

A van Dijkman: I got the impression from inoculation experiments that the resistant reaction is somewhat faster than the reactions which occur in the compatible combination. You see the chlorotic spots in an incompatible combination somewhat earlier than the spread of the mycelium and the formation of the conidia.

Dr E. Hislop: If you add sucrose to your fungal extract and infiltrate your tissues with this, do the cells still die? Do they still leak? In other words, does a plasmolysing solution protect them, in the same way that it does from pectic enzymes?

Dr Sijpesteijn: We have never tried.

A. van Dijkman: To try out the best buffer to use I included sucrose, and sucrose + albumen, and that with the lowest basic leakage was the tris-HCl buffer, pH 6. I have not tried a toxin and sucrose together. Why do you think they will not leak? At what concentration?

Dr Hislop: I wondered whether it was an effect on the wall or the membrane and whether perhaps one could separate the effects by using a strength of medium which would plasmolyse the cells while they are being treated with the fungal extract.

A. van Dijkman: But that is covered by the cross-relations we have. An R and an S and the opposite, an S and an R.

Dr Sijpesteijn: That is, the same fungal filtrate or preparation causes one tomato to leak but not another.

Dr Hislop: I accept that, but I was just wondering if this will give any indication of the mechanism by which you are stimulating leakage.

Professor P. W. Brian: I think the point which Dr Hislop is making is that you can protect a cell from a pectic enzyme, and thus prevent leakage by osmotica, whereas you cannot protect a cell, shall we say, from a specific toxin.

Dr Sijpesteijn: Yes, but we do not have the idea that the leakage could be caused by a pectic enzyme. I think it is a different type of compound.

V.4 Role of Lysosomal Enzymes in Pathogenicity

D. PITT AND MARY GALPIN

Department of Biological Sciences, University of Exeter, Devon, England

INTRODUCTION

The term lysosome was first introduced by de Duve *et al.* (1955) to describe a group of membrane-bound sub-cellular particles rich in acid hydrolases found in animal cells. Since that time appreciable effort has been directed towards determining the role of these particles in healthy and diseased cells and the extensive literature that has accumulated is reviewed in two recent volumes (Dingle and Fell, 1969). In addition the refinement of cell fractionation techniques has led to the discovery of other sub-cellular particles containing different enzymes e.g. peroxisomes (de Duve and Baudhuin, 1966) and permitted an extension of the concept of cellular compartmentalization of enzymes.

Although, for many years, spherosomes have been recognized in plants as organelles associated with lipid metabolism it is only comparatively recently that lysosome-like particles have been isolated from higher plant tissues (Matile *et al.*, 1965), and the evidence for lysosomal compartments in such cells has been thoroughly reviewed by Matile (1969). Since the experimental evidence indicates that lysosomes may be important physiologically as components of the intracellular digestive system, close attention has been paid in medical research to the possibility that a malfunctioning of these organelles could result in disruption of the normal controlled cellular lytic process with consequent autolysis and cell death. Although much evidence suggests that lysosomal disorganization may precede cell death there are no conclusive reports that this is so.

Pitt and Coombes (1968, 1969) showed that lysosomal disruption may be involved in fungal diseases of plants; the present paper describes experiments which support this view and also examines the possible role of lysosomal enzymes in the pathology of diseased tissues.

Materials and Methods

ORGANISMS

Callus tissue of potato tuber was grown and inoculated as described by Pitt and Coombes (1969). Tubers (cv. Majestic was used throughout these experiments) were inoculated and incubated according to Pitt and Coombes (1969). *Fusarium caeruleum* (Lib.) Sacc. was isolated from potato tubers which showed symptoms of dry rot disease and maintained in culture with occasional passage through the host.

PREPARATION OF ENZYMES FROM POTATO TUBERS

Acid phosphomonoesterase (E.C. 3.1.3.2)

This was obtained commercially (Boehringer, Mannheim), and was found to give elution patterns on gel filtration and profiles on polyacrylamide gel disk electrophoresis that were similar to this enzyme in crude potato homogenates.

Phosphodiesterase (E.C. 3.1.4.1)

This was a highly purified preparation from potato tubers (3 kg) obtained by isoelectric precipitation, DEAE-cellulose batch extraction followed by CM-cellulose column chromatography of the fluid fraction with a final separation on Sephadex G150. The enzyme was freeze dried in 1% (w/v) glycerol and stored in evacuated vials at -20° C. As with the commercial preparations the product contained slight acid phosphomonoesterase activity but was free from ribonuclease (RNase) and deoxyribonuclease activities.
Ribonuclease was obtained from potato tubers (3 kg) and contained two RNase antigens and a single acid phosphomonoesterase antigen (Pitt, 1971).

ENZYME ASSAYS

Acid phosphomonoesterase, acid phosphodiesterase and acid RNase activities were determined as previously described (Pitt and Galpin, 1971). The unit of phosphomonoesterase or phosphodiesterase activity is that amount of enzyme/mg protein which liberates 1.0 μmole of *p*-nitrophenol from appropriate substrates (*p*-nitrophenyl phosphate or *bis*-nitrophenyl phosphate, respectively) in 10 min at 37° C. A unit of RNase is that amount of enzyme causing ΔE_{260} of 1.0/h/mg protein.

GEL FILTRATION ON SEPHADEX G100

This was done by the method of Pitt and Galpin (1971) with elution by 0.02 M acetate buffer, pH 5.0, containing 0.05 M KCl in the cold.

PROTEIN DETERMINATIONS

Soluble protein was determined by the method of Lowry *et al.* (1951). Aliquots from column effluents were used directly, but all other determinations were carried out after the removal of interfering substances by protein precipitation with 25 vol. of cold acetone.

IMMUNOLOGICAL METHODS

Preparation of antisera

Antibodies to RNase from potato tubers were raised in rabbits as reported by Pitt (1971). Antiserum to acid phosphomonoesterase (Boehringer, Mannheim) was a gift from J. A. Lucas.

Double immunodiffusion

The technique of Ouchterlony (1953) was used as described by Pitt (1971).

Immunoelectrophoresis

This was carried out on agar-covered slides by the technique of Graber and Williams (1955) in a commercial apparatus (Shandon Scientific Co. Ltd., London) using Owen's quarter-strength agar according to the procedure used by Pitt (1971) with runs lasting 4 h at 30 mA.

Single radial immunodiffusion

The basic method used was that of Mancini *et al.* (1965) modified according to Pitt (1971) using agar containing final antisera concentrations of one-sixth of undiluted antisera.

Quantitative immunoelectrophoresis (antigen-antibody crossed electrophoresis)

This was basically the modification of Laurell's technique devised by Clarke and Freeman (1968). The first dimension separation was done by the Graber and Williams method with the second run at right angles to the first into 1.5% (w/v) agarose in 0.06 M barbitone-HCl buffer, pH 8.6, for 24 h at 2.5 V/cm. Antibody concentrations were devised for each batch of antiserum by trial, but usually the second dimension gel contained 9% (v/v) antiserum and the wells contained volumes of homogenate containing 4.5-9.0 μg of protein.

RESULTS

DISRUPTION OF LYSOSOMES OF CELLS OF *SOLANUM TUBEROSUM* DURING INFECTION BY TUBER-ROTTING FUNGI

Established histochemical methods were used by Pitt and Coombes (1968) to demonstrate the existence in fresh and fixed tuber tissues of sub-cellular particles containing a number of acid hydrolases normally located within animal lysosomes and the lysosome-like particles of plants (Fig. 1). It was also possible to show that these particles fulfilled several of the criteria listed by Gahan

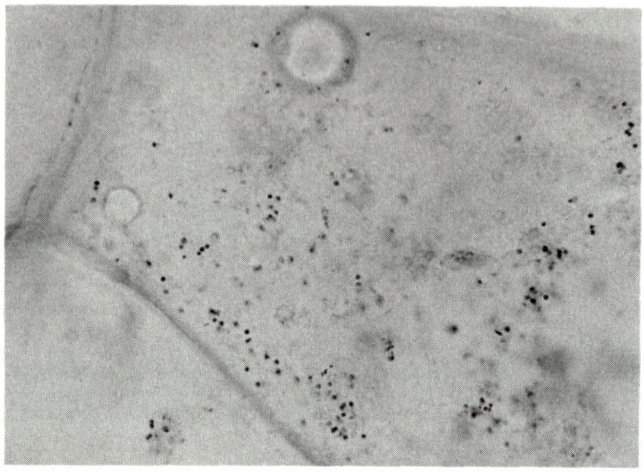

Fig. 1. Section of healthy potato tuber tissue stained for acid phosphomonoesterase by the standard coupling azo dye method after fixation in formol-calcium. The enzyme is localized in many small particles 0.2 μ–1.0 μ in diameter. x370 (From Pitt and Coombes, 1968).

(1967) with respect to the uptake of vital dyes, such as neutral red; and of fluorochromes, paticularly acridine dyes, and were subject to disruption by Triton X-100 and by freezing and thawing. As suggested by Matile (1969), the conflicting opinions on whether lysosomes exist in plants derive from the particular definitions adopted. Generally, however, the biochemical, histochemical and ultrastructural evidence for the existence of these structures in plants is strong and the present tendency is to refer to lysosomes instead of lysosome-like bodies for this group of particles in plants.

During infection of potato tuber tissue by *Phytophthora erythroseptica* there is swelling and disruption of host cytoplasmic particles which is revealed when sections of fresh or fixed material are stained for acid phosphomonoesterase activity. Of particular interest is the widespread and heavy cytoplasmic staining of this enzyme in infected tissues (Fig. 2). It is assumed since such diffuse cytoplasmic staining is not a normal feature of parenchymatous tissue that this enzyme had originated from particles following their disruption. Similar observations made by Pitt and Coombes (1969) on potato tuber tissues infected with *P. infestans* and *Fusarium caeruleum,* were extended to include other hydrolases believed to have a lysosomal localization including carboxylic esterases, β-galactosidase and an aminopeptidase. However, cytoplasmic staining for each of these was less than with the acid phosphomonoesterase procedure. In spite of extensive efforts to prepare sub-cellular fractions from potato tuber tissue, it has been impossible, so far, to isolate a particle-rich preparation containing significant amounts of hydrolases even by using the grinding and fractionation procedures which have proved successful for other tissues. However, callus tissue showed histochemical localization similar to that found in tubers and was used to obtain biochemical support for these histochemical

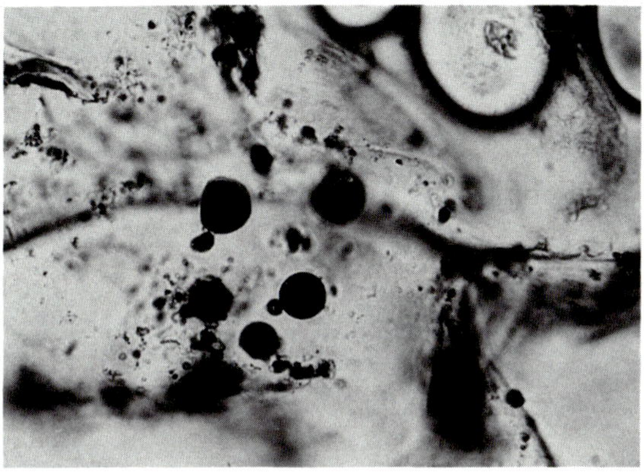

Fig. 2. Section of potato tuber tissue 4 days after infection with *Phytophthora erythroseptica,* fixed and stained as in Fig. 1. Relatively few particles are present with the remaining particles enlarged and surrounded by diffuse cytoplasmic stain. x370 (From Pitt and Coombes, 1968).

observations. A decreased activity of acid phosphomonoesterase and RNase in the particulate fractions of infected callus cell homogenates was accompanied by increases in the activities of these enzymes in the supernatant fluid fractions (Table I).

The esterase activity of the particulate fractions of infected cells was greater than that of the healthy controls suggesting the possibility that this enzyme was

TABLE I

Acid phosphomonoesterase activity in particulate (P) and supernatant fluid (S) fractions of potato callus tissue using β-glycerophosphate as substrate (after Pitt and Coombes, 1969).

Treatment	Activity of fractions:– inorganic phosphate released (μg P_i/ 20 min/mg protein)		% total activity in P + S fractions	
	P	S	P	S
P. erythroseptica				
Uninfected	3.1	2.3	57.2	42.8
4-day infected	1.0	2.3	31.0	69.0
P. infestans				
Uninfected	5.3	3.9	57.4	42.6
5½-day infected	2.6	9.0	22.5	77.5
F. caeruleum				
Uninfected	3.6	1.4	68.1	31.9
4½-day infected	2.0	4.9	28.9	71.1

not released during infection. These data contradicted the histochemical evidence, although it is possible that some of the remaining esterase activity of infected cells may reside in a particulate form which was not resolved by the light microscope. The behaviour of lysosomal esterase during cell fractionation (Matile *et al.,* 1965), and during lysosomal staining (Holt, 1963) has long remained a matter of conjecture since it has been suggested that this enzyme may not be liberated on lysosomal damage as it may be a structural component of the lysosome and is sedimented with the rest of the lysosomal debris. Furthermore, hydrolysis of the α-naphthyl acetate substrate by lipase, which is not believed to be a lysosomal enzyme, could explain the soluble esterase activity in fractionated healthy seedlings of corn and maize (Matile *et al.,* 1965). A recent view (de Duve, 1969) indicates a microsomal location for esterases.

Although Matile *et al.* (1965) have successfully demonstrated such activity in plant lysosomes, we have not detected proteolytic enzyme activity by assay procedures using callus tissue homogenates in spite of the good cytochemical localization of these enzymes.

An additional point of interest was the consistent apparent excess recovery of RNase from homogenates of infected cells when the activity of this enzyme within the supernatant-fluid fractions of callus cells infected with *P. infestans* and *F. caeruleum* exceeded by many times the total activity of healthy tissues. The possible origin of this increased RNase activity during such infections was examined further.

CHANGES IN HYDROLASE ACTIVITY DURING FUNGAL INFECTIONS

Although it is known that infection of both animal and plant tissues is linked with disruption of host lysosomes there is no evidence to indicate whether the increased cytoplasmic staining of enzymes which results from this process is due to liberation and activation of pre-existing enzyme or to enzyme synthesis *de novo.*

Much is known about the nature of hydrolase changes during tissue infection by bacteria (Farkas and Lovrekovich, 1965; Rudolph and Stahmann, 1966) and in fungi (Stahmann, 1967). In rust infections, available evidence suggests that increased acid-phosphomonoesterase activity appearing in the host–parasite complex may be contributed by both the host and the pathogen (Williams and Staples, 1964). There is relatively little information concerning the changes in these enzymes during infection by necrotrophic fungi, although Pitt (1970) has shown, by using polyacrylamide gel disk electrophoresis, that infection of potato tuber by *Phytophthora erythroseptica* produces increases in enzyme activities corresponding to those found in both the uninfected host and the pathogen.

Increase in ribonuclease activity in potato tuber callus during infection with F. caeruleum.

Ribonuclease assay by spectrophotometric determination of acid soluble nucleotides produced from the RNA substrate is the most convenient, cheap and sensitive method available, but it is subject to interference by other enzymes which also hydrolyse nucleotides. Phosphomonoesterase and phosphodiesterase are two such enzymes found abundantly in potato tubers and this material is frequently chosen for the commercial preparation of the former. Thus, the lack of specificity of the RNase assay procedure is a considerable source of error when used with crude homogenates.

This interaction of the various nucleolytic enzymes *in vitro* was demonstrated by using highly-purified enzymes from potato tuber tissues. Phosphomonoesterase was a commercial product, RNase was purified as described earlier (Pitt, 1971) and the phosphodiesterase was obtained by the procedure outlined in 'Materials and Methods'. Table II shows that hydrolysis of RNA (highly polymerized from yeast, B.D.H.), by a mixture of these three enzymes in physiological concentrations, is considerably more than the sum of the activity of each measured singly. Enzyme interactions of this type are complex and are frequently encountered during structural determination of nucleic acids and nucleotide sequencing and depend on the specificity of the enzymes and the nature of the substrates (Schmidt, 1957).

We believe that such interactions of enzymes are likely to occur in crude homogenates subjected to the RNase assay and within cells where lysosomal disruption has occurred, allowing for the limits of controlling factors, e.g. pH, ionic strength. Evidence of a comparable interaction was presented by Kuć (1962) in the pectolysis associated with infections by *Cladosporium*

TABLE II

Hydrolysis of RNA (yeast) by various combinations of purified nucleolytic enzymes of *Solanum.*

Treatment	E_{260}/reaction mixture
RNase	1.7
Phosphodiesterase	0.65
Phosphomonoesterase	nil
RNase + phosphodiesterase	2.8
RNase + phosphomonoesterase	2.0
Phosphodiesterase + phosphomonoesterase	0.38
RNase + phosphodiesterase + phosphomonoesterase	3.35

Units of enzyme/reaction mixture:
RNase, 6.75; phosphodiesterase, 0.08; phosphomonoesterase, 1.5.

cucumerinum. Infection is likely to result in extremely complex interactions between enzymes and substrates, and investigators need to consider such multicomponent systems in addition to single enzyme activity against purified substrates.

Owing to the heat labile nature of potato RNase, we could not adopt the usual techniques for determination of heat stable RNases which involves a preliminary heat treatment to destroy interfering non-specific phosphatases, a method not open to us. Therefore, the interfering phosphatases were removed by prior separation of homogenates by gel filtration on Sephadex G100 as a routine procedure. The apparent RNase increase of *Fusarium*-infected callus noted by Pitt and Coombes (1969) was examined in detail by this procedure because such increases in lysosomal RNase activity, if real, may be of particular interest in view of recent attention focused on this enzyme as a possible genetic inducer (Hadwiger and Schwochau, 1969) or in a postulated role in inducing immunity in sweet potatoes, infected by *Ceratocystis fimbriata* (Weber and Stahmann, 1966; Stahmann *et al.,* 1968). Figures 3a and b reveal clearly the

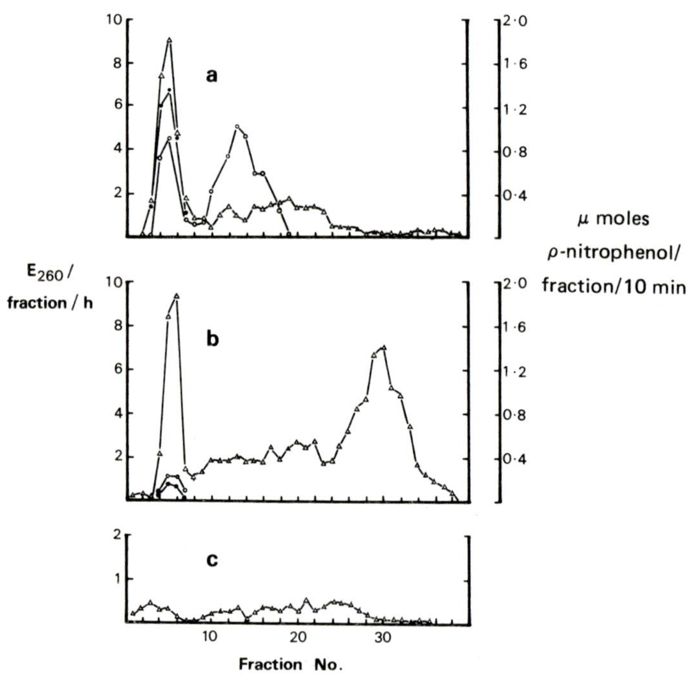

Fig. 3. (a). Enzyme activity of fractions from gel filtration of homogenates of healthy callus tissue. Ribonuclease (E_{260}) △——△; acid phosphomonoesterase ○–○; acid phosphodiesterase ●–●. (Column load 3 ml containing 6.6 mg protein). (b) As 3(a) but using homogenates of callus 4 days after infection with *Fusarium caeruleum.* (c) Ribonuclease activity (E_{260}) of homogenates of mycelial mats of *Fusarium caeruleum* grown on potato broth. (Column load of 3 ml containing 2.06 mg protein.)

decrease in phosphomonoesterase and phosphodiesterase activities and the very large increase in RNase activity associated with infection. The RNase content of a homogenate derived from mycelial mats of *F. caeruleum* grown on potato broth revealed no activity (Fig. 3c), in fractions equivalent to those in which healthy callus RNase was eluted, and there was negligible activity of phosphodiesterase and phosphomonoesterase. It is likely that the fungus in intimate contact with the host may produce enzymes which are not found in pure culture, but it will remain difficult to determine the extent of such subtle interactions until pathogens can be separated from the host-parasite combination.

Increased hydrolysis of ribonucleic acid during tuber infection by F. caeruleum.
The extent and nature of the increase in RNase activity in callus cells prompted us to examine the changes in nucleolytic enzymes in the zone immediately ahead of the fungal rot into which mycelium had not penetrated but which is subject to lysosomal disruption and enzyme release as judged by cytochemical enzyme localization studies. As *F. caeruleum* is a pathogen which causes latent disease development in the spring following harvest time infections, we examined the development of infections established in February and incubated for one month at 20° C. Potato tubers were wound-incubated at the 'heel' end with a pure culture of the fungus grown on agar. The rotted zone was removed and the zone 1.0 cm (Fl) ahead of the rot was homogenized in a reducing buffer (Pitt and Galpin, 1971). A further sample of tissue was removed 1.0-2.0 cm beyond the rot (F2) and similarly homogenized, centrifuged and stored under nitrogen at –30° C until required. Control tissue (C1), from wounded but uninoculated tubers, was similarly treated. Determinations of enzyme activities were carried out on aliquots of crude homogenates and Table III shows the large increases in apparent RNase activity accompanied by increased phosphodiesterase activity. Relatively small increases were found in phosphomonoesterase activity.

On gel filtration through Sephadex G100 columns (40 cm x 2.5 cm), (whereby good recovery of all enzymes was achieved if reducing agents were

TABLE III

Specific activity of enzymes in crude homogenates of healthy and *Fusarium*-infected tubers.

Treatment	Phosphodiesterase	Enzyme activity Phosphomonoesterase	RNase (E_{260})
Control	0.30	2.60	19.0
F1	0.44	2.73	53.6
F2	0.45	3.24	28.6

included in the homogenization buffer) the elution patterns shown in Figs 4 and 5 were obtained. These show increases in the activity of molecular forms of phosphodiesterase which was well separated from the RNase and increases in some peaks of phosphomonoesterase whilst others were reduced on infection. The peak of RNase activity was eluted with the low mol. wt. acid phosphomonoesterase but as the results (Table II) show that combining these

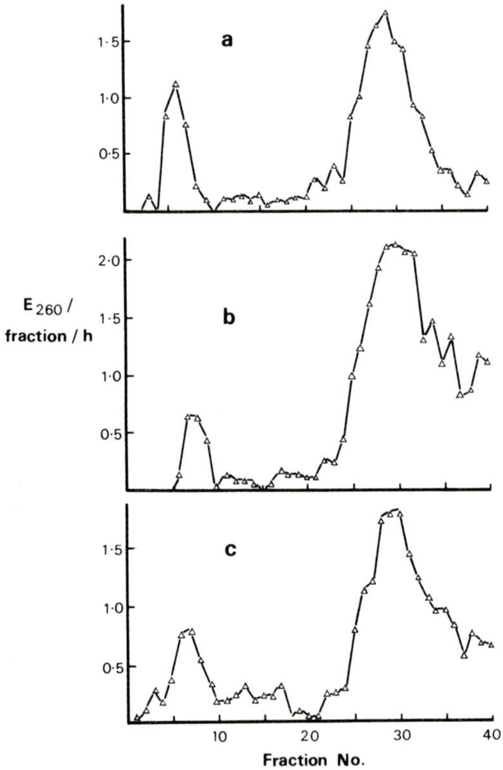

Fig. 4. (a) Enzyme activity of fractions from gel filtration of homogenates of healthy tuber tissue (C1). Ribonuclease activity (E_{260}) △——△ (Column load 3 ml containing 9.65 mg protein.) (b) As (a) but using homogenate (F1) from *Fusarium*-infected tubers. (c) As 4(a) but using homogenate (F2) from *Fusarium*-infected tubers.

enzymes has a very small effect on increased RNA hydrolysis it is unlikely that much interference has occurred in the assay and the peaks represent true RNase activity. The area under the RNase curve in sample F1 is approximately double that of the healthy tissues indicating that the value for crude homogenates was inexplicably high. There was a smaller (20-30%) increase in the activity of this enzyme in sample F2. Therefore infection has increased enzyme activity and since these increases may be associated with peaks having gel-filtration characteristics of enzymes of known host origin, it would seem that these increases in activity could be due to synthesis of new host enzyme or to the activation of pre-formed enzyme. There are appreciable changes in the elution pattern of the low mol. wt. forms of acid phosphomonoesterase but the nature of these changes has not yet been fully examined. The exact components giving rise to the high mol. wt. peak of apparent RNase activity (fractions 5-8 in Fig. 5)

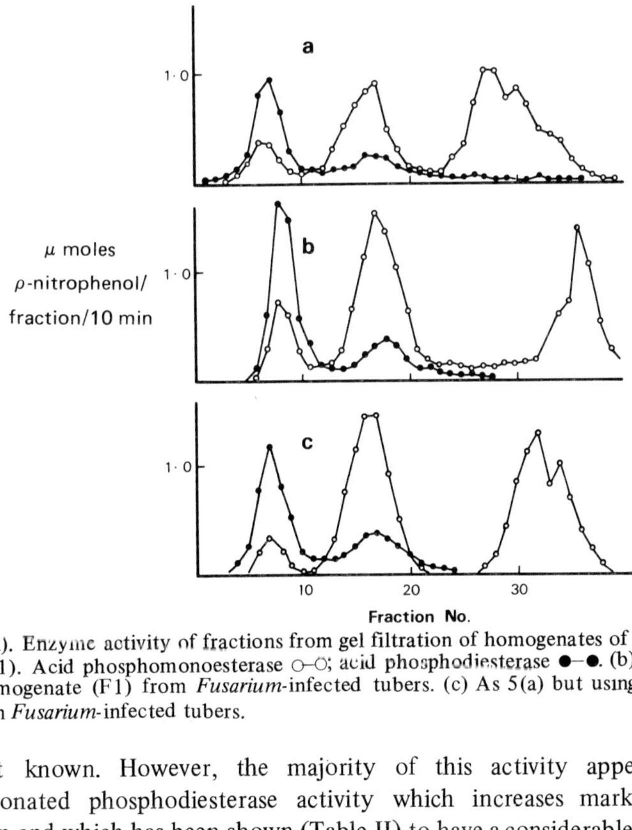

Fig. 5. (a). Enzymic activity of fractions from gel filtration of homogenates of healthy tuber tissue (C1). Acid phosphomonoesterase ○–○; acid phosphodiesterase ●–●. (b) As 5(a) but using homogenate (F1) from *Fusarium*-infected tubers. (c) As 5(a) but using homogenate (F2) from *Fusarium*-infected tubers.

are not known. However, the majority of this activity appears due to unfractionated phosphodiesterase activity which increases markedly during infection and which has been shown (Table II) to have a considerable capacity for hydrolysing RNA.

The large increase in RNase activity during infection by *F. caeruleum* is particularly interesting in the light of the interrelationship between RNase activity and RNA metabolism in *Phaseolus vulgaris* infected with *Uromyces phaseoli* (Heitefuss, 1968). The exact significance of such changes is not yet clear but Quick and Shaw (1966) followed the qualitative and quantitative changes in nucleotides in rust-infected wheat leaves and suggested that nucleotides derived from the host may eventually pass to the parasite. Perhaps more significant are the findings by Reddi (1968) that degradation products of tobacco leaf RNA are utilized in the synthesis of viral nucleic acid mediated by RNase I, RNase II and phosphomonoesterase which leads to the final production of ribonucleotides 5′-phosphate via the action of ribonucleoside phosphokinase. However, it is more difficult to envisage such a degree of sophistication in tissue soft-rots when the extent and speed of rotting suggests rapid and extensive macromolecular hydrolysis.

Lysosomes of animal cells are involved in a wide range of disease symptoms of animals, e.g. necrosis, virus infection and congenital disease which are associated with varying degrees of lysosomal damage—from complete disruption to controlled leakage and even enzyme deficiency.

Atkinson and Shaw (1955) observed increased acid phosphatase staining of haustoria in epidermal cells of wheat leaves infected with powdery mildew. This suggests that the enzyme may be involved in biotrophic infections as well as in the tissue soft-rots.

Quantitative immunoelectrophoresis of RNase during tuber damage and infection with F. caeruleum.

Extensive literature records the increased activities of RNase and other enzymes in various plant tissues following mechanical damage and various forms of stress. Opinion is divided as to whether this is a result of enzyme synthesis *de novo* or activation of preformed enzymes. The results of Pitt and Galpin (1971) dealing with the large RNase increases in damaged potato tuber and leaf tissues derived from experiments with inhibitors of protein synthesis and deuterium oxide labelling using the ultra-centrifuge expose the limitations of the use of inhibitors for this type of work. The immunochemical observations of Pitt (1971) have shown that the large increases in RNase activity of damaged tubers are not accompanied by increases in total ribonuclease protein in these tissues. Indeed, 48 h after tissue damage there was a significant decrease in this antigen content although RNase activity was still high. It is concluded that such large increases in RNase activity could be due to activation of pre-formed enzyme rather than to new protein synthesis. The use of the single radial immunodiffusion technique with samples F1 and F2 and the control showed no significant differences in the content of the two RNase antigens measurable by this method suggesting that the increase in activity of these enzymes is not associated with increased synthesis of the enzyme protein having immunological characteristics of the uninfected host. Additional confirmation has been obtained by use of the antigen-antibody crossed electrophoresis technique in which the concentrations of both RNase antigens may be assayed independently along with contaminating phosphomonoesterase present in the original RNase preparation (Pitt, 1971). The results (Figs 6 and 7) compare the RNase antigen content of tuber tissue initially and 48 h after damage.

Negligible quantitative differences in the areas of the precipitin arcs confirm the conclusion of Pitt (1971) on the origin of RNase increases in damaged potato tuber. Similarly, the results in Figs 8 and 9 show no significant differences in the concentrations of RNase antigens in homogenates from control and *Fusarium*-infected (F1) tubers although the activity of this enzyme(s) increases markedly on infection. In order to give a sufficiently large phosphomonoesterase peak in the second-dimension gel the volume of homogenate in the wells was doubled, and Figs 10 and 11 show how this peak changes during infection, with a large decrease in concentration in the homogenate which is antigenic towards the antibodies in the antiserum. However, as the immunological affinities of the various molecular forms of phosphomonoesterase of *Solanum* are not known the changes in this peak cannot be related to the enzyme activities of the other peaks eluted by gel filtration or to the cross-reaction obtained using antibodies raised against the commercial phosphomonoesterase which contained multiple molecular forms of this enzyme. These complexities associated with the immunological assay of

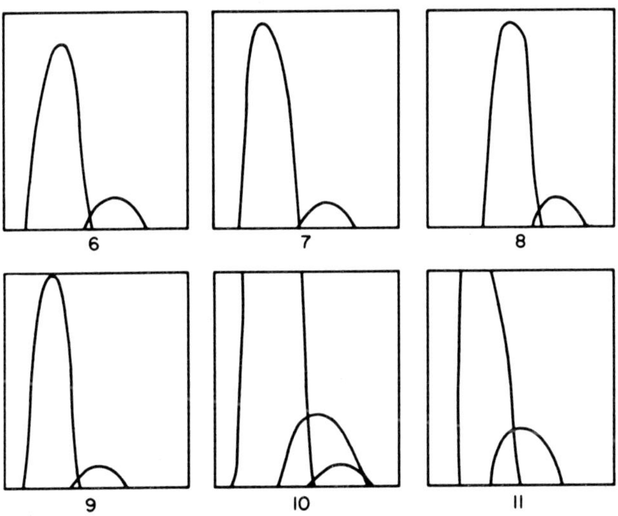

Fig. 6. Quantitative immunoelectrophoresis of 2 μl of homogenate of healthy tuber cv. Majestic containing 4.5 μg of soluble protein showing the two RNase precipitin peaks in zero time (undamaged) controls.

Fig. 7. As Fig. 6 but homogenates from tubers 22 h after mechanical damage by slicing.

Fig. 8. Quantitative immunoelectrophoresis of 2 μl of homogenate of healthy tubers containing 4.5 μg of soluble protein showing precipitin peaks of the two RNase antigens.

Fig. 9. As Fig. 8 but using homogenate F1 from *Fusarium*-infected tubers.

Fig. 10. As Fig. 8 but using 4 μl of homogenate C1 containing 9.0 μg of soluble protein, showing the peak due to acid phosphomonoesterase and the peak due to the RNase antigens increased in proportion.

Fig. 11. As Fig. 10 but using homogenate from *Fusarium*-infected tubers (F1).

phosphomonoesterase are not apparent with the simpler RNase assay which showed no increase in RNase protein to match the increase in activity of this enzyme which occurred during infection. Therefore, it is concluded that there is no new synthesis of these RNase antigens by the host during infection.

The antigenic properties of enzymes may change on infection or the increases in activity of the molecular form of RNase separated by gel filtration may be due to a new form of protein which does not cross-react with the antigens derived from healthy tissues. Since there is no evidence of such new forms in infected tissues using both gel filtration and agar gel electrophoresis carried out according to Pitt (1971) there is no evidence for such doubts at present. A further possibility, however, is that the increased enzyme activity may be due to enzymes secreted by the parasite because it is known (Pitt and Walker, 1967; Pitt, 1968) that fungi contain these hydrolases localized in fungal lysosomes (Fig. 12) which are thought to be secretory (Matile, 1969). However, there was no cross-reactivity between the antisera used in this work and the homogenates derived from the fungal pathogens. Since it is now believed that mechanical damage to potato tuber tissue can activate preformed RNase, it is possible that the increased enzyme activity found in infections by *F. caeruleum* may be part of a similar host response. Alternatively, the pathogen in the presence of the host may have a remarkable capacity for synthesis of molecular forms of enzymes with characteristics of those of the uninfected host.

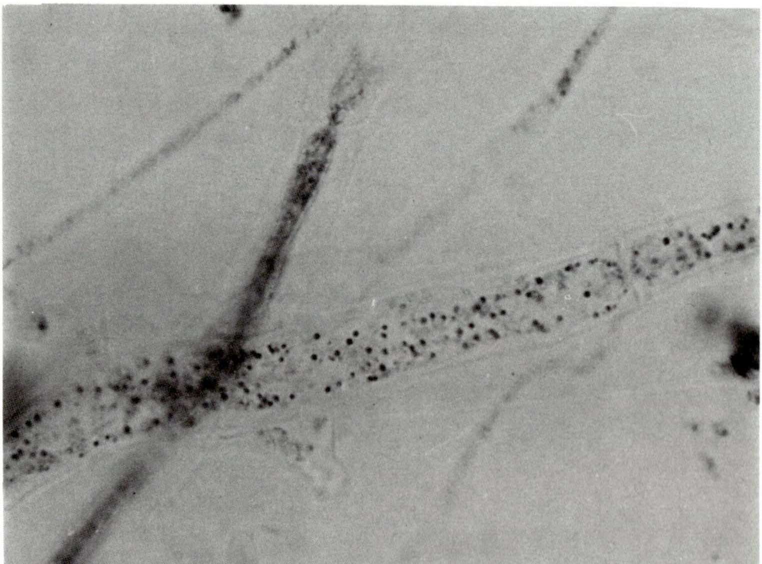

Fig. 12. Particulate localization of acid phosphomonoesterase in *Botrytis cinerea* revealed by the Gomori lead salt method. ×2000. (From Pitt, 1968).

Although the increased RNase activity associated with infection by *F. caeruleum* is not as great as that arising in tissue damage, the results further support the hypothesis that disease and mechanical damage may be due to similar biochemical changes. It is also interesting that current biochemical work, recently reviewed by Marcus (1971), suggests that enzyme activation may be more important in regulation in eucaryotic organisms than was hitherto recognized.

COMMENTS

Although it is almost 20 years since lysosomes were first discovered it is still not known if damage to these organelles is a cause or a consequence of cell death. Malfunctioning of the lysosome system is known to be associated with many diseases of animals and with plant diseases caused by soft-rot fungi; but it is not yet known if these structures are also involved in diseases caused by obligate plant parasitic fungi or plant viruses. In working with plant lysosomes, the principal difficulty is that inherent in isolating particles from tissues requiring high shearing forces for their disintegration which also damage cell contents. Even the best preparations of these particles obtained so far, from seedlings, show relatively large amounts of acid hydrolase activity in the supernatant fluid fractions. With the gradual improvement of plant cell fractionation techniques other groups of particles are now being discovered e.g. peroxisomes and glyoxysomes, and the role of these particles in plant cell metabolism has been reviewed by Tolbert (1971). Another outstanding problem concerns those factors causing disruption of membranes at sites in the host remote from the pathogen. Although it is possible to envisage many factors which could influence membrane stability and hence lead to a breakdown in compartmentalization within cells, it is difficult to prove the involvement of any particular factor or, even if known, to modify its action in disease, although some progress has been made on this aspect in the field of medicine.

ACKNOWLEDGEMENT

We wish to thank the Agricultural Research Council for financial support during this work.

REFERENCES

Atkinson, T. G. and Shaw, M. (1955). Occurrence of acid phosphatase in association with the haustoria of powdery mildew on barley. *Nature, Lond.* **175**, 993-995.

Clarke, H. G. M. and Freeman, T. (1968). Quantitative immunoelectrophoresis of human serum proteins. *Clin. Sci.* **35**, 403-413.

de Duve, C. (1969). The lysosomes in retrospect. *In* 'Frontiers of Biology, 14A. Lysosomes in Biology and Pathology (eds J. T. Dingle and H. B. Fell), Vol. 1, Chap. 1, 3-37. North Holland Publishing Co., Amsterdam and London.

de Duve, C., Pressman, B. C., Gianetto, R., Wattiaux, R. and Appelmans, F. (1955). Tissue fractionation studies 6. Intracellular distribution patterns of enzymes in rat-liver tissue. *Biochem. J.* **60**, 604-617.

de Duve, C. and Baudhuin, P. (1966). Peroxisomes (Microbodies and related particles). *Physiol. Rev.* **46**, 323-357.

Dingle, J. T. and Fell, H. B. (ed.) (1969). 'Frontiers of Biology, 14A & 14B. Lysosomes in Biology and Pathology', 2 vols. North Holland Publishing Co. Amsterdam and London.

Farkas, G. L. and Lovrekovich, L. (1965). Enzyme levels in tobacco leaf tissues affected by the wildfire toxin. *Phytopathology* **55**, 519-524.

Gahan, P. B. (1967). Histochemistry of lysosomes. *Int. Rev. Cytol.* **21**, 1-63.

Graber, P. and Williams, C. A., Jun. (1955). Méthode immunoélectrophoretique d'analyse des mélanges de substances antigénique. *Biochim. biophys. Acta* **17**, 67-74.

Hadwiger, L. A. and Schwochau, M. E. (1969). Host resistance responses—an induction hypothesis. *Phytopathology* **59**, 223-227.

Heitefuss, R. (1968). Regulation of host-parasite relations in obligate parasitism. *In* 'Biochemical regulation in diseased plants or injury' (ed. T. Hirai), pp. 223-231. Phytopathological Society of Japan, Tokyo.

Holt, S. J. (1963). Some observations on the occurrence and nature of esterases in lysosomes. *In* 'The Lysosomes' (ed. A. V. S. de Reuck and M. P. Cameron), p. 114. Churchill, London.

Kuć, J. (1962). Production of extracellular enzymes by *Cladosporium cucumerinum*. *Phytopathology* **52**, 961-963.

Lowry, O. H., Rosebrough, N. J., Farr, A. L. and Randall, R. J. (1951). Protein measurement with the Folin phenol reagent. *J. biol. Chem.* **193**, 265-275.

Mancini, G., Carbonara, A. O. and Heremans, J. F. (1965). Immunological quantitation of antigens by single radial immunodiffusion. *Immunochemistry* **2**, 235-254.

Marcus, A. (1971). Enzyme induction in plants. *A. Rev. Pl. Physiol.* **22**, 313-336.

Matile, P., Balz, J. P., Semadeni, E. and Jost, M. (1965). Isolation of spherosomes with lysosome characteristics from seedlings. *Z. Naturforsch.* **20b**, 693-698.

Matile, P. (1969). Plant Lysosomes. *In* 'Frontiers of Biology, 14A. Lysosomes in Biology and Pathology' (ed. J. T. Dingle and H. B. Fell), Vol. 1 Ch. 15, 406-430. North Holland Publishing Co. Amsterdam and London.

Ouchterlony, O. (1953). Antigen antibody reactions in gel. IV. Types of reactions in coordinated systems of diffusion. *Acta path. microbiol. Scand.* **32**, 231-240.

Pitt, D. and Walker, P. J. (1967). Particulate localization of acid phosphatase in fungi. *Nature, Lond.* **215**, 783-784.

Pitt, D. (1968). Histochemical demonstration of certain hydrolytic enzymes within cytoplasmic particles of *Botrytis cinerea* Fr. *J. gen. Microbiol.* **52**, 67-75.

Pitt, D. and Coombes, C. (1968). The disruption of lysosome-like particles of *Solanum tuberosum* cells during infection by *Phytophthora erythroseptica* Pethbr. *J. gen. Microbiol.* **53**, 197-204.

Pitt, D. and Coombes, C. (1969). Release of hydrolytic enzymes from cytoplasmic particles of *Solanum* tuber tissue during infection by tuber-rotting fungi. *J. gen. Microbiol.* **56**, 321-329.

Pitt, D. (1970). Changes in hydrolase activity of *Solanum* tuber tissues during infection by *Phytophthora erythroseptica. Trans. Br. mycol. Soc.* **55**, 257-266.

Pitt, D. (1971). Purification of a ribonuclease from potato tubers and its use as an antigen in the immunochemical assay of this protein following tuber damage. *Planta* **101**, 333-351.

Pitt, D. and Galpin, M. (1971). Increase in ribonuclease activity following mechanical damage to leaf and tuber tissues of *Solanum tuberosum* L. *Planta* **101**, 317-332.

Quick, W. A. and Shaw, M. (1966). The physiology of host-parasite relations. XVII. Acid-soluble nucleotides in rust-infected and senescing wheat leaves. *Can. J. Bot.* **44**, 777-788.

Reddi, K. K. (1968). Biochemical events within the cell following infection with tobacco mosaic virus. *In* 'Biochemical regulation in diseased plants or injury' (ed. T. Hirai), pp. 79-90. Phytopathological Society of Japan, Tokyo.

Rudolph, K. and Stahmann, M. A. (1966). Multiple hydrolases in bean leaves (*Phaseolus vulgaris* L.) and the effect of the halo blight caused by *Pseudomonas phaseolicola* (Burkh) Dowson. *Pl. Physiol., Lancaster* **41**, 389-394.

Schmidt, G. (1957). Chemical and enzymatic methods for the identification and structural elucidation of nucleic acids and nucleotides. *In* 'Methods in Enzymology' (eds S. O. Colowick and N. O. Kaplan), Vol. 3, pp. 747-774. Academic Press, New York.

Stahmann, M. A. (1967). Influence of host-parasite interactions on proteins, enzymes and resistance. *In* 'The dynamic role of molecular constituents in plant-parasite interaction' (eds C. J. Mirocha and I. Uritani), pp. 357-369. American Phytopathological Society, St. Paul.

Stahmann, M. A., Woodbury, W., Lovrekovich, L. and Macko, V. (1968). The role of enzymes in the regulation of disease resistance and host-pathogen specificity. *In* 'Biochemical regulation in diseased plants or injury' (ed. T. Hirai), pp. 263-274. Phytopathological Society of Japan, Tokyo.

Tolbert, N. E. (1971). Microbodies–peroxisomes and glyoxysomes. *A. Rev. Pl. Physiol.* 22, 45-74.

Weber, D. J. and Stahmann, M. A. (1966). Induced immunity to *Ceratocystis* infection in sweet potato root tissue. *Phytopathology* **56**, 1066-1070.

Williams, P. H. and Staples, R. C. (1964). Acid phosphatase from healthy and rust infected pinto bean leaves. *Contr. Boyce Thompson Inst. Pl. Res.* 22, 269-282.

DISCUSSION

Professor J. Friend: There is published evidence to show that *P. infestans* produces an extracellular RNase.

Dr D. Pitt: Page finds that *P. infestans* can hydrolyse RNA as the sole nutrient source, at least for a fairly limited time. This need not necessarily be by an

RNase, but by a combination of nucleolytic enzymes, but certainly fungi do produce these enzymes. Our *Fusarium* produces these in small quantities, and even if we fractionated some of these on gels, we might see that the RNase from this *Fusarium caeruleum* is a different molecular form from that normally occurring in the host tissue. Incidentally, we are not claiming that the fungus does nothing in all this, we just say that there can be other mechanisms whereby hydrolysis may be achieved.

Dr E. Hislop: Do active RNase and heat-inactivated RNase give the same ring diameter in the diffusion assay?

Dr Pitt: We have not looked at this. We do not know, for example, whether the RNase we extract from healthy tissues is antigenically the same as that which is activated in healthy tissues or the one which turns up in infected tissues. I do not think anyone knows. No one has examined, for instance, the differences in response of rabbits to the active enzyme and an inactive form. Now I know you get different molecular forms of enzymes, and there are some rather interesting relationships between these, but I think that the immunologists are working on this, and on what determines antigenic capacity, but I do not know that we are in a position even to speculate on whether activated or inactivated forms are antigenically similar or different.

Professor P. W. Brian: I was intrigued by your remark that you were not very satisfied with the results you got with your experiments with inhibitors. I wonder if you would tell us a bit about them.

Dr Pitt: We put actinomycin into our system as a transcriptional inhibitor, and we found very little effect of this, on increases in enzyme activity, and so we used a number of other inhibitors, and we got all sorts of queer and variable results, which were totally inexplicable. Some of our conclusions are based on the use of cycloheximide, which seemed to kill the tissue with remarkable speed, and one wonders about the effects of the others. I think one of the classic examples is the effect of puromycin on phosphodiesterase. It just inhibits the enzyme and sets off a whole series of chain reactions within the cell resulting in the activation of a number of enzymes, particularly in tadpoles, where you ultimately get glycogen synthetase being activated by administration of puromycin. Superficially this inhibitor seemed to be affecting transcription-translation, but it was enzyme activation via a very complex system (Blatt *et al.* (1969). *Biochem. biophys. Acta* **177**, 553).

Professor P. H. Williams: In plant cells there are known to be a number of organelles, such as lysosomes, microbodies, sphaerosomes, and lipid bodies. Could you characterize some of the staining products which you showed in Fig. 1?

Dr Pitt: We called these lysosomes because we can show that they contain a number of hydrolytic enzymes which are located in lysosomes, by definition. Mostly we found hydrolytic enzymes such as esterases, proteases, acid hydrolases, e.g. phosphodiesterase, phosphomonoesterase. But a number of other particles do exist, as you know: glyoxysomes; peroxisomes; sometimes they are grouped together, but some people think that they are separate in that they each contain a different set of enzymes, others think that glyoxisomes are the same as peroxisomes. It depends upon the tissue you look at. Microbody is to some people another term for peroxisome, but in this proliferation people are beginning to look very seriously at subcellular compartmentalization, and I think we are in for a rash of new particles when people find that their particular enzyme is located in a special particle which is different from an already named particle. You have to isolate these particles to look at them critically, and this, of course, can be extremely difficult.

Professor Williams: Do you know whether your lysosomes are membrane-bound?

Dr Pitt: Their response to the classic treatments with detergents, osmotic changes, and heat treatment suggests that they are membrane-bound.

Dr R. C. Hignett: I wonder if you could say anything about the numbers of lysosomes involved in the autolysis of a single cell, and whether it is only necessary just to prick one in order to get a tremendous snowball effect?

Dr Pitt: I do not know. This is, of course, very interesting. The people who worked on animals seem to think that you can get a snowballing type of effect once you initiate the sequence, but here I am talking about mainly necrotrophic infections. I am not thinking in terms of biotrophs and more sophisticated control mechanisms as these are rather more delicate system altogether. Mine is very much a sledgehammer effect, and one would think that it might well snowball, but we are concerned about what causes these things to disintegrate. There are many candidates.

Dr Hignett: I was thinking that it might be just the sort of trigger people are looking for in the case of hypersensitivity, where a slight amount of mechanical damage to membrane-bound lysosomes, just one or two, may start something that continues.

Dr Pitt: This is something that had crossed our minds, but to examine it is extremely difficult, as you are very limited in what you can do histochemically. You have to be able to isolate these particles to look at them seriously. But I agree with you, it is an interesting possibility that if this could be localized in a few cells, you have got your hypersensitive reaction.

Concluding Remarks

PROFESSOR P. W. BRIAN F.R.S.

Department of Botany, University of Cambridge, England
Honorary Director of the A.R.C. Unit of Developmental Botany

Of the various impressions which I am taking away, and I think there are seven of them, the first is this: listening to the discussion it seems to me that we are all far too prone to forget the fact that a higher plant, even if it is only a small annual weed, and even more if it is a perennial tree, is very complex indeed. It always has a massive number of physical and chemical events going on at the same time and following one another all the time, and events taking place in one part of this complex organism can have many different kinds of effect in other parts. Accompanying this complexity there is an equally complex set of control systems, control systems at various levels, at genetic level, at enzyme level, at hormonal level, and so on. We are continually learning how much more important these controls are than we at one time thought, and we are finding that any one type of control has a far more pervading influence than we suspected. So, for instance, considering hormonal control mechanisms which in the past we have tended to associate most with growth and morphogenesis, we now find that they affect other quite different sorts of activities, such as sexuality or photosynthetic carbon assimilation. I have in mind, for example, the control of the synthesis of RuDP-carboxylase by gibberellins or cytokinins; or the effect of abscisic acid on stomatal opening and consequently on water movement. As a result of this complexity of control mechanisms, there are many ways in which an invading parasite can mess things up, quite apart from crude things like destruction of tissue. So, just to consider a few examples, in the wilt diseases, one knows how increasing resistance to the flow of water in the stem xylem leads to all the symptoms of water stress. One knows now how pathways of translocation can be altered in diseases such as cereal smuts and rusts, about which Dr Myers spoke (III.4), or in clubroot infection. As a result of this rechannelling of pathways of translocation, assimilates, already perhaps reduced in quantity, are distributed to places where they are not needed, and that particular part of the plant which is to be harvested gets little or none. We know, now, how invading parasites can activate biosynthetic pathways in various ways, and we have had many examples of this during the last few days. Turning to cruder effects, we know how in the case of rust infection of a cereal, once the uredial pustules burst through the epidermis, there is, at the same time, a consequent loss of water, so that the plant suffers water stress, and this has secondary effects on the rate of photosynthesis. A further consequence of this complexity is that there are always several potential ways in which a given effect, accompanying parasitic attack, can be produced. So, for instance, in the case discussed by Dr Myers, where you get changes in the rate of photosynthesis, there are a very large number of possibilities which would have to be investigated before we really know what the answer to the problem is. So, that is my first impression—one of the complexity of organization of higher plants which is reflected in the difficulties we encounter in explaining the course of pathogenesis.

The second impression, and I must add that I am giving these in random order, is the remarkable extent to which old problems are still unsolved. A striking example is the cell-killing effect of the action of macerating enzymes produced by invading fungi. We know a lot more now than we did even ten years ago, of the nature of the activities and of the specificity of the enzymes involved. But the mechanism of cell-killing, as we have seen in the discussions we have had, is still in many respects mysterious. It is also becoming clear that this is a problem which is no longer a private problem of plant pathologists, but one of increasing importance to plant physiologists, and once we really do understand this phenomenon, we shall know far more about the interrelations between cytoplasm, plasmalemma and cell wall than we do now.

My third impression, which I am sure everyone here must share, is of the great complexity of the events set in motion by the entry of a parasite into the tissues of a plant. We have talked about cell death and necrosis, enhanced protein synthesis, including a good deal of *de novo* synthesis of new enzymes. We have seen how some of this production of new enzymes is involved in the production of phytoalexins, on the one hand, or of the new isoenzymes of peroxidase and other enzymes discussed by Professor Stahmann (V.1) We have seen how entry of the parasite into the plant tissue can lead to quite radical changes in hormone balance in different parts of the plant. This complexity makes interpretation of observations very difficult for several reasons. As I have already suggested, a single event may have quite a number of apparently unrelated consequences. So, for instance, it is a matter of observation that an increase in indolyl acetic acid level, or of cytokinin level, particularly if you increase these levels by exogenous application, is frequently responsible for increased ethylene production. This may, in turn, induce the formation of all sorts of enzymes in host tissues, and we have heard mention in the course of our discussions of phenylalanine ammonia lyase, peroxidase, chitinase, cellulase, glucanases, and so on. You can make the story even more complex, because an increase in gibberellin level is almost always accompanied by an increase in auxin level, and all these things follow on from that. So, as a consequence of a single event, all sorts of different things happen, and happen very quickly after one another. This occurrence of so many events, more or less at once, makes it very difficult to separate cause and effect. This is a point which has been mentioned by quite a number of speakers; this is a real difficulty. The work which was reported by Professor Williams (III.2) illustrated very nicely indeed how very rapid are some of the changes consequent on infection. He gave us some data showing how you can get the formation of a papilla within three minutes. One knows of even more rapid occurrences, where one can detect changes in the host cell while the fungal cell is just approaching, and has not actually got in. It therefore seems to me that in order to understand fully the sequence of events we shall need to carry out time-course experiments on a very short time scale. This, of course, will inevitably necessitate improvements in methods of detecting small metabolic changes, and it will all depend on the elaboration of new techniques. One can see examples of how new techniques have made a difference. For many years it was thought that the relationship of the respiratory climacteric of apples to ethylene production was that first you got the climacteric, and then the ethylene production. As methods for detecting low levels of ethylene developed, we found that the reverse, in fact, was true, showing that experimental truth depends to a very great extent on the sensitivity of experimental technique. Professor Wood made the point that we have to look more and more to detecting things that happen very quickly, and I am absolutely sure that this is right. I thought that, in this connection, a point made by Professor Burnett is well worth thinking about: he said that the first thing the invaded plant cell feels is the protein on the outside of a fungal hypha. In this situation also we have got to work on a very much smaller time scale than we have been used to. I do not want to give the impression that progress has not been made. Professor Williams' contribution (III.2) showed what can be done; again in some recent work by Hess, Hadwiger and Schwochau, they have shown that *de novo* synthesis of phenylalanine ammonia lyase (PAL), does in fact precede the formation of phaseollin in *Phaseolus.* We have known for some time that both phaseollin and PAL are produced, and we have assumed that there may be a causal connection between them, but the proof depends upon showing a time sequence, and this has now been done. This is the sort of thing which we have got to do more and more. In this connection, it is obvious to all of us from the papers which have been presented, that there is an immense value in combining the biochemical approach with fine-structure observation in these time-course studies.

These remarks arose out of my saying that we must all have been impressed by the complexity of the events that happen upon infection. I think that we should also be impressed by the fact, which is in some ways rather surprising, that in the majority of cases the reactions are much more intense in a resistant combination than in a susceptible one.

This brings me to my fourth impression, which was stimulated by the papers given by Drs Bailey and Smith (IV.1 and IV.2); that is, that the formation of phytoalexins is not so much a highly specific defence reaction, as we at one time thought, as a consequence of a general expansion or activation of secondary metabolic pathways. One notes that in an infection, not all the phenolics involved are in fact phytoalexins, in the sense that they are anti-fungal. For example, one can consider the infection of some albino-type snapdragons by *Botrytis,* where, in the white corolla, formation of anthocyanins is blocked. Around the points of the infection anthocyanins are produced. I do not believe that this has any function in the protection of the corolla from the *Botrytis,* though I may be wrong about that, but let us assume that it has not. This is a perfect analogy of the formation of phytoalexins, but it has not got the same biological significance. As has been pointed out, it is becoming clearer and clearer that not only are the so-called phenolics involved, but also aliphatic acetylenic compounds, terpenoids and all sorts of compounds; the more we look at more families of flowering plants the greater the variety of secondary metabolic products which will be found to be involved as phytoalexins. As Dr Martin said, sometimes completely new compounds are formed as a response to infection, and at other times it is just a more rapid production, or a quantitatively greater production, of substances which are there in the first place. So, although distinctions have been drawn between preformed resistance factors and ones formed as a response to infection, to my mind the distinction does not exist. The two phenomena glide into one another. Pisatin is, perhaps, a genuinely new compound; on the other hand, gossypol in cotton plants is a normal secondary metabolite of the cotton plant, and all that happens in response to an infection is that an earlier production occurs, and in a greater concentration. We should also bear in mind, and this relates to the complexity of which I spoke earlier, that many of these phenolics and secondary metabolites which accumulate after infection, have got functions other than preventing infection. They may do nothing at all, or they may influence the activity of pectic enzymes, or peroxidases, etc., and indeed one has to see this whole complex of events taking place as related, as Professor Friend showed (IV.4), to such well known processes as lignification.

I do not want to over-emphasize this point. There is evidence of some compartmentation of the pathways stimulated on infection, but in general I think that phytoalexin response is part of a wider phenomenon.

My fifth impression, also mentioned by several contributors, is that we have great difficulty in disentangling the activities of the parasite and of the host in an infected plant. It could be said that it is not very important that we should do this, but it is a question that one does ask from time to time. When a new compound accumulates, one wonders if it is a host product, a parasite product, or a product of a combination of the two metabolic systems. Sometimes you can give one answer, sometimes another. Consider, for example the very interesting work of Evans and Wilson: an accumulation of indole aceto-nitrile occurs in a caryophyllaceous plant, and you know that the substance has never before been observed in such plants; you cannot find it in this one when it is healthy, but you do find that the infecting fungus, in this instance a smut, can produce it; you can then be reasonably sure that when it turns up in an infected plant, it is a fungal product. Also when you get polyols accumulating, you can usually be fairly sure that this is a fungal product. On the other side, we can be almost certain that phytoalexins are, generally speaking, host products. Sometimes it is fairly obvious that products are the result of the interlocking of the two systems, as was shown particularly clearly in Dr Lund's explanation of the way in which pectic enzymes induce ethylene biosynthesis (II.1). But all too often it is very difficult indeed to disentangle the responsibility of the host and parasite.

This leads me on to make another related observation, that we know very little about what happens to the fungus in many infections. We devote all our time to looking at what happens to the host tissue, and we do not know so much about what happens to the fungus—we just assume that it is doing fine, except in cases of resistance, where it obviously is not. We do not really have any reliable methods of determining the mass of the fungal parasite in most infected plants, and it would be very nice if we did. We do know that obligate parasites get something valuable from the relationship, which allows protein synthesis to go ahead, whereas this cannot take place if the appropriate host is not available. But we do not know how the secondary metabolism of the fungus is affected in this partnership. We do not even know such simple things such as what ethylene does to a fungus; when it is produced so frequently as a response to infection, we ought to know a good deal more about its effects. So much then for allocating blame or credit to the partners in the parasitic relationship.

Let me come to my sixth impression. I have always thought, in the past, that as a resistance mechanism the phytoalexin response was highly unspecific. However, the work which Dr Bailey presented (IV.1), and other recent work, does indicate that they have an important part to play in an understanding of hypersensitive responses, which are, of course, far more specific reactions. This is another way in which our concept of phytoalexins is changing considerably. I agree with what Professor Wood said in his Opening Address about the understanding of the specificity of host–parasite relationships, the specificity of the hypersensitive response being one of our central problems today, if not indeed the central problem. I therefore found the contribution we had from Dr Kaars Sijpesteijn (V.3) very exciting. The host-specific toxins of *Helminthosporium victoriae* and those other organisms which Professor Wood talked about in his Opening Address have to most of us seemed most interesting, and the first real explanation of specificity and host–parasite relationships that one has encountered. Unfortunately, these particular diseases are just a bit off-beat, in the sense that they are all fairly recently discovered parasites, and in each case, they are weak parasites, almost verging on saprophytic activity; they did not really seem to be typical cases. But if it can be shown that in yet other diseases, where there is a real, well-known specificity (as in the case of the *Cladosporium* infection of tomato), the trigger is indeed provided by host-specific toxins of this kind, then we are going to make a very big step forward indeed.

My seventh impression is shared by several people during the course of the Symposium, and I think they are right: that it is very difficult indeed to distinguish wound reaction from infection reaction. Are they the same, are they distinct, or do they overlap? My opinion is that there is a certain degree of similarity, but that there are differences, and that they do overlap in nature. This is a topic we shall know far more about in a few years' time.

That really concludes the list of impressions which I am going to take away; you may like to compare my list with yours. I think it is clear to all of us that we are in a completely new era of plant pathology; that in our investigations of the biochemical and physiological basis of plant disease we are rapidly moving out of the phase where too many of us are amateur biochemists, that we are now at just the same advancing frontier as the molecular biologists, as the plant biochemists, as the plant physiologists, and that their problems are our problems. As Dr Myers said, many of our problems will not be solved without a general advance in knowledge of plant function. I think we can comfort ourselves, in a sense, with the thought that our task is a good deal more difficult than that of simple plant biochemists and plant physiologists, in that we are dealing not merely with one complex organism, but with at least two, in a complex relationship. So my feeling is that we are going to be very much more concerned with the advancing frontiers of biological science in the next few years than we have been in the past.

Finally, I should like to say that those who organized this Symposium showed great imagination in arranging the different topics which have come up before us. It has shown the great vigour and the great breadth of this new kind of plant pathology.

Somebody, and I think it was Dr Myers, drew attention to the way in which, in the past, advancing control methods depended upon empirical approaches. I hope that in the future we can base more logical approaches to control on our growing knowledge of the host–parasite relationship. We must always recognize the extent to which we are indebted to empirical approaches; all the antibiotics, with their use in medicine, and their still more interesting use in molecular biology, were first discovered by empirical methods. But one must retain the belief that investigations of the kind that have been reported here will in due course lead to completely new approaches to the control of plant disease.

Author Index

Numbers in italics refer to the page on which the reference is listed

C

I

J

K

L

T

U

V

W

Subject Index

This index is a guide to main arguments and topics of special interest. Numbers in italics refer to pages which show micrographs.

D

E